In-vitro Maturation of Human Oocytes

REPRODUCTIVE MEDICINE & ASSISTED REPRODUCTIVE TECHNIQUES SERIES

Series Editors

David K Gardner DPhil
Colorado Center for Reproductive Medicine, Englewood, CO, USA

Jan Gerris MD PhD
Professor of Gynecology, University Hospital Ghent, Ghent, Belgium

Zeev Shoham MD
Director, Infertility Unit, Kaplan Hospital, Rehovot, Israel

Published Titles

1. Gerris, Delvigne and Olivennes: Ovarian Hyperstimulation Syndrome
2. Sutcliffe: Health and Welfare of ART Children

Forthcoming Titles

1. Keck, Tempfer and Hugues: Conservative Infertility Management
2. Pellicer and Simón: Stem Cells in Reproductive Medicine
3. Elder and Cohen: Human Embryo Evaluation and Selection
4. Tucker and Liebermann: Vitrification in Assisted Reproduction

In-vitro Maturation of Human Oocytes
Basic science to clinical application

Edited by

Seang Lin Tan MBBS FRCOG FRCSC FACOG MMed (O&G) MBA

James Edmund Dodds Professor and Chair
Department of Obstetrics and Gynecology
McGill University
Obstetrician and Gynecologist in Chief
McGill University Health Centre
Medical Director
McGill Reproductive Centre
Montreal, QC
Canada

Ri-Cheng Chian MSc PhD

Scientific Director
McGill Reproductive Centre
Assistant Professor
Department of Obstetrics and Gynecology
McGill University, Royal Victoria Hospital
Montreal, QC
Canada

William M Buckett MB ChB MD MRCOG

Assistant Professor
Department of Obstetrics and Gynecology
McGill University, Royal Victoria Hospital
Montreal, QC
Canada

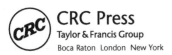

CRC Press
Taylor & Francis Group
Boca Raton London New York

CRC Press is an imprint of the
Taylor & Francis Group, an **informa** business

CRC Press
Taylor & Francis Group
6000 Broken Sound Parkway NW, Suite 300
Boca Raton, FL 33487-2742

First issued in paperback 2020

© 2007 by Taylor & Francis Group, LLC
CRC Press is an imprint of Taylor & Francis Group, an Informa business

The Editors have asserted their right under the Copyright, Designs and Patents Act 1988 to be identified as the Editors of this Work.

No claim to original U.S. Government works

ISBN-13: 978-0-367-45324-4 (pbk)
ISBN-13: 978-1-84214-332-2 (hbk)

Visit the Taylor & Francis Web site at
http://www.taylorandfrancis.com

and the CRC Press Web site at
http://www.crcpress.com

A CIP record for this book is available from the British Library.

Library of Congress Cataloging-in-Publication Data

Data available on application

Contents

Contributors

Ronit Abir PhD
IVF and Infertility Unit
Department of Obstetrics and Gynecology
Helen Schneider Hospital for Women
Israel and Sackler Faculty of Medicine
Tel Aviv University
Tel Aviv
Israel

Nelly Achour-Frydman PhD
Service de Gynécologie-Obstétrique
Hôpital Antoine Béclère (AP-HP) and
Service d'Histologie-Embryologie-
Cytogénétique à orientation Biologique et
Génétique de la Reproduction
Clamart
France

Hanadi Ba-Akdah MD
Department of Obstetrics and Gynecology
McGill University
Royal Victoria Hospital
Montreal, QC
Canada

Adam H Balen MD FRCOG
Unit of Reproductive Medicine and Surgery
Leeds General Infirmary
Leeds
UK

Frank L Barnes PhD
IVF Labs, LLC
Salt Lake City, UT
USA

Aykut Bayrak MD
Division of Reproductive Endocrinology
and Infertility
Department of Obstetrics and Gynecology
University of Southern California
Keck School of Medicine
Los Angeles, CA
USA

Avi Ben-Haroush MD
IVF and Infertility Unit
Department of Obstetrics and Gynecology
Helen Scheider Hospital for Women
Israel and Sackler Faculty of Medicine
Tel Aviv University
Tel Aviv
Israel

Frank J Broekmans MD PhD
Department of Reproductive Medicine and
Gynecology
University Medical Center
Utrecht
The Netherlands

William M Buckett MB ChB MD MRCOG
Department of Obstetrics and Gynecology
McGill University
Royal Victoria Hospital
Montreal, QC
Canada

Inger Britt Carlsson MD
Karolinska Institutet
Department of Clinical Science
Intervention and Technology
Division of Obstetrics and Gynecology
Fertility Unit
Karolinska University Hospital
Stockholm
Sweden

Ri-Cheng Chian MSC PhD
Department of Obstetrics and Gynecology
McGill University
Royal Victoria Hospital
Montreal, QC
Canada

Ezgi Demirtas
Department of Obstetrics and Gynecology
McGill University
Royal Victoria Hospital
Montreal, QC
Canada

Ursula Eichenlaub-Ritter PhD
Universität Bielefeld
Fakultät für Biologie
Gentechnologie/Mikrobiologie
Bielefeld
Germany

Renato Fanchin MD
Service de Gynécologie-Obstétrique
Hôpital Antoine Béclère (AP-HP) and
Service d'Histologie-Embryologie-
Cytogénétique à orientation Biologique et
Génétique de la Reproduction
Clamart
France

Bart CJM Fauser MD PhD
Department of Reproductive Medicine and
Gynecology
University Medical Center
Utrecht
The Netherlands

Estelle Feyereisen MD
Service de Gynécologie-Obstétrique
Hôpital Antoine Béclère (AP-HP) and
Service d'Histologie-Embryologie-
Cytogénétique à orientation Biologique et
Génétique de la Reproduction
Clamart
France

Benjamin Fisch MD PhD
IVF and Infertility Unit
Department of Obstetrics and Gynecology
Helen Scheider Hospital for Women
Israel and Sackler Faculty of Medicine
Tel Aviv University
Tel Aviv
Israel

Amanda L Fortier MD MSC
McGill University – Montreal Children's
Hospital Research Institute and
Departments of Paediatrics and Human
Genetics
McGill University
Montreal, QC
Canada

Réné Frydman MD
Service de Gynécologie-Obstétrique
Hôpital Antoine Béclère (AP-HP) and
Service d'Histologie-Embryologie-
Cytogénétique à orientation Biologique et
Génétique de la Reproduction
Clamart
France

David K Gardner PhD
Colorado Center for Reproductive
Medicine
Englewood
Colorado, CO
USA

Bulent Gulekli MD
Department of Obstetrics and Gynecology
Dokuz Eylul University
Izmir
Turkey

Sarah E Harris PhD
Research Fellow
Reproduction and Early Development
Research Group
Department of Obstetrics and Gynaecology
University of Leeds
UK

Hananel EG Holzer MD
Department of Obstetrics and Gynecology
McGill University
Royal Victoria Hospital
Montreal, QC
Canada

Outi Hovatta MD PhD
Karolinska Institutet
Department of Clinical Science
Intervention and Technology
Division of Obstetrics and Gynecology
Fertility Unit
Karolinska University Hospital
Stockholm
Sweden

Julius Hreinsson PhD
Karolinska Institutet
Department of Clinical Science
Intervention and Technology
Division of Obstetrics and Gynecology
Fertility Unit
Karolinska University Hospital
Stockholm
Sweden

Jiann-Loung Hwang MD
Department of Obstetrics and Gynecology
Shin Kong Wu Ho-Su Memorial Hospital
Shih Lin District
Tapei
Taiwan

Ping Jin PhD
Reproduction and Early Development
Research Group
Department of Obstetrics and Gynaecology
University of Leeds
UK

Gabor Kovacs MD
Monash IVF
Department of Obstetrics and Gynaecology
Monash University
Victoria
Australia

Jin-Ho Lim MD
Maria Infertility Hospital
Dongdaemun-Gu
Seoul
South Korea

Kyung-Sil Lim MD
Maria Infertility Hospital
Dongdaemun-Gu
Seoul
South Korea

Yu-Hung Lin MD
Department of Obstetrics and Gynecology
Shin Kong Wu Ho-Su Memorial Hospital
Shin Lin District
Taipei
Taiwan

Jiayin Liu MD PhD
IVF Center
Department of Obstetrics and Gynecology
The First Affiliated Hospital of Nanjing
Medical University
The People's Republic of China

Julie Lukic MD
Department of Obstetrics and Gynecology
McGill University
Royal Victoria Hospital
Montreal, QC
Canada

Anne Lis Mikkelsen MD PhD
The Fertility Clinic
Herlev University Hospital
Herlev
Denmark

Wanzirai Muruvi PhD
Reproduction and Early Development
Research Group
Department of Obstetrics and Gynaecology
University of Leeds
UK

Shmuel Nitke PhD
IVF and Infertility Unit
Department of Obstetrics and Gynecology
Helen Schneider Hospital for Women
Israel and Sackler Faculty of Medicine
Tel Aviv University
Tel Aviv
Israel

Seo-Yeong Park MD
Maria Infertility Hospital
Dongdaemun-Gu
Seoul
South Korea

Richard J Paulson MD
Division of Reproductive Endocrinology
and Infertility
Department of Obstetrics and Gynecology
University of Southern California
Keck School of Medicine
Los Angeles, CA
USA

Helen M Picton PhD
Reproduction and Early Development
Research Group
Department of Obstetrics and Gynaecology
University of Leeds
UK

Jeffrey B Russell MD
Delaware Institute for Reproductive
Medicine
Newark, DE
USA

Mark Sedler PhD
Unit of Reproductive Medicine and
Surgery
Leeds General Infirmary
Leeds
UK

Gary D Smith PhD
Department of Obstetrics and Gynecology
University of Michigan
Ann Arbor, MI
USA

Anne-Maria Suikkari MD PhD
The Family Federation of Finland
Infertility Clinic
Helsinki
Finland

Jason E Swain PhD
Department of Molecular and Integrated
Physiology
University of Michigan
Ann Arbor, MI
USA

Seang Lin Tan MBBS FRCOG FRCSC FACOG MMed
(O&G) MBA
Department of Obstetrics and Gynecology
McGill University
Royal Victoria Hospital
Montreal, QC
Canada

Fiona H Thomas PhD
Department of Cellular and Molecular
Medicine
University of Ottawa
Centre for Cancer Therapeutics
Ottawa Health Research Institute
Ottawa, ON
Canada

Antoine Torre MD
Service de Gynécologie-Obstétrique
Hôpital Antoine Béclère (AP-HP) and
Service d'Histologie-Embryologie-
Cytogénétique à orientation Biologique et
Génétique de la Reproduction
Clamart
France

Jacquetta M Trasler MD PhD
McGill University – Montreal Children's
Hospital Research Institute and
Departments of Paediatrics, Human
Genetics, and Pharmacology and
Therapeutics
McGill University
Montreal, QC
Canada

Barbara C Vanderhyden PhD
Department of Cellular and Molecular
Medicine
University of Ottawa
Centre for Cancer Therapeutics
Ottawa Health Research Institute
Ottawa, ON
Canada

Seong-Ho Yang MSC
Maria Infertility Hospital
Dongdaemun-Gu
Seoul
South Korea

San-Hyun Yoon PhD
Maria Infertility Hospital
Dongdaemun-Gu
Seoul
South Korea

Foreword

In-vitro maturation comes of age

Since its clinical outset 30 years ago, human in-vitro fertilization (IVF) has depended on expensive gonadotrophins to induce ovarian stimulation and oocyte maturation, at prices virtually one-half of total costs for this infertility treatment. The in-vitro maturation of human oocytes (IVM) now offers a much cheaper alternative. Invented more than 60 years ago, it has recently been developed as a far simpler approach to IVF, preimplantation diagnosis (PGD) and the preparation of embryo stem cells (ES cells). Indeed, it is already used in some IVF clinics and will doubtless spread to others. Clinical and scientific aspects of this advance, presented in this book, are published at a most opportune moment. It will be welcomed by investigators worldwide, as successive chapters describe background endocrinology, developmental biology of the ovarian follicles, the formation, growth and maturation of oocytes and modifications of well-tested IVF techniques to suit the needs of IVM. The First World Congress on In Vitro Maturation, held in Montreal in 2004, and a new Society will doubtless give a further stimulus to clinics assessing the role of IVM.

Writing a Foreword for this book is not easy in view of its size and contents. Successive well-written and informative chapters are so detailed that each of them can be mentioned only briefly,

so I will divide chapters into successive sections for discussion. An excellent opening chapter by Thomas and Vanderhyden covers oocyte growth and developmental competence, which are essential to understand IVM. They discuss follicle formation during human gestation, fundamental aspects of oocyte growth, and the metabolism of oocytes during growth and maturation, how primordial germ cells enter the fetal ovary, enter meiosis I then arrest in diplotene as their germinal vesicle is formed. The follicular pool thus consists of oocytes arrested in diplotene, which is basically a meiotic I arrest that persists throughout succeeding growth stages until just before ovulation. The authors offer a welter of knowledge on later follicular stages including the biochemistry of oocytes and follicles and their interactions with various hormones and cytokines as they enter their growth stages. They exit the follicular pool, apparently re-awoken under the control of regulatory proteins such as p34cdc2 and cyclin B, to enter their growth stages, which vary metabolically. For example, growth recommences as levels of the oocyte proteins Gpr3 and its receptor decline. Several weeks of growth under the partial control of granulosa cells maintains diplotene oocytes via cAMP and PKA pathways as they synthesise mRNAs and zona proteins. Fully-grown oocytes enter their maturation phase driven by the LH surge, and meiosis resumes as chromosomes enter diakinesis and complete metaphase I and extrude the first polar body. Active agents during these stages include kit ligand, its receptor, GDF (growth differentiation factor) and BMP-15 (bone morphogenic protein-15). These authors stress the importance of FSH and LH, gap junctions and transzonal factors during these stages of development.

Genetics and biochemistry of oocyte growth and maturation are covered in Chapters 2 and 3. Harris and Picton initially assess the metabolic activities in oocytes and follicles which is essential when devising specific culture media. Little is known about primordial stages, although glycolysis is essential for later stages. Glucose breakdown forms ATP via the reduction of NAD, itself formed via the conversion of pyruvate and an active Krebs cycle. Oocytes of most mammalian species require pyruvate and a little glucose, and their oxidative energy depends on mitochondria inherited from the primodial germ cell. These organelles initially aggregate to form the Balbiani body before dispersing in ooplasm. The authors describe the increasing sensitivity of oocytes to FSH and LH, the former determining varying levels of kit ligand. Preovulatory follicles consume glucose and produce lactate, and accumulate stable RNA species and proteins. These topics are also discussed by Picton et al. in Chapter 3. This team assesses oocyte/follicle interactions and how various nutrients including pyruvate especially and a little glucose supply the great majority of the oocyte's needs. Mitochondria are hence essential for their energy source. Attention also concentrates on the role of gap junctions in coordinating follicle growth and differentiation, and their connexins which are seemingly phosphorylated by LH. Differing connexion subgroups characterise thecal and granulosa compartments, and their knockout arrests follicles in antral stages. Increasing numbers of granulosa cells cross-talk with oocytes via paracrines maintaining extracellular matrices, together with

GDF-9, anti-Mullerian hormone, basic FGF, retinoblastoma protein, myc oncogene and c-kit and KL/CSF. Picton et al. stress how oocytes become meiotically competent, gap junctions lose their properties, and cAMP levels decline, perhaps regulated by agents such as 3-isobutyl-1-methylxanthine. All this information is essential to understand how granulosa cell properties are modified, luteinisation commences, hyaluronidase is secreted, prostaglandins are released and intracellular calcium is mobilised.

Genetic and developmental factors unique to oocytes must be understood when practising IVM. Ursula Eichenlaub-Ritter provides a stage-by-stage description of biochemical patterns in growing and mature oocytes. She describes in detail the massive increases in mitochondrial numbers, chromatin remodelling, and various forms of RNA and protein synthesis. In oocytes, MPF and cytostatic factor regulate development to metaphase II which is very different to mitotic cells where anaphase is triggered as chromosomes attach to the spindle. Errors in the complex factors controlling the synaptonemal complex, gene recombination and DNA repair must be understood to understand, and perhaps one day control, chromosomal non-disjunction which leads to embryonic aneuploidy and the death of many fetuses. In these stages, ribosomal and other RNAs are synthesised together with transcription factors such as the homeobox gene *Nobox* which sustains downstream developmental genes such as *Oct-4, BMP15*. Post-translational mechanisms are involved as polyadenylated mRNA is translated and numerous mRNAs are recruited. Continuing these themes, Swain and Smith identify successive mechanistic events as oocytes mature such as meiotic I resumption, polar body extrusion, meiotic II re-arrest, and chromatin condensation. They relate to the actions of developmental factors such as laminin proteins, cAMP and protein kinase C, aurora A kinase, protein phosphatase-1, Cdc25 and p34cdc2 kinase and cyclin B with the roles of granulosa cells. Fortier and Trasler are concerned with a detailed analysis of epigenetic phenomena during oocyte growth. Uniparental mouse embryos, for example, are nonviable because their disordered epigenesis can impair placental and embryonic development. They are formed as methylated sites decline in primordial germ cells migrated to the genital ridge, single-copy genes being rapidly demethylated in both sexes to make them epigenetically equivalent. Reports have appeared of imprinting syndromes in rare IVF children, which may be due to the imbalanced methylation of maternal but not paternal genes. For example, parthenogenetic mice may die in utero through variations in methylation, which can be overcome by isolating the large chromosomal domain between *H19* and *Igf2*. Such defects in the maternal component may also account for human hydatidiform moles and teratomas. Fortier and Trasler are intent on describing how imprints involve DNA methyltransferases (DNMT) which are absent in fertilised eggs and appear in the 8-cell stage. They take us even deeper into the mysteries of methylation by analysing the roles of isoforms, including DNMT1 which is expressed at day 11.5, as imprints are being erased. They also describe two variant DNMT3s; namely, 3a and 3b, with differing activities; e.g., the former possessing methyltransferase activity but not the latter. All this knowledge is essential to understand how the inclusion of various sera in culture media may modify demethylation and remethylation in fertilised eggs and produce children with imprinting syndromes such as Angelman's. Brief mention is finally made of sperm imprinting which may reduce sperm counts, and on imprinting defects in infertile patients with Angelman syndrome.

Three chapters on the physiology of IVM are opened as Ronit Abir et al. concentrate on successive development stages in primordial human follicles which peak at 7×10^6 by mid-pregnancy. These early aspects of follicular development are highly significant for understanding the formation of the ovary when considering oocyte and ovarian donation. Both tissues can be cryopreserved and thawed, although poor results to date indicate the need for greater knowledge on growth factors and endocrinology in fetal stages. Hreinsson et al. stress that live young have nevertheless been born in certain mammalian species, and human births from ovarian grafts have been reported. They consider strategies for preserving female fertility, and again stress the need for improved knowledge on the formation and growth of follicles. Various technical details are also discussed such as using FSH to reduce atresia in vitro, GDF-9 and insulin-like growth factors to promote follicle growth, and designing optimal culture media. New therapies for various afflictions, and the restoration of fertility to cancer patients and post-menopausal women depend on such improvements in this field.

Endocrinology is a basic aspect of ovarian and follicular development. Six chapters are devoted to it, covering ovarian hyper- and hypostimulation and the polycystic ovary. Broekmans and Fauser review ovarian endocrinology in detail, with attention to the roles of gonadotrophins and steroids and the roles of receptors expressed in thecal and granulosa cells as follicles grow and mature. They describe the role of TGF in sustaining germ cells in the yolk sac and their migration to the genital ridge. They stress how 2 mm follicles can respond to FSH to form Graffian and dominant follicles highly responsive to gonadotrophins. The roles of FSH and LH in follicular recruitment must obviously be understood together with the roles of granulosa cells in steroidogenesis. They also stress how intraovarian modulators of follicle growth; for example, IGF and EGF, regulate the ovarian follicular pool and the selection of a dominant follicle in association with factors such as GDF and BMP-15. Clinical implications such as the polycystic ovary syndrome and malfunctions in these development systems are discussed by Jeffrey Russell. Research in the 19th and 20th centuries produced the Stein-Leventhal operation in 1935, and a better understanding of effects of diminishing levels of ovarian androgens. They draw attention to the thin layer of hundreds of small follicles just below the ovarian surface in PCOS patients and their endocrinology. PCOS occurs in 3-7% of women as assessed by diagnoses based on FSH, LH and steroids, and providing that similar symptoms such as premature ovarian failure are excluded. They describe the use of the free testosterone index as a measure of PCOS, stress that obesity is common but not atypical of PCOS cases, that ultrasound helps to assess follicle numbers, and assess the significance of ovarian volume, blood flow and other characteristics. Studies on insulin resistance have led to work on metformin, and letrozole, an inhibitor of aromatase, may also assist with induced ovulation. Despite these findings, OHSS remains today a serious risk for patients and their pregnancies, with serious side-effects leading to hospitalisation.

Adam Balen discusses the diagnostic value of ultrasound in detecting PCOS and hyperstimulation and concludes that it is highly significant. Somewhat in contrast, a recent consensus on PCOS concluded that ultrasound, Doppler and MRI should be restricted to research. Bayrak and Paulson concentrate on methods aimed at predicting and preventing OHSS, and dealing with serious side effects such as ischaemic stroke, myocardial infarction and even death. Pathophysiological studies clarified rises in vascular permeability, capillary leakage and pleural or pericardial effusion, among others. They stress the need for tight controls, since increased permeability may involve oestrogens, histamine, serotonin, prolactin, angiogenic factors and possibly angiotensin. They caution that hCG must be given carefully, whether for ovarian stimulation or to sustain early pregnancy, OHSS may be alleviated by aspirating follicles, administering albumin, maintaining doses of GnRH agonists, and giving methylprednisolone. Unfortunately, many such tests have failed in controlled trials. Kovacs then lists IVF-associated clinical problems other than OHSS, such as errors in FSH dosage, the need for luteal support and continu-

ous ultrasound monitoring of follicles in the follicular phase. He stresses how IVM could help to avoid OHSS. In a final chapter on managing OHSS, Sedler and Balen assess its prevalence and define its mild, moderate and severe forms. For example, VEGF may be a risk factor enhancing capillary permeability, and younger ages involve greater responsiveness to gonadotrophins. Other preventive strategies include aspirating follicles, delaying hCG injections (coasting), abandoning the treatment cycle, and cryopreserving all embryos; and more unusual treatments include antihistamines, inhibitors of prostaglandin synthesis, diuretics and dopamine. Aspirating ascitic fluid may reduce symptoms including pleural effusion in severe cases.

The penultimate section of this book covers details of oocyte maturation. To this end, Ba-Akdah et al. stress the value of various IVM protocols for women with PCOS, and other wishing to avoid treatment with hCG or LH when promoting oocytes maturation. They clarify the benefits of IVM when treating PCOS patients with considerable numbers of small antral follicles. Persisting risks of PCOS may be offset by reducing gonadotrophin dosages or by ultrasound between days 2 and 5 of the menstrual cycle to measure factors such as ovarian volume, the velocity of ovarian stromal blood flow, counts and sizes of follicles, and endometrial thickness. They comment on how a dominant follicle present during IVM does not prevent the aspiration of many oocytes. They also assess the benefits for IVM of small FSH doses in early follicular stages, rapid rates of maturation and its shorter duration, and permitting oocytes to mature in vitro for 24 h or longer. Administering hCG 36 h prior to oocyte collection is also effective, reaching pregnancy rates of >35% per cycle in women <35 years of age when the development of oocytes and endometrium are synchronised. Other technical advances include finer needles for aspiration via the vagina, although they can be blocked by blood, and reducing the need for multiple punctures. Sufficient oocytes can be aspirated, immature oocytes being matured in maturation medium with FSH and LH, and those with a first polar body being inseminated immediately.

Applied aspects of IVM are now discussed, beginning as Frank Barnes describes the history of IVM from the days of Pincus, Enzmann and Saunders. Early errors delayed progress, although slow but deliberate investigations began as clinical IVF was introduced. Anne Mikkelesen assesses the benefits of FSH priming with 150 IU daily for 3 days before oocyte collection, and confirms high pregnancy rates of 29%, and implantation rates per embryo of 29% (versus 0% in controls). Such advances may have emerged through increased follicular sizes or plateauing FSH levels, and hCG injections (10,000 IU) at 36 h before oocyte retrieval could have raised pregnancy rates by hastening maturation in vitro. She concludes that IVM may replace ovarian stimulation in IVF. Hwang and Lin also discuss the advantages of FSH and hCG stimulation, querying the value of FSH priming but stressing the beneficial effects of hCG despite its misuse in some clinics. FSH coasting seems to be more acceptable. They stress the differences between IVM, routine gonadotrophin stimulation and 'rescue' IVF, especially the timing of hCG injections which are usually given during IVM when follicles reach 12 mm, versus ca. 18 mm for IVF. Despite such differences, IVM has already led to >500 babies free of anomalies. Bulent Gulekli et al. stress the widening use of transvaginal aspirations with spinal or epidural anaesthesia and the continued value of ultrasound for visualisation. They stress again how mature oocytes can be aspirated from small follicles during IVM, using 19-20G needles and strict asepsis. Anne-Maria Suikkari assesses varying methods for endometrial preparation in IVM which differ from those applied during IVF, oocyte donation and transfers of frozen-thawed embryos. Endometrial proliferation must be achieved quickly, oestrogens are delayed and oestrogens plus progesterone are given over weeks 7-12 of gestation for IVM. Laboratory aspects of IVM, natural cycle IVF and

IVF with ovarian stimulation are compared by Ri-Cheng Chian who reports that IVM culture media demand attention to serum additives, gonadotrophins, steroids and growth factors. He also stresses that IVM must be timed to particular stages of the menstrual cycle to avoid exposing oocytes to androgens, although, overall, side effects are fewer than with ovarian stimulation.

Embryonic growth, pregnancies and social aspects of IVM are discussed in the final section. Several contributors cover pregnancy rates, opening with David Gardner's review on embryo culture. He describes numerous factors, including media composition, problems with static cultures, the values of various supplements, gas phases, the size of culture droplets, the overlying paraffin oil and quality control. Significant aspects also include embryo grading, sequential scoring, the optimal day for transfer, and attention to embryonic arrest at the 8-cell stage. William Buckett attends to neonatal outcomes after IVM, especially pregnancy complications and neonatal health. He stresses that, despite the risk of imprinting syndromes, multiple pregnancies and low weight for gestational age, overall, current data are reassuring. Antoine Terré and his colleagues from France comment on improved implantation rates when IVM is used for patients with PCOS, IVF failure, oocyte donation, and previous chemotherapy. Their many PCOS patients have poor rates of embryonic growth in vitro, low implantation rates and high rates of loss in early and later pregnancy, some of it ascribed to lifestyle and other matters. Benefits include avoiding OHSS, lower costs, and a simpler treatment. Jiayan Liu and colleagues identify benefits of IVM to patients with diminished ovarian reserve, few small follicles and weak responses to gonadotrophins. Even so, IVM pregnancy rates nevertheless reach 20% and further advantages include the lack of need for high gonadotrophin doses when treating poor responders. Over-responders to hormones who are sensitive to OHSS are discussed by Kyung-Sil Lim and colleagues who conclude that IVM offers new approaches to the care of patients and that disorders may be preventable. Jin-Ho Lim et al. report on combining natural cycle IVF and IVM. For IVM, they administer 10,000 IU hCG then aspirate follicles of <12 mm diameter to collect mature and immature oocytes simultaneously. Mature oocytes with a first polar body are inseminated immediately, whereas unripe oocytes with germinal vesicles are matured in vitro and inseminated in vitro 3-4 days later to produce implantation rates of 10% per embryo and pregnancy rates of 30%. The final chapter of the book is given to Holzer et al. who discuss IVM and fertility preservation after therapies for malignancies, lupus and premature ovarian failure. They stress again how the reproductive period can be extended through ovarian or oocyte cryopreservation, and how IVM oocytes can also assist this purpose.

It has not been easy to summarise the considerable information in this book. It is spiced with information and provides the personal views of leading investigators. IVM is clearly a new branch of IVF, with special advantages and disadvantages. A book such as this is urgently needed to reveal variations between laboratories, the application of current techniques and the chances of establishing pregnancies. Differences between individual authors are apparent, although there is little doubt that optimal techniques will emerge with further research. In this and other ways, this book is also reminiscent of the early days of IVF when a series of conferences extended the technique worldwide, and we will watch with interest for a similar expansion of IVM.

I have little doubt that IVM will extend to many clinics. The numerous small follicles in most patients can be aspirated for mature oocyte without any need for massive forms of ovarian stimulation as practised with IVF. Enormous advantages could flow; for example working with immature oocytes should avoid the risks of cryopreservation damage which was a serious and long-term impediment to oocyte freezing for IVF. New classes of patients could well be attracted to cryopreserve their immature oocytes for their older ages. It may be much safer to cryopreserve immature oocytes than those which are fully mature. The ability to extract dozens of oocytes, especially in PCOS patients, will also open possibilities of detailed research using enormous banks of oocytes (or follicles). Research such as this should help those patients recovering from cancer therapies or an innate loss of oocytes. The causes of meiotic errors due to anomalies in chromosome pairing in diakinesis, or in the attachment of chromosomes to the meiotic spindle should be assessed. Such knowledge could help to avoid these anomalies, so that embryos are free of aneuploidies or polyploidies without any need for FISH as used today. Lastly, research will be opened into the hidden nature of primordial germ cells and follicles to uncover the fundamentals of early development. In short, scientists and clinicians could be presented with enormous opportunities at present denied to them.

To finish, let me compliment the Editors planning and publishing this book. It is certain to carry IVM into many more clinics.

Dr Robert G Edwards
Emeritus Professor
University of Cambridge
Chief Editor
Reproductive BioMedicine Online
Cambridge
UK
September 2006

Preface

An introduction to in-vitro maturation of human oocytes

Seang Lin Tan, Ri-Cheng Chian, and William M Buckett

The clinical use of in-vitro matured (IVM) oocytes has come a long way since the initial work of Robert Edwards in the United Kingdom in the 1960s[1-3] and the early clinical successes of Kwang Yul Cha et al.[4] in South Korea and Alan Trounson et al.[5] in Australia in the early 1990s. There are now successful clinical IVM programs around the world and nearly a thousand children have been born as a result of clinical IVM treatment. In fact the contributing authors to this book are testament to the geographic spread of IVM.

Although the world's first IVF baby, Louise Brown, was conceived within an unstimulated menstrual cycle[6], it soon became obvious that if IVF was to progress from a research tool to a clinical treatment, the use of ovarian stimulation would be necessary. The principle was that ovarian stimulation recruited more of the developing primary follicles to progress to maturation rather than atresia and thus generated more oocytes and ultimately more embryos for transfer. Ovarian stimulation is responsible for IVF reaching the success rate which has enabled it to be readily available throughout the world[7,8]

However, ovarian stimulation also has a cost. Stimulation protocols are associated with side-effects and risks, including ovarian hyper stimulation syndrome (OHSS), as well as with increased direct and indirect costs. The develop ment of IVM allows the benefits of ovarian stimu lation – namely more oocytes and more embryos – without these additional risks and costs. IVM appears particularly suited to women with poly cystic ovaries (PCO) and polycystic ovary syn drome (PCOS), who seem to do well with IVM treatment and who are at significantly increased risk of OHSS following ovarian stimulation[9,10]

Following the First World Congress on In-Vitro Maturation held in Montreal in 2004 and the establishment of the International Society for the In-Vitro Maturation of Human Oocytes, it became apparent as IVM is increasingly prac ticed throughout the world that there is a real need for a comprehensive IVM textbook. We hope that this volume will fulfill this need!

We have endeavored to collect contributors with international expertise in all aspects of IVM from the basic scientific teams to the clinical treatment programs from around the world. The book is divided into four parts.

Part I covers the scientific rationale for IVM by outlining the normal oocyte growth, interac tion, and maturation in vivo and how these have led to the current understanding and develop ment of protocols for oocyte maturation in vitro. We have also sought to determine possible future scientific developments in IVM and scientific concerns regarding the effect of IVM on oocyte and later embryo development. Here we have to mention that follicular maturation and oocyte maturation are two totally different concepts. Follicular maturation refers to the process from primordial follicle to preovulatory follicle, in other words it reflects follicular growth. Oocyte maturation refers to the development of the fully grown oocyte from germinal vesicle (GV) to metaphase II (MII) stage, in order to receive sperm at fertilization. Oocyte maturation is triggered by the LH surge in vivo, and occurs spontaneously in vitro with suitable culture conditions. IVM mentioned in this book mainly refers to oocyte maturation in vitro, not follicular development in vitro.

Part II covers the normal ovarian function and the clinical, ultrasound, and biochemical features of PCO and PCOS. It also covers the risks of ovarian stimulation for conventional IVF and the prevention and treatment of OHSS.

Part III covers the clinical application of IVM. It aims to cover all aspects including patient selection, current treatment protocols (including the various priming protocols), immature oocyte retrieval, endometrial preparation, embryo development, all laboratory aspects, and the pregnancy and neonatal outcome following IVM.

Finally, Part IV covers possible new developments – such as how to improve IVM success rates – and also new treatment directions for IVM – such as those with previous poor conventional IVF treatments, the development of natural cycle IVF/IVM, and the use of IVM in fertility preservation.

Although IVM is still relatively new amongst assisted reproductive technologies (ART), we hope that this textbook will contribute towards its increased availability. We all believe that IVM offers many advantages over conventional IVF and that couples who would benefit from this treatment modality should be able to do so.

REFERENCES

1. Edwards RG. Maturation *in vitro* of mouse, sheep, cow, pig, rhesus monkey and human ovarian oocytes. Nature 1965; 208: 349–51.

2. Edwards RG. Maturation *in vitro* of human ovarian oocytes. Lancet 1965; 286: 926–9.

3. Edwards RG, Bavister BD, Steptoe PC. Early stages of fertilization *in vitro* of human oocytes matured *in vitro*. Nature 1969; 221: 632–5.

4. Cha KY, Koo JJ, Ko JJ et al. Pregnancy after *in vitro* fertilization of human follicular oocytes collected from nonstimulated cycles, their culture *in vitro* and their transfer in a donor oocyte program. Fertil Steril 1991; 55: 109–13.

5. Trounson A, Wood C, Kausche A. *In vitro* maturation and fertilization and developmental competence of oocytes recovered from untreated polycystic ovarian patients. Fertil Steril 1994; 62: 353–62.

6. Steptoe PC, Edwards RG. Successful birth after IVF. Lancet 1978; 312: 366.

7. Tan SL, Royston P, Campbell S et al. Cumulative conception and live birth rates after in vitro fertilisation. Lancet 1992; 339: 1390–4.

8. Engmann L, Maconochie N, Bekir JS et al. Cumulative probability of clinical pregnancy and live birth after a multiple cycle IVF package: a more realistic assessment of overall and age-specific success rates? Br J Obstet Gynecol 1999; 106: 165–70.

9. Chain RC, Guleki B, Buckett WM et al. Priming with Human Chorionic Gonadotropin before Retrieval of Immature Oocytes in Women with Infertility Due to the Polycystic Ovary Syndrome. N Engl J Med 1999; 341: 1624–6.

10. Tan SL, Child TJ, Gulekli B. In-vitro maturation and fertilization of oocytes from unstimulated ovaries: Predicting the number of immature oocytes retrieved by early follicular phase ultrasonography. Am J Obstet Gynecol 2002; 186: 684–9.

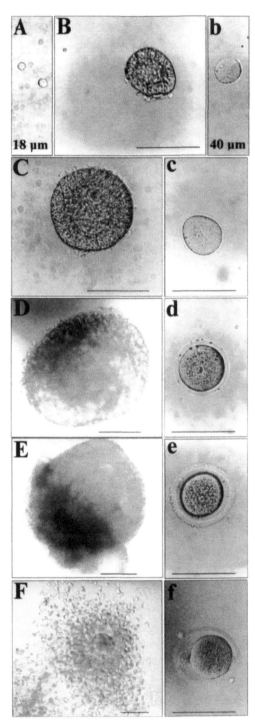

A
18 µm
B
b
40 µm
C
c
D
d
E
e
F
f

Bar represents 100 µm

Figure 2.2 Mouse oocyte and follicle development. (A) Primordial follicle consisting of an immature oocyte enclosed by a single layer of pregranulosa cells; (B) primary follicle showing an immature, growing oocyte (b) within approximately two layers of granulosa cells; (C) late primary/early secondary preantral follicle showing a growing, immature oocyte (c) surrounded by 3–4 layers of granulosa cells and an incomplete layer of theca cells; (D) early antral follicle showing an oocyte (d) at the center of a multilaminar follicle showing pockets of follicular fluid; (E) antral follicle showing an oocyte–cumulus complex (e) suspended in the follicular antrum; (F) ovulated oocyte–cumulus complex; and (f) ovulated, denuded, metaphase II oocyte with visible first polar body

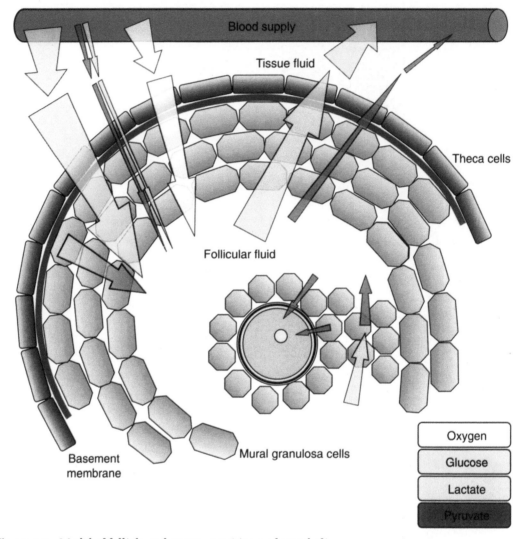

Figure 2.6 Model of follicle and oocyte nutrition and metabolism

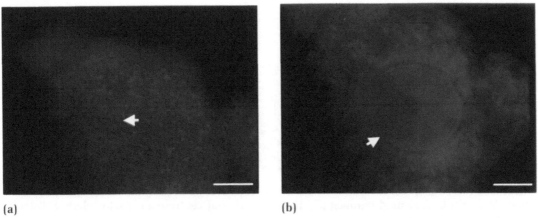

(a)   (b)

Figure 3.1 Fluorescent staining of f-actin in an unexpanded bovine cumulus oocyte complex. An example of the close proximity of the many adjacent cumulus cells (arrowhead) which facilitate cell–cell communication in the cumulus complex is shown in (a). The close association between the oocyte (arrowhead) and the companion cumulus cells is shown in (b) oocyte. Scale bars = 50 µm

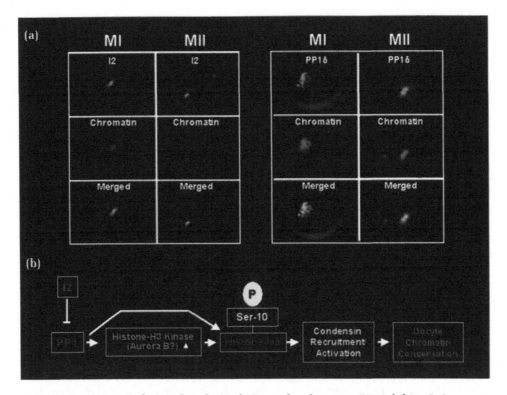

Figure 5.5 (a) Immunocytochemical analysis of $PP1_\delta$ and endogenous PP1 inhibitor I2 in mouse metaphase I and metaphase II oocytes. Both $PP1_\delta$ and I2 localize with condensed chromatin. (b) Proposed mechanism of how PP1 may regulate oocyte histone phosphorylation and chromatin condensation. During times of oocyte chromatin condensation, chromatin associated I2 may inhibit PP1 activity. This decrease in chromatin associated PP1 activity results in increased histone-H3 phosphorylation through direct effects, or via possible activation of a histone-H3 kinase (aurora B). This increased histone-H3 phosphorylation leads to chromatin condensation, possibly through recruitment and/or activation of condensation factors, such as the condensin complex

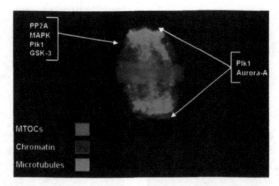

Figure 5.6 Micrograph of a mouse oocyte metaphase I meiotic spindle displaying microtubules (green/β-tubulin), condensed chromatin (blue/Hoescht), and centrosomes (red/γ-tubulin). Potential regulators of spindle component phosphorylation and activity are listed

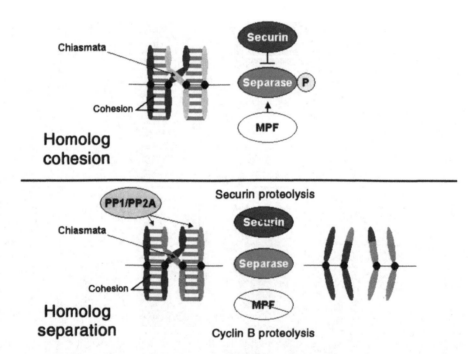

Figure 5.7 Proposed mechanism of control of homolog cohesion and separation during meiosis I of oocyte maturation. The cohesion complex (red) maintains cohesion between sister chromatids, while homologous chromosomes are connected at chiasmata. Separase activity is inhibited through the action of securin and phosphorylation of separase by MPF. Homologs separate when securin and the MPF component, cyclin B, undergo proteolysis, resulting in separase activity. Separase activity, along with desphosphorylation of cohesin complex components by PP1 and/or PP2A, allows for separation of sister chromatids, resolution of chiasmata, and separation of homologs

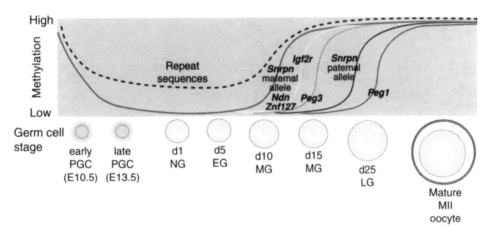

Figure 6.2 Methylation dynamics of imprinted genes and repeat sequences during female germ line development. The lower panel illustrates the stages of germ cell development shown in the top panel. The top panel illustrates the methylation dynamics of imprinted genes in the developing oocyte, beginning with the demethylation of imprinted and single copy genes in the primordial germ cells (red line). At this early stage, repeat sequences are not demethylated to the same extent as the single copy genes (dotted line). During oocyte growth, single copy genes become hypermethylated throughout the growth stages. Imprints are established asynchronously in the oocyte, with the latest imprints being established in the late growing stages. PGC: primordial germ cell; NG: non-growing oocyte; EG: early growing oocyte; MG: mid growth oocyte; LG: late growing oocyte; MII: metaphase II. Adapted from references 4 and 32

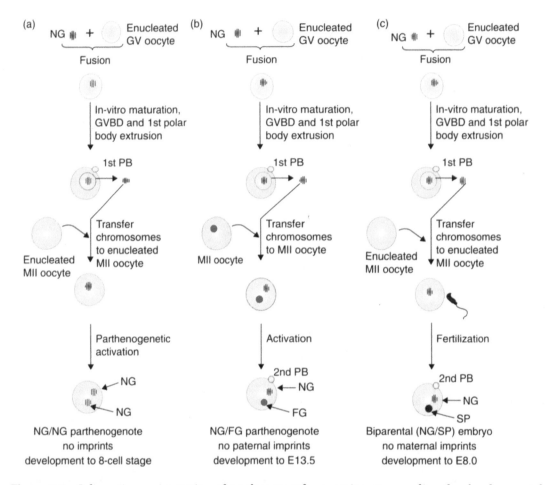

Figure 6.3 Schematic representation of nuclear transfer experiments revealing the developmental potential of oocytes at different stages of growth and maturation. Non-growing oocytes have not estab lished maternal imprints (pink hatched nuclei). (a) When non-growing oocytes are used in nuclear transfer experiments followed by parthenogenetic activation of the oocyte, development stalls at the 8-cell stage. (b) When the nucleus of a non-growing oocyte is transferred to a mature MII oocyte which retains its nucleus (red nucleus) development proceeds to E13.5. (c) When the nucleus of a non-grow ing oocyte is transferred to an enucleated MII oocyte and fertilized with a normal spermatozoon (blue nucleus) development stalls at E8.0. NG: non-growing oocyte; GV: germinal vesicle stage oocyte; PB: polar body; MII: metaphase II; FG: fully grown (mature) oocyte; SP: sperm. Adapted from references 27 and 29

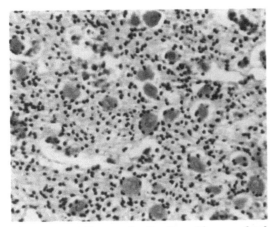

Figure 7.1 Micrograph of cultured human fetal follicles[9]. Section of human ovarian fetal follicles after 3 weeks in culture, stained for bromodeoxy-uridine (BrdU) incorporation (DNA division). The tissue was taken from a 33 GW fetus with achondroplasia. Note the normal primordial follicles, lack of brown BrdU staining in the GCs indicating no proliferation, and brown staining only in the oocytes. Background blue staining is hematoxylin. Magnification × 400

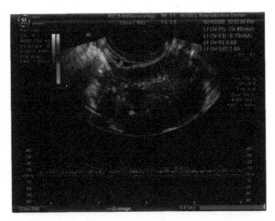

Figure 15.3 Stromal blood flow in polycystic ovary

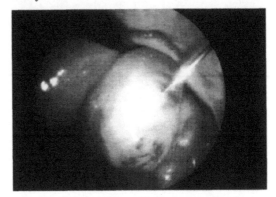

Figure 19.1 Laparoscopic oocyte retrieval

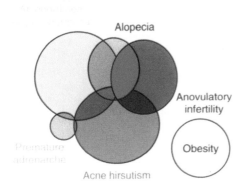

Figure 15.1 The spectrum of presentation in polycystic ovary syndrome

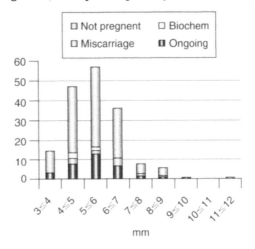

Figure 20.1 Protocol for endometrial preparation in IVM cycle

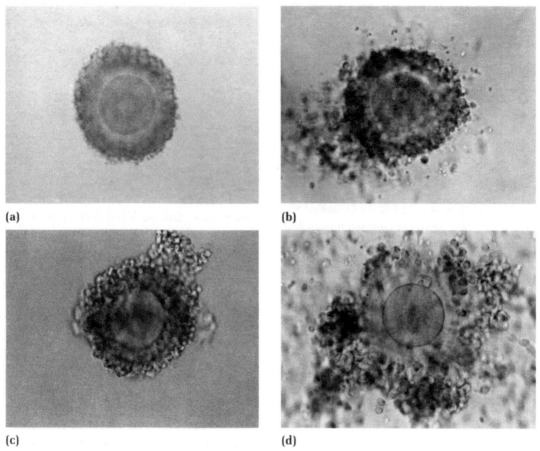

(a)

(b)

(c)

(d)

Figure 21.5 During COC sliding, it is possible to observe clearly whether or not the oocyte cytoplasm contains a germinal vesicle (GV) (a and b) or whether the oocyte has extruded a first polar body (1PB) into the perivitelline space (PVS) (c). If neither a GV is seen in the oocyte cytoplasm nor a 1PB is found in the PVS, then the oocyte is defined as germinal vesicle breakdown (GVBD) or metaphase I stage (MI) (d)

CHAPTER 1

Oocyte growth and developmental competence

Fiona H Thomas and Barbara C Vanderhyden

INTRODUCTION

While great progress has been made in the treatment of infertility by assisted reproduction technologies (ART), the quality of human oocytes retrieved for infertility treatment is still surprisingly low, with only 10–20% of human eggs producing pregnancy. In order to improve treatment, we must better understand how healthy oocytes develop and what can go wrong during oocyte growth and maturation. The ability to grow mature oocytes from immature oocytes in vitro would mean that women would not require the expensive drug regime and monitoring that they currently have to undergo, as this could all be controlled in vitro. However, progress has been slow in developing these techniques for use in women, with the major problem being a lack of knowledge of how the oocyte acquires developmental competence during its growth within the follicle. The overall aim of current research should be to gain an understanding of how to produce quality oocytes and to elucidate the consequences of impaired oocyte health. The key processes required to produce healthy mature oocytes should be identified, as well as the identification of non-invasive markers to distinguish healthy from unhealthy oocytes. Once we have a better understanding of the factors that

are required during development to make a good oocyte, then perhaps we will be able to develop in-vitro growth systems for clinical application.

OVERVIEW OF OOCYTE DEVELOPMENT

Ovarian follicles begin their development as primordial structures, which consist of an oocyte arrested at the diplotene stage of the first meiotic division, surrounded by a few flattened granulosa cells. Once the pool of primordial follicles has been established, and in response to an unknown signal, follicles are gradually and continuously recruited to grow. This initial growth is independent of the pituitary gonadotropins. During early follicular development, the oocyte grows and the granulosa cells proliferate to form a multi-laminar structure called a preantral follicle. Once the follicle reaches a species-specific size, it forms a fluid-filled space called an antrum. When this stage has been reached, follicles become acutely dependent on gonadotropins for further growth and development.

The growth phase of the oocyte allows development of the zona pellucida and production of mRNA and proteins required for subsequent fertilization and early embryonic development.

These factors must be stored within the oocyte, as resumption of meiosis results in transcriptional silencing[1]. Oocyte developmental competence, defined as the ability of the oocyte to resume and complete meiosis, and support preimplantation embryonic development after fertilization, is acquired gradually during folliculogenesis, and oocytes must grow in order to become competent (Figure 1.1). During growth, oocytes also differentiate; a complex cytoplasmic organization is required, dependent on production of new gene products and organelles and the modification and redistribution of existing ones[2]. Since the oocyte chromosomes and cytoplasm have many roles during this process, functional distinctions between nuclear, cytoplasmic, and molecular maturation have been made[3]. Nuclear maturation reflects the transformation of chromatin status from dictyate (germinal vesicle, GV) to metaphase II stage, whereas cytoplasmic maturation encompasses changes in the distribution and organization of the individual organelles such as the cortical granules from germinal vesicle to metaphase II stages. Lastly, molecular maturation can be described as the legacy of the instructions accumulated during the GV stage that control both nuclear and cytoplasmic progression[3].

Oocytes may reach a diameter of approximately 120 μm in early antral follicles of humans, while in rodents, the maximum diameter of 70 μm has already been reached at the end of the preantral stage and the oocyte acquires the competence to resume meiosis. Once competence is achieved, the oocyte remains in meiotic arrest until the preovulatory gonadotropin surge. The competence of an oocyte to resume and complete meiosis and, after fertilization, to develop into a blastocyst is markedly increased during preovulatory development through a process called oocyte capacitation[4]. Thus, after termination of oocyte transcription, the oocyte does not enter quiescence but prepares itself for a possible continued development as an embryo after fertilization.

MAINTENANCE OF OOCYTE MEIOTIC ARREST

Throughout oocyte growth, prophase arrest is thought to be maintained by inherent factors in

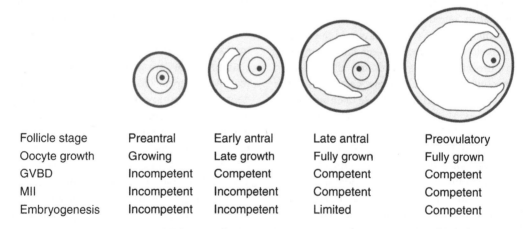

Follicle stage	Preantral	Early antral	Late antral	Preovulatory
Oocyte growth	Growing	Late growth	Fully grown	Fully grown
GVBD	Incompetent	Competent	Competent	Competent
MII	Incompetent	Incompetent	Competent	Competent
Embryogenesis	Incompetent	Incompetent	Limited	Competent

Figure 1.1 Oocyte developmental competence is defined as the ability of the oocyte to resume and complete meiosis, i.e. to undergo germinal vesicle breakdown (GVBD) and progression to metaphase II (MII), and to support preimplantation embryonic development after fertilization. This acquisition of oocyte developmental competence is acquired gradually during follicular development

the oocytes, and is correlated with low levels of cell cycle regulatory proteins such as p34[cdc2] and cyclin B[5]. Once oocytes become meiotically competent, maintenance of meiotic arrest requires the activity of signaling molecules within the oocyte such as the heterotrimeric G protein, Gs[6,7]. A G protein-coupled receptor, named Gpr3, which is present in oocytes, has recently been identified as a negative regulator of meiotic resumption[7]. A high proportion of oocytes within antral follicles in mice lacking Gpr3 contained metaphase chromosomes, indicating the resumption of meiosis. The predominant expression of Gpr3 mRNA in the oocyte, compared with somatic cells, and the dependence of meiotic arrest on Gs, supports the conclusion that the Gpr3 receptor in the oocyte is required to maintain meiotic arrest[7] (Figure 1.2). However, the putative ligand for the Gpr3 receptor remains unidentified, but may be produced by the granulosa cells, since competent oocytes

spontaneously resume meiosis upon removal from the surrounding granulosa cells[8].

The level of cyclic adenosine monophosphate (cAMP) in the oocyte plays a critical role in resumption of meiotic maturation, as pharmacologic manipulation to increase cAMP levels in competent mammalian oocytes results in inhibition of meiosis[9]. It has been hypothesized that a breakdown in gap junctional communication between the oocyte and granulosa cells at the time of the preovulatory LH surge results in a decrease in cAMP levels within the oocyte, leading to the inactivation of the PKA pathway[10] (Figure 1.2). However, germinal vesicle breakdown (GVBD), the first stage of meiotic resumption, occurs prior to any detectable ionic or metabolic uncoupling between the oocyte and cumulus cells, supporting the idea that a cumulus or granulosa cell factor could override the inhibitory effects of cAMP and promote meiotic resumption[11]. On

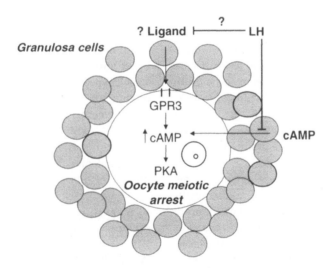

Figure 1.2 The level of cyclic adenosine monophosphate (cAMP) in the oocyte plays a critical role in resumption of meiotic maturation. Breakdown in gap junctional communication between the oocyte and granulosa cells at the time of the preovulatory LH surge is thought to result in a decrease in cAMP levels within the oocyte, leading to the inactivation of the PKA pathway. The Gpr3 receptor in the oocyte has been recently identified and is required to maintain meiotic arrest. However, the putative ligand for the Gpr3 receptor remains unidentified, but may be produced by the granulosa cells, since competent oocytes spontaneously resume meiosis upon removal from the surrounding granulosa cells

the other hand, the oocyte and granulosa cells may respond separately to LH in terms of their production of cAMP. This idea is supported by experiments using cell type-specific phosphodiesterase (PDE) inhibitors, where inhibition of PDE3A, expressed exclusively in oocytes, completely blocks oocyte maturation in vitro and in vivo[12,13], whereas inhibition of PDE4, restricted to granulosa cells, has no effect[12,14,15].

IN-VITRO MODELS FOR THE STUDY OF OOCYTE GROWTH AND DEVELOPMENTAL COMPETENCE

Culture systems for preantral follicles, or their oocyte–granulosa cell complexes (OGCs), are important for studying oocyte development, as well as for analysis of follicular development and function. Techniques for isolation of immature follicles and OGCs have been established in rodent and domestic animal species, as well as in humans[16–18]. The viability of the rodent systems has been demonstrated by the production of live offspring from in-vitro grown OGCs from preantral follicles[19] and from the culture of whole preantral follicles[20]. More recently, oocytes from primordial follicles activated in vitro have acquired competence to be matured and fertilized, resulting in the production of live offspring[21,22].

The limited success of these rodent systems has resulted in attempts to develop similar methods to be applied in humans[23–25]. Less densely packed follicles, fibrous stromal tissue, larger follicles, and slow follicular growth have all played a role in delaying a successful system for isolation and culture of preantral follicles from women. In addition, difficulty in obtaining a sufficient amount of quality human ovarian material has limited the progress of development of culture systems for human follicles. Both mechanical[24] and enzymatic isolation techniques[23,26] have been applied to human preantral follicles. Another potential method of obtaining human

follicles is the use of aspirates obtained during oocyte retrieval for IVF, as has been reported by Zhang et al.[27]. However, the number of follicles recovered was low, and it was concluded that this was not a useful source of human follicles[27]. Thus, research should focus on improving techniques for the isolation and growth of human follicles. Another potential option for the preservation of fertility in women at risk of premature ovarian failure, such as those about to undergo chemotherapy, is the cryopreservation and subsequent transplant of ovarian tissue. Ten years after the first demonstration of restoration of fertility in sheep[28], a healthy child was born after transplant of a frozen-thawed ovarian autograft into a woman cured of Hodgkin's disease[29]. However, despite further success in this area[30], this technology is still very much at an early stage and more research is required to improve clinical outcome. In addition, as the risk of reseeding cancer cells from the graft poses a serious problem, research should focus on improving in-vitro methods for growing and maturing early stage follicles present in the cryopreserved ovarian tissue.

In-vitro systems for rodent and domestic animal species have been instrumental in the progression of knowledge of oocyte growth and developmental competence. This review will highlight some of the factors that have been shown to participate in oocyte development in animal models, as well as the relevance to human fertility.

PARACRINE CONTROL OF OOCYTE DEVELOPMENT

Within the follicle, the three-dimensional organization of the cells and the paracrine interactions between the oocyte and surrounding granulosa cells are critical for normal cell development and function[31–33] (Figure 1.3). Intrafollicular paracrine factors mediate oocyte–granulosa cell interactions and are essential for the production of healthy oocytes. The importance of some of these factors is described in the following sections.

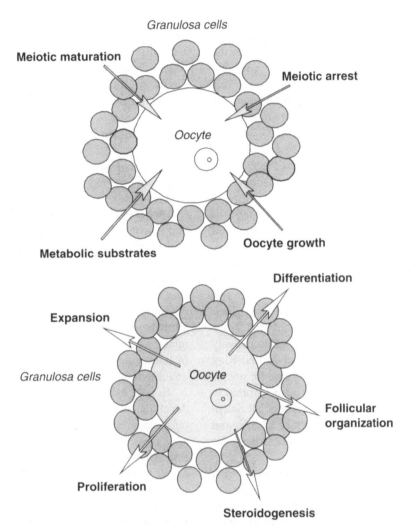

Figure 1.3 Within the follicle, the three-dimensional organization of the cells and the paracrine interactions between the oocyte and surrounding granulosa cells are critical for normal cell development and function. Via gap junctions and paracrine factors, granulosa cells influence a number of oocyte activities (upper diagram), while oocytes are capable of controlling and/or influencing several granulosa cell functions (lower diagram)

Granulosa cell factors

Kit ligand

The tyrosine kinase receptor Kit and its ligand, Kit ligand (KL; also known as KitL and SCF), have been localized to oocytes and granulosa cells, respectively[34]. KL has been shown to stimulate oocyte growth[35,36], and increased KL in follicular fluid in in-vitro fertilization (IVF) patients has been correlated with successful pregnancies[37]. KL is expressed in granulosa cells as either membrane-bound or soluble proteins arising from alternatively spliced mRNAs[38].

Soluble KL (KL-1) can be cleaved due to the presence of an 84 base pair exon (exon 6), which encodes a proteolytic cleavage site, allowing the extracellular domain to be released as a soluble product. Membrane-bound KL (KL-2) lacks this exon, is not efficiently cleaved, and thus remains more stably on the membrane[38]. The ratio of KL-1/KL-2 mRNA differs between tissues[38], between ovaries of mice of different ages[39], and between granulosa cells of preovulatory and ovulatory rat follicles[40], suggesting that these transcripts are differentially regulated.

Kit, the receptor for KL, is expressed in oocytes at all stages of follicular development in the mouse ovary[41], and several studies have demonstrated that female mice with naturally occurring mutations in KL or Kit are infertile due to developmental abnormalities[41,42]. For example, mice homozygous for the *Sld* allele, which only produce KL-1, are sterile due to a deficiency in germ cells[43]. However, mice that exclusively produce KL-2 are fertile[44], suggesting that KL-2 may be the principal isoform required for oocyte development. Indeed, KL-2 has been reported to induce a more persistent activation of Kit receptor kinase than the soluble form of KL[45,46], and thus is likely to be the more potent isoform for regulation of oocyte growth.

In order to determine the specific role of each KL isoform in promoting murine oocyte growth and maintenance of meiotic arrest in vitro, experiments using oocytes in co-culture with fibroblasts expressing either KL-1 or KL-2 have been performed in our laboratory. The data suggest that KL-2 is the principal isoform required to regulate oocyte growth and prevent spontaneous GVBD in isolated growing oocytes[47]. In addition, using immunofluorescence, it was found that KL-2 maintained the expression of Kit on the oocyte surface, whereas treatment with soluble KL-1 resulted in downregulation and/or internalization of the Kit receptor[47]. This phenomenon has previously been shown in mast cells[48]. Previous data from our laboratory have also shown that, in response to human chorionic gonadotropin

(hCG), there is a shift in steady-state mRNA from KL-2 to KL-1 in rat mural granulosa cells[40], and a rapid depletion of both isoforms in cumulus cells, which suggests differential functions of the KL isoforms during oocyte development and meiotic progression.

Oocyte factors

Growth/differentiation factor-9 (GDF-9)

GDF-9 has been shown to be expressed in human and mouse ovaries, and appears to be localized exclusively to oocytes at all stages of follicular growth, except primordial follicles, in neonatal and adult mice[49]. The pattern of GDF-9 expression as well as results from GDF-9 gene knock-out studies suggest that this factor may play an autocrine role in the regulation of oocyte development and maturation and/or a paracrine role in the regulation of granulosa cell proliferation and differentiation[50,51].

In GDF-9-deficient mouse ovaries, follicular development does not progress beyond the primary stage, but the oocytes within these follicles grow larger than normal[50,52]. In addition, oocytes from GDF-9-deficient mice do not acquire full developmental competence[51]. Interestingly, these mutant mice also have elevated levels of KL mRNA[51,52], which suggests that GDF-9 regulates KL expression. Differential regulation of the two KL transcripts is likely to be a vital component of regulation of KL expression during oocyte and follicular development. Since downregulation of KL-2 expression coincides with the cessation of oocyte growth[36], oocytes in GDF-9-deficient mice may exceed the normal maximum diameter due to continued elevation of KL-2 expression. Thus, a failure to downregulate KL-2 at the appropriate stage of development may impair oocyte growth and acquisition of developmental competence.

With respect to human fertility, a decrease in GDF-9 mRNA expression has been reported in human polycystic ovaries[53], thus deregulation of GDF-9 expression may contribute to aberrant folliculogenesis in women with polycystic ovary syndrome (PCOS). In addition, recombinant GDF-9 has been shown to promote the development of human primordial follicles to the secondary stage in culture, as well as improving follicular survival[54]. However, more studies are required to determine the significance of GDF-9 for oocyte growth and developmental competence in humans.

Bone morphogenetic protein-15 (BMP-15)

BMP-15 is an oocyte-specific homolog of GDF-9, and has been cloned in mice[55]. In sheep, where this factor has been well studied, the Inverdale fecundity gene (FecX) carries an inactivating mutation in BMP-15[56], implicating this factor in the control of ovulation rate. In rodents, both GDF-9 and BMP-15 promote proliferation of granulosa cells from small antral follicles[57–59], and BMP-15 has been reported to inhibit FSH-stimulated progesterone production by rat granulosa cells[58]. Evidence of interactions between GDF-9, BMP-15, and KL in vitro has been reported[60,61]. For example, recombinant GDF-9 inhibits KL mRNA expression in mouse preantral granulosa cells[60], whereas BMP-15 promotes KL expression in monolayers of granulosa cells from rat early antral follicles[61] (Figure 1.4). Recently, work in our laboratory has provided evidence of communication between BMP-15 and KL at the molecular level in intact murine OGCs in vitro[36]. By inhibition of Kit activity within OGCs in vitro, we are able to propose a mechanism whereby FSH regulates BMP-15 expression in a dose-dependent manner via Kit signaling. Thus interactions between these oocyte and granulosa cell factors, regulated by FSH, are likely to play a role in oocyte development (Figure 1.5).

The relevance of BMP-15 in human ovarian development remains unclear; one study has reported no aberrant BMP-15 mRNA expression

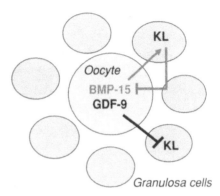

Figure 1.4 Interactions between GDF-9, BMP-15, and KL in vitro. Recombinant GDF-9 has been shown to inhibit KL mRNA expression in mouse preantral granulosa cells, whereas BMP-15 promotes KL expression in monolayers of granulosa cells from rat early antral follicles. In addition, a negative feedback loop can be proposed, as an increase in KL expression results in suppression of BMP-15 in mouse oocyte–granulosa cell complexes grown in vitro

in human polycystic ovaries[53], whereas preliminary data have recently been presented showing a loss of BMP-15 protein expression in ovaries from women with PCOS[62]. Significant species differences may exist in the relative importance of BMP-15, and much remains to be elucidated about the roles of BMP-15 and GDF-9 in the human ovary.

THE ROLE OF FSH IN OOCYTE DEVELOPMENT

Endocrine control of follicular development by FSH rests on a network of intrafollicular paracrine interactions[63]. For example, FSH promotes proliferation and differentiation of preantral follicles via paracrine factors such as IGF-1 and activin[64,65]. In addition, FSH regulates KL expression in granulosa cells from murine preantral follicles[66]. We have recently investigated the role of FSH in the regulation of KL

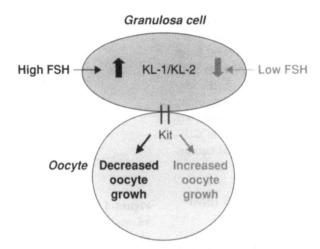

Figure 1.5   The correct concentration of FSH is required to modulate intrafollicular levels of KL mRNA, which subsequently controls oocyte growth. Low concentrations of FSH promote oocyte growth by increasing KL-2 expression, thereby reducing the ratio of KL-1/KL-2. Increased KL-1/KL-2 expression, stimulated by high concentrations of FSH, enhances follicle development but impairs oocyte growth

expression during the development of mouse preantral oocyte–granulosa cell complexes in vitro[36]. It was demonstrated that a low concentration of FSH decreased the ratio of steady-state KL-1/KL-2 mRNA by increasing KL-2 mRNA levels, and this was associated with increased oocyte growth in culture[36] (Figure 1.5). These results suggest that the correct balance of KL-1/KL-2 production is necessary for optimum oocyte growth in vitro. In addition, the correct concentration of FSH is crucial for appropriate regulation of paracrine factors to promote oocyte development. In granulosa-luteal cells obtained after oocyte harvest from patients undergoing IVF, a decrease in KL mRNA expression was reported in response to FSH and hCG in a time- and concentration-dependent manner in vitro[67], suggesting that KL is hormonally regulated in humans, and is likely to participate in follicular function during the human menstrual cycle.

Several studies provide evidence that a cautious approach is required when using FSH to stimulate oocyte and granulosa cell development. For example, repeated ovarian stimula-

tion of mice with gonadotropins in vivo has been reported to reduce subsequent in-vitro meiotic competence of oocytes[68]. Eppig et al.[69] reported that a relatively high concentration of FSH, in the presence of insulin, promoted precocious differentiation of granulosa cells within cultured preantral OGCs. These OGCs were also found to contain oocytes with reduced competence to undergo fertilization and preimplantation development[69] (Figure 1.6). A subsequent study by the same authors used a much lower concentration of FSH during follicular growth in vitro, and the rate of oocyte fertilization and blastocyst development was significantly improved[22]. Therefore, FSH is important for the acquisition of oocyte developmental competence, but the correct concentration of FSH is required to prevent premature follicle differentiation that would impair oocyte developmental competence. Recently, Roberts et al.[70] demonstrated that FSH impaired metaphase I chromosome alignment and increased aneuploidy in oocytes from mouse antral follicles matured in vitro, and these abnormalities were exacerbated

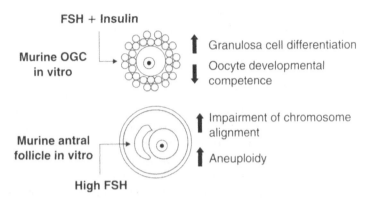

Figure 1.6 Murine oocyte–granulosa cell complexes (OGC) and antral exposed to high concentrations of FSH in vitro result in aberrant granulosa cell differentiation and oocyte development

with increased concentrations of FSH (Figure 1.6). Interestingly, the authors hypothesized that exposure of oocytes to high levels of FSH during meiotic maturation increases PKB/Akt phosphorylation, resulting in global phosphorylation and inactivation of spindle GSK-3. The resulting increased spindle stability provides an explanation for the greater chromosomal dispersion in oocytes exposed to high concentrations of FSH[70]. Importantly, the need for appropriate use of FSH in the treatment of human infertility has been demonstrated by Leader et al. (unpublished observations), who have shown that follicular growth and ovulation rate are increased using a low-dose FSH protocol for ovulation induction in women with anovulatory infertility, compared with a higher dose of FSH.

The association between oocyte and embryo culture and fetal abnormalities in animal models[71,72] is a growing cause for concern. The increasing trend to culture embryos for longer periods of time before uterine transfer so that the 'best' embryos can be used for transfer could also pose a problem[73]. The contribution of embryo culture to perturbations in metabolism and gene expression and the long-term consequences on development and behavior have been examined by Ecker et al.[73], who demonstrated that adult mice derived from cultured embryos exhibited specific behavioral alterations in anxiety/

locomotor activity, as well as spatial memory. Another study also demonstrated that specific culture conditions have the ability to change the pattern of gene expression in preimplantation mouse embryos[74]. It is therefore of the utmost importance to investigate this phenomenon during the growth and maturation of immature oocytes in vitro, as well as during embryo culture, if in-vitro technology is to be applicable to the preservation of human fertility.

GAP JUNCTIONS AND TRANSZONAL PROCESSES (TZPS) PARTICIPATE IN THE CONTROL OF OOCYTE DEVELOPMENT

Efficient delivery of factors to and from the oocyte at critical stages of development is essential for the coordination of oogenesis and folliculogenesis. Gap junctions, a form of oocyte–granulosa cell communication mediated by connexins, are also necessary for normal follicular development. A stage-specific pattern of distribution of different types of connexins during murine follicle development has been established[75]. Another study has shown that KL induces the onset of in-vitro growth of isolated fetal mouse oocytes, in the absence of gap junctional communication with granulosa cells[76]. However, these oocytes were unable to progress to the final stages of growth, and there was a lack of synchrony between nuclear and cytoplasmic maturation. It was noted that these oocytes had characteristics resembling oocytes from connexin-43- and -37-deficient mice, which have impaired follicular development beyond the preantral and early antral stages, respectively[77,78]; thus it was hypothesized that the preantral/antral transition is a critical stage of oocyte development requiring the coordinated differentiation of the oocyte with the granulosa cells[76]. The maintenance of adequate communication between these two cell types during the preantral and early antral stages is therefore necessary to ensure subsequent oocyte developmental competence. Gittens et al.[79] have provided evidence for interplay between paracrine signaling and gap junctional communication. In that study, expression of KL, Kit, and GDF-9 were analyzed in connexin-43-deficient mice, and the expression of connexin 43 was analyzed in GDF-9-deficient mice. The results suggest that, although gap junctional coupling among granulosa cells is not required to sustain expression of these paracrine factors, and GDF-9 is not required to sustain gap junctional coupling among granulosa cells, granulosa cells must be coupled via connexin 43 gap junctions in order to optimally respond to GDF-9[79].

As discussed earlier, paracrine factors secreted by oocytes and somatic cells regulate many important aspects of oocyte and follicular development, and there is substantial evidence which supports a model for bi-directional paracrine communication, based on the developmental regulation of the delivery and reception of paracrine factors at the oocyte–granulosa cell interface[80]. TZPs, which are granulosa cell extensions that traverse the zona pellucida and terminate on the oocyte cell surface, have been characterized in many mammals by electron microscopy[80,81]. These TZPs have been shown to undergo dynamic alterations in form and number during the course of follicular development[81]. TZPs are

most numerous at the preantral stage, forming adhesive and gap junctional contacts at the oolemma. During peak periods of oocyte growth, TZPs extend as deep invaginations, impinging on the oocyte germinal vesicle[81]. FSH has recently been shown to regulate the ability of granulosa cells to make connections with the oocyte[82]. In that study, it was shown that FSH treatment of prepubertal or FSHβ-knockout mice decreased the density of TZPs, which coincided with changes in chromatin remodeling and acquisition of oocyte meiotic competence[82]. Given the importance of oocyte–somatic cell interactions during early follicular development, investigation into regulation of the structural integrity of this interface during growth in vitro is required if culture systems for the production of competent oocytes are to improve significantly.

CONCLUSIONS

At present, the major barrier to developing and optimizing in-vitro techniques for alleviation of infertility in women is our lack of knowledge of how the oocyte acquires developmental competence during its growth within the follicle. The overall aim of current research should be to gain an understanding of how to produce quality oocytes and to elucidate the consequences of impaired oocyte health. Currently, research is under way to identify cross-species (including human) determinants of oocyte quality using a variety of techniques, from culture systems to animal models of infertility. Once we have a better understanding of the factors that are required during development to make a good oocyte in these animal models, then perhaps we will be able to develop in-vitro growth systems for clinical application. Importantly, any factors identified that promote oocyte health, or are indicators of oocyte quality, will be investigated in humans with correlations to pregnancy outcome and offspring health.

ACKNOWLEDGMENTS

FHT is partly funded by a fellowship from the Canadian Institutes of Health Research (CIHR) Strategic Training Initiative in Research in the Reproductive Health Sciences. BCV is a Project Leader of the Program on Oocyte Health funded under the Healthy Gametes and Great Embryos Strategic Initiative of the CIHR, Institute of Human Development, Child and Youth Health, Grant number HGG62293.

REFERENCES

1. Bouniol-Baly C, Hamraoui L, Giubert J et al. Differential transcriptional activity associated with chromatin configuration in fully grown mouse germinal vesicle oocytes. Biol Reprod 1999; 60: 580–7.

2. Picton H, Briggs D, Gosden R. The molecular basis of oocyte growth and development. Mol Cell Endocrinol 1998; 145: 27–37.

3. Sirard MA. Resumption of meiosis: mechanism involved in meiotic progression and its relation with developmental competence. Theriogenology 2001; 55: 1241–54.

4. Van den Hurk R, Zhao J. Formation of mammalian oocytes and their growth, differentiation and maturation within ovarian follicles. Theriogenology 2005; 63: 1717–51.

5. Kanatsu-Shinohara M, Schultz RM, Kopf GS. Acquisition of meiotic competence in mouse oocytes: absolute amounts of p34(cdc2), cyclin B1, cdc25C, and wee1 in meiotically incompetent and competent oocytes. Biol Reprod 2000; 63: 1610–16.

6. Mehlmann LM, Jones TLZ, Jaffe LA. Meiotic arrest in the mouse follicle maintained by a Gs protein in the oocyte. Science 2002; 297: 1343–5.

7. Mehlmann LM, Saeki Y, Tanaka S et al. The Gs-linked receptor GPR3 maintains meiotic arrest in mammalian oocytes. Science 2004; 306: 1947–50.

8. Erickson GF, Sorensen RA. In-vitro maturation of mouse oocytes isolated from late, middle and preantral graafian follicles. J Exp Zool 1974; 190: 123.

9. Conti M, Andersen CB, Richard F et al. Role of cyclic nucleotide phosphodiesterases in resumption of meiosis. Mol Cell Endocrinol 1998; 145: 9–14.

10. Dekel N. Cellular, biochemical and molecular mechanisms regulating oocyte maturation. Mol Cell Endocrinol 2005; 234: 19–25.

11. Homa ST. Calcium and meiotic maturation of the mammalian oocyte. Mol Reprod Dev 1995; 40: 122–34.

12. Conti M. Specificity of the cyclic adenosine 3′,5′-monophosphate signal in granulosa cell function. Biol Reprod 2002; 67: 1653–61.

13. Duckworth BC, Weaver JS, Ruderman JV. G2 arrest in xenopus oocytes depends on phosphorylation of cdc25 by protein kinase A. Proc Natl Acad Sci 2002; 99: 16794–9.

14. Tsafriri A, Chun SY, Zhang R et al. Oocyte maturation involves compartmentalization and opposing changes of cAMP levels in follicular somatic and germ cells: studies using selective phosphodiesterase inhibitors. Devel Biol 1996; 178: 393–402.

15. Conti M, Andersen CB, Richard F et al. Role of cyclic nucleotide signaling in oocyte maturation. Mol Cell Endocrinol 2002; 187: 153–9.

16. Cortvrindt R, Smitz J. In-vitro follicle growth: achievements in mammalian species. Reprod Domest Anim 2001; 36: 3–9.

17. Vanderhyden BC. Oocyte–granulosa cell interactions. In: Fleming TP, ed. Cell–Cell Interactions A Practical Approach. Oxford University Press, Oxford, 2002: 177–201.

18. Thomas FH, Walters KA, Telfer EE. How to make a good oocyte: an update on in-vitro models to study follicle regulation. Hum Reprod Update 2003; 9: 1–15.

19. Eppig JJ, Schroeder AC. Capacity of mouse oocytes from preantral follicles to undergo embryogenesis and development to live young after growth, maturation, and fertilization in-vitro. Biol Reprod 1989; 41: 268–76.

20. Spears N, Boland NI, Murray AA et al. Mouse oocytes derived from *in-vitro* grown primary ovarian follicles are fertile. Hum Reprod 1994; 9: 527–32.

21. Eppig JJ, O'Brien MJ. Development in-vitro of mouse oocytes from primordial follicles. Biol Reprod 1996; 54: 197–207.

22. O'Brien MJ, Pendola JK, Eppig JJ. A revised protocol for in-vitro development of mouse oocytes from primordial follicles dramatically improves their developmental competence. Biol Reprod 2003; 68: 1682–6.

23. Roy SK, Treacy BJ. Isolation and long-term culture of human preantral follicles. Fertil Steril 1993; 59: 783–90.

24. Abir R, Franks S, Mobberley MA et al. Mechanical isolation and in vitro growth of preantral and small antral human follicles. Fertil Steril 1997; 68: 682–8.

25. Wright CS, Hovatta O, Margara R et al. Effects of follicle-stimulating hormone and serum substitution on the in-vitro growth of human ovarian follicles. Hum Reprod 1999; 14: 1555–62.

26. Roy SK, Terada DM. Activities of glucose metabolic enzymes in human preantral follicles: in-vitro modulation by follicle-stimulating hormone, luteinizing hormone, epidermal growth factor, insulin-like growth factor I, and transforming growth factor beta1. Biol Reprod 1999; 60: 763–8.

27. Zhang P, Hreinsson JG, Telfer E et al. Few instead of many: human follicle collection from follicular aspirates at oocyte retrieval. Hum Reprod 2002; 17: 3190–2.

28. Gosden RG, Baird DT, Wade JC et al. Restoration of fertility to oophorectomized sheep by ovarian autografts stored at –196 degrees C. Hum Reprod 1994; 9: 597–603.

29. Donnez J, Dolmans MM, Demylle D et al. Livebirth after orthotopic transplantation of cryopreserved ovarian tissue. Lancet 2004; 364: 1405–10.

30. Meirow D, Levron J, Eldar-Geva T et al. Pregnancy after transplantation of cryopreserved ovarian tissue in a patient with ovarian failure after chemotherapy. N Engl J Med 2005; 353: 318–21.

31. Buccione R, Schroeder AC, Eppig JJ. Interactions between somatic cells and germ cells throughout mammalian oogenesis. Biol Reprod 1990; 43: 543–7.

32. Vanderhyden BC, Caron PJ, Buccione R et al. Developmental pattern of the secretion of cumulus expansion-enabling factor by mouse oocytes and the role of oocytes in promoting granulosa cell differentiation. Devel Biol 1990; 140: 307–17.

33. Vanderhyden BC, Telfer EE, Eppig JJ. Mouse oocytes promote proliferation of granulosa cells from preantral and antral follicles in-vitro. Biol Reprod 1992; 46: 1196–204.

34. Motro B, Bernstein A. Dynamic changes in ovarian c-kit and Steel expression during the estrous reproductive cycle. Devel Dyn 1993; 197: 69–79.

35. Packer AI, Hsu YC, Besmer P et al. The ligand of the c-kit receptor promotes oocyte growth. Devel Biol 1994; 161: 194–205.

36. Thomas FH, Ethier JF, Shimasaki S et al. Follicle-stimulating hormone regulates oocyte growth by modulation of expression of oocyte and granulosa cell factors. Endocrinology 2005; 146: 941–9.

37. Smikle CB, Dandekar PV, Schriock ED et al. Elevated ovarian follicular fluid stem cell factor concentrations are associated with improved pregnancy rates in in-vitro fertilization cycles. Fertil Steril 1998; 69: 70–2.

38. Huang EJ, Nocka KH, Buck J et al. Differential expression and processing of two cell associated forms of the Kit-Ligand: KL-1 and KL-2. Mol Biol Cell 1992; 3: 349–62.

39. Manova K, Huang EJ, Angeles M et al. The expression pattern of the c-kit ligand in gonads of mice supports a role for the c-kit receptor in oocyte growth and in proliferation of spermatogonia. Devel Biol 1993; 157: 85–99.

40. Ismail RS, Dube M, Vanderhyden BC. Hormonally regulated expression and alternative splicing of Kit Ligand may regulate Kit-induced inhibition of meiosis in rat oocytes. Devel Biol 1997; 184: 333–42.

41. Manova K, Nocka K, Besmer P et al. Gonadal expression of c-kit encoded at the W locus of the mouse. Development 1990; 110: 1057–69.

42. Driancourt MA, Reynaud K, Cortvrindt R et al. Roles of Kit and Kit Ligand in ovarian function. Rev Reprod 2000; 5: 143–52.

43. Flanagan JG, Chan DC, Leder P. Transmembrane form of the kit ligand growth factor is determined by alternative splicing and is missing in the Sld mutant. Cell 1991; 64: 1025–35.

44. Tajima Y, Moore MA, Soares V et al. Consequences of exclusive expression in vivo of kit ligand lacking the major proteolytic cleavage site. Proc Natl Acad Sci USA 1998; 95: 11903–8.

45. Miyazawa K, Williams DA, Gotoh A et al. Membrane-bound steel factor induces more persistent tyrosine kinase activation and longer life span of c-kit gene-encoded protein than its soluble form. Blood 1995; 85: 641–9.

46. Kurosawa K, Miyazawa K, Gotoh A et al. Immobilized anti-Kit monoclonal antibody induces ligand-independent dimerization and activation of steel factor receptor: biologic similarity with membrane-bound form of steel factor rather than its soluble form. Blood 1996; 87: 2235–43.

47. Thomas FH, Vanderhyden BC. KL-2 is the principal KL isoform for the promotion of murine oocyte growth and maintenance of meiotic arrest in-vitro. Biol Reprod 2005 (special issue): abstract 76.

48. Yee NS, Hsiau C-WM, Serve H et al. Mechanism of down-regulation of c-kit receptor: roles of receptor tyrosine kinases, phosphatidylinositol 3′-kinase, and protein kinase C. J Biol Chem 1994; 269: 31991–8.

49. McGrath SA, Esquela AF, Lee SJ. Oocyte-specific expression of growth/differentiation factor-9. Mol Endocrinol 1995; 9: 131–6.

50. Dong J, Albertini DF, Nishimori K et al. Growth differentiation factor-9 is required during early ovarian folliculogenesis. Nature 1996; 383: 531–5.

51. Elvin JA, Yan C, Wang P et al. Molecular characterization of the follicular defects in the growth differentiation factor 9-deficient ovary. Mol Endocrinol 1999; 13: 1018–34.

52. Ethier JF, Thomas FH, Vanderhyden BC. Initiation of oocyte growth in growth and differentiation factor-9 (GDF-9) deficient mice precedes both initiation of follicle development and the increase in Kit ligand (KL) mRNA expression. Biol Reprod 2005 (special issue): abstract 420.

53. Filho FLT, Baracat EC, Lee TH et al. Aberrant expression of growth/differentiation factor-9 in oocytes of women with polycystic ovary syndrome. J Clin Endocrinol Metab 2002; 87: 1337–44.

54. Hreinsson JG, Scott JE, Rasmussen C et al. Growth differentiation factor-9 promotes the growth, development, and survival of human ovarian follicles in organ culture. J Clin Endocrinol Metab 2002; 87: 316–21.

55. Dube JL, Wang P, Elvin J et al. The bone morphogenetic protein 15 gene is X-linked and expressed in oocytes. Mol Endocrinol 1998; 12: 1809–17.

56. Galloway SM, McNatty KP, Cambridge LM et al. Mutations in an oocyte-derived growth factor gene (BMP15) cause increased ovulation rate and infertility in a dosage-sensitive manner. Nat Genet 2000; 25: 279–83.

57. Hayashi M, McGee EA, Min G et al. Recombinant growth differentiation factor-9 (GDF-9) enhances growth and differentiation of cultured early ovarian follicles. Endocrinology 1999; 140: 1236–44.

58. Otsuka F, Yao Z, Lee T et al. Bone morphogenetic protein-15. Identification of target cells and biological functions. J Biol Chem 2000; 275: 39523–8.

59. Vitt UA, Hayashi M, Klein C et al. Growth differentiation factor-9 stimulates proliferation but suppresses the follicle-stimulating hormone-induced differentiation of cultured granulosa cells from small antral and preovulatory rat follicles. Biol Reprod 2000; 62: 370–7.

60. Joyce IM, Clark AT, Pendola FL et al. Comparison of recombinant growth differentiation factor-9 and oocyte regulation of Kit Ligand messenger ribonucleic acid expression in mouse ovarian follicles. Biol Reprod 2000; 63: 1669–75.

61. Otsuka F, Shimasaki S. A negative feedback system between oocyte bone morphogenetic protein 15 and granulosa cell Kit Ligand: its role in regulating granulosa cell mitosis. Proc Natl Acad Sci USA 2002; 99: 8060–5.

62. Stubbs SA, Al-Qahtani A, Laitinen M et al. Bone morphogenetic protein-15 (growth differentiation factor 9B) protein expression is reduced in human polycystic ovaries. Abstracts of ESHRE Campus Mammalian Oogenesis and Folliculogenesis 2005: abstract 7.

63. Hillier SG. Gonadotropic control of ovarian follicular growth and development. Mol Cell Endocrinol 2001; 179: 39–46.

64. Adashi EY, Resnick CE, Hurwitz A et al. Insulin-like growth factors: the ovarian connection. Hum Reprod 1991; 6: 1213–19.

65. Miro F, Hillier SG. Modulation of granulosa cell deoxyribonucleic acid synthesis and differentiation by activin. Endocrinology 1996; 137: 464–8.

66. Joyce IM, Pendola FL, Wigglesworth K et al. Oocyte regulation of Kit Ligand expression in mouse ovarian follicles. Devel Biol 1999; 214: 342–53.

67. Laitinen M, Rutanen EM, Ritvos O. Expression of c-kit ligand messenger ribonucleic acids in human ovaries and regulation of their steady state levels by gonadotropins in cultured granulosa-luteal cells. Endocrinology 1995; 136: 4407–14.

68. Combelles CMH, Albertini DF. Assessment of oocyte quality following repeated gonadotropin stimulation in the mouse. Biol Reprod 2003; 68: 812–21.

69. Eppig JJ, O'Brien MJ, Pendola FL et al. Factors affecting the developmental competence of mouse oocytes growth in-vitro: follicle stimulating hormone and insulin. Biol Reprod 1998; 59: 1445–53.

70. Roberts R, Iatropoulou A, Ciantar D et al. Follicle-stimulating hormone affects metaphase I chromosome alignment and increases aneuploidy in mouse oocytes matured in vitro. Biol Reprod 2005; 72: 107–18.

71. Young LE, Sinclair KD, Wilmut I. Large offspring syndrome in cattle and sheep. Rev Reprod 1998; 3: 155–63.

72. McEvoy TG, Robinson JJ, Sinclair KD. Developmental consequences of embryo and cell manipulation in mice and farm animals. Reproduction 2001; 122: 507–18.

73. Ecker DJ, Stein P, Xu Z et al. Long term effects of culture on preimplantation mouse embryos on behaviour. Proc Natl Acad Sci 2003; 101: 1595–600.

74. Rinaudo P, Schultz RM. Effects of embryo culture on global pattern of gene expression in preimplantation mouse embryos. Reproduction 2004; 128: 301–11.

75. Wright CS, Becker DL, Lin JS et al. Stage-specific and differential expression of gap junctions in the mouse ovary: connexin-specific roles in follicular regulation. Reproduction 2001; 121: 77–88.

76. Klinger FG, De Felici M. In vitro development of growing oocytes from fetal mouse oocytes: stage-specific regulation by stem cell factor and granulosa cells. Devel Biol 2002; 244: 85–95.

77. Simon AM, Goodenough DA, Li E et al. Female infertility in mice lacking connexin 37. Nature 1997; 385: 525–9.

78. Juneja SC, Barr KJ, Enders GC et al. Defects in the germ line and gonads of mice lacking connexin43. Biol Reprod 1999; 60: 1263–70.

79. Gittens JEI, Barr KJ, Vanderhyden BC et al. Interplay between paracrine signaling and gap junctional communication in ovarian follicles. J Cell Sci 2005; 118: 113–22.

80. Albertini DF, Combelles CM, Benecchi E et al. Cellular basis for paracrine regulation of ovarian follicle development. Reproduction 2001; 121: 647–53.

81. Motta PM, Makabe S, Naguro T et al. Oocyte follicle cells association during development of human ovarian follicle. A study by high resolution scanning and transmission electron microscopy. Arch Histol Cytol 1994; 57: 369–94.

82. Combelles CM, Carabatsos MJ, Kumar TR et al. Hormonal control of somatic cell oocyte interactions during ovarian follicle development. Mol Reprod Dev 2004; 69: 347–55.

CHAPTER 2

Metabolism of follicles and oocytes during growth and maturation

Sarah E Harris and Helen M Picton

INTRODUCTION

The current repertoire of human assisted reproduction therapies is undergoing constant development and improvement. In-vitro maturation (IVM) of near-grown oocytes and in-vitro growth (IVG) of follicles from early developmental stages are two such technologies, with much clinical potential for several groups of patients.

The success of both technologies is dependent on optimized culture conditions and development of a complete understanding of the metabolic and molecular processes occurring during growth initiation, development, and maturation. So far, efforts to elucidate and understand metabolic dynamics and nutritional requirements during folliculogenesis and oocyte growth, particularly in humans, have been small and investigations have largely focused on the metabolism of fully grown and maturing oocytes in rodent and ruminant species. It is becoming increasingly clear, however, that metabolic processes play complex roles in development, in addition to energy generation. The benefits of studying metabolism patterns during folliculogenesis and oogenesis are 2-fold. Firstly, a fuller understanding of the nutrient metabolism, energy demands, and nutrition of the follicle and oocyte during development will contribute to the improvement of systems for their growth and maturation in vitro. Secondly, metabolic profiling has attracted much interest as a potential non-invasive strategy for assessment of developmental competence in humans and other mammalian species[1,2]. Very little effort has been expended on characterizing the nutritional and metabolic profiles of mammalian follicles and oocytes, especially at stages prior to meiotic resumption, yet metabolic processes and nutrition play key roles in determining the developmental capacity and fate of the growing oocyte. Studies of the mature mammalian oocyte indicate that its metabolism is unique compared to most other tissues. Study of the follicular oocyte, however, is complicated by the functional and metabolic interaction of oocytes with companion granulosa cumulus cells. Metabolism of the whole oocyte–cumulus complex masks metabolism of the oocyte within it and removal of the oocyte from the oocyte–cumulus complex subjects the oocyte to additional culture stresses and deprivation of nutrients and signaling molecules. However, metabolic analysis of denuded oocytes isolated from staged follicles gives a useful indication of nutrient consumption and energy requirements at different developmental stages, but it is difficult to quantify and account for nutrients taken up by the oocyte via cytoplasmic bridges to granulosa cells.

This chapter will focus on pathways for energy production and nutrition of the mammalian oocyte and explore changes in energy requirements and metabolic patterns during growth and maturation.

BASIC ASPECTS OF CELLULAR ENERGY PRODUCTION

Cellular adenosine triphosphate (ATP) can be generated via several nutrient metabolism pathways (Figure 2.1). Glycolysis is the stepwise breakdown of the six-carbon sugar glucose to two molecules of the α-keto acid pyruvate. Associated with this pathway is the direct (substrate level) net phosphorylation of two molecules of adenosine diphosphate (ADP), forming two ATPs (Table 2.1) and the reduction of two molecules of the coenzyme nicotinamide adenine dinucleotide (NAD; oxidized form), forming two molecules of NADH (reduced form). Regeneration of NAD is critical for continued glycolysis and can be achieved in two ways. Firstly, in conditions of

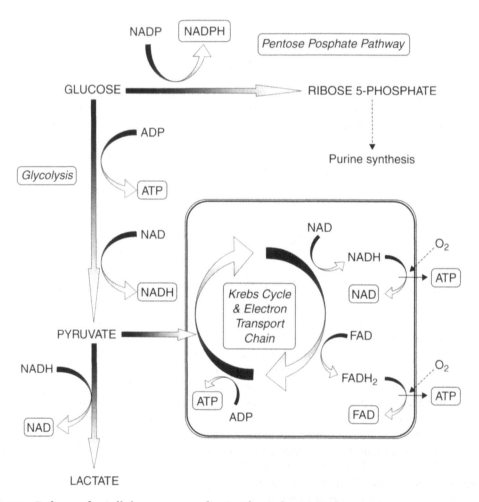

Figure 2.1 Pathways for cellular energy production from glucose and pyruvate

Table 2.1 Energy production from glucose and pyruvate

Nutrient	Metabolic pathway	Oxygen required (moles)	ATP produced (moles)
Glucose	Complete oxidation	6	31
Glucose	Glycolysis	0	2
Pyruvate	Complete oxidation	2.5	12.25

limited oxygen availability or where oxygen must be conserved for other processes, oxygen-independent regeneration of NAD from NADH is achieved by the lactate dehydrogenase (LDH) catalyzed conversion of pyruvate to lactate. Although glycolysis provides a means of rapid ATP generation, glycolytic metabolism of glucose to lactate is rather inefficient, resulting in a net gain of just two molecules of ATP. Secondly, during oxidative glucose metabolism NADH can be re-converted to NAD via the mitochondrial electron transport chain with co-production of ATP. When oxygen is plentiful, more efficient glucose metabolism is possible, whereby the two molecules of pyruvate produced by glycolysis are then further metabolized through the Krebs cycle. This is also associated with reduction of the coenzymes NAD and flavin adenine dinucleotide (FAD) to NADH and $FADH_2$. The electron transport chain uses molecular oxygen to re-oxidize the glycolysis and Krebs cycle derived NADH and $FADH_2$, re-forming NAD and FAD with the co-production of ATP. Oxidative metabolism is around 15-fold more efficient than simple substrate level ATP formation.

ROLE OF MITOCHONDRIA IN OOCYTE ENERGY PRODUCTION AND QUALITY

Oocytes of many mammalian species, including human and mouse, are unusual in their absolute requirement for oxidizable energy substrates, in particular pyruvate[3–5], and typically consume little glucose for energy production[6–8]. Mouse primordial germ cells and primordial oocytes without an intact genetic template for the glycolysis pathway are still competent to complete growth and can be fertilized[9], but when oxidative phosphorylation is inhibited or when in-vitro culture is under anaerobic conditions rodent oocyte development is prevented[10,11]. Oocyte glycolysis is limited by low activities of key glycolytic enzymes[12,13] and a lack of glucose transporters in the plasma membrane, making the oocyte reliant upon an adequate complement of mitochondria for oxidative energy production.

While oxidative energy production is very efficient there are toxic consequences in the generation of reactive oxygen species (ROS), such as the superoxide anion ($O^{·-}$), hydrogen peroxide (H_2O_2), and the hydroxyl radical ($HO^·$), formed when up to 2% of electrons leak from the transport chain and interact with molecular oxygen. ROS can have devastating effects, reacting with mitochondrial and nuclear DNA, proteins, and lipids, causing structural and functional instability, and can ultimately lead to apoptosis. Mitochondrial DNA is particularly vulnerable to oxidative stress[14] due to its close proximity to the electron transport chain, which is compounded by a lack of histones[15] and defense and repair systems[16]. The mitochondrial genome has a high exon content, so mutations are more likely to exert a detrimental effect on gene function. It is therefore not surprising that the mutation rate of mitochondrial genes is nearly 20 times that of nuclear DNA[15]. Mitochondria are critical elements in the process of aging[17,18] and impaired mitochondrial function is a factor in the age-related decline in oocyte quality, through (1) insufficient mitochondrial energy production[19,20] and (2) overwhelming free radical production[21].

In most cell types mitochondria carry multiple copies of their genome, which compensates for loss in function of damaged genes. Differences in DNA sequences can therefore occur between mitochondria and between copies of the genome within the same mitochondrion, resulting in heteroplasmy. Mitochondrial proliferation is by genome replication and fission, making mutations susceptible to inheritance. To counter the problem of inheriting a lethal load of mutations and to maintain the quality of mitochondrial DNA passed on to successive generations, a mitochondrial 'bottleneck' occurs during oocyte formation, severely restricting the number of mitochondria entering the germ line[22]. Clonal expansion of the very small number of 'pure' mitochondria inherited by the primordial germ cell forms the entire mitochondrial population of the oocyte and potential offspring. The very small initial population of mitochondria increases the chances that those mitochondria inherited by the primordial germ cell are homoplasmic and that mitochondria with function-impairing mutations are not transferred. Additionally, mitochondria which remain in the germ line of each generation remain haploid[23], presumably to reduce the risk of heteroplasmy.

During oogenesis, the number, distribution, and activity of mitochondria within the developing oocyte change to reflect growth and alterations in energy demand at different locations within the ooplasm. The newly formed population of human primordial germ cells in the yolk sac of the early embryo contains around 100 cells, each containing a cohort of only around 10 mitochondria[24]. Primordial germ cell proliferation forms a population of around 7 million oogonia in humans, while replication of the original mitochondria cohort forms a population of hundreds of mitochondria in an oogonium. The human primordial oocyte is thought to contain between 6 and 10 thousand mitochondria[23], which replicate further during oogenesis to finally number 100 000–400 000 in the mature oocyte[25].

During oocyte growth, the distribution of mitochondria within the ooplasm changes. In the primordial oocyte, mitochondria and other organelles are clustered around the nucleus, forming the 'Balbiani body'. As growth proceeds, a group of mitochondria remain close to the nucleus whilst other groups colonize the oocyte periphery or form clusters near energy-demanding processes, for example during spindle, polar body[26], and pronuclei formation[27]. In addition to changes in their number and distribution, mitochondrial activity changes markedly during development. The human primordial germ cell has a large store of glycogen and few mitochondria[23], suggesting that glycolysis might be an important contributor to energy production. Mitochondria in the oocyte are small and spherical with few cristae[28] and have a predominantly perinuclear location[29]. The morphology of oocyte mitochondria at this stage would suggest rather sluggish metabolic activity, but the oocyte compensates for this by being comparatively mitochondria dense[28]. Upon oocyte growth, initiation, and development up to the secondary follicle stage, mitochondria become progressively more elongated[29], suggestive of increased activity. Similar changes can be observed in the early embryo, where elongated mitochondria with increased numbers of cristae are observed during early embryogenesis; these morphologic changes are associated with the increased oxygen consumption seen in the later stages of preimplantation embryo development[30]. Low oocyte mitochondrial activity has been linked to poor oocyte morphology in the cow[31] and slow human preimplantation embryo development[19]. These data point to the number and quality of the mitochondrial complement of the oocyte as being a major selection pressure during oogenesis. Oocytes with defective mitochondria may be selected against at several points during their development, starting at the oogonia stage[32], helping to distill the population of germ cells with healthy mitochondria. The absolute reliance of the oocyte upon mitochondrial energy production ensures that oocytes become developmentally competent only if they carry a mitochondrial cohort producing energy above a threshold level needed to survive, and producing ROS below a threshold level needed to survive.

Metabolic interactions between follicular oocytes and surrounding granulosa cells are essential throughout oocyte growth and maturation. Gap junctions permit transfer of small molecules from somatic cells to the oocyte[33], including ATP[34]. This may mask mitochondrial insufficiency, which becomes apparent only when gap junction connections are severed during maturation, and may partially explain why some oocytes with defective mitochondria reach maturation but post-fertilization development is impaired. While threshold mitochondrial activity is necessary, excessive activity is disadvantageous: in addition to ROS generation, overactive mitochondria can become overwhelmed with crystals of divalent cations and inorganic phosphate and in mouse embryos this causes arrest during preimplantation development[35]. Advanced human maternal age has frequently been associated with reduced oocyte quality and the mitochondrial cohort is an important factor in this decline[19]. While mitochondrial quality cannot be improved per se, oocytes of advanced reproductive age have been rejuvenated by mitochondrial or cytoplasmic transfer[36]. However, while there appear to be benefits of this procedure in the short term, the long-term consequences of this controversial approach have not been identified.

OOCYTE REDOX STATE

ROS generation is an inevitable consequence of oxidative metabolism. The effects of ROS can be kept in check by cellular antioxidant defense systems including enzymes, vitamins, and metabolites. Superoxide dismutase (SOD) reduces superoxide radicals to H_2O_2 and hydroxyl radicals, which are then detoxified to water by catalase (CAT) and glutathione peroxidase (GPX). Glucose contributes to maintenance of the redox state via production of NADPH through the pentose phosphate pathway. NADPH is a potent reducing agent, and one of its myriad roles is pushing the reduction of oxidized glutathione. Other energy metabolites, like pyruvate and the α-keto acids[37], are also very important free radical scavengers, which spontaneously decarboxylate in the presence of free radicals. In culture, mammalian cells secrete pyruvate until a balance between intra- and extracellular levels is achieved[37]. If the culture medium concentration of pyruvate is low during IVM and the culture volume is high, intracellular pyruvate becomes excessively depleted, resulting in metabolic stress in the oocyte which will be manifested in the form of stunted ATP production and skewed redox potential[37]. Altered redox state appears to be a common occurrence after exposure of mammalian oocytes and embryos to the culture environment, affected by inappropriate levels and balance of culture medium components[38,39], oxygen[40], and oxidative stress[41,42].

METABOLISM DURING FOLLICULOGENESIS

The primordial follicle

The primordial follicle (Figure 2.2) is the most abundant follicle type within the ovary, but much of its biology remains something of an enigma. The population of primordial follicles represents a limited pool of female germ cells, with infertility and menopause the consequences of critical levels of depletion. The ovarian load of primordial follicles peaks during the fifth month of human fetal development, but by

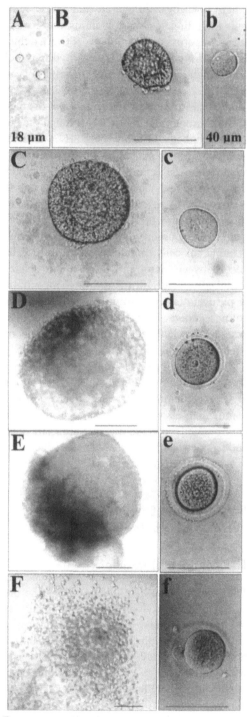

A 18 μm **B** **b** 40 μm **C** **c** **D** **d** **E** **e** **F** **f**

Bar represents 100 μm

birth numbers have declined from upwards of 5 million to around 1 million. A further substantial loss is seen between birth and menarche, when the population typically numbers 400 000. The etiology of this drastic atresia is unclear but it is possible that strict selection processes are operating, targeting defective or substandard germ cells for destruction. Primordial follicles and the oocytes within them appear to remain in a state of suspended development, sometimes for many years, and are thought to be relatively metabolically quiescent. Their very nature, however, implies that certain subcellular activities must occur, not least to maintain general 'housekeeping'. Follicular metabolism is the sum of the net metabolism of the oocyte and surrounding somatic cells. The combination of glucose and pyruvate consumption with lactate production indicates that both glycolytic and aerobic metabolism pathways are operating. Glycolysis is the major fate of the glucose taken up by the primordial follicle. However, lactate production exceeds that which could be generated from the glucose being taken up. Therefore, additional energy substrates must be metabolized, possibly glycogen[43].

Figure 2.2 Mouse oocyte and follicle development. (A) Primordial follicle consisting of an immature oocyte enclosed by a single layer of pregranulosa cells; (B) primary follicle showing an immature, growing oocyte (b) within approximately two layers of granulosa cells; (C) late primary/early secondary preantral follicle showing a growing, immature oocyte (c) surrounded by 3–4 layers of granulosa cells and an incomplete layer of theca cells; (D) early antral follicle showing an oocyte (d) at the center of a multilaminar follicle showing pockets of follicular fluid; (E) antral follicle showing an oocyte–cumulus complex (e) suspended in the follicular antrum; (F) ovulated oocyte–cumulus complex; and (f) ovulated, denuded, metaphase II oocyte with visible first polar body (see color plate section)

It has long been thought that the primordial follicle is relatively metabolically quiescent, as some primordial oocytes may wait up to 50 years to be recruited into the growing pool. This presumption is probably inaccurate as data from murine primordial follicles show that, for their size, primordial follicles have relatively high metabolism of energy substrates[44]. Glucose is consumed at an average rate of 14 +/– 6 fmoles/ follicle per hour and pyruvate at a rate of 28 +/– 9 fmoles/follicle per hour, while relatively large amounts of lactate are produced at a rate of 58 +/– 23 fmoles/follicle per hour.

The growing follicle

Glucose is the key nutrient consumed by the preantral follicle at the primary[44] and secondary[44,45] stages. During growth in vitro, the quantity of glucose consumed and lactate produced by preantral follicles steadily increases[44,45] (Figure 2.3)

as the follicle grows in size[45]. By analyzing the proportion of glucose consumed that accounts for lactate production, the contribution of glycolysis to glucose metabolism can be revealed; purely glycolytic metabolism of one molecule of glucose produces two molecules of lactate. At the late primary/early secondary preantral stage, 27% of glucose is metabolized glycolytically by mouse follicles (Figure 2.3), suggesting that the remaining glucose consumed has another metabolic fate. Some of this glucose may be used for glycogen synthesis, but it is likely that the majority is used for oxidative energy production. At the primary/secondary follicle stage, the oocyte is surrounded by only two to four layers of cells and the low proportion of glycolytic glucose metabolism implies that sufficient oxygen is reaching the developing oocyte. As the granulosa and theca cells continue to proliferate, there is a consequent increase in follicle size and an increased distance between the oocyte and

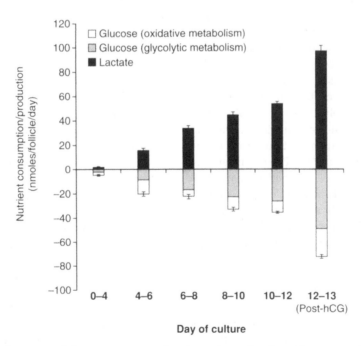

Figure 2.3 Development of glucose consumption (negative values) and lactate production (positive values) during growth of mouse follicles in culture

the follicle surface. This in turn means that an adequate oxygen supply must reach the growing oocyte, whose metabolism is obligately aerobic. To accommodate the metabolic demands of both the oocyte and somatic compartments, the follicle switches to a metabolic strategy more reliant upon glycolytic glucose breakdown[11,44–46]. The oocyte plays a key role in pushing this follicular metabolic switch[47]. Antrum formation appears to be a tactic to increase the available surface area for diffusion of nutrients while increasing the follicular mass. Sampling of human follicular fluid glucose and lactate concentrations supports the model of glycolytic glucose metabolism[48,49], with levels of these two nutrients being inversely related[48,49], and granulosa cells isolated from rat follicles produce large amounts of lactate[50]. In the late antral mouse follicle, the contribution of anerobic glycolysis to glucose metabolism reaches 76–100%[44,45]. Eppig and colleagues[47,51–53] have elegantly shown that the oocyte is a major driving force in the differentiation of granulosa cell metabolism phenotype. Metabolic pressure experienced by the oocyte may induce its stimulation of glycolytic metabolism and inhibition of oxidative metabolism in cumulus cells[47], thereby conserving the oxygen supply. The oocyte even goes so far as to promote cumulus cell uptake of certain amino acids (including glutamate, histidine, and alanine)[53] which may then be transferred to the oocyte via gap junctions[33,53]. The competence to adjust follicular glucose metabolism is acquired by the oocyte in the later stages of follicle development[47], presumably at a point when oxygen tension in follicular fluid becomes critically low. Healthy human oocytes are retrieved from follicles in which the oxygen tension is high (4–5%), and when oxygen availability is low (1–2%) oocyte viability is severely compromised[54]. When mouse follicles are cultured in low oxygen, the oocyte maturation rate is lower with a higher incidence of unaligned chromosomes[55]. This is likely due to inadequate oxidative energy production, resulting in metabolic stress and

insufficient ATP for processes involved in cytoplasmic and meiotic maturation.

Glucose is taken up by the follicle via facilitated transport systems[56] which are sensitive to glucose availability and endocrine stimuli. We have shown that mouse preantral follicles cultured in 5.5 mM glucose have glucose consumption rates approximately 4-fold higher than mouse follicles at comparable stages in another study in which 1–2 mM glucose was used[11]. The magnitude in the difference in glucose consumption rates paralleled the magnitude of the difference in glucose availability. Furthermore, insufficient glucose hinders growth and steroidogenesis of mouse follicles growing in vitro[45] and limits glucose consumption by cow oocyte–cumulus complexes[57]. Even 5.5 mM glucose may be suboptimal for mouse follicle culture. Follicles in vivo are exposed to glucose concentrations close to those observed in plasma, which can be as high as 11.0 mM[58]. Endocrine signaling also plays a major role in regulation of follicle glucose consumption. FSH promotes metabolism in rat granulosa cultures[50], and mouse[59] and bovine[57] oocyte–cumulus complexes, and metabolism of intact mouse follicles increases in response to ovulation induction[44,46,60]. Gonadotropin-stimulated glucose metabolism is subject to influence by insulin[61,62] and ovarian growth factors[63–66]. Endocrine effects are mediated by altered expression of glucose transporters[65] and their translocation to the cell membrane[67], and increased activity of glucose metabolism pathways[59,68].

In addition to their consumption of glucose, ovarian follicles produce large quantities of lactate. Secretion of lactate is higher by more developed follicles (Figure 2.3) and, like glucose consumption, peaks during the peri-ovulatory period in response to ovulation induction (Figure 2.3). During antral development, the contribution of glycolytic energy metabolism increases, causing a relative increase in lactate output. The appearance of high quantities of lactate as a byproduct of glycolytic glucose consumption may also influence processes occurring in the peri-ovulatory oocyte–cumulus complex. An increased lactate output would increase the lactate concentration in follicular fluid, so pushing down the pH. It has previously been shown that meiotic maturation of the mouse oocyte–cumulus complex is suppressed in more acidic conditions[69].

In conditions affecting aspects of metabolism, such as diabetes or polycystic ovarian syndrome, follicle metabolism may be perturbed. Hexokinase normally phosphorylates glucose forming glucose-1-phosphate, which can then be metabolized through glycolysis or through the pentose phosphate pathway. During hyperglycemia, hexokinase becomes saturated, forcing glucose along alternative metabolism pathways, generating molecules which suppress meiotic maturation in mouse oocyte–cumulus complexes[70]. FSH-stimulated pentose phosphate pathway activity is also compromised in oocyte–cumulus complexes from diabetic mice, reducing purine and ATP production[71]. Another observation is perturbed cell–cell coupling in oocyte–cumulus complexes from diabetic mice[71] and this has implications for normal oocyte development. In culture, bovine follicles deprived of insulin have impaired maturation rates compared to their insulin-treated counterparts[72].

The ovulatory follicle

In vivo, ovarian glucose uptake is augmented during the peri-ovulatory period, a phenomenon known as the 'metabolic shift'[73]. In vitro, follicle glucose consumption and lactate production are enhanced by up to 2-fold prior to ovulation (Figure 2.3). The exact reasons for this are unclear, but it is likely that several energy-demanding processes become operational after maturation induction. Firstly, synthesis of estrogens increases[74], with the dominant follicle producing up to 95% of circulating estradiol, and greater ATP availability would be needed to sustain estrogen output. Secondly, increased activity of the pentose phosphate pathway[75] is

necessary for generation of precursors for molecules which either suppress[76] or stimulate[77] resumption of meiosis in the oocyte. Thirdly, the process of ovulation itself is unlikely to be passive. The production of follicular fluid is driven by accumulation of salts and water in the antrum[78], with sodium appearing to be actively accumulated in the later stages of development[79]. This may go some way to explain the increase in intrafollicular pressure observed prior to ovulation in the hamster[80] and other species[81]. Lastly, it has recently been shown that the increase in glucose consumption by cow oocyte–cumulus complexes during maturation can, in part, be explained by the synthesis of hyaluronic from glucose metabolites, which facilitates cumulus expansion[57].

Cumulus cells from many mammalian species have been demonstrated to produce pyruvate from glucose[82]. This increases the availability of pyruvate in the vicinity of the oocyte. Secretion of pyruvate by cumulus cells is stimulated by gonadotrophins[59]. Ovulation induction signals the disruption of cytoplasmic contacts between the oocyte and cumulus cells, and the increase in pyruvate may serve two purposes, namely to ensure that an adequate supply of energy substrate is available to the oocyte and to reduce oxidative stress.

METABOLISM DURING OOGENESIS

The primordial germ cell

The primordial germ cell contains few mitochondria[24] and a store of glycogen[83], suggesting that glycolysis may contribute to energy production. There are many energetic demands within these cells, with cytoplasmic blebbing and pseudopodia formation[84] aiding movement of the primordial germ cell along the gonadal ridge. Mouse oocyte metabolism of radiolabeled pyruvate and glucose indicates that the CO_2 formation from pyruvate oxidation is in the region of 7.85×10^{-14}

moles/hour[84], equivalent to 0.026 pmoles of pyruvate oxidized per hour. CO_2 formation from glucose is 0.73×10^{-14} moles per hour[84], which is equivalent to 0.00121 pmoles of glucose oxidized per hour. This forms a ratio of pyruvate oxidation to glucose oxidation of 21.5:1. The potential ATP generation from pyruvate oxidation would be in the region of 0.32 pmoles per hour, while ATP from glucose oxidation would be about 0.0375 pmoles per hour, thus the proportion of ATP generated by pyruvate oxidation is 89%. Pyruvate oxidation therefore appears to be a major pathway for energy production. This is surprising in view of the low numbers in the mitochondrial cohort. However, glycolytic glucose consumption has not yet been analyzed. The primordial germ cell also contains glycogen, an endogenous energy source, but ATP generation from glycolytic or oxidative metabolism of this fuel has not yet been investigated. When its cytoplasmic volume is accounted for, pyruvate oxidation by the mouse primordial germ cell is high in comparison to pyruvate consumption at later stages of mouse oocyte and embryo development. While the high oxidative capacity of the mouse primordial germ cell is surprising, it is clear that the pathway for oocyte pyruvate oxidation has been laid down by the earliest stage of oogenesis.

The primordial oocyte

Nutrient consumption by oocytes during development has been largely underinvestigated and work in this area has concentrated on the mouse oocyte as a model[44,85]. As discussed above, pyruvate is consumed by the mouse primordial follicle at a rate of 26 fmoles per hour. This value is very close to the 26 fmoles of pyruvate oxidized per hour by mouse primordial germ cells[84] and the 28 fmoles oxidized per hour by denuded primordial oocytes. The primordial oocyte occupies a large volume within the whole primordial follicle and, in light of this, it is tempting to speculate that it is the oocyte that drives the majority

of pyruvate consumed by the primordial follicle and that the fate of this pyruvate is oxidation. The potential ATP produced by oxidation of this pyruvate would more than cover the energy demands of protein synthesis at this stage, but numerous other subcellular energy-consuming processes are operating, including transcription[86] and sodium pumping. Recent presentation of a selection of primate primordial oocyte-expressed genes involved in the cell cycle, signal transduction[87], transport[87], the cytoskeleton[87], transcription factors[86,87], immune responses[86], production of auto/paracrine factors[88], apoptosis[89,90], and RNA processing[86] indicates that the primordial oocyte is far from quiescent. When oocyte volume is taken into account, pyruvate consumption by the primordial oocyte is higher than during the latest stages of development (Figure 2.4).

The growing oocyte

Investigation of pyruvate[44,85] and oxygen[44] consumption by developing mouse oocytes reveals a steady increase in demand, in tandem with increasing oocyte size (Figures 2.4 and 2.5). This consumption peaks during the resumption of meiosis[44]. It is apparent that the template for oxidative pyruvate metabolism by the early preimplantation embryo is laid down during oogenesis and energy production from glucose is limited by low glycolytic activity[12]. The assumption that growing oocytes are metabolically quiescent has probably arisen after comparison of mature oocytes with blastocysts. It is true that after their arrest in the second meiotic metaphase oocyte nutrient consumption is relatively low, but during growth the oocyte has a comparatively high demand for pyruvate[44,85] and oxygen[44] to support protein[91,92] and RNA synthesis[93,94]. Throughout development the oocyte not only synthesizes molecules to support its own growth, but it must also synthesize and accumulate molecules in preparation for fertilization and postfertilization development[95-97]. In support of this notion, high

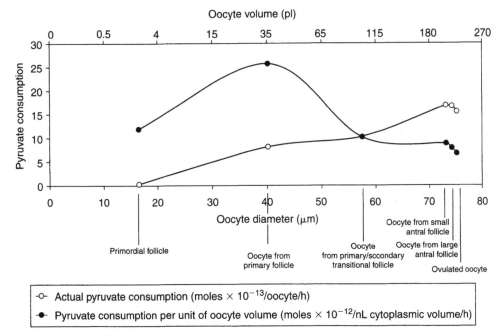

Figure 2.4 Pyruvate consumption by non-growing, growing, and mature mouse oocytes

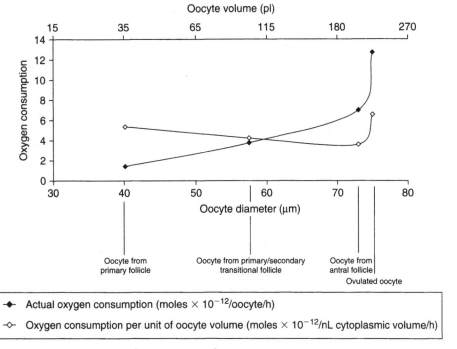

Figure 2.5 Oxygen consumption by growing and mature mouse oocytes

rates of oocyte metabolic activity are observed when metabolism profiles are adjusted for oocyte size (Figures 2.4 and 2.5). Oocyte pyruvate and oxygen consumption per unit of oocyte volume are highest during the earliest stages of development, pinpointing the primary follicle stage as a hotspot of metabolic activity within the oocyte. Demand for pyruvate, per unit of oocyte volume, is 4-fold greater during the primary follicle stage compared to the ovulated oocyte.

Comparison of pyruvate with oxygen consumption allows an estimate of maximum potential ATP production from pyruvate oxidation to be made. One mole of pyruvate requires 2.5 moles of oxygen for complete oxidation producing a maximum of 12.25 moles of ATP. The potential rates of ATP synthesis from pyruvate oxidation are shown in Table 2.1. Again, when oocyte volume is accounted for, the potential rate of ATP generation is much greater in the early stages of oogenesis. In the latter stages of oocyte development, consumption of oxygen exceeds that necessary for oxidation of pyruvate. While it is possible that some oxygen is used for oxidation of endogenous energy substrates, for example glycogen or triglyceride, convincing data have been published suggesting that there is a high rate of ROS generation by mouse zygotes[98], with up to 70% of oxygen being used for processes other than energy production[98]. High rates of ROS generation are likely a culture artefact of exposure to oxygen levels found in air rather than a more physiologic 5%[99]. On the other hand, ROS generation is a normal consequence of mitochondrial activity and H_2O_2 influences gene expression, including glucose metabolism genes[42]. In addition to pyruvate, other nutrients are known to be taken up by the growing oocyte to supplement energy production and to be used as building blocks for growth. The oocyte can take up many nutrients directly and follicle cells mediate mouse oocyte uptake of other nutrients[100], including the amino acids alanine[53,101], lysine[101], choline[101], glycine[101], and histidine[53].

Nutrient metabolism is not exclusively for energy production. Analysis of enzyme activity reveals that metabolic pathways can be suppressed or enhanced at different time points during development. Glucose-6-phosphate dehydrogenase (G6PDH) activity is greater in follicular mouse oocytes compared to ovulated oocytes[102], possibly reflecting differential requirements for NADPH or purine precursors between the different developmental stages. Interestingly, G6PDH activity is greater in follicular oocytes from adult mice than follicular oocytes of both prepubertal and aged mice[102]. The reason for this is unclear but may reflect alterations in redox state. There are also considerable differences in oocyte enzyme activities between different species. Even when the differences in volume are accounted for, large differences in the activities of the metabolic enzymes hexokinase, phosphofructokinase, pyruvate kinase, G6PDH, and glutamate dehydrogenase can be seen in human compared to mouse oocytes[103]. Glucose-6-phosphate dehydrogenase activity has been reported to be 285-fold higher in mouse compared to Tammar wallaby oocytes, while LDH activity is 10-fold higher[104]. Data from three decades ago indicated that primordial and growing mouse oocytes had very active rates of protein synthesis. As with pyruvate consumption, a development-related decline in protein synthesis per unit of volume was observed, with the primordial oocyte (1.22 fmoles/follicle per hour), which dropped sharply after growth initiation and proceeded to steadily decline during development to 0.14 fmoles/follicle per hour in the fully grown oocyte[92].

The preovulatory oocyte

Once the oocyte has grown to full size and has gathered stable mRNA species and proteins for continued development, it becomes competent to undergo maturation, encompassing the processes of meiotic resumption and cytoplasmic maturation. For some time prior to ovulation the oocyte is capable of resuming meiosis, but this is suppressed by interactions within the follicular cells until the gonadotropin surge.

The oocyte–cumulus complex

Glucose has multiple metabolic fates in the oocyte–cumulus complex and is essential for both maintenance of meiotic arrest and hormone-stimulated meiotic maturation[59,105,106]. Its metabolism through the cumulus cell pentose phosphate pathway provides ribose-5-phosphate, a precursor of phospho-ribosyl-pyrophosphate (PRPP), an essential metabolite for de novo purine synthesis. The meiosis-suppressing purines[107] adenosine and hypoxanthine have been identified in follicular fluid and granulosa-derived cAMP is maintained in the oocyte via gap junctions[108], where it contributes to meiotic suppression.

FSH and LH are known to stimulate glucose consumption in mouse[109] and cow[110] oocyte–cumulus complexes, an interaction which is directly related to the ability of the oocyte–cumulus complex to promote oocyte meiotic resumption[59]. Translocation of GLUT4 to the cell membrane[67] and hexokinase translation, and hence activity, are also known to increase in response to FSH, providing intermediates for glycolysis, the Krebs cycle, and the pentose phosphate pathway[59]. During the final phases of oocyte development, oxygen consumption by the mouse oocyte–cumulus complex drops[111,112] while glycolytic activity increases substantially[109], suggesting that the oocyte–cumulus complex becomes more reliant upon glycolytic, rather than oxidative, glucose metabolism. This phenomenon has also been noted in the cow, where glucose metabolism through glycolysis and the pentose phosphate pathway increases, but the proportion of glucose metabolized glycolytically decreases[57]. After endocrine induction of oocyte maturation, cumulus cell pentose phosphate pathway activity is involved in promoting meiosis in the oocyte[109].

The availability of appropriate levels of glucose and pyruvate is very important during oocyte maturation and the concentrations and combinations of these nutrients are known to affect meiotic progression in both mouse[106,112] and cow[113] oocyte–cumulus complexes. Glucose metabolites are also directly involved in hyaluronic acid synthesis[57], with low glucose impairing cumulus expansion in non-human primates[114]. Thus, glucose metabolism is also involved in disruption of oocyte–cumulus gap junctions during maturation. Furthermore, reduced glucose consumption and lactate production by cumulus cells are associated with lower rates of oocyte maturation[67]. Oocyte–cumulus complexes showing enhanced pyruvate production from glucose in response to FSH, which is modulated by EGF and IGF1[115], have been shown to yield oocytes with better maturation rates[67].

The oocyte

While high intraoocyte cAMP suppresses meiosis, decreased cAMP and ATP enable maturation to progress. During maturation, pyruvate remains the preferred energy substrate of mouse and human oocytes and its uptake over the plasma membrane is mediated by the monocarboxylate transporter family[116]. The stage of meiosis, i.e. prophase I, metaphase I, and metaphase II, affects pyruvate and amino acid consumption in many species[117–121]. Upon resumption of meiosis, an increase in consumption of oxidizable energy substrates has been observed in mouse[117] and cow[119,120,122] oocytes. This is coincident with activation of metabolically demanding processes, including microtubule-mediated spindle formation, chromosome condensation and segregation, protein synthesis, and polar body formation. Once it has reached metaphase II, the metabolic needs of the oocyte appear to drop, with a coincident reduction in pyruvate consumption. Investigation of oxygen consumption by mouse oocytes during growth (Figure 2.5) shows that there is an almost

2-fold increase in the consumption rate between fully grown, but immature, oocytes from antral follicles and oocytes at metaphase II, while pyruvate consumption is very similar at all stages. At the antral stage, enough oxygen is consumed for complete pyruvate oxidation, so the cause of this apparent increase in demand is unclear.

Metabolic profiling has attracted some interest as a potential measure of cytoplasmic maturation and developmental competence. While pyruvate metabolism is not a definitive indicator of either of these processes, human oocytes with low rates of pyruvate consumption are more likely to arrest during preimplantation development[123]. Mouse oocyte glucose consumption tends to be many fold lower than pyruvate, but is stimulated upon fertilization[6] and has been related to the number of pronuclei formed after polyspermy[124]. In cat oocytes, glycolytic and oxidative glucose metabolism increases during in-vitro maturation[1] have been shown to be predictive of embryo development to blastocyst stage.

NUTRITION OF THE FOLLICLE AND OOCYTE IN VIVO AND IN VITRO

During normal growth in vivo, the follicle is exposed to tissue fluid, largely composed of plasma transudate, containing physiologic concentrations of nutrients, oxygen, and macromolecules such as albumin. The outer layers of the follicle are vascularized and the follicle promotes angiogenesis and increased vascular porosity through secretion of vascular endothelial growth factor[125], thus regulating its blood supply. Follicles failing to develop an adequate blood supply become underoxygenated which has serious consequences for the follicular oocyte[54], whose energy production becomes compromised, leading to cytoplasmic and nuclear abnormalities[54]. As folliculogenesis progresses, the distance between the oocyte and blood supply increases. Nutrients and oxygen must diffuse over a greater distance before reaching the oocyte, first passing through the granulosa cell compartment. Granulosa cell metabolism produces a marked change in concentrations of nutrients and oxygen between the blood and follicular fluid, with consumption of glucose and amino acids and production of pyruvate, lactate, and other amino acids. Differential concentrations of electrolytes also exist between the plasma and follicular fluid compartments[126], with the follicle accumulating salts[79] and therefore water, which follows osmotically. The oocyte and cumulus complex is thus bathed in a unique fluid, which can be modeled as shown in Figure 2.6. Concentrations of glucose are markedly lower in follicular fluid, compared to plasma, while pyruvate and lactate are much higher. Table 2.2 shows concentrations of some important nutrients in human and mouse plasma and follicular fluids.

Many different culture media formulations exist which are used to support the in-vitro development of follicles and oocytes, however no medium has been designed specifically for these tissues. Most commercially available media that are commonly used, for example Minimum Essential medium and Tissue Culture medium-199, were originally formulated for optimum culture of somatic cancer cells[127]. Glucose concentration has a marked effect on follicle survival in culture, with reduced growth and steroidogenesis when glucose availability is low[45]. Media composition appears to have marked effects upon development in vitro. Most work in this area has focused on embryo culture, with media composition affecting blastocyst formation[128], cell number[129], implantation rate[130], and embryo metabolism[131]. When the concentrations of culture medium nutrients deviate further away from physiologic ranges, increasing stress responses can be observed. While this has been demonstrated in mouse embryos[132], there has been little investigation into the effects of culture medium composition on follicle and oocyte culture; however, during mouse follicle culture, low glucose is known to reduce the capacity for follicle glucose consumption and

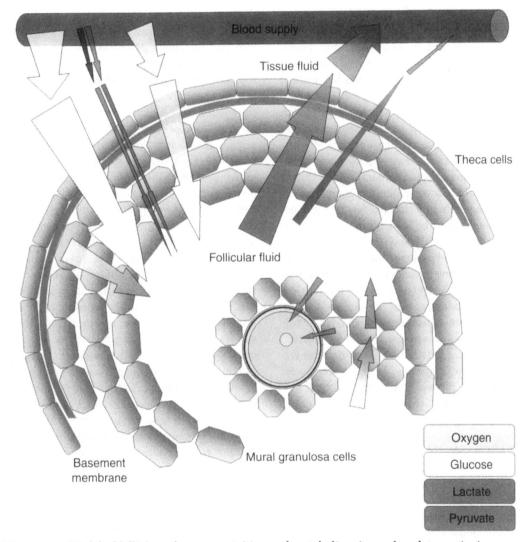

Figure 2.6   Model of follicle and oocyte nutrition and metabolism (see color plate section)

Table 2.2   Concentrations of nutrients in mouse and human plasma and follicular fluid

Nutrient (mM)	Mouse plasma	Mouse follicular fluid	Human plasma	Human follicular fluid
Glucose	11.71 ± 0.76[58]	0.46 ± 0.08[58]	3.9–6.1	3[48,49]
Pyruvate	0.157 ± 0.02[58]	0.38 ± 0.03[58]	0.03–0.1	0.26[48]
Lactate	4.77 ± 0.43[58]	17.34 ± 1.1[58]	0.3–2.2	3.4–6.3[48,49]
Glutamine	0.907[58]	0.032[58]	0.372[137]	0.411[137]

steroidogenesis[45]. Oocyte–cumulus maturation medium composition is also known to influence maturation rate and subsequent embryo development in the cow[128]. Additionally, maturation of pig oocytes in a variety of media has yielded mature oocytes with different intracellular concentrations of glutathione, which were all much lower than observed in pig oocytes matured in vivo[133]. While certain nutrients are preferred by the follicle and oocyte, their appropriate concentrations and combinations are important. During maturation of oocyte–cumulus complexes in unphysiologically high oxygen tension, glucose concentration must be lowered to reduce excessive ROS generation[134], and the ratio of nutrients such as lactate and pyruvate must be balanced so as to avoid altering the oocyte redox state. It may thus be prudent to expose follicles to nutrient levels found in plasma, as they are exposed to near-plasma nutrient concentrations in vivo, while oocyte–cumulus complexes should be exposed to media similar to follicular fluid. Another factor to consider is species; marked interspecies differences in plasma, follicular fluid, and oviduct fluid have been observed[58,135].

METABOLISM IN VITRO VS. EX VIVO

It is perhaps not surprising that altered metabolism occurs as a consequence of exposure to the culture environment. This has been demonstrated in mouse embryos[132,136] but is also true of in-vitro grown mouse oocytes which have lower pyruvate consumption compared to their in-vivo grown counterparts[44]. Similarly, in human oocytes undergoing in-vitro maturation the specific culture medium used affects rate of pyruvate consumption and lactate production[118].

CONCLUSIONS

Metabolic processes play diverse roles in oocyte growth and maturation, from fueling energy pro-

duction to providing intermediates for a variety of biosynthetic processes. It is not surprising therefore that metabolic processes may be expected to play a significant part in the selection and rejection of oocytes for continued development. Oocyte metabolic competence is a major factor in the age-related decline in oocyte quality through accumulation of oxidative damage and impaired mitochondrial function. Limited investigations of metabolism during oogenesis reveal that the growing oocyte is metabolically active, with high demands for oxidizable energy substrates during early stages of development. In addition to energy generation, metabolites such as pyruvate and amino acids serve many subcellular roles as free radical scavengers, osmolytes, toxin chelators, and regulators of intracellular pH. More than this, the energy-generating capacity of mitochondria appears to significantly contribute to oocyte quality. In vitro, culture medium composition can have a marked, negative bearing upon the capacity of an oocyte to undergo the final steps of meiosis and subsequently on its competence to undergo preimplantation development, as well as altering redox state and elevating levels of oxidative stress to varying degrees. These factors must be considered when optimizing culture systems for oocyte growth and maturation. The prospects for long-term culture of oocytes from early stages to maturity will depend on replicating the in-vivo environment more closely and on developing a more sympathetic understanding of the metabolic and molecular processes that define oocyte quality.

REFERENCES

1. Spindler R, Pukazhenthi B, Wildt D. Oocyte metabolism predicts the development of cat embryos to blastocyst *in vitro*. Mol Reprod Dev 2000; 56: 163–71.

2. Krisher RL, Bavister BD. Enhanced glycolysis after maturation of bovine oocytes *in vitro* is associated with increased developmental competence. Mol Reprod Dev 1999; 53: 19–26.

3. Biggers J, Whittingham D, Donahue R. The pattern of energy metabolism in the mouse oocyte and zygote. Proc Natl Acad Sci USA 1967; 58: 567.

4. Eppig J. Analysis of mouse oogenesis *in vitro*. Oocyte isolation and the utilization of exogenous energy sources by growing oocytes. J Exp Zool 1976; 198: 375–82.

5. Tsutsumi O, Yano T, Satoh K et al. Studies of hexokinase activity in human and mouse oocyte. Am J Obstet Gynecol 1990; 162: 1301–4.

6. Saito T, Hiroi M, Kato T. Development of glucose utilization studied in single oocytes and pre-implantation embryos from mice. Biol Reprod 1994; 50: 266–70.

7. Pantaleon M, Harvey MB, Pascoe WS et al. Glucose transporter GLUT3: ontogeny, targeting, and role in the mouse blastocyst. Proc Natl Acad Sci USA 1997; 94: 3795–800.

8. Pantaleon M, Kaye PL. Glucose transporters in preimplantation development. Rev Reprod 1998; 3: 77–81.

9. Kelly A, West JD. Survival and normal function of glycolysis-deficient mouse oocytes. Reproduction 2002; 124: 469–73.

10. Zeilmaker GH, Verhamme CM. Observations on rat oocyte maturation *in vitro*: morphology and energy requirements. Biol Reprod 1974; 11: 145–52.

11. Boland NI, Humpherson PG, Leese HJ et al. Characterization of follicular energy metabolism. Hum Reprod 1994; 9: 604–9.

12. Barbehenn EK, Wales RG, Lowry OH. The explanation for the blockade of glycolysis in early mouse embryos. Proc Natl Acad Sci USA 1974; 71: 1056–60.

13. Barbehenn EK, Wales RG, Lowry OH. Measurement of metabolites in single preimplantation embryos; a new means to study metabolic control in early embryos. J Embryol Exp Morphol 1978; 43: 29–46.

14. Kowaltowski AJ, Vercesi AE. Mitochondrial damage induced by conditions of oxidative stress. Free Radic Biol Med 1999; 26: 463–71.

15. Wallace DC, Ye JH, Neckelmann SN et al. Sequence analysis of cDNAs for the human and bovine ATP synthase beta subunit: mitochondrial DNA genes sustain seventeen times more mutations. Curr Genet 1987; 12: 81–90.

16. Avise JC. Ten unorthodox perspectives on evolution prompted by comparative population genetic findings on mitochondrial DNA. Annu Rev Genet 1991; 25: 45–69.

17. Ozawa T. Genetic and functional changes in mitochondria associated with aging. Physiol Rev 1997; 77: 425–64.

18. De Grey AD. A proposed refinement of the mitochondrial free radical theory of aging. Bioessays 1997; 19: 161–6.

19. Wilding M, Dale B, Marino M et al. Mitochondrial aggregation patterns and activity in human oocytes and preimplantation embryos. Hum Reprod 2001; 16: 909–17.

20. Van Blerkom J, Davis P, Lee J. ATP content of human oocytes and developmental potential and outcome after in-vitro fertilization and embryo transfer. Hum Reprod 1995; 10: 415–24.

21. Tarin J, Perez-Albala S, Cano A. Oral antioxidants counteract the negative effects of female aging on oocyte quantity and quality in the mouse. Mol Reprod Dev 2002; 61: 385–97.

22. Bergstrom CT, Pritchard J. Germline bottlenecks and the evolutionary maintenance of mitochondrial genomes. Genetics 1998; 149: 2135–46.

23. Jansen RP, de Boer K. The bottleneck: mitochondrial imperatives in oogenesis and ovarian follicular fate. Mol Cell Endocrinol 1998; 145: 81–8.

24. Jansen RP. Germline passage of mitochondria: quantitative considerations and possible embryological sequelae. Hum Reprod 2000; 15(Suppl 2): 112–28.

25. Steuerwald N, Barritt JA, Adler R et al. Quantification of mtDNA in single oocytes, polar bodies and subcellular components by real-time rapid cycle fluorescence monitored PCR. Zygote 2000; 8: 209–15.

26. Calarco PG. Polarization of mitochondria in the unfertilized mouse oocyte. Devel Genet 1995; 16: 36–43.

27. Sun QY, Wu GM, Lai L et al. Translocation of active mitochondria during pig oocyte maturation, fertilization and early embryo development *in vitro*. Reproduction 2001; 122: 155–63.

28. Makabe S, Van Blerkom J. An Atlas of Human Female Reproduction:Ovarian Development to Embryogenesis In Vitro. Taylor and Francis Books, London, UK. 2004.

29. Fair T, Hulshof SC, Hyttel P et al. Oocyte ultrastructure in bovine primordial to early tertiary follicles. Anat Embryol (Berl) 1997; 195: 327–36.

30. Houghton FD, Thompson JG, Kennedy CJ et al. Oxygen consumption and energy metabolism of the early mouse embryo. Mol Reprod Dev 1996; 44: 476–85.

31. Stojkovic M, Machado S, Stojkovic P et al. Mitochondrial distribution and adenosine triphosphate content of bovine oocytes before and after *in vitro* maturation: correlation with morphological criteria and developmental capacity after *in vitro* fertilization and culture. Biol Reprod 2001; 64: 904–9.

32. Krakauer DC, Mira A. Mitochondria and germcell death. Nature 1999; 400: 125–6.

33. Anderson E, Albertini DF. Gap junctions between the oocyte and companion follicle cells in the mammalian ovary. J Cell Biol 1976; 71: 680–6.

34. Heller DT, Schultz RM. Ribonucleoside metabolism by mouse oocytes: metabolic cooperativity between the fully grown oocyte and cumulus cells. J Exp Zool 1980; 214: 355–64.

35. Ginsberg L, Hillman N. ATP metabolism in tn/tn mouse embryos. J Embryol Exp Morphol 1975; 33: 715–23.

36. Van Blerkom J, Sinclair J, Davis P. Mitochondrial transfer between oocytes: potential applications of mitochondrial donation and the issue of heteroplasmy. Hum Reprod 1998; 13: 2857–68.

37. O'Donnell-Tormey J, Nathan CF, Lanks K et al. Secretion of pyruvate. An antioxidant defense of mammalian cells. J Exp Med 1987; 165: 500–14.

38. Ludwig TE, Squirrell JM, Palmenberg AC et al. Relationship between development, metabolism, and mitochondrial organization in 2-cell hamster embryos in the presence of low levels of phosphate. Biol Reprod 2001; 65: 1648–54.

39. Barnett DK, Bavister BD. Inhibitory effect of glucose and phosphate on the second cleavage division of hamster embryos: is it linked to metabolism? Hum Reprod 1996; 11: 177–83.

40. Tarin JJ. Potential effects of age-associated oxidative stress on mammalian oocytes/embryos. Mol Hum Reprod 1996; 2: 717–24.

41. Thouas GA, Trounson AO, Wolvetang EJ et al. Mitochondrial dysfunction in mouse oocytes results in preimplantation embryo arrest *in vitro*. Biol Reprod 2004; 71: 1936–42.

42. Hashimoto S, Minami N, Takakura R et al. Low oxygen tension during *in vitro* maturation is beneficial for supporting the subsequent development of bovine cumulus–oocyte complexes. Mol Reprod Dev 2000; 57: 353–60.

43. Cran DG, Hay MF, Moor RM. The fine structure of the cumulus oophorus during follicular development in sheep. Cell Tissue Res 1979; 202: 439–51.

44. Harris SE. Experimental and Clinical Investigation into Mammalian Oocyte Metabolism, Nutrition and Fertility. PhD Thesis, University of Leeds, 2002.

45. Boland NI, Humpherson PG, Leese HJ et al. The effect of glucose metabolism on murine follicle development and steroidogenesis *in vitro*. Hum Reprod 1994; 9: 617–23.

46. Boland NI, Humpherson PG, Leese HJ, Gosden RG. Pattern of lactate production and steroidogenesis during growth and maturation of mouse ovarian follicles *in vitro*. Biol Reprod 1993; 48: 798–806.

47. Sugiura K, Pendola FL, Eppig JJ. Oocyte control of metabolic cooperativity between oocytes and companion granulosa cells: energy metabolism. Dev Biol 2005; 279: 20–30.

48. Leese HJ, Lenton EA. Glucose and lactate in human follicular fluid: concentrations and interrelationships. Hum Reprod 1990; 5: 915–19.

49. Gull I, Geva E, Lerner-Geva L et al. Anaerobic glycolysis. The metabolism of the preovulatory human oocyte. Eur J Obstet Gynecol Reprod Biol 1999; 85: 225–8.

50. Hillier SG, Purohit A, Reichert LE, Jr. Control of granulosa cell lactate production by follicle-stimulating hormone and androgen. Endocrinology 1985; 116: 1163–7.

51. Eppig JJ, Chesnel F, Hirao Y et al. Oocyte control of granulosa cell development: how and why. Hum Reprod 1997; 12(Suppl): 127–32.

52. Eppig JJ, Wigglesworth K, Pendola FL. The mammalian oocyte orchestrates the rate of ovarian follicular development. Proc Natl Acad Sci USA 2002; 99: 2890–4.

53. Eppig JJ, Pendola FL, Wigglesworth K et al. Mouse oocytes regulate metabolic cooperativity between granulosa cells and oocytes: amino acid transport. Biol Reprod 2005; 73: 351–7.

54. Van Blerkom J. Epigenetic influences on oocyte developmental competence: perifollicular vascularity and intrafollicular oxygen. J Assist Reprod Genet 1998; 15: 226–34.

55. Hu Y, Betzendahl I, Cortvrindt R et al. Effects of low O_2 and ageing on spindles and chromosomes in mouse oocytes from pre-antral follicle culture. Hum Reprod 2001; 16: 737–48.

56. Zhou J, Bievre M, Bondy CA. Reduced GLUT1 expression in Igf1–/– null oocytes and follicles. Growth Horm IGF Res 2000; 10: 111–17.

57. Sutton-McDowall ML, Gilchrist RB, Thompson JG. Cumulus expansion and glucose utilisation by bovine cumulus–oocyte complexes during in vitro maturation: the influence of glucosamine and follicle-stimulating hormone. Reproduction 2004; 128: 313–19.

58. Harris SE, Gopichandran N, Picton HM et al. Nutrient concentrations in murine follicular fluid and the female reproductive tract. Theriogenology 2005; 64: 992–1006.

59. Downs SM, Humpherson PG, Martin KL et al. Glucose utilization during gonadotropin-induced meiotic maturation in cumulus cell-enclosed mouse oocytes. Mol Reprod Dev 1996; 44: 121–31.

60. Tsafriri A, Lieberman ME, Ahren K et al. Dissociation between LH-induced aerobic glycolysis and oocyte maturation in cultured Graafian follicles of the rat. Acta Endocrinol (Copenh) 1976; 81: 362–6.

61. Lin Y, Fridstrom M, Hillensjo T. Insulin stimulation of lactate accumulation in isolated human granulosa-luteal cells: a comparison between normal and polycystic ovaries. Hum Reprod 1997; 12: 2469–72.

62. Carvalho CR, Carvalheira JB, Lima MH et al. Novel signal transduction pathway for luteinizing hormone and its interaction with insulin: activation of Janus kinase/signal transducer and activator of transcription and phosphoinositol 3-kinase/Akt pathways. Endocrinology 2003; 144: 638–47.

63. Nilsson L. Acute effects of gonadotrophins and prostaglandins on the metabolism of isolated ovarian follicles from PMSG-treated immature rats. Acta Endocrinol (Copenh) 1974; 77: 540–58.

64. Hillensjo T. Oocyte maturation and glycolysis in isolated pre-ovulatory follicles of PMS-injected immature rats. Acta Endocrinol (Copenh) 1976; 82: 809–30.

65. Kol S, Ben-Shlomo I, Ruutiainen K et al. The midcycle increase in ovarian glucose uptake is associated with enhanced expression of glucose transporter 3. Possible role for interleukin-1, a putative intermediary in the ovulatory process. J Clin Invest 1997; 99: 2274–83.

66. Chen HF, Shew JY, Chao KH et al. Luteinizing hormone up-regulates the expression of interleukin-1 beta mRNA in human granulosa-luteal cells. Am J Reprod Immunol 2000; 43: 125–33.

67. Roberts R, Stark J, Iatropoulou A et al. Energy substrate metabolism of mouse cumulus–oocyte complexes: response to follicle-stimulating hormone is mediated by the phosphatidylinositol 3-kinase pathway and is associated with oocyte maturation. Biol Reprod 2004; 71: 199–209.

68. Roy SK, Terada DM. Activities of glucose metabolic enzymes in human preantral follicles: in vitro modulation by follicle-stimulating hormone, luteinizing hormone, epidermal growth factor, insulin-like growth factor I, and transforming growth factor beta1. Biol Reprod 1999; 60: 763–8.

69. Downs SM, Mastropolo AM. Culture conditions affect meiotic regulation in cumulus cell-enclosed mouse oocytes. Mol Reprod Dev 1997; 46: 551–66.

70. Colton SA, Downs SM. Potential role for the sorbitol pathway in the meiotic dysfunction exhibited by oocytes from diabetic mice. J Exp Zoolog A Comp Exp Biol 2004; 301: 439–48.

71. Colton SA, Humpherson PG, Leese HJ et al. Physiological changes in oocyte–cumulus cell complexes from diabetic mice that potentially influence meiotic regulation. Biol Reprod 2003; 69: 761–70.

72. Landau S, Braw-Tal R, Kaim M et al. Preovulatory follicular status and diet affect the insulin and glucose content of follicles in high-yielding dairy cows. Anim Reprod Sci 2000; 64: 181–97.

73. Armstrong DT, Greep RO. Effect of gonadotrophic hormones on glucose metabolism by luteinized rat ovaries. Endocrinology 1962; 70: 701–10.

74. Spears N, Murray AA, Allison V et al. Role of gonadotrophins and ovarian steroids in the development of mouse follicles in vitro. J Reprod Fertil 1998; 113: 19–26.

75. Downs SM, Humpherson PG, Leese HJ. Meiotic induction in cumulus cell-enclosed mouse oocytes: involvement of the pentose phosphate pathway. Biol Reprod 1998; 58: 1084–94.

76. Shim C, Lee DK, Lee CC et al. Inhibitory effect of purines in meiotic maturation of denuded mouse oocytes. Mol Reprod Dev 1992; 31: 280–6.

77. Downs SM. Adenosine blocks hormone-induced meiotic maturation by suppressing purine de novo synthesis. Mol Reprod Dev 2000; 56: 172–9.

78. Rondell PA. Follicular fluid electrolytes in ovulation. Proc Soc Exp Biol Med 1964; 116: 336–9.

79. Wise T. Biochemical analysis of bovine follicular fluid: albumin, total protein, lysosomal enzymes, ions, steroids and ascorbic acid content in relation to follicular size, rank, atresia classification and day of estrous cycle. J Anim Sci 1987; 64: 1153–69.

80. Talbot P. Intrafollicular pressure promotes partial evacuation of the antrum during hamster ovulation in vitro. J Exp Zool 1983; 226: 129–35.

81. Rondell P. Follicular pressure and distensibility in ovulation. Am J Physiol 1964; 207: 590–4.

82. Leese HJ, Barton AM. Production of pyruvate by isolated mouse cumulus cells. J Exp Zool 1985; 234: 231–6.

83. De Felici M, Scaldaferri ML, Lobascio M et al. Experimental approaches to the study of primordial germ cell lineage and proliferation. Hum Reprod Update 2004; 10: 197–206.

84. Brinster RL, Harstad H. Energy metabolism in primordial germ cells of the mouse. Exp Cell Res 1977; 109: 111–17.

85. Eppig J. Analysis of mouse oogenesis in vitro. Oocyte isolation and the utilization of exogenous energy sources by growing oocytes. J Exp Zool 1976; 198: 375–82.

86. Arraztoa JA, Zhou J, Marcu D et al. Identification of genes expressed in primate primordial oocytes. Hum Reprod 2005; 20: 476–83.

87. Bayne RAL, Martins da Silva SJ, Anderson RA et al. Increased expression of the FIGLA transcription factor is associated with primordial follicle formation in the human fetal ovary. Mol Hum Reprod 2004; 10: 378–81.

88. Rodriguez GC, Nagarsheth NP, Lee KL et al. Progestin-induced apoptosis in the Macaque ovarian epithelium: differential regulation of transforming growth factor-beta. J Natl Cancer Inst 2002; 94: 50–60.

89. Lee CJ, Park HH, Do BR et al. Natural and radiation-induced degeneration of primordial and primary follicles in mouse ovary. Anim Reprod Sci 2000; 59: 109–17.

90. Depalo R, Nappi L, Loverro G et al. Evidence of apoptosis in human primordial and primary follicles. Hum Reprod 2003; 18: 2678–82.

91. Schultz RM, Wassarman PM. Biochemical studies of mammalian oogenesis: protein synthesis during oocyte growth and meiotic maturation in the mouse. J Cell Sci 1977; 24: 167–94.

92. Schultz RM, Letourneau GE, Wassarman PM. Program of early development in the mammal: changes in the patterns and absolute rates of tubulin and total protein synthesis during oocyte growth in the mouse. Devel Biol 1979; 73: 120–33.

93. Oakberg EF. Relationship between stage of follicular development and RNA synthesis in the mouse oocyte. Mutat Res 1968; 6: 155–65.

94. Moore GP, Lintern-Moore S. A correlation between growth and RNA synthesis in the mouse oocyte. J Reprod Fertil 1974; 39: 163–6.

95. Christmann L, Jung T, Moor RM. MPF components and meiotic competence in growing pig oocytes. Mol Reprod Dev 1994; 38: 85–90.

96. Chesnel F, Eppig JJ. Synthesis and accumulation of p34cdc2 and cyclin B in mouse oocytes during acquisition of competence to resume meiosis. Mol Reprod Dev 1995; 40: 503–8.

97. Rosner MH, De Santo RJ, Arnheiter H et al. Oct–3 is a maternal factor required for the first mouse embryonic division. Cell 1991; 64: 1103–10.

98. Trimarchi JR, Liu L, Porterfield DM et al. Oxidative phosphorylation-dependent and -independent oxygen consumption by individual preimplantation mouse embryos. Biol Reprod 2000; 62: 1866–74.

99. Orsi NM, Leese HJ. Protection against reactive oxygen species during mouse preimplantation embryo development: role of EDTA, oxygen tension, catalase, superoxide dismutase and pyruvate. Mol Reprod Dev 2001; 59: 44–53.

100. Colonna R, Mangia F. Mechanisms of amino acid uptake in cumulus-enclosed mouse oocytes. Biol Reprod 1983; 28: 797–803.

101. Haghighat N, Van Winkle L. Developmental change in follicular cell-enhanced amino acid uptake into mouse oocytes that depends on intact gap junctions and transport system Gly. J Exp Zool 1990; 253: 71–82.

102. de Schepper G, van Noorden C, Houtkooper J. Age-related changes of glucose–6-phosphate dehydrogenase activity in mouse oocytes. Histochem J 1987; 19: 467–70.

103. Chi M, Manchester J, Yang V et al. Contrast in levels of metabolic enzymes in human and mouse ova. Biol Reprod 1988; 39: 295–307.

104. Briscoe D, Robinson E, Johnston P. Glucose-6-phosphate dehydrogenase and lactate dehydrogenase activity in kangaroo and mouse oocytes. Comp Biochem Physiol – B: Comp Biochem 1983; 75: 685–8.

105. Fagbohun CF, Downs SM. Requirement for glucose in ligand-stimulated meiotic maturation of cumulus cell-enclosed mouse oocytes. J Reprod Fertil 1992; 96: 681–97.

106. Downs SM, Mastropolo AM. The participation of energy substrates in the control of meiotic maturation in murine oocytes. Devel Biol 1994; 162: 154–68.

107. Downs SM. Uptake and metabolism of adenosine mediate a meiosis-arresting action on mouse oocytes. Mol Reprod Dev 1999; 53: 208–21.

108. Downs S. The influence of glucose, cumulus cells, and metabolic coupling on ATP levels and meiotic control in the isolated mouse oocyte. Devel Biol 1995; 167: 502–12.

109. Downs S, Utecht A. Metabolism of radiolabeled glucose by mouse oocytes and oocyte–cumulus cell complexes. Biol Reprod 1999; 60: 1446–52.

110. Zuelke K, Brackett B. Effects of luteinizing hormone on glucose metabolism in cumulus-enclosed bovine oocytes matured in vitro. Endocrinology 1992; 131: 2690–6.

111. Billig H, Magnusson C. Gonadotropin-induced inhibition of oxygen consumption in rat oocyte–cumulus complexes: relief by adenosine. Biol Reprod 1985; 33: 890–8.

112. Downs SM, Houghton FD, Humpherson PG et al. Substrate utilization and maturation of cumulus cell-enclosed mouse oocytes: evidence that pyruvate oxidation does not mediate meiotic induction. J Reprod Fertil 1997; 110: 1–10.

113. Iwata H, Hashimoto S, Ohota M et al. Effects of follicle size and electrolytes and glucose in maturation medium on nuclear maturation and developmental competence of bovine oocytes. Reproduction 2004; 127: 159–64.

114. Zheng P, Bavister B, Ji W. Energy substrate requirement for in vitro maturation of oocytes from unstimulated adult rhesus monkeys. Mol Reprod Dev 2001; 58: 348–55.

115. Rieger D, Luciano A, Modina S et al. The effects of epidermal growth factor and insulin-like growth factor I on the metabolic activity, nuclear maturation and subsequent development of cattle oocytes in vitro. J Reprod Fertil 1998; 112: 123–30.

116. Herubel F, El Mouatassim S, Guerin P et al. Genetic expression of monocarboxylate transporters during human and murine oocyte maturation and early embryonic development. Zygote 2002; 10: 175–81.

117. Downs SM, Humpherson PG, Leese HJ. Pyruvate utilization by mouse oocytes is influenced by meiotic status and the cumulus oophorus. Mol Reprod Dev 2002; 62: 113–23.

118. Roberts R, Franks S, Hardy K. Culture environment modulates maturation and metabolism of human oocytes. Hum Reprod 2002; 17: 2950–6.

119. Rieger D, Loskutoff N. Changes in the metabolism of glucose, pyruvate, glutamine and glycine during maturation of cattle oocytes in vitro. J Reprod Fertil 1994; 100: 257–62.

120. Steeves T, Gardner D. Metabolism of glucose, pyruvate, and glutamine during the maturation of oocytes derived from pre-pubertal and adult cows. Mol Reprod Dev 1999; 54: 92–101.

121. Zuelke K, Brackett B. Increased glutamine metabolism in bovine cumulus cell-enclosed and denuded oocytes after in vitro maturation with luteinizing hormone. Biol Reprod 1993; 48: 815–20.

122. Gandolfi F, Milanesi E, Pocar P et al. Comparative analysis of calf and cow oocytes during in vitro maturation. Mol Reprod Dev 1998; 49: 168–75.

123. Hardy K, Hooper MA, Handyside AH et al. Non-invasive measurement of glucose and pyruvate uptake by individual human oocytes and pre-implantation embryos. Hum Reprod 1989; 4: 188–91.

124. Pantaleon M, Ryan J, Gil M et al. An unusual subcellular localization of GLUT1 and link with metabolism in oocytes and preimplantation mouse embryos. Biol Reprod 2001; 64: 1247–54.

125. Ancelin M, Buteau-Lozano H, Meduri G et al. A dynamic shift of VEGF isoforms with a transient and selective progesterone-induced expression of VEGF189 regulates angiogenesis and vascular permeability in human uterus. Proc Natl Acad Sci USA 2002; 99: 6023–8.

126. Gosden RG, Hunter RH, Telfer E et al. Physiological factors underlying the formation of ovarian follicular fluid. J Reprod Fertil 1988; 82: 813–25.

127. Eagle H. Amino acid metabolism in mammalian cell cultures. Science 1959; 130: 432–7.

128. Rose-Hellekant T, Libersky-Williamson E, Bavister B. Energy substrates and amino acids provided during in vitro maturation of bovine oocytes alter acquisition of developmental competence. Zygote 1998; 6: 285–94.

129. Van Soom A, Boerjan M, Ysebaert MT et al. Cell allocation to the inner cell mass and the trophectoderm in bovine embryos cultured in two different media. Mol Reprod Dev 1996; 45: 171–82.

130. Barak Y, Goldman S, Gonen Y et al. Does glucose affect fertilization, development and pregnancy rates of human in vitro fertilized oocytes? Hum Reprod 1998; 13(Suppl 4): 203–11.

131. Conaghan J, Handyside AH, Winston RM et al. Effects of pyruvate and glucose on the development of human preimplantation embryos in vitro. J Reprod Fertil 1993; 99: 87–95.

132. Gardner DK, Leese HJ. Concentrations of nutrients in mouse oviduct fluid and their effects on embryo development and metabolism in vitro. J Reprod Fertil 1990; 88: 361–8.

133. Brad AM, Bormann CL, Swain JE et al. Glutathione and adenosine triphosphate content of in vivo and in vitro matured porcine oocytes. Mol Reprod Dev 2003; 64: 492–8.

134. Hashimoto S, Minami N, Yamada M et al. Excessive concentration of glucose during in vitro maturation impairs the developmental competence of bovine oocytes after in vitro fertilization: relevance to intracellular reactive oxygen species and glutathione contents. Mol Reprod Dev 2000; 56: 520–6.

135. Orsi NM, Gopichandran N, Leese HJ et al. Fluctuations in bovine ovarian follicular fluid composition throughout the oestrous cycle. Reproduction 2005; 129: 219–28.

136. Fleming TP, Kwong WY, Porter R et al. The embryo and its future. Biol Reprod 2004; 71: 1046–54.

137. Jimena P, Castilla JA, Peran F et al. Distribution of free amino acids in human preovulatory follicles. Horm Metab Res 1993; 25: 228–30.

CHAPTER 3

Interaction of oocyte and somatic cells

Helen M Picton, Wanzirai Muruvi, and Ping Jin

INTRODUCTION

Throughout growth and maturation the production of a fertile oocyte requires the maintenance of a two-directional communication between the multicellular follicle and the germ cell it contains. From the primordial stage, oocytes are invested in follicular cells which not only produce growth factors and hormones but provide the oocyte with physical support, nutrients (such as pyruvate), metabolic precursors (such as amino acids and nucleotides), and other small molecules which can equilibrate between the cellular compartments without affecting the distinctive macromolecular phenotype of either cell type. Granulosa cells can be considered to provide the oocyte with the majority of its nutritional requirements while at the same time the oocyte helps coordinate growth and differentiation of the follicle which houses it. Additionally, specific molecules produced by the somatic cells have been identified as taking part in the mechanism for the maintenance of meiotic arrest in the oocyte. It can therefore be considered that the growth of ovarian follicles is dependent upon the presence of an oocyte and vice versa.

It is generally agreed that the interdependency of the germ cells and the companion somatic cells of the follicle is coordinated by the passage of signals from the germ cell to the follicle cells and back. The bi-directional communication between oocytes and somatic cells is mediated by two distinct mechanisms: (1) intercellular signals pass between oocytes and granulosa cells via paracrine factors that may trigger different signaling pathways; and (2) small molecules pass directly between the oocytes and somatic cells via specialized membrane channels or gap junctions. Heterologous gap junctions form between the oocyte and granulosa cells or cumulus cells whereas homologous gap junctions maintain cumulus–cumulus cell contacts and granulosa–granulosa cell junctions. This chapter aims therefore to review the current state of knowledge of the cell–cell interactions and communication which occur between oocytes and somatic cells throughout their development and which act as a vehicle for oocyte metabolism (discussed in detail in Chapter 2) and which underpin the processes of oocyte growth and maturation (discussed in Chapters 1 and 4).

GAP JUNCTIONS AND OOCYTE DEVELOPMENT

A series of complex cell-to-cell interactions coordinate the development of mammalian oocytes.

Cellular communication in ovarian follicles is achieved by a combination of endocrine, paracrine, and autocrine pathways and through gap junctions. Follicular gap junctions take the form of clusters of intercellular channels between the oocyte and surrounding somatic cells (heterologous junctions), or collections of channels between granulosa cells (homologous gap junctions) (Figure 3.1). Functional gap junctions connect the cytoplasm of adjacent cells and permit the passage of inorganic ions, second messengers, and small metabolites of <1 kDa, between adjoining cells[1,2].

The primary unit of a gap junction is the connexon – a cylindrical organelle with a hexamer of connexin (Cx) protein subunits which form a hemichannel in the plasma membrane of the cell. The end-to-end docking of two connexons from adjacent cells forms the intercellular gap junction[3–5]. Connexins which make up the connexons are members of a closely related family of integral membrane proteins in which at least 20 members have been identified in the mammalian genome[6]. While different connexins can associate to form connexons, each connexin conveys unique biophysical properties to the gap junction channel, thereby influencing both its permeability properties[7] and the types of molecules which can be transmitted via the junction[8].

To date at least three members of the Cx family have been recorded in follicular cells. Connexin 43 (Cx43: molecular mass 43 kDa), which is the most abundant in the ovary[9,10], is a multi-phosphorylated protein whose phosphorylated status has been shown to moderate both the conductance and permeability of the gap junctions it forms[11]. Interestingly, ovarian Cx43 appears to be phosphorylated in response to LH[12]. The network of gap junctions in the follicle contains two other members of the connexin family – connexin 37 (Cx37) a 37-kDa protein and connexin 45, a 45-kDa protein. Confocal microscopy studies of rat and mouse ovarian cells has localized Cx37 to heterologous gap junction plaques between granulosa cells and the oocyte, whereas Cx43 and Cx45 have been co-localized in homologous gap junctions between adjacent granulosa cells[2;13].

Communication via intercellular membrane channels feature prominently in mammalian oogenesis as gap junctions are known to be responsible for the timely transfer of nutrients,

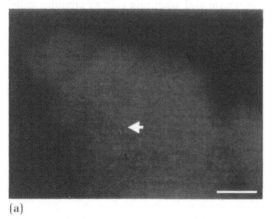 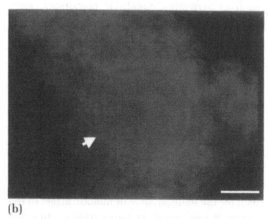

(a) (b)

Figure 3.1 Fluorescent staining of f-actin in an unexpanded bovine cumulus oocyte complex. An example of the close proximity of the many adjacent cumulus cells (arrowhead) which facilitate cell–cell communication in the cumulus complex is shown in (a). The close association between the oocyte (arrowhead) and the companion cumulus cells is shown in (b) oocyte. Scale bars = 50 μm (see color plate section)

nucleotides, and amino acids between the different cellular compartments of the follicle[14,15]. For example, ribonucleoside triphosphates which are required to support RNA synthesis in the oocyte are supplied to the oocyte via gap junctions[16]. Functional gap junctions in the granulosa cells have been shown to regulate the internal pH of growing oocytes until the oocyte reaches a developmental stage where it becomes capable of independent homeostasis[17]. Conversely, the internal pH of the oocyte and surrounding granulosa cells is thought to modulate gap junction permeability[5].

Metabolic cooperation between the oocyte and follicular cells provides growing oocytes with biosynthetic substrates. Although the oocyte can take up some nutrients directly via membrane-based transporters, granulosa cell–oocyte gap junctions offer the most efficient conduit for the uptake of nutrients and other small molecules such as sugars, amino acids, and ribonucleosides, required to fulfill the metabolic needs of the oocyte[18]. It has been estimated that granulosa cells, via gap junctions, allow the transfer of around 85% of the metabolic need of the oocyte[14]. The amounts of labeled uridine, choline, 2-deoxyglucose, and some amino acids incorporated into oocytes have been shown to vary with the numbers of attached granulosa cells[19,20]. Notwithstanding the significant role played by gap junctions in supporting the metabolic needs of the oocyte, it is important to remember that discrete biochemical differences exist between the different cellular compartments of the follicle. For example: as outlined in detail in Chapter 2 of this volume, granulosa cells preferentially metabolize glucose to pyruvate, whereas oocytes lack the cellular machinery to utilize this energy source with the result that pyruvate derived from granulosa cells is the primary energy substrate utilized by oocytes[21]. Similarly, oocytes have a low ability to incorporate and use cystines. The cumulus granulosa cells therefore convert cystines to cysteines to enable the oocyte to utilize the cysteines for glu-tathione synthesis[22]. Glutathione is required to both protect the oocyte against the destructive effects of free radicals during growth and maturation[23] and to contribute to nuclear decondensation in the fertilizing sperm in mature oocytes – a process which is a prerequisite for male pronucleus formation[24].

Gap junctions between oocytes and granulosa cells appear to have an important role in the cross-talk between the two cell types during both oocyte growth and meiotic maturation. For example, granulosa cell gap junctions have been shown to modulate oocyte transcriptional activity and chromatin remodeling[25] and to induce post-translational modification of several oocyte proteins[26,27]. Furthermore, heterologous gap junctions between the oocyte and granulosa cells have been widely implicated in the regulation of meiotic maturation late in oogenesis when follicle-derived meiosis inhibiting factors[28-31], which maintain the oocyte in prophase I, are replaced by maturation promoting factors (see Chapter 5 for more details). This hypothesis has been supported by chimeric re-aggregation experiments using mouse ovaries which demonstrate that the absence of Cx43 from granulosa cells and Cx37 from oocytes is sufficient to compromise both oocyte and follicle development[8]. Furthermore, wild type oocytes paired with Cx37-deficient granulosa cells generate antral follicles containing fertile oocytes that developed to at least the two-cell embryo stage following fertilization. These results indicate that murine oocytes do not need to express Cx43 in order to develop into meiotically competent, fertile gametes, but they must express Cx37 for communication with granulosa cells as this requirement is fundamental for oogenesis to occur[8].

The importance of functional gap junctions throughout oocyte and follicle development and the role of Cx in these processes have been demonstrated in gene knockout experiments in mice. Connexin 37 is expressed by oocytes throughout all stages of folliculogenesis; without this protein there is no oocyte–granulosa cell gap junctional communication. Connexin molecules have also been shown to be essential for the growth and expansion of the granulosa compartment early on in folliculogenesis[32]. Targeted deletion of *Gja4*, the gene encoding Cx37, results in the production of infertile mice which lack granulosa-oocyte gap junctions[32,33]. The severe phenotype associated with *Gja4^null* mice is characterized by arrested follicle development at the preantral stages, failure to ovulate, and luteinization of the retained follicular structures[33], together with incomplete oocyte growth and meiotic incompetence as manifest by asynchrony between nuclear and cytoplasmic maturation in the oocyte[31]. Coupling between granulosa cells is however maintained in *Gja4^null* mice[33]. In contrast, the ovaries of *Gja1^null* mice which lack Cx43 are larger than those of *Gja4^null* mice and contain follicles which fail to develop beyond preantral stages as granulosa–granulosa cell coupling is prevented, and although meiotic maturation of oocytes in vitro is inhibited[32], oocyte–granulosa cell gap junctional coupling is maintained in these animals[13]. These data reinforce the idea that gap junctions which couple the oocyte to the surrounding granulosa cells have a different function to those that couple granulosa cells to each other. Granulosa–oocyte junctions therefore primarily function to support oocyte growth, regulate meiotic maturation, and regulate granulosa differentiation[15], whereas granulosa-granulosa junctions serve to optimize the proliferative response of granulosa cells to paracrine signals emitted from the oocyte[34]. Interestingly, different types of Cx are found in different parts of the follicle; for example, Cx32 (β1) is found in theca cells while Cx43 (α1) is present in the granulosa compartment[35]. This differential pattern of connexin expression may be important during the selective disconnection of gap junctions in certain parts of the follicle during meiotic resumption. In pigs, for example, cumulus–oocyte connections are disrupted during the transition between metaphase I and II, even though cumulus–cumulus connections remain intact[36].

CELL INTERACTIONS DURING OOCYTE GROWTH AND DEVELOPMENT

Commencing with follicle formation and continuing throughout folliculogenesis, bi-directional cell–cell interactions between oocytes and their companion granulosa cells are essential for the coordinated development of both the germs cells and the somatic compartments of the follicle. Indeed, it is now well established that oocytes and granulosa cells are dependent on each other for growth and survival throughout the different stages of follicular development as normal oocyte development cannot take place without the supporting somatic cells of the follicle and visa versa[37,38]. Furthermore, the rate of oocyte growth in vitro appears to be directly correlated to the number of granulosa cells surrounding it[39]. This is a possible reflection of the amount of uridine, choline, and amino acids incorporated into the oocyte, which also varies with the number of attached supporting cells[19,20]. However, while it also appears that different types of communication-competent somatic cells can support oocyte survival in vitro, the great majority of evidence indicates that oocytes are dependent on secreted soluble growth factors, meiotic inhibitors, and stimulators from the granulosa cells for their growth and development. For example, Cecconi et al.[40] demonstrated that granulosa cell conditioned medium could support limited growth of denuded mouse oocytes cultured on mouse fibroblasts cells. Interestingly, the same authors also detected oocyte growth when Sertoli cell conditioned medium was used, suggesting either that Sertoli cells share a common origin with granulosa cells, or that gonadal somatic cells secrete similar growth factors to support germ cell growth. In contrast, other authors have shown that denuded murine oocytes do not grow if cultured on Sertoli cells, 3T3 cells, primary mouse fibroblast cells, L-cells, Chinese hamster ovarian cells, and mouse hepatoma cells[38–40], whereas co-culture with granulosa cells has been consistently shown to induce phosphorylation of specific proteins in the oocyte[41]. Furthermore, maximal oocyte growth is obtained when denuded oocytes are in direct contact with granulosa cells[42], whereas denuded oocytes co-cultured with, but not in direct contact with, follicle cells had a 60% reduced growth rate compared to their direct contact counterparts.

CELL INTERACTIONS DURING FOLLICULOGENESIS

Each mature ovarian follicle is composed of an oocyte surrounded by a stratified series of granulosa and theca cells. Heterologous gap junctions are formed between oocytes and granulosa cells before deposition of the zona pellucida proteins[1]. After the zona pellucida is formed between the oocyte and the innermost layer of granulosa cells contact is maintained with cytoplasmic processes which extend from the granulosa cells, penetrate the zona pellucida, and establish/maintain junctional contact with the surface of the cell membrane of the oocyte (Figure 3.2).

While oocyte growth is clearly moderated by granulosa cells and/or their derivatives, the relationship between oocytes and granulosa cells is reciprocal as granulosa cell division and differentiation appear to be influenced by the oocyte[43,44]. Evidence suggests that oocytes can produce paracrine factors to regulate dissolution of extracellular matrix[14,45] and tPA production[46]. Oocytes are also thought to participate in the moderation of follicular steroidogenesis by maintaining estradiol production and inhibiting progesterone production by the granulosa cells[47]. Granulosa cell proliferation also appears to be accelerated in the presence of oocytes[48],

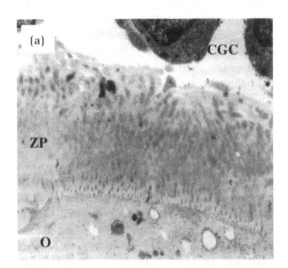
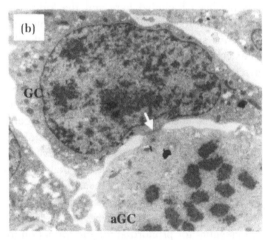

Figure 3.2 Transmission electron micrograph showing the homologous and heterologous contacts between sheep oocytes and their companion granulosa cells. (a) Cumulus granulosa cells (CGC) are in contact with the surface of the oocyte (O) via cytoplasmic processes which extend through the zona pellucida (ZP) and contact the surface of the oolemma. (b) Gap junctional contact between two adjacent granulosa cells; the arrow identifies the point of contact between a healthy granulosa cell (GC) and an apoptotic granulosa cell (aGC). The gap junctions cannot be seen at this magnification but they are present between the tips of the granulosa projections and the oolemma in (a) and between the two granulosa cells at the point of cell membrane contact in (b).

whereas the expression of LH receptor mRNA is inhibited by oocytes[49]. Furthermore, recent evidence suggests that paracrine factors from fully grown oocytes exhibited greater ability than those from growing oocytes to promote the expression of genes encoding glycolytic enzymes and glycolysis on the granulosa cells of preantral murine follicles[50]. These data also suggest that oocytes regulate glycolysis and the TCA cycle in granulosa cells by regulating the expression of the genes encoding glycolytic enzymes in a manner specific to the population of the granulosa cell and to the stage of growth and development of the oocyte.

Numerous endocrine and paracrine factors including cytokines, growth factors, and neuro-peptidergic substances have been identified as important moderators of follicle and hence oocyte development. Of these factors FSH has been most extensively studied (as reviewed in Chapters 7, 8, and 9 in this volume), in the interests of brevity further information on FSH has not been included here and the following account will focus on the less well documented paracrine signals from the oocyte which facilitate cell–cell interactions and regulate key events such as follicle formation, growth initiation, growth, and maturation[51]. In the context of follicle formation, this phenomenon cannot occur in the absence of germ cells, which confirms that signals from the oocyte are required for follicle assembly in the presumptive fetal ovary. Murine studies have shown that expression of the oocyte-derived transcription factors such as factor in the germ line alpha (Figla)[52], WNT4[53], as well as the c-kit proto-oncogene[54], are essential for primordial follicle formation to occur.

Until recently the identity of many of the putative oocyte derived factors thought to modulate early follicle growth had remained elusive, but persuasive evidence is now emerging to suggest that growth differentiation factor 9 (GDF-9)[55,56], KL[54] (see later), anti-Müllerian hormone[57], basic fibroblastic growth factor[58], reti-

noblastoma protein, and *myc* oncogene may be involved. For example, studies of *Gdf-9null* mice show that granulosa cell proliferation is inhibited and follicle development is arrested at the primary stage of development[55]. However, a possible role for *Gdf-9* in the later stages of follicle development cannot be excluded as it is synthesized throughout oocyte growth and can be detected in all stages of follicle development in some species[55], and it has been implicated in the mechanism for cumulus cell expansion and mucification during oocyte maturation[59].

A well documented example of the paracrine cross-talk between early oocytes and the somatic cells of the follicle which surround them is provided by the c-kit proto-oncogene and the genes encoding the ligand for c-kit – KL or stem cell factor (SCF)[54]. Oocyte-derived c-kit is a member of the tyrosine kinase receptor family, whereas KL/SCF is a membrane-spanning protein synthesized from two alternatively spliced forms of KL mRNA isoforms which lead to the production of a soluble form KL-1 and a membrane-bound form KL-2 in the granulosa cells[60]. The ratio of KL-1 and KL-2 mRNA expressed by granulosa cells alters during follicle development and is regulated by the oocyte[61]. Since KL is too large a molecule to be transmitted through gap junctions, it must necessarily be released in the extracellular environment before binding to its receptor c-kit which is present on the oocyte membrane. Receptors for c-kit are also thought to promote the adhesiveness of oocytes to follicle cells[54] which appears central to primordial follicle activation. Granulosa-cell-derived KL may also be partly responsible for the formation of the theca cell layer which encloses the developing follicle from the secondary stage of development onwards[62]. The two-way communication between granulosa cells and oocytes is further illustrated by the study by Otsuka and Shimasaki[63], who demonstrated a feedback loop between oocyte-derived BMP-15 and granulosa cell expressed KL using oocyte–granulosa cell co-cultures of rat preantral follicles. These authors showed that both BMP-15 and KL stimulated granulosa cell mitotic activity in vitro. However, while KL suppressed *bmp-15* mRNA expression in the oocytes, BMP-15 stimulated *kl* mRNA expression in the granulosa cells. The mechanism by which KL stimulates granulosa cell proliferation remains unknown.

CELL INTERACTIONS DURING OOCYTE MATURATION

The cellular interactions between the somatic cells of the follicle and the oocyte are critical for completion of the final stages of oocyte maturation[64]. As soon as the oocyte has acquired meiotic competence, a shift in the balance of the inhibitory and stimulatory interactions between oocytes and somatic cells contributes to the maintenance of meiotic arrest or the resumption of meiosis following the surge of LH. In mice, for example, studies have shown that signaling from the fully grown oocyte is responsible for the functional differentiation of the mural and cumulus granulosa cells[65]. Furthermore, the preovulatory gonadotropin surge, which is a prerequisite for the ovulation of a fertile oocyte, is known to induce a series of marked changes in both follicular cells and oocytes such that the specialized signals required for the completion of oocyte maturation can be generated and read by both cell types. The loss of gap junctional contacts between the oocyte and cumulus cells which occurs consequent to the preovulatory LH surge is a key event in this cascade which has been proposed to be the physiologic mechanism which drives the resumption of oocyte meiosis[66]. Members of the mitogen activated protein kinase (MAPK) family (P44[mapk] and P42[mapk]) are thought to mediate the disruption of the cell–cell communication induced by the LH surge in rat ovarian follicles[67].

Control of the resumption of meiosis in the oocyte is believed to be due in part to changes in the intraoocyte concentrations of the cyclic nucleotide cAMP. While it is generally acknowledged that high tonic levels of cAMP must be maintained in the oocyte to keep the meiotic cycle on hold and that a drop in oocyte cAMP levels is required to drive the resumption of meiosis, the source of the inhibitory cAMP signal remains a matter of some controversy. A number of studies suggest that cAMP is generated within the oocyte itself[68,69]. According to this theory, oocytes produce cAMP in response to an as yet unidentified ligand which is continually generated by the granulosa cells and which in turn activates an oocyte membrane bound Gs protein which stimulates adenylate cyclase in the oocyte[69]. Release of the oocyte from the ovarian follicle through the loss of gap junctional contact therefore terminates the exposure of the oocyte to the granulosa-cell-derived Gs-activating ligand, which in turn results in the resumption of meiosis. The alternative theory which embodies the great majority of the published literature on this subject supports the hypothesis that high levels of cAMP produced by the granulosa cell mass are transferred to the oocyte via gap junctions in order to maintain meiotic arrest. Thus, LH-induced oocyte maturation occurs as a consequence of the LH surge-induced loss of gap junctional contacts between the oocyte and cumulus cells[67]. This latter suggestion is supported by evidence from the studies which have used cAMP analogs such as dibutyryl cAMP, forskolin, and inhibitors of phosphodiesterases (PDE) such as hypoxanthine and 3-isobutyl-1-methylxanthine (IBMX) to maintain high intraoocyte cAMP levels and so inhibit GVBD in cultured rodent oocytes[70,71], or conversely to instigate a drop in intraoocyte cAMP levels[66]. Evidence also suggests that a change in the relative proportions of PDE type 4 in the granulosa cells and PDE type 3 in the oocyte may contribute to the maintenance of high cAMP levels and meiotic arrest in oocytes[70]. In mice, IBMX is used to prevent GVBD in oocytes whereas specific inhibitors of PDE3, such as cilostamide and milrinone, are effective in preventing meiotic resumption of oocytes[70,72]. Further strong support for the second theory is provided by the recent demonstration that cAMP transported from granulosa cells to the oocyte via gap junctions is subjected to negative regulation by the gonadotropins[73].

Interactions between oocyte- and granulosa-derived paracrine factors have been shown to play a role in regulating cumulus cell expansion and mucification and the resumption of meiosis by the oocyte. KL and bone morphogenetic protein 15 (BMP-15) from the granulosa cells cooperate with oocyte derived GDF-9 to regulate oocyte maturation[59]. Further evidence of the putative role of members of the TGF-β superfamily in the regulation of oocyte maturation is provided from studies of a dominant activating mutation in the receptor ALK6. This mutation is responsible for the increased ovulation rates and litter sizes in Booroola sheep[74]. However, the importance of this receptor in GDF-9 and BMP-15 signaling pathways has yet to be established. There is also evidence that granulosa-derived activin A may signal to the oocyte as gene expression studies and immunostaining localized activin receptors in oocytes of mouse, human, and bovine follicles[75,76]. Furthermore, oocytes have been shown to contain binding sites for the granulosa cell derived epidermal growth factor (EGF), consequently EGF is often added to medium designed to support oocyte maturation in vitro as it has been reported to promote cytoplasmic maturation[77].

It is not just the maintenance of cumulus contacts with the oocyte that is important in the regulation of the meiotic progression in secondary oocytes, paracrine factors secreted by the oocyte are becoming increasingly relevant to studies of cell–cell interactions during the terminal stages of oogenesis. Oocyte secreted factors have been shown to affect the patterns of gene expression in granulosa cell populations. For example, via secretion of GDF-9 fully grown murine oocytes suppress *kl* and *Lhr* mRNA in cumulus granulosa cells[59]. Oocyte-derived factors have been found to: (1) stimulate mitosis in granulosa cells; (2) promote the cumulus cell phenotype[59,61]; (3) stimulate prostaglandin and progesterone synthesis and/or signaling in pre-ovulatory cumulus cells; (4) prevent premature luteinization of the granulosa cells and elevated progesterone secretion; (5) inhibit LH receptor expression in cumulus granulosa cells; (6) regulate the expansion of additional functional genes in the cumulus cell mass by inducing cumulus granulosa cells to secrete hyaluronan synthase 2, pentraxin 3, and tumor necrosis induced factor 6, while at the same time suppressing urokinase plasminogen activator[61,78,79]; (7) mediate prostaglandin and progesterone production pathways, e.g. CCAAT/enhancer binding protein b, cyclooxygenase 2 and progesterone receptor 9; and (8) promote alterations in subcellular functions, such as calcium release from intracellular stores, and redistribute cellular organelles such as the mitochondria and cortical granules. All of these events are required to drive the oocyte towards completion of meiosis and to prepare the oocyte for fertilization.

PERSPECTIVE

The discussion presented here clearly indicates that bi-directional communication between oocytes and their surrounding somatic cells is vital to support normal oocyte and follicle growth and development. Furthermore, complex cell–cell interactions are an integral part of the process of oocyte maturation leading to the production of a fertile gamete in vivo. It is essential, therefore, that we not only understand the complexity and nature of these cellular interactions and associated signaling pathways but also that we try to replicate the conditions needed to support them in vitro if we are to fully exploit IVM of oocytes as an alternative to conventional assisted reproduction technologies.

REFERENCES

1. Anderson E, Albertini DF. Gap junctions between the oocyte and companion follicular cells in the mammalian ovary. J Cell Biol 1976; 71: 680–6.

2. Kidder GM, Mhawi AA. Gap junctions and ovarian folliculogenesis. Reproduction 2002; 123: 613–20.

3. White TW, Paul DL. Genetic diseases and gene knockouts reveal diverse connexin functions. Annu Rev Physiol 1999; 61: 283–310.

4. Bruzzone R, White W, Paul DL. Connections with connexins: the molecular basis of direct intercellular signalling. Eur J Biochem 1996; 238: 1–27.

5. Sosinsky GE, Nicholson BJ. Structural organisation of gap junction channels. Biochim Biophys Acta 2005; 1711(2): 99–125.

6. Willecke K, Eiberger J, Degen J et al. Structural and functional diversiy of connexin genes in the mouse and human genome. Biol Chem 2002, 383: 725–37.

7. Elfgang C, Eckert R, Linchtenberg-Frate H et al. Specific permeability and selective formation of gap junctional channels in connexin-transfected HeLa cells. J Cell Biol 1995; 129: 805–17.

8. Gittens GE, Kidder GM. Differential contributions of connexin37 and connexin43 to oogenesis revealed in chimeric reaggregated mouse ovaries. J Cell Sci 2005; 118: 5071–8.

9. Beyer EC, Kistler J, Paul DL et al. Anisera directed against connexin43 peptides react with a 43-KD protein localised to gap junction in myocardium and other tissues. J Cell Biol 1989; 108: 595–605.

10. Grazul-Bilska AT, Reynolds LP, Redmer DA et al. Gap junctions in the ovaries. Biol Reprod 1997; 57: 947–57.

11. Lampe PD, Lau AF. The effects of connexin phosphorylation on gap junctional communication. Int J Biochem Cell Biol 2004; 36: 1171–86.

12. Granot I, Dekel N. Phosphorylation and expression of connexin-43 ovarian gap junction protein are regulated by luteinizing hormone. J Biol Chem 1994; 269: 30502–9.

13. Veitch GI, Gittens JE, Shao Q et al. Selective assembly of connexin37 into heterocellular gap junctions at the oocyte/granulosa cell interface. J Cell Sci 2004; 117: 2699–707.

14. Buccione R, Schroeder AC, Eppig JJ. Interactions between somatic cells and germ cells throughout mammalian oogenesis. Biol Reprod 1990; 43: 543–7.

15. Eppig JJ. Intercommunication between mammalian oocytes and companion somatic cells. Bioessays 1991; 13: 569–74.

16. Heller DT, Schultz RM. Ribonucleoside metabolism by mouse oocytes: metabolic cooperativity between granulosa cells and growing mouse oocytes. Devel Biol 1980; 84: 455–64.

17. FitzHarris G, Baltz JM. Granulosa cells regulate intracellular pH of murine growing follicles via gap junctions: development of independent homeostasis during oocyte growth. Development 2005; 133: 591–9.

18. Senbon S, Hirao Y, Miyano T. Interactions between the oocyte and surrounding somatic cells in follicular development: lessons from in vitro culture. J Reprod Dev 2003; 49: 259–69.

19. Heller DT, Schultz RM. Ribonucleoside metabolism by mouse oocytes: metabolic cooperativity between the fully grown oocyte and cumulus cells. J Exp Zool 1980; 214: 355–64.

20. Haghighat N, van Winkle LJ. Developmental change in follicular cell-enhanced amino acid uptake into mouse oocytes that depends on intact gap junctions and transport system Gly. J Exp Zool 1990; 253: 71–82.

21. Biggers JD, Whittingham DG, Donahue RP. The pattern of energy metabolism in the mouse oocyte and zygote. Proc Natl Acad Sci USA 1967; 58: 560–7.

22. de Matos DG, Furnus CC, Moses DF. Glutathione synthesis during in vitro maturation of bovine oocytes: role of cumulus cells. Biol Reprod 1997; 57: 1420–5.

23. Meister A. Selective modification of glutathione metabolism. Science 1983; 220: 472–7.

24. Perreault SD, Barbee RR, Slott VL. Importance of glutathione in the acquisition and maintenance of sperm nuclear decondensing activity in maturing hamster oocytes. Devel Biol 1988; 125: 181–6.

25. De la Fuente R, Eppig JJ, Transcriptional activity of the mouse oocyte genome: companion granulosa cells modulate transcription and chromatin remodelling. Devel Biol 2001; 229: 224–36.

26. Colonna R, Ceccioni S, Tatone F et al. Somatic cell–oocyte interactions in mouse oogenesis: stage specific regulation of mouse oocyte protein phosphorylation by granulosa cells. Devel Biol 1989; 133: 305–8.

27. Cecconi S, Tatone C, Buccione R et al. Granulosa cell–oocyte interactions: the phosphorylation of specific proteins in mouse oocytes at the germinal vesicle stage is dependent upon the differentiative state of companion somatic cells. J Exp Zool 1991; 258: 249–54.

28. Motlik J, Sutovsky P, Kalous J et al. Co-culture with pig membrane granulosa cells modulates the activity of cdc2 and MAP kinase in maturing cattle oocytes. Zygote 1996; 4: 247–56.

29. Thibault C, Szollosi D, Gerard M. Mammalian oocyte maturation. Reprod Nutr Dev 1987; 27: 865–96.

30. Downs SM, Coleman DL, Eppig JJ. Maintenance of murine oocyte meiotic arrest: uptake and metabolism of hypoxanthine and adenosine by cumulus cell-enclosed and denuded oocytes. Devel Biol 1986; 117: 174–83.

31. Carabatsos MJ, Sellitto C, Goodenough DA et al. Oocyte–granulosa cell heterologous gap junctions are required for the coordination of nuclear and cytoplasmic meiotic competence. Devel Biol 2000; 226: 167–79.

32. Ackert CL, Gittens JE, O'Brien MJ et al. Intercellular communication via connexin43 gap junctions is required for ovarian folliculogenesis in the mouse. Devel Biol 2001; 233: 258–70.

33. Simon AM, Goodenough DA, Li E et al. Female infertility in mice lacking connexin 37. Nature 1997; 385: 525–9.

34. Gittens JE, Barr KJ, Vanderhyden BC et al. Interplay between paracrine signalling and gap junctional communication in ovarian follicles. J Cell Sci 2005; 118: 113–22.

35. Wright CS, Becker DL, Lin JS et al. Stage-specific and differential expression of gap junctions in the mouse ovary: connexin-specific roles in follicular regulation. Reproduction 2001; 121: 77–88.

36. Suzuki H, Jeong BS, Yang XZ. Dynamic changes of cumulus–oocyte cell communication during the in vitro maturation of porcine oocytes. Biol Reprod 2000; 63: 723–9.

37. Rankin T, Familari M, Lee E et al. Mice homozygous for an insertional mutation in the Zp3 gene lack a zona pellucida and are infertile. Development 1996; 122: 2903–10.

38. Bachvarova R. Gene expression during oogenesis and oocyte development in mammals. In: Browder LW, ed. Developmental Biology. A Comprehensive Synthesis, Volume 1, Oogenesis. Plenum, New York, 1985: 453–524.

39. Brower PT, Schultz RM. Intercellular communication between granulosa cells and mouse oocytes: existence and possible nutritional role during oocyte growth. Devel Biol 1982; 90: 144–53.

40. Cecconi S, Colonna R, Rossi G et al. Influence of granulosa cells and of different somatic cell types on mammalian oocyte development in vitro. Zygote 1996; 4: 305–7.

41. Colonna R, Cecconi S, Tatone C et al. Somatic cell–oocyte interactions in mouse oogenesis: stage-specific regulation of mouse oocyte protein phosphorylation by granulosa cells. Devel Biol 1989; 133: 305–8.

42. Bachvarova R, Baran MM, Tejblum A. Development of naked growing mouse oocytes in vitro. J Exp Zool 1980; 211: 159–69.

43. Eppig JJ, Wigglesworth K, Pendola FL. The mammalian oocyte orchestrates the rate of ovarian follicular development. Proc Natl Acad Sci USA 2002; 99: 2890–4.

44. Matzuk MM, Burns KH, Viveiros MM et al. Intercellular communication in the mammalian ovary: oocytes carry the conversation. Science 2002; 296: 2178–80.

45. Salustri A, Yanagishita M, Hascall VC. Mouse oocytes regulate hyaluronic acid synthesis and mucification by FSH-stimulated cumulus cells. Devel Biol 1990; 138: 26–32.

46. Canipari R, Epifano O, Siracusa G et al. Mouse oocytes inhibit plasminogen actvator production

by ovarian granulosa cells. Devel Biol 1995; 167: 371–8.

47. Vanderhyden BC, Tonary AM. Differential regulation of progesterone and estradiol production by mouse cumulus cells and mural granulosa cells by a factor(s) secreted by the oocyte. Biol Reprod 1995; 53: 1243–50.

48. Vanderhyden BC, Telfer EE, Eppig JJ. Mouse oocytes promote proliferation of granulosa cells from preantral and antral follicles in vitro. Biol Reprod 1992; 46: 1196–204.

49. Eppig JJ, Wigglesworth K, Pendola FL et al. Murine oocytes suppress expression of luteinizing hormone receptor messenger ribonucleic acid by granulosa cells. Biol Reprod 1997; 56: 976–84.

50. Sugiura K, Pendola FL, Eppig JJ. Oocyte control of metabolic cooperativity between oocytes and companion granulosa cells: energy metabolism. Devel Biol 2005; 279: 20–30.

51. Eppig JJ. Oocyte control of ovarian follicular development and function in mammals. Reproduction 2001; 122: 829–38.

52. Soyal SM, Amleh A, Dean J. FIGalpha, a germ cell-specific transcription factor required for ovarian follicle formation. Development 2000; 127: 4645–54.

53. Vainio S, Heikkila M, Kispert A et al. Female development in mammals is regulated by Wnt-4 signalling. Nature 1999; 397: 405–9.

54. Clark DE, Tisdall DJ, Fidler AE et al. Localisation of mRNA encoding c-kit during the initiation of folliculogenesis in ovine fetal ovaries. J Reprod Fertil 1996; 106: 329–35.

55. Dong J, Albertini DF, Nishimori K et al. Growth differentiation factor-9 is required during early ovarian folliculogenesis. Nature 1996; 383: 531–5.

56. Vitt UA, McGee EA, Hayashi M et al. In vivo treatment with GDF-9 stimulates primordial and primary follicle progression and theca cell marker CYP17 in ovaries of immature rats. Endocrinology 2000; 141: 3814–20.

57. Durlinger AL, Gruiters MJ, Kramer P et al. Anti-Mullerian hormone inhibits initiation of primordial follicle growth in the mouse ovary. Endocrinology 2002; 143: 1076–84.

58. Nilsson E, Parrott JA, Skinner MK. Basic fibroblast growth factor induces primordial follicle development and initiates folliculogenesis. Mol Cell Endocrinol 2001; 175: 123–30.

59. Giu LM, Joyce IM. Interference evidence that growth differentiation factor-9 mediates oocyte regulation of cumulus expansion in mice. Biol Reprod 2005; 72: 195–9.

60. Manova K, Huang EJ, Angeles M et al. The expression pattern of the c-kit ligand in gonads of mice supports a role for the c-kit receptor in oocyte growth and in proliferation of spermatogonia. Devel Biol 1993; 157: 85–99.

61. Joyce IM, Clark AT, Pendola FL et al. Comparison of GDF-9 and oocyte regulation of kit ligand expression in mouse ovarian follicles. Biol Reprod 2000; 63: 1669–75.

62. Parrott JA, Skinner MK. Kit ligand actions on ovarian stromal cells: effects on theca cell recruitment and steroid production. Mol Reprod Dev 2000; 55: 55–64.

63. Otsuka F, Shimasaki S. A negative feedback system between oocyte bone morphogenetic protein 15 and granulosa cell kit ligand: its role in regulating granulosa cell mitosis. Proc Natl Acad Sci USA 2002; 99: 8060–5.

64. Canipari R. Oocyte–granulosa cell interactions. Hum Reprod Update 2000; 6: 279–89.

65. Vanderhyden BC, Caron PJ, Buccione R et al. Developmental pattern of the secretion of cumulus expansion-enabling factor by mouse oocytes and the role of oocytes in promoting granulosa cell differentiation. Devel Biol 1990; 140: 307–17.

66. Sela-Abramovich S, Edry I, Galiani D et al. Disruption of gap junctional communication within the ovarian follicle induces oocyte maturation. Endocrinology 2006; 147(5): 2280–6.

67. Sela-Abramovich S, Chorev E, Galiani D et al. Mitogen-activated protein kinase mediates luteinizing hormone induced breakdown of communication and oocyte maturation in rat ovarian follicles. Endocrinology 2005; 146: 1236–44.

68. Horner k, Livera G, Hinckley M et al. Rodent oocytes express an active adenylate cyclase required for meiotic arrest. Devel Biol 2003; 258: 385–96.

69. Mehlmann LM, Saeki Y, Tanaka S et al. The Gs-linked receptor GPR3 maintains meiotic arrest in mammalian oocytes. Science 2004; 306: 1947–50.

70. Tsafriri A, Chun SY, Zhang R et al. Oocyte maturation involves compartmentalization and opposing changes of cAMP levels in follicular somatic and germ cells: studies using selective phosphodiesterase inhibitors. Devel Biol 1996; 178: 393–402.

71. Chesnel F, Wigglesworth K, Eppig JJ. Acquisition of meiotic competence by denuded mouse oocytes: participation of somatic-cell product(s) and cAMP. Devel Biol 1994; 161: 285–95.

72. Conti M, Andersen CB, Richard FJ et al. Role of cyclic nucleotide phosphodiesterases in resumption of meiosis. Mol Cell Endocrinol 1998; 145: 9–14.

73. Webb RJ, Marshall F, Swann K et al. Follicle stimulating hormone induces a gap junction-dependent dynamic change in [cAMP] and protein kinase a in mammalian oocytes. Devel Biol 2002; 246: 441–54.

74. Souza CJ, Campbell BK, McNeilly AS et al. Bone morphogenetic proteins and folliculogenesis: lessons from the Booroola mutation. Reprod Suppl 2003; 61: 361–70.

75. Hulshof SCJ, Figueiredo JR, Beckers JF et al. Bovine preantral follicles and activin: Immunohistochemistry for activin and activin receptor and the effect of bovine activin A in-vitro. Theriogenology 1997; 48: 133–42.

76. Sidis Y, Fujiwara T, Leykin L et al. Characterization of inhibin/activin subunit, activin receptor, and follistatin messenger ribonucleic acid in human and mouse oocytes: evidence for activin's paracrine signaling from granulosa cells to oocytes. Biol Reprod 1998; 59: 807–12.

77. Driancourt MA, Thuel B. Control of oocyte growth and maturation by follicular cells and molecules present in follicular fluid. A review. Reprod Nutr Dev 1998; 38: 345–62.

78. Elvin JA, Yan C, Matzuk MM. Oocyte-expressed TGF-beta superfamily members in female fertility. Mol Cell Endocrinol 2000; 159: 1–5.

79. Varani S, Elvin JA, Yan C et al. Knockout of pentraxin 3, a downstream target of growth differentiation factor-9, causes female subfertility. Mol Endocrinol 2002; 16: 1154–67.

CHAPTER 4

Gene expression in oocytes during growth and maturation

Ursula Eichenlaub-Ritter

INTRODUCTION: RELEVANCE OF EXPRESSION PATTERNS STAGE-BY-STAGE

Mammalian oocytes are exceptional cells. Unlike male germ cells they are extremely long-lived and initiate the meiotic program during fetal development in the embryonic ovary. Much unlike most other cell types, they arrest for long periods at the G2-phase of the cell cycle and thus undergo a discontinuous meiosis. Their development is associated with major starts and stops in meiotic progression as well as major changes in gene expression patterns during transitional phases of oogenesis, e.g. when oocytes complete the first stages of prophase of meiosis I[1], when oocytes become meiotically arrested, or when follicles and oocytes become recruited from the resting to the growing pool[2]. Before resumption of maturation oocytes undergo extensive growth, accompanied by high transcription rates. However, fully mature oocytes subsequently become transcriptionally repressed[3,4], whereas specific stored messages are recruited by polyadenylation to be translated during maturation or early embryogenesis[5,6].

With respect to cell cycle progression, S-phase, chromatin condensation, pairing, and recombination take place during meiotic prophase I of oogenesis within the fetal ovary, followed by a long meiotic arrest phase with decondensed chromatin in the G2-phase of the cell cycle (dictate or dictyate stage), in which the oocyte is surrounded by a single layer of squamous non-proliferating granulosa cells within a primordial follicle[7]. Oocytes have an intact nucleus (germinal vesicle, GV) throughout this arrest period and remain quiescent, up to decades in humans, before growth is initiated and the transition from the resting primordial to the primary stage of folliculogenesis is initiated. However, during the arrest oocytes may be more 'active' in expression than previously anticipated[8]. Primary follicle development is followed by development from the preantral to the large antral, preovulatory stage, and finally, oocyte meiotic resumption and ovulation.

To acquire full maturational and developmental competence the oocyte has to undergo an extensive growth phase. This is associated with an accumulation of components for nuclear maturation, dramatic increases in numbers of cell organelles like mitochondria, chromatin remodeling, and rises in protein and RNA content. Most mammalian oocytes mature to metaphase II, in response to activation of maturation promoting factor (MPF)[9]. Most protein is subsequently synthesized in the mammalian oocyte[10,11] as an essential component of the cytostatic factor (CSF) that arrests oocytes with well aligned chromosomes in metaphase II (for reviews see references 12 and 13). This is much unlike the situation in mitotic cells, that trigger anaphase once chromosomes are stably attached to spindle fibers and aligned at the spindle equator (termed: congression) (e.g. reference 14). Meiosis is completed after fertilization and inactivation of maturation promoting factor (MPF) downstream from calcium oscillations[15-17]. Subsequently, ooplasmic factors mediate chromatin remodeling and male pronuclear formation. Global changes in methylation imprinting are initiated by oocyte derived factors (e.g. references 18 and 19 and Chapter 6). Importantly, maternal and paternal imprinting marks acquired during gametogenesis have to be established and oocytes conditioned such that specific marks maintained during maturation and early embryogenesis for mono-allelic gene expression (e.g. references 20 and 21 and Chapter 6).

The oocyte provides all proteins, especially transcription factors, mRNA, tRNA, and ribosomal RNA, as well as cell organelles like mitochondria to support the first mitotic divisions and early embryogenesis. It has to provide for initiation of zygotic gene activation until full zygotic gene expression is achieved. All the information obtained by genetic models and observations on correlations between oocyte quality and developmental competence in assisted reproduction thus support the notion that embryogenesis is governed by and begins during oogenesis[22,23] and is dependent on timed expression during oogenesis. The continued development and maturation of the oocyte within the ovarian follicle in vivo facilitates the production of oocytes of the highest developmental potential. Up to now, in-vitro conditions do not fully support the process of oocyte growth and maturation as effectively. This may relate to deficiencies in the extracellular milieu, or result from the suboptimal quality of the oocyte at the beginning of and during culture, especially in primates (e.g. reference 24).

TEMPORAL AND SUSTAINED EXPRESSION OF EARLY MEIOTIC GENES FOR GENOMIC INTEGRITY

The early stages of oocyte development in the fetal ovary, prior to birth, are characterized by the expression of genes that are necessary for chromosome pairing, homologous recombination, and DNA repair. This accounts for the requirement of meiotic exchange to establish physical attachments between homologous chromosomes and the formation of chiasmata. The latter are required for reductional division, to help chromosomes orient properly on the spindle and to segregate from each other at meiosis I (for discussion see references 25–27). For instance, genes expressed in recombination encode proteins of the synaptonemal complex and chromosome cohesion like SCP1, SCP 3, REC 8, and SMC1 beta[28-30], as well as genes involved in recombination and DNA repair such as Atm, Spo11, Dmc1, Msh2, Msh 3, Msh 4, Msh 5, and Mlh 1[31-37]. Reduced expression, mutation, or knockout of such genes can have long lasting effects and severe implications for fertility in the female, causing death of oocytes[38,39] and/or affecting the ability of the oocyte to faithfully segregate chromosomes at meiosis I and ovulate metaphase II oocytes with normal chromosomal constitution (for review see references 26 and 40).

The relevance of stage-specific regulation of gene expression by transcription factors and factors in initiation of translation at this early meiotic stage can be deduced from knockout models. For instance, the gene for CPEB (cytoplasmic polyadenylation element binding protein) is a sequence-specific RNA binding protein that is involved in translation initiation during vertebrate oogenesis. Ablation of CPEB expression causes arrest at the pachytene stage in female meiosis of the mouse. Synaptonemal complexes that mediate efficient pairing and recombination do not form, presumably because expression of mRNAs with cytoplasmic polyadenylating elements (CPE), binding sites for CPEB, that encode synaptonemal complex proteins, is reduced[41]. However, translation of CPE-containing mRNA is also required at resumption of meiosis. Regulation at pachytene appears to rely on phosphorylation of CPEB by kinase Aurora A followed by dephosphorylation when oocytes enter dictyate stage[42]. Differential phosphorylation also modulates transcription of polyadenylated mRNAs at resumption of maturation and at early development (see below).

Genetic models demonstrate how a disturbed expression of meiotic genes at early stages of oogenesis like Mlh1 affects pool size and leads to premature ovarian failure, but also causes predisposition to non-disjunction (errors in chromosome segregation) in oocytes at early maternal ages[28,30,34,43]. Interestingly, ceasing of expression of the gene for synaptonemal complex protein 1 (SCP1) is implicated in formation of primordial follicles in the mouse[1]. Most genes in meiotic recombination are no longer expressed at the end of meiotic prophase I, when nuclear maturation becomes arrested in the G2-phase. In contrast, genes that apparently remain to be expressed at low levels up to meiotic resumption are ones that mediate chromatid cohesion, like Smc1β. Usually, sister chromatids stay attached to each other until anaphase I, when chiasmata are resolved synchronously by the loss of cohesion between arms of sister chromatids (reviewed in references 44 and 45). Reduced Smc1β expression may be one of the conditions responsible for premature loss of sister chromatid cohesion and chiasma resolution that predispose to random segregation of chromosomes and aneuploidy in aged oocytes[43]. Once chromatids lose cohesion, there may be no possibility of re-attachment. Although it has been claimed that the ooplasm of fully grown GV-stage or metaphase II oocytes is capable of expressing genes that induce reductional segregation of somatic chromosomes, the lack of coordinated expression of prophase I-specific recombination genes at postnatal stages of oogenesis and the absence of a physical connection between homologous parental chromosomes render it rather unlikely that the ooplasm is able to promote normal chromosome segregation. In fact, random segregation was observed in oocyte reconstitution approaches[46–48], although meiosis-like spindles may be formed after somatic cell nuclear transfer[49]. This appears to be different for oocytes derived by in-vitro development from ES cells in animal models, which exhibit stage-specific expression of meiotic markers and develop within a follicle-like somatic compartment[50]. It will be of great interest to assess their stage-specific gene expression patterns to identify essential pathways regulating early and late meiotic events and, particularly, chromatin remodeling and chromosome separation at oogenesis. This may also be useful in improving future in-vitro maturation (IVM) approaches.

GENE EXPRESSION AT RECRUITMENT OF PRIMORDIAL FOLLICLES AND THROUGHOUT FOLLICLE AND OOCYTE GROWTH

Oocyte survival at the dictyate stage initially depends on follicle assembly, and primordial follicle formation prior to birth as in humans[51,52] or shortly after birth as in rodents (e.g. references 53 and 54), depending on species (see reference 55). At this and later stages, oocyte and follicular health or atresia rely on complex interactions of oocytes with somatic cells, e.g. through interactions via growth and survival factors and later via gap junctional communication[56,57] (see Chapter 3). For instance, failure of expression of Foxl2 encoding a transcription factor in mice results in impaired follicle formation and deregulated oocyte growth[58,59]. Oocytes in primordial follicles express Gdf9 precociously to induce folliculogenesis shortly after birth and this causes atresia and premature ovarian failure. Early stages mainly depend on locally produced intercellular signaling and regulatory feedback signaling between the germ cell compartment and the oocyte (e.g. reference 60).

Later, additional feedback signaling with the neuroregulatory axis is essential for normal follicular development and differentiation, and for oocyte growth (see Chapter 2). As an example, female mice lacking FSHβ are infertile and follicular development is arrested at the preantral stage of folliculogenesis[61].

Multiple gene products act on the oocyte or are expressed by oocytes at several distinct stages of folliculogenesis and during oocyte growth, having distinct and diverse functions. For example, Factor in the Germaline alpha (FIG-α), a basic helix-loop-helix transcription factor, is initially required for primordial follicle formation, but also regulates expression of zona proteins during oocyte growth[62,63]. Other factors expressed in oocytes at primordial follicle formation include, for example, neurotrophins and their receptors, like the tyrosine kinase B receptor (TrkB receptor)[64,65].

Cohorts of primordial follicles are continuously recruited from the resting into the growing phase throughout reproductive life. This is accompanied by differentiation of flattened granulosa cells into large cuboidal granulosa cells of the primary follicle by still largely unknown factors. Anti-Müllerian hormone (AMH), a member of the TGF (β) family that signals through a bone morphogenetic protein (BMP)-like signaling pathway is expressed in the granulosa cells of growing and preovulatory follicles and appears to play a role in inhibiting primordial follicle recruitment. It is also expressed in oocytes of preantral and preovulatory oocytes and may enhance survival and growth of follicles at these later stages of oocyte and follicle development[66–69]. Expression of AMH and levels of AMH in serum are inversely proportional to follicle pool size and can possibly be used to assess physiologic age[70]. Thus AMH may present a marker of aging and thus may be predictive of the success of IVM.

The length of the oocyte growth phase differs between species from about 20 days in small rodents like the mouse to months in larger mammals (e.g. references 71 and 72). Oocyte growth and follicular development to the preovulatory stage lasts several months in the human. The volume of the oocyte increases 100-fold during this period and oocyte diameter expands from about 35 to 120 μm[73,74]. In the mouse the diameter of the oocyte increases from about 10–15 μm in the primordial follicle to about 80 μm in the preovulatory antral follicle[75]. Accordingly, oocyte volume also increases about 150-fold between primordial and large antral stage[2]. Most proteins and RNAs are produced during the oocyte's growth phase, when rapid divisions of granulosa cells commence and the oocyte significantly increases in volume. RNA content rises by about 300% during the 2–3 weeks of oocyte growth in the mouse. The meiotically competent, fully grown mouse oocyte contains about 200 times more RNA than a typical somatic cell[76]. About 20–25% of total RNA accounts for tRNA. About 60–65% of the total RNA comprises ribosomal RNA, and 10–15% represents heterogeneous RNA. About 8% of the latter is polyadenylated. While RNA synthesis is high at the early and middle growth phase, it is already reduced during the late growth period of the oocyte. Ribosomal RNA synthesis reaches highest levels at the beginning of follicular antrum formation.

Unlike in other vertebrate species (e.g. *Xenopus*) there is no amplification of ribosomal DNA for efficient rRNA synthesis in mammalian oogenesis[77]. However, there is a steady and rapid increase in RNA due to active transcription with peak values of 0.175 pg/h and a rise in protein content due to translation of mainly polyadenylated mRNA. Over 90% of the egg's ribosomes are already present in the mouse oocyte at 14 days of oocyte growth, although the oocyte has by then only reached 60–70% of its final size[78]. The nucleolus enlarges and nuclear proteins like fibrillarin, nucleoplasmin, nucleolin, and RNA polymerase I as well as nucleolar upstream binding factor are constantly synthesized. In fact, gene expression at the transition from the primordial to primary stage particularly involves genes in protein synthesis, ribosome biosynthesis and assembly, and translation to support oocyte growth[2]. Interestingly, Pan and co-workers also detected a significant increase in expression of mRNA of genes coding for proteins in DNA repair and chromatin conformation in mouse oocytes at this stage of folliculogenesis[2]. The latter may protect from mutation but may also preset the pattern of expression at later stages. For instance, expression of DNA damage factors like murine HR6A from maternal stores may be essential for development since oocytes of mHR6A–/– knockout mice do not develop beyond the embryonic two-cell stage[79].

There are two major transitions in the follicular and oocyte growth phase that correspond to steps in acquisition of maturational and developmental competence in oocytes, respectively, in association with characteristic changes in expression. Oocytes initially gain the competence to resume nuclear maturation although they may not be capable to support development after fertilization. At a later stage, full developmental competence is acquired. In the mouse, maturational competence is reached by the secondary to small antral follicle stage. Only afterwards do oocytes become fully competent for supporting embryogenesis to the blastocyst stage, corresponding to the transition from the small antral to the large antral stage of folliculogenesis in the mouse[80–82]. Analysis of genes that are up- or downregulated at these transition stages should help to identify critical factors in oocytes that support full cytoplasmic and developmental competence[2].

Acquisition of full meiotic competence coincides with a markedly decreased rRNA transcriptional activity. Fully mature oocytes of several species examined so far become transcriptionally quiescent when they reach full nuclear and developmental competence[3,4]. This is associated with characteristic alterations in nuclear and nucleolar morphology[83,84]. In pig oocytes it was shown that pocket protein, p130, is involved in the downregulation of rRNA transcription at the end of the oocyte growth phase through an inhibition of the activity of upstream binding factor (UBF). The latter protein is necessary for the function of RNA polymerase I (RNA Pol I), which is the actual enzyme driving rRNA gene transcription[85]. Ribosomal RNA genes are re-activated only at zygotic gene activation. Messenger RNA synthesis inevitably ceases in oocytes when they resume maturation and undergo germinal vesicle breakdown (GVBD).

At the end of the growth period, the oocyte is packed with ribosomes, mitochondria, protein, tRNA, and mRNA, which are maternally provided for the resumption of meiotic division, for fertilization, and for the rapid divisions and early stages of development of the preimplantation embryo. All of this requires substantial gene expression in a temporally and quantitatively controlled fashion at the transcriptional and translational level. Identification of key factors expressed in oocytes to initiate and promote oocyte and follicle growth and oocyte maturation to provide a high quality egg supporting embryonic development has been greatly facilitated in recent years by the analysis of transgenic mouse models[86], characterization of expression libraries, and analysis of differential expression patterns of oocyte-specific genes throughout oogenesis and at transition from early to advanced stages of folliculogenesis in several species, e.g. by transcript profiling using microarray analysis, in silico analysis, etc.[2,8,87–97].

Growth and survival factors and signaling pathways

Many locally produced factors promote the primordial to primary follicle transition, for instance, growth factors such as kit ligand (KL), leukemia inhibitory factor (LIF), bone morphogenetic proteins (BMPs), keratinocyte growth factor (KGF), and basic fibroblast growth factor (bFGF) (for reference see Picton and Harris, Chapter 2). Primary oocytes in primordial follicles and granulosa cells express the ligand for the c-kit gene for a tyrosine kinase receptor, kit ligand (KL), while c-kit mRNA concentration increases during oocyte growth in the mouse[98]. FSH-stimulated oocyte growth is inhibited by Gleevec, an inhibitor of kit activity, suggesting that the correct concentration of FSH is crucial for appropriate modulation of expression of KL and also of BMP15 to support oocyte growth[99]. Autocrine and paracrine signaling by c-kit/KL may be important for oocyte survival and transition from primordial to primary stage, as is leukemia inhibitory factor[100]. Basic fibroblast growth factor increases KL expression, and together they are believed to promote primary follicle formation[101]. Keratinocyte growth factor appears to be a mesenchymal factor, produced by progenitor theca cells, that promotes the primordial to primary follicle transitions with unknown downstream targets for altered gene expression in oocytes[102].

Several recent studies addressed the characteristic changes in expression patterns during primordial follicle assembly and in oocytes progressing from primordial to primary to preantral and large antral stages in rodents using microarray analysis, analyzing expression in either follicles or isolated oocytes (e.g. references 2 and 102). Several mRNAs for steroidal enzymes as well as inhibin, Müllerian inhibiting substance (MIS, another term for AMH), and all three zona genes appear unregulated at primordial follicle formation in the rat ovary[102]. As expected, genes encoding proteins of the synaptonemal complex are downregulated in the oocytes. About 15% of all the genes upregulated at the transcriptional level at the primordial to primary stage of follicle formation comprise metabolic enzymes. Endocrine factors inhibin and AMH appear downregulated at the transition from primordial to primary stage, in contrast to their increased expression at primordial follicle formation. In the experimental approach by Pan et al. using mRNA from mouse oocytes, one third of all genes identified by gene chip analysis to be expressed in oocytes of primordial follicles

changed 2-fold in expression at the transition to the primary stage[2]. About every second gene appeared to be either up- or downregulated at this stage, as may be expected by initiation of oocyte growth. At the protein level, the dramatic increase in growth is associated with transitions in transcription accompanied by major increases in RNA polymerase activity at the progression from primordial to growing oocytes[103]. The final acquisition of competence to undergo nuclear maturation and to support embryonic development is accompanied by global, characteristic changes in protein synthesis, first shown in the mouse[75].

Apart from supporting development after fertilization, the oocyte is by itself the major driving force in the development, organization, and function of the somatic cells of ovarian follicles[104–106]. Growth differentiation factor 9 (GDF-9), one of the members of the TGF-β growth factor family, is a key regulatory oocyte synthesized and secreted molecule that contributes to oocyte mediated differentiation of granulosa cells and differential expression patterns in the somatic compartment of the follicle. For instance, it is required for the survival and growth of follicle cells, suppresses apoptosis, and is involved in cumulus expansion[107–109] (see Chapter 3). Follicular development from the primary stage of growth is accordingly disturbed in homozygous mutations for GDF-9 in sheep, in specific GDF-9 RNAi-microinjected hamster oocytes, and in GDF-9-/- knockout mice[108,110]. Both GDF-9 and BMP-15 proteins are secreted proteins in follicular fluid. Type II and type I activin receptor-like kinase (ALK) receptors in granulosa cells like ALK-6 signaling appear to be downstream from the receptor-mediated BMP signaling since the ability of BMPs to inhibit differentiation of follicular cells was decreased in the presence of ALK-6 mutations. Messenger RNA for ALK-6 together with related genes for cell-surface receptors such as ALK-5 and BMP-RII mRNA is also present in oocytes at most, if not all, stages of follicular growth. In sheep carrying the ALK-6 mutation, ovarian follicles undergo precocious maturation. Three to seven follicles are ovulated, mostly with a smaller diameter. BMP-15 and GDF-9 mutations in sheep are thought to result in reduced levels of mature protein or altered binding to cell-surface receptors. Sheep heterozygous for mutations in BMP-15 or GDF-9 or homozygous for an ALK-6 mutation have higher ovulation rates (up to 10 times higher) than wild-type animals. In sheep, GDF-9 mRNA is present in oocytes before and after follicle formation as well as throughout follicular growth, whereas BMP-15 appears expressed only from the primary stage of growth. In mouse, both orthologs, GDF-9 and BMP-15, as well as other members of the TGF-β superfamily, BMP-5 and BMP-6, are highly expressed at the primordial and primary follicle stage.

Expression is reduced at the mRNA levels from the small antral stage[2]. Although expression patterns of BMPs may differ slightly between species, possibly related to mono- or multi-ovular species, the necessity of BMP-15 for folliculogenesis in humans has been recently supported by the discovery of a BMP-15 mutation that is associated with ovarian dysgenesis (for review see reference 111). The list of oocyte-controlled signaling pathways during follicular development includes also Sonic hedgehog (Shh) signaling, signaling through epidermal growth factor (EGF), and transforming growth factor alpha (TGF-α) as well as their respective ligands that are highly expressed at primordial to primary follicle stage[2,97]. For instance, Deltex2 coding for a cytoplasmic SH3-ring finger gene that mediates Notch receptor signaling is expressed in oocytes (see reference 97). Components of Notch pathway were also identified in cDNA clones from human primordial follicles[8]. Interestingly, there was an abundance of retroviral elements and transcriptional repressor in the cDNA library from human primordial follicles, suggesting that they could contribute to the maintenance of this stage and to meiotic arrest.

With respect to essential oocyte–granulosa cell signaling, expression of connexins that form gap junctions between the oocyte and granulosa cells is necessary to allow for development of the follicle beyond the secondary follicle stage[112] (see also Chapter 3). The family of 2′,5′oligoadenylate synthasc 1 (OAS1) proteins was originally recognized by its involvement in the control of the interferon/OAS/RNase L pathway of degradation of viral double stranded RNAs (dsRNAs) in host defense against viral infection. OAS1D has recently been identified in the cytoplasm of growing and maturing oocytes and may protect from loss of oocytes in response to viral infection. OAS1D–/– mice are subfertile, revealing the significance of expression of this gene in mammalian oogenesis[113]. In conclusion, it is far beyond the scope of this review to list all regulatory components that are expressed in growing oocytes and their signaling pathways. The significance of expression of the plethora of known and novel oocyte and germ cell specific genes encoding growth and survival factors and their ligands that appear up- or downregulated at oocyte growth is awaiting further analysis.

Transcription factors in oocyte growth and developmental competence

The homeobox gene Nobox (newborn ovary homeobox-encoding gene), first identified in a cDNA library of the mouse ovary[114], is expressed in mouse oocytes from primordial follicles through antral stages and appears essential for progression from primordial to primary stage of oogenesis[115], possibly because downstream expression of genes like mos, oct-4, rfl4, fgf8, zar1, dnmtlo, gdf9, bmp15, and H1oo is regulated. The gene for oocyte-specific mammalian H1 linker histone, H1FOO, is exclusively expressed during oocyte growth and maturation. The message is alternatively spliced, and protein synthesis coincides with recruitment of resting primordial follicles into a developing primary follicular cohort. Association with perinucleolar heterochromatin suggests a role in restructuring chromatin at the transition to oocyte growth[115].

The transcription factor Oct-4 that is involved in maintaining pluripotency in stem cells and the embryo may have two additional roles in oogenesis: in the recruitment of oocytes for initiating growth and in the selection of oocytes for ovulation[116]. Messenger RNA for Oct-4 is transcribed during oocyte growth but is not present in oocytes at the primordial follicle stage. Oogenesin-1 is a recently recognized oocyte-specific transcription factor that is expressed in mouse oocytes from primordial to preovulatory follicles, while related family members of the transcription factor oogenesin 2–4 appear first expressed in primary but not in primordial follicles[117]. Thus, expression of these factors may contribute to the transition in stage-specific gene expression in oocytes. The functional significance of oocyte-specific homeobox transcription factors like obox-1, 2, 3, and 6, whose mRNAs were detected in mouse oocytes, is still unclear – they may contribute to transcriptional activation at initiation of and during oocyte growth (for discussion see reference 118). The obox-5 gene that may be central to initiation of oocyte growth, is markedly increased at primordial to primary follicle transition as well as the transcription factors Mrg1, Tcfap2e, and Gli3[2]. The latter may regulate transcription of target genes like the BMPs[119], coinciding with the increase in their expression in the growing oocyte. Mrg1 may stimulate expression of multiple other transcription factors[2]. Zfp37 codes for a KRAB-box zinc finger protein that was inferred to be expressed preferentially in growing oocytes[97]. Expression of Sox8 transcription factor was found only in the oocytes of preantral follicles and in the oocytes, cumulus cells, and mural granulosa cells of preovulatory follicles. Initially Sox8 was believed to affect expression of AMH, but this could be disproved experimentally, so that its oocyte-specific function is still unclear[67].

Major increases in expression of some genes at early stages of mouse oocyte growth are followed by substantial reductions in mRNA levels in oocytes when folliculogenesis progresses to the antral stage. Such patterns of expression are characteristic for Polr2h and j, Tafl1, Cebpb, and Cebpd genes. Downregulation at antral stages is also characteristic for genes like Sp4, Crebbp, and Tcfl2, which are implicated in reduced activity of RNA polymerase II. Sp4 mRNA is reduced by 33%, and Tcf12 decreases by 12.5% at small to large antral follicle stage in the mouse oocyte[2] concomitantly with cessation of oocyte growth and acquisition of maturational competence.

Many transcripts have to remain dormant until their products are spatially and temporally required in development. Clast-4 is a homolog of the Drosophila Cup protein, a translational repressor during female germ line development in the fruit fly. Clast-4 mRNA and protein are highly expressed within the cytoplasm of growing oocytes. The mouse Clast-4 protein is stable during this developmental window and post-translationally modified by phosphorylation upon oocyte meiotic maturation[120]. This might release translational repression in order to synthesize maturation proteins that are required for oocyte and embryo development (see below).

Oocyte growth, and chromatin structure and remodeling in control of expression

Histone mRNAs are the only metazoan mRNAs that are not polyadenylated. Instead, they end with a conserved stem-loop structure, which is recognized by the stem-loop binding protein (SLBP)[121]. Histone synthesis in immature and maturing mammalian oocytes appears governed by a translational control mechanism that is directly regulated by changes in the amount of SLBP. SLBP binds to the highly conserved sequence in the 3′-untranslated region of the non-polyadenylated histone mRNAs. Unlike in somatic cells where SLBP is expressed during S-phase, SLBP is expressed in growing oocytes of the mouse at the G2-phase of the cell cycle and further accumulates substantially during meiotic maturation. Ablation of expression of SLBP causes a significant decrease in pronuclear size and in the amount of acetylated histone detectable on the chromatin of fertilized zygotes of SLBP-depleted mouse oocytes. This supports the concept of a tight link between oocyte quality and developmental potential. The competence to control chromatin constitution during oocyte growth impinges on expression patterns at early embryogenesis[122].

DNA methylation (for review see reference 18 and Chapter 6), histone post-translation modifications, e.g. acetylation[123], and changes in chromatin organization and nuclear structure[124,125] are all involved in global and specific changes in gene expression and represent epigenetic mechanisms in control of gene expression. Chromatin structure and imprinting involving methylation at GpG islands at promoters of developmentally expressed genes is intimately involved in programming expression, and this is particularly important during oocyte growth and after fertilization, e.g. when oocytes are matured in vitro (e.g. references 21 and 126 to 128, and Chapter 6). This review will not focus in detail on such regulatory mechanism in gene expression in oocytes but it is of interest that expression profiles of oocytes developing in vitro to metaphase II either from mouse oocytes obtained from primordial follicles or from the secondary follicle stage are quite similar. However, some genes differ in expression profile, possibly reflecting the lower developmental competence when culture was from the primordial follicle stage. Of note, these may be relevant for epigenetic modulation of gene expression. It is remarkable that Ctcf, coding for a protein that blocks methylation of specific DNA sequences[129], as well as Dnmt-3a, coding for an active de novo DNA methyltransferase required for development[130], appear upregulated in the metaphase II mouse oocytes that have a reduced developmental potential[2]. Increased repression by methylated DNA due to increased expression of these genes has therefore been discussed in respect to critical changes in the growing oocytes that could contribute to

reduced size characteristics for in-vitro grown and matured oocytes[131,132]. It could also critically affect expression patterns at embryogenesis. Alterations in expression of genes in chromatin conformation and imprinting, e.g. in association with IVM or adverse exposures, might therefore be of high relevance for developmental potential as well as for genetic disease in the offspring (discussed in Chapter 6).

Screening ovarian libraries by in-silico subtraction approaches as well as by differential display identified new oocyte-specific genes that are expressed in a temporally controlled fashion. Interestingly, there is increasing evidence that some of the oocyte-specific genes are either up- or downregulated in a coordinate fashion[2] as they are transcribed from specific chromosome domains in clusters[133]. For instance, the clusters on mouse chromosome 9 comprise the oogenesin genes, those on chromosome 7 the Obox genes, and another cluster on chromosome 7 the Nalp family of genes, related to Mater, a maternal effect gene that is essential for embryogenesis. Tcl1 genes are in a cluster on mouse chromosome 9, shown to have human orthologs expressed in oocytes. The F-box genes (FBO12) on mouse chromosome 9 belong to a family of proteins that serve as link between target proteins and ubiquitin-ligases such as early mitotic inhibitor 1 (Emi-1), an inhibitor of anaphase promoting complex that prevents MPF inactivation (see below)[134]. Other genes may code for proteins that interact with the cytoskeleton (e.g. actin/dynein) and other proteins that may help to reorganize the chromatin[133]. Finally, some genes on mouse chromosome 12 encode known oocyte-specific genes (e.g. oocyte secreted protein 1, Oosp-1) with zona protein-like domains that may be involved in zona formation. It has been suggested that the clustering of expressed genes reflects coordinated gene regulation in oocytes by large-scale genome organization and oocyte-specific regulation of chromatin constitution[2,133]. Pan et al. suggested that local differences in histone modifications are involved[2].

Spatial organization of telomeres and chromatin domains within the nucleus during oogenesis may also play a role[133]. This suggests that spatial-temporal changes in the cytoskeleton, nucleus, and cellular organization may affect efficiency and control of expression as well as the quality of the oocyte.

A major change in chromatin/DNA configuration in the GV is characteristic for the acquisition of meiotic competence[135]. While DNA is diffusely distributed within the nucleus of meiotically incompetent oocytes, termed non-surrounded nucleolus (NSN), condensation of DNA in a rim-like fashion is characteristic for fully mature oocytes (termed surrounded nucleolus, NS)[81,136] that are transcriptionally suppressed[31,83]. In NSN oocytes ribosomal transcripts are accumulated within the nuclear matrix with nucleolus organizing regions (NORs) within the nucleolus. In contrast, NORs are in the nucleolar periphery in the mature SN oocytes[136]. The expression of histone deacetylase 4 (HDAC4) mRNA appears low in growing oocytes, but to be characteristic for fully grown oocytes. The HDAC4 protein has been implicated in transcriptional repression but is also associated with the chromosomes at resumption of maturation. Message decreases sharply after fertilization[137]. Currently it is unclear in which way chromatin reorganization contributes to transcriptional silencing in mature GV stage oocytes because mouse oocytes deficient in nucleoplasmin 2 (Npm2) do not develop to the SN stage but are still transcriptionally repressed. Also, chromatin hyperacetylation due to Trichostatin A (a deacetylase inhibitor) exposure does not release from the transcriptionally repressed state, although it induces chromatin decondensation[4]. In contrast, core histone deacetylation is associated with the modification of chromatin and termination of RNA synthesis from blastomere nuclei when they are exposed to cytoplasm of mature, fully grown oocytes[138]. ATRX, a member of the SNF2 family of helicase/ATPases, that is associated with chromosomes, may also critically affect chromatin constitution.

Expression appears to be required for chromosome alignment and meiotic spindle organization in metaphase II stage mouse oocytes[4]. The regulatory mechanisms for transcriptional silencing and spatio-temporal regulation of chromatin conformation have still to be uncovered and the functional significance of the silencing is still an enigma in oogenesis research.

There may be also a link between gene expression in oocytes, the presence of maternal mRNA and protein at early embryogenesis, and changes in chromatin organization that facilitate zygotic gene expression and nuclear reprogramming. Mouse nucleoplasmin (Npm2) protein accumulates in oocyte nuclei and persists in preimplantation embryos. Npm2−/− knockout females have fertility defects owing to failed preimplantation embryo development[139]. Experimental data showed that pretreatment of mouse somatic nuclei with Npm2 facilitated activation of oocyte-specific genes from somatic cell nuclei injected into *Xenopus laevis* oocytes[140]. Zygote arrest 1 (Zar1 and ZAR1 in mouse and human, respectively), the first identified oocyte-specific maternal-effect gene, is also transcribed during oocyte growth. Maternal and paternal genomes remain separate in Zar1−/− mutants and there is a marked reduction in the synthesis of the transcription-requiring complex Zar1, suggesting that the protein is required for zygotic gene activation[141]. The role of MATER (maternal antigen that embryos require) and other members of the NACHT NTP family of proteins that are expressed during oocyte growth and required for early embryogenesis[142,143] is still under investigation. MATER protein was detected in mitochondria and nucleoli, suggesting that it may participate in both cytoplasmic and nuclear events during early development[143].

Notably, among approximately 11 000 genes whose transcripts were detected in mouse oocytes by microarray, about 5% showed statistically significant expression changes with advanced maternal age, including members of the NALP gene family and genes involved in chromatin structure, DNA methylation, genome stability, and RNA helicases[144]. It remains to be determined whether optimizing oocyte growth and maturation in vivo or in vitro may reduce or prevent age-associated changes in expression of such genes, in particular, when they are involved in nuclear remodeling and zygotic gene activation at embryogenesis in order to obtain healthy oocytes with high developmental potential. Polycomb group (Pc-G) gene products that are expressed in growing and mature oocytes are essential to maintain stable repression of homeotic (HOM C) genes during development. Messenger RNA of members of the Pc-G like Yin Yang 1 (YY1), Enhancer of Zeste (EZH2), and Early Ectoderm Development (EED) are involved in X-chromosome inactivation[145]. Their deregulation in ART or, possibly, in IVM could contribute to disturbances in epigenetic regulation with adverse effects on embryo health (see reference 145 and Chapter 6).

DIFFERENTIAL EXPRESSION OF GENES REQUIRED FOR OOCYTE MATURATION AND EARLY EMBRYOGENESIS

The fate of mRNAs can differ depending on the need to provide proteins for metabolic activities associated with growth and acquisition of meiotic competence of the oocyte, or processes essential for meiotic progression or early embryogenesis[146]. For instance, housekeeping genes like β-actin are actively transcribed and translated during murine oocyte growth, accounting for 1% of the total protein synthesized. The store of mRNA rises to 2×10^4 molecules, then decreases by 50% at metaphase II and becomes further reduced to 10% of the initial amount by the two-cell stage. The zona proteins ZP-1, ZP-2, and ZP-3 are coordinately expressed, predominantly during oocyte growth under the control of Fig-α transcription factor[62,147]. At mid growth phase they represent a large fraction, 1.5% of the total polyadenylated RNA. At ovulation mRNA is substantially lower (5% of peak values) and is undetectable in the embryo. Other mRNAs like that encoding lactate dehydrogenase (LDH-β) are more stable in mature oocytes and embryos. The synthesis of LDH protein reaches high levels, comprising up to 2–5% of the totally synthesized protein or 200–400 pg in murine oocytes[148]. However, it only recently became obvious that the relative rate of expression of genes, for instance as in metabolism, is influenced by oocyte–granulosa cell cooperativity, which may have a major impact on egg quality (for discussion, see reference 106 and Chapter 2).

Regulation of translation by polyadenylation

Generally, most mRNAs are immediately polyadenylated within the nucleus and then transcribed in the cytoplasm of the growing oocyte (Figure 4.1). Abundant mRNAs for typical housekeeping genes with long poly(A) tails actively transcribed during oocyte growth include actin and globin mRNAs. However, others are temporarily stored and expressed at distinct times during maturation or in early development in a temporally coordinated fashion. Stored mRNAs especially abundant in fully grown mouse oocytes are, for instance, those encoding c-kit, zona protein ZP-3, lactate dehydrogenase, and the product of the c-mos proto-oncogene[76,149]. Control of expression was first extensively studied for genes like tissue plasminogen activator, tPA, and hypoxanthine phosphoribosyltransferase (HPRT) in the mouse[148], and mRNA for the spindle associated protein spindlin[150], and notably, cell cycle regulatory components like cyclins A1 and B2[151–153], Mos[154,155], and Cdc25 [156] in several species. Maturation dependent polyadenylation associated with translational initiation and expression was earlier also described for mRNAs of antioxidant enzymes, glutathione peroxidase (GPX), and Mn-superoxide dismutase (Mn-SOD)[157].

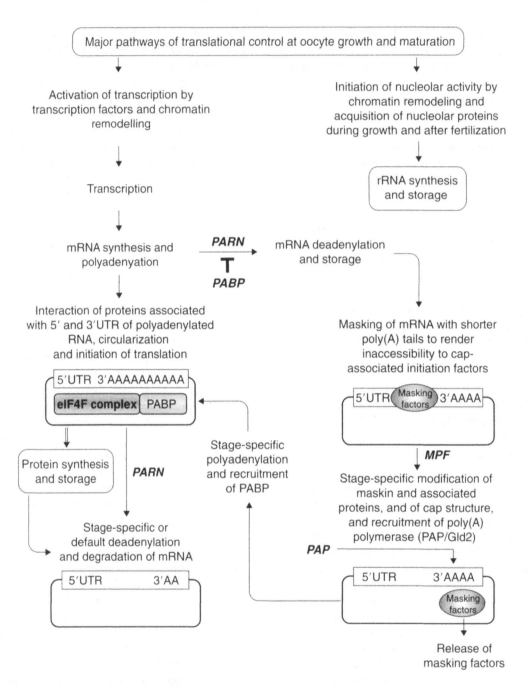

Figure 4.1 Overview of storage, recruitment, and translation initiation of mRNAs in growing and maturing oocytes. PAP: poly(A) polymerase; PARN: poly(A) RNase; PABP: cytoplasmic poly(A) binding protein; MPF: maturation promoting factor. For further explanation see text. (Modified from reference 179)

Prior to maturation, repression of a large number of these mRNA species is controlled by deadenylation of the 3' end of the untranslated region (3'UTR) of the mRNA, usually to about 20 nucleotides[146]. Messages with a short poly(A) tail are much less susceptible to degradation[150]. For translation, polyadenylation by poly(A) polymerases (PAPs) is required (see Figure 4.1). The core factors that control adenylation and translational initiation in vertebrate oocytes and embryos include key components like the cytoplasmic polyadenylation element binding protein (CPEB), an RNA binding protein with recognition motif and zinc finger, associated with the cytoplasmic polyadenylation element on the mRNA (CPE) that specifies which mRNAs undergo polyadenylation[158,159] (Figure 4.2a). Furthermore, cleavage and polyadenylation specificity factor (CPSF) is a multi-factor complex that interacts with a conserved, ubiquitous hexanucleotide AAUAAA of the 3'UTR of the mRNA[160] (Figure 4.2a). In addition, symplectin, believed to be a scaffolding protein that anchors the CPEB and CPSF proteins, may help to position the poly(A) polymerase to prolong the poly(A) tail[161,162] (Figure 4.2c). In contrast, Maskin, a CPEB and initiation factor (eIF4E) binding protein, prevents polyadenylation[163,164] and inhibits the association of the mRNA with ribosomes (Figures 4.1, 4.2b, and 4.2c). The masking inhibits not only polyadenylation but also the recruitment of the eIF4F elongation initiation complex to the 3'UTR of the mRNA by preventing ring formation of the mRNA required for interactions between the 3' and 5' UTR of the mRNA. Ring formation for initiation of translation is achieved by association of the elongation initiation complex at the 5'UTR cap structure with the poly(A) binding protein (PABP) that is itself associated with the 3'UTR of polyadenylated mRNAs (Figure 4.1). This requires a long poly(A) tail for PABPs to interact with the mRNA (about 100–150 nucleotides)[165]. Therefore, it is mainly the regions at

the 3' untranslated end of the mRNA (Figure 4.2a) and the presence/release of maskin or related proteins allowing or preventing polyadenylation (Figure 4.2c) that direct storage, masking, and recruitment of mRNAs[6,161,166,167].

Deadenylation is catalyzed by a poly(A)-specific ribonuclease (PARN; Figure 4.1). When oocytes re-enter the meiotic cycle, removal of masking factors occurs downstream from inactivation of protein kinase A[164] and activation of MPF[166,167] (Figure 4.2c), by displacement of masking factors and recruitment and activation of poly(A) polymerases (PAP or Gld2) by CPEB/CPSF. Stage-specific post-translational modifications of proteins like maskin and CPEB (Figure 4.2c) then contribute together with the poly(A) binding protein (PABP) to recruit the eIF4F initiation complex to the 5'UTR and cap structure of the mRNA and to initiate translation (Figures 4.1 and 4.2b).

At resumption of meiosis and at fertilization there are major switches for control of polyadenylation of mRNAs that greatly affect translational initiation and/or mRNA stability[168]. The timing of adenylation/deadenylation depends on the specific cis sequences in the 3'UTP of the message and their relative distance on the mRNA for deadenylation and polyadenylation at the appropriate time (Figure 4.2a) (e.g. reference 155). During oocyte maturation it is predominantly the cytoplasmic polyadenylation elements on the 3'UTP (CPEs or adenylation control element, ACE), and the canonical AAUAAA hexamer of the premRNA in the 3'UTR that associate with proteins like CPEB, and CPSF, respectively (Figure 4.2a). They direct polyadenylation by influencing activity of RNA PAP (or rather Gld2 PAP in oocytes), or poly(A) deadenylases (PARN), respectively (Figure 4.2c). Screening by microarray analysis showed that in *Xenopus* oocytes more than 500 mRNAs from 3000 in an array were regulated at the post-transcriptional level during oocyte maturation and early embryogenesis[169].

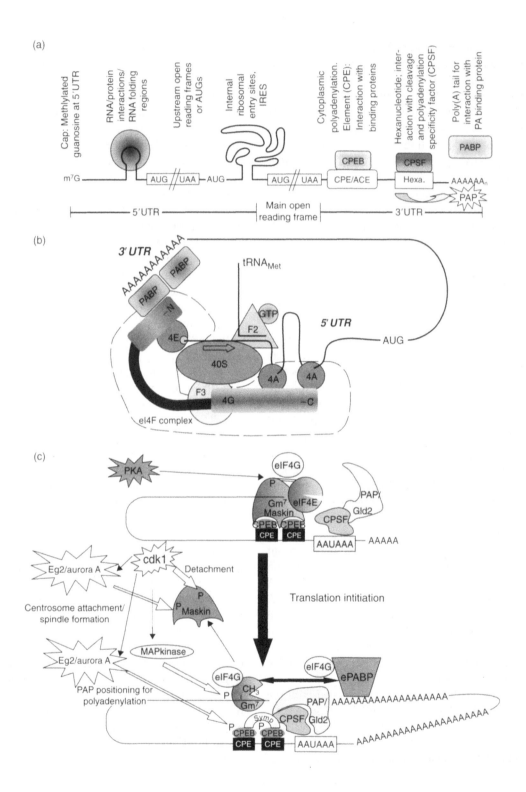

Translational inactivation of mRNA

Messenger RNAs in growing mouse oocytes that contain a short poly(A) tail (<90 residues) are much more stable compared to those with longer poly(A) tails. Those with about 150 residues are immediately translated[150]. Messenger RNA can be stored in the mouse oocyte for long periods during the growth phase with half-life times of approximately 28 days[170]. In *Xenopus* some messages without poly(A) tails are stable up to the mid-blastula transition[171,172]. Microinjection of RNAs containing long poly(A) tails (100–200 As) into mouse oocytes has shown that PARN reduces the length of the poly(A) tail of injected, foreign cytoplasmic mRNAs efficiently to about 20 to 50 adenosines at the 3'UTR of the mRNA during oocyte growth. A message with a short poly(A) tail is not only more stable, but initiation of translation is repressed by the de-

adenylation[173], as shown above. Thus, poly(A) tail removal is the initial and rate-limiting step in mRNA turnover that controls storage as well as decay. Deadenylation is the main mechanism responsible for translational silencing of maternal mRNAs during oocyte maturation and early development to cause translational repression or save them for their timed recruitment at a specific stage of maturation or development, depending on the 3'UTRs[172]. Most mRNAs, especially those of housekeeping genes like actin, appear deadenylated at GVBD as shown in the mouse[174], and this requires the activity of poly(A)-specific ribonuclease (PARN, or deadenylating nuclease, DAN)[175]. PARN is a member of the RNaseD family of RNA deadenylating nucleases. Interestingly, disturbances in default deadenylation and enhanced, untimely expression appear characteristic for bovine oocytes with low developmental potential[176]. Thus it

Figure 4.2 Messenger RNA sequences and RNA-binding proteins in regulation of circularization and initiation of translation of mRNAs during oocyte maturation and early development (modified from references 197, 224, and 246). (a): Modulation of expression of mRNAs by elements in RNA and binding of conserved proteins. CPEB and CPSF influence targeting of PAP to elongate the poly(A) tail for binding of PAPB. (b) Model of circularization of the mRNA. The N-terminal domain of elF4G adapter protein (hook-shaped gray structure, 4G) of the el4F complex (indicated by strippled line) is associated with the elFE cap binding protein (4E) to mediate binding to the PABP while the C-teminal domain of the elF4G protein of the elF4F complex is associated with the helicases elF4A (4A) and recruits the 40S ribosomal subunit with elF3 (F3) and the methyl tRNA with elF2 (triangle F2) to initiate RNA translation. (c) Upper part: masking of mRNAs with short poly(A) tail by binding to Maskin or related proteins to the CPEB, thus preventing tight interaction between CPEB and CPSF to position PAP/Gld2 poly(A) polymerase to elongate the poly(A) tail. Maskin phosphorylated by PKA when bound to elF4E excludes the elF4G protein from the complex and prevents ring formation by attachment to PABP. Lower part: upon resumption of maturation and activation of MPF/cdk1, Maskin is phosphorylated by cdk1 and this releases its interaction with elF4G (and possibly CPEB). Further phosphorylation by Eg2/aurora A kinase may facilitate centrosome attachment and regulation of microtubule length by maskin. Downstream from synthesis of Mos and activation of MAP kinases, phosphorylation of elF4E by kinases facilitates binding to the methylated cap mRNA at the 5'UTR and interaction with ePABP in circularization. Phosphorylation of CPEB by Eg2/aurora A kinase may induce conformational changes that promote tight interaction between CPEB, CPSF, and symplekin to position the PAP/Gld2 poly(A) polymerase at the 3'UTR to induce polyadenylation. In turn, this provides sites for attachment of embryonic PABP (ePAB) for ring formation and association of the ePAB with the elF4G adapter protein of the el4F initiation complex. For further explanation and references, see text

is feasible that overexpression of genes due to insufficient deadenylation in not fully developmentally competent oocytes such as derived from a suboptimal follicular environment might contribute to reduced quality.

Microinjection of PARN antibodies into *Xenopus* oocytes resulted in untimely overexpression of housekeeping genes[175]. Overexpression of PABP also prevented translational silencing[177] (Figure 4.1), suggesting that the relative abundance of PARN, PAP/Gld2, and PABP affects temporal control of expression at oogenesis. Alizadeh et al. showed, by subtractive cDNA analysis of oocytes and one-cell embryos, that H1oo, c-mos, tPA (tissue type plasminogen activator gene), and Gdf-9 transcripts underwent rapid degradation after fertilization of mouse oocytes[178]. This appeared associated with the presence of CPEs near a poly(A) signal in the 3'UTR of all of these mRNA species, suggesting that polyadenylation, translation, and subsequent degradation of these stage-specifically expressed genes may have occurred.

Cell cycle control and translation of genes for maturation

Before discussing cytoplasmic polyadenylation it is necessary to understand the salient features of cell cycle regulation in mammalian oocytes. Resumption of maturation is species-specifically regulated. In vertebrates like *Xenopus*, the signaling by progesterone initially induces translation of the Mos protein, which then triggers increases in expression of the catalytic subunit of maturation promoting factor (MPF) and MPF activation (for review see references 146, 172, and 179). In mammals like the mouse, protein synthesis is not required for initial resumption of maturation. The G-protein coupled receptors rendering adenylate cyclase active[180–182] and the cAMP transmitted by gap junctions from the cumulus to the oocyte retain high cAMP and, accordingly, high activity of the cAMP-dependent protein kinase A (PKA) in meiotically arrested oocytes (for review

see reference 183). The latter inhibits activation of preMPF, the complex of inactive cdc2/cdk1 (cyclin dependent kinase 1) and cyclin B, that is already present in sufficient concentrations to induce resumption of maturation in meiotically competent oocytes, until inactivation of PKA has occurred (Figure 4.3). PKA mediates meiotic arrest by phosphorylation and inactivation of the cdc25 phosphatase[184–186], concomitantly with the phosphorylation and activation of the Wee1 kinase (Figure 4.3). The latter renders MPF inactive by phosphorylation of the catalytic subunit of MPF, the cdc2 kinase (also termed cyclin dependent kinase 1, cdk1) on a regulatory site in the meiotically blocked, maturation competent oocyte[187]. Resumption of maturation is mediated by activation of phosphodiesterase 3 (PDE3), causing reduction in cAMP levels[188,189] (Figure 4.3). Moreover, downstream from the LH surge, Leydig insulin-like 3 protein (INSL3) appears to activate inhibitory G proteins, thereby decreasing cAMP production and initiating resumption of meiosis[190]. Inactivation of PKA changes the balance between activity of the phosphatase Cdc25 and the kinase Wee1. Eventually, removal of inhibitory phosphorylation on residues of the cdk1 kinase will activate MPF (Figure 4.3). In species like the mouse, no new protein synthesis is required for meiotic resumption, e.g. after removal of cumulus, whereas oocytes of other species like the pig still require synthesis of Cdc25C phosphatase from stored mRNA for GVBD[176]. Accordingly, in mouse and most other oocytes the key factors in cell cycle control that mediate initial resumption of meiosis are already present in fully grown oocytes. However, progression to metaphase II and meiosis II arrest depend on synthesis of several additional key proteins in cell cycle control and maturation (Figure 4.3), and this appears to be conserved between vertebrate oocytes. For instance, new protein synthesis of the regulatory subunit of MPF, cyclin B, is required after GVBD throughout oocyte maturation. Accordingly, the relative rate of cyclin B synthesis may influence the kinetics of meiotic progression[191]

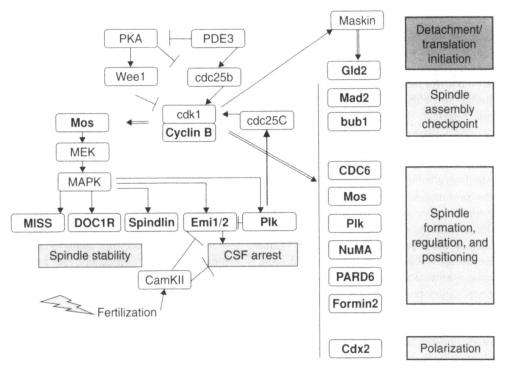

Figure 4.3 Major pathways in cell cycle control and regulation of maturation and early development by post-translational mechanisms involving newly synthesized proteins. Gene products that are synthesized at maturation are printed in bold letters; boxes indicate function of newly synthesized proteins at maturation or in the preimplantation embryo. Arrows and T lines indicate activation or inactivation, respectively, by post-translational modification; double arrows symbolize induction of synthesis as a consequence of activation of kinases, e.g. MPF (cdk1/CyclinB). For further explanation, see text

Acquisition of meiotic competence in the mouse is accompanied by characteristic changes in expression of genes engaged in regulation of maturation. Proteins like the catalytic and regulatory subunits of maturation promoting factor, CDC2/CDK1, and cyclin B, as well as their activating/inactivation phosphatase/kinase Cdc25 and Wee1, respectively, change in subcellular distribution and expression[192]. Accordingly, mouse cyclin cdcnb1 mRNA and phosphatase cdc25b mRNA are already upregulated at the primordial to primary stage of folliculogenesis, while cdc2a mRNA encoding the catalytic subunit of MPF increases at the small antral to large

antral stage. Wee1 is downregulated at the transcriptional level concomitantly, presumably in preparation for decreased activities at resumption of maturation[2]. Acquisition of meiotic competence in the mouse coincides with an increase in cdc25c transcription, probably supporting the enhanced synthesis of this protein that induces activation of preMPF at resumption of maturation in an autocatalytic loop by dephosphorylating preMPF at the regulatory site of cdk1 (Figure 4.3). Active MPF in turn is required for inducing polyadenylation of c-mos mRNA, thus initiating translation of Mos protein and the downstream activation of MAP kinases in mammalian oocytes (e.g. reference 193). Selective ablation of cyclin B expression by RNAi in GV stage mouse oocytes thus results in low MPF activity and prevents polyadenylation of c-mos mRNA.

After oocytes have undergone GVBD, formed a spindle, and aligned all chromosomes at the equator (termed chromosome congression), entry into anaphase I is initiated by activation of APC/C, the anaphase promoting complex[45]. This complex is present and induces degradation of the regulatory subunit of MPF, cyclin B, as well as the protein securin. Securin is associated with separin, a protease, up to metaphase, thus rendering it inactive. Upon release of securin, separase is free to proteolytically cleave proteins of the meiotic cohesin complex that hold sister chromatid arms attached to each other before anaphase, thus preventing chiasma resolution (for review, see references 179 and 194). Upon APC/C activation cohesins are cleaved by separase and cohesion is lost between the arms of sister chromatids, so that homologs separate. MPF is also transiently inactivated by degradation of cyclin B[45]. The sustained synthesis of cyclin B from mRNA stores and recruitment of protein from the cytoplasm restores MPF activity and is also required for sustained cytostatic arrest at metaphase II, in the presence of aligned chromosomes[195,196]. Timed translation of cyclin B has been studied extensively in oocytes, revealing regulatory regions in the 3′ untranslated part of the mRNAs that are responsible for regulation (see below). Ret finger protein-like 4 (Rfpl4) was discovered during an in silico search for germ cell specific genes. RFPL4 mRNA accumulates in all growing oocytes and rapidly disappears at early embryogenesis. Downstream from recognition and initiation of polyubiquinylation by APC/C it appears to target proteins like cyclin B for degradation at anaphase of meiotic divisions as a component of the ubiquitin–degradation pathway[197].

Another key factor that is essential for meiotic cell cycle regulation in mammalian oocytes is Mos kinase. Mos mRNA is translated at resumption of maturation. It is an essential component of cytostatic factor (CSF) (for discussion, see references 13, 198, and 199). The kinase phosphorylates MEK and MAP kinases in a phosphorylation cascade together with several other substrates, which contribute to meiotic arrest at metaphase II (Figure 4.3). Mos protein can also bind to tubulin and regulates spindle formation and positioning of the spindle for unequal division at first polar body formation[13,200]. In effect, Mos translation is required for normal cell cycle regulation and CSF arrest in oocytes, although the pivotal factor in CSF is probably the Emi2 meiotic inhibitor of APC/C (see below).

At the transition from meta- to anaphase the so-called spindle attachment checkpoint (SAC) is expressed in oocytes (see references 201–204). Initially believed to be a component of CSF, it is now clear that SAC senses attachment of spindle fibers to chromosomes and tension on centromeres by bipolar attachment of chromosomes at mitosis and meiosis I and II[202]. Several essential proteins involved in checkpoint control are synthesized from mRNA after resumption of maturation as suggested by RNAi approaches. For instance, knockdown of the checkpoint component Mad2 in oocytes[45,203,204] by injection of specific small interfering RNAs may speed up meiotic resumption and ablate checkpoint control at meiosis, showing the significance of timed synthesis for ordered chromosome segregation in oocytes and for maturation kinetics (Figure 4.3). Indeed, checkpoint control may be essential for prevention of aneuploidy when there are disturbances in spindle formation[45,203,204]. Emi1, another essential component of cell cycle control in oogenesis, is expressed throughout meiosis, albeit the protein is rather unstable (Figure 4.3). Emi1 is an inhibitor of the APC/C. Ablation by RNAi in mouse oocytes results in spontaneous activation, suggesting that it is a pivotal CSF component[205]. Possibly, Emi2 represents the major and most important component of CSF as an inhibitor of the APC at meiosis II[17]. Emi2 is more stable compared to Emi1 and was the first component identified to be a direct target of the calcium calmodulin kinase II (CamKII) (Figure 4.3). This calcium activated kinase is induced by fertilization and mediates CSF inactivation[206–208]. Emi2 is also a target of polo-like kinase 1[207] that marks it for destruction by phosphorylation. As long as Emi2 concentration is high, oocytes remain arrested at metaphase II by inhibition of APC/C. It was earlier shown that levels of polo-like kinase protein increase at GVBD (plk in Figure 4.3) and the kinase associates initially with the spindle poles, depending on phosphorylation by MAP kinases[209,210], downstream from Mos kinase. Polo-like kinase 1 (plk1) has multiple tasks. It appears involved in an autocatalytic loop between CDC25C phosphatase and M-phase promoting factor (MPF), supporting the conversion of pre-MPF to active MPF by dephosphorylation of cdk1 (Figure 4.3). Plk1 is activated before MPF in maturing porcine oocytes[211]. Destruction of Emi2 is triggered in coordination with fertilization events. Activation of CamKII leads initially to phosphorylation of Emi2 at a specific motif (Figure 4.3). This then enables Plk1 to strongly interact with Emi2, and, in turn, phosphorylate and target it for destruction[207] (as indicated in Figure 4.3). Comparable to fertilization, ablation of Emi2 by RNAi causes exit from CSF-mediated metaphase II arrest[17]. The experimental data thus suggest that key components of cell cycle regulation, including Emi2, need to be synthesized from a pre-existing message at maturation to mediate normal meiotic progression as well as arrest at meiosis II (Figure 4.3).

Mouse meiotic mutants as well as ablation of expression of genes by degradation and inactivation of translation by introduction of anti-sense RNA, double-stranded RNA, or RNAi into oocytes have revealed that several other genes involved in regulation of the cell cycle, spindle formation, and early development need to be synthesized from mRNAs during maturation (Figure 4.3). For instance, DOC1R (deleted oral cancer 1 related), initially described as a tumor proto-oncogene, has been identified as a MAP kinase substrate

that is synthesized during oocyte maturation and that, when knocked down, will result in spindle deregulation and random microtubule aster formation in mouse oocytes[212]. DOC1R protein increases during maturation whereas MISS protein (MAP kinase-interacting and spindle stabilizing protein), another MAP kinase substate, is unstable in meiosis I, and only stably associates with the meiosis II spindle[213] (Figure 4.3). PARD6A is a protein that is apparently synthesized at resumption of meiosis, concentrated on the spindle half that will attach to the cell cortex, and is essential for unequal division at meiotic anaphase in oocytes[214]. Formin 2 encodes an actin-polymerizing protein involved in spindle migration to the oolemma that needs to be synthesized at oocyte maturation[215]. Furthermore, ablation of expression of CDC6, a checkpoint component in S-phase in mitosis, showed that translation of mRNA is essential for spindle formation at meiosis I and thus constitutes another essential oocyte factor for maturation that is synthesized stage-specifically[211]. Finally, several mRNAs translated after resumption of maturation or in early embryogenesis are essential maternal components for meiosis and/or early development. For instance, it appears that NuMA (nuclear mitotic apparatus antigen) needs to be synthesized during maturation[179]. This protein is required for spindle formation and function in meiosis. In addition, it is one of the maternal products that are transiently enriched at the meiotic metaphase II spindle, subsequently transits to the female and male pronucleus after fertilization, and is required for normal development[216]. Spindlin (Spin) is another maternal effect gene expressed from maternal mRNA stores at maturation. It is associated with the spindle at metaphase II when it is phosphorylated by MAP kinase[217,218]. The message for Spin encoding the 30-kDa protein is highly expressed in mature oocytes (Figure 4.3).

Differential polyadenylation and translation occurs at two critical points: upon oocyte maturation and after fertilization. While the message is diminished in meiosis II, the protein level is high in the zygote and may play an important role in zygotic gene activation (ZGA)[219]. Depletion of oocytes of maternally expressed spindle-associated proteins like NuMA and spindlin by removal of chromosomes and the spindle before somatic cell nuclear transfer in cloning may be one etiologic factor in the failure to obtain viable embryos[179,220]. The apolar localization and recruitment of proteins by the spindle may also facilitate their targeting to specific sites in the embryo (e.g. pronuclei or mitotic spindles) such that disturbances due to oocyte freezing or suboptimal conditions at maturation might adversely affect development. Several studies support the notion that not only control of timely expression but also spatial distribution of gene products influence development (e.g. references 221 and 222). For instance, Cdx2 mRNA coding for a transcription factor is localized toward the vegetal pole in the mammalian oocyte. The message reorients after fertilization and mRNA and protein become concentrated in the late-dividing, two-cell-stage blastomere that defines the lineage to trophectoderm[223]. In conclusion, many proteins that are cell cycle dependently synthesized during maturation are pivotal in the control of cytoskeletal, chromatin, and embryonal regulation in mammalian oocytes and in polarization of the embryo (Figure 4.3).

Translation of polyadenylated mRNA

Initiation of translation is a complex multi-step process that requires a large number of protein factors and multi-protein complexes, in addition to ribosomes[165] (Figure 4.2b). Cap-dependent translational initiation in eukaryotes requires a methylated guanosine residue at the 5'untranslated region of the mRNA (m7GpppN) (Figure 4.2a and b). The 5'cap structure attracts the eukaryotic initiation factor eIF4F complex (indicated by strippled lines in Figure 4.2b) to recruit it to the mRNA. The eIF4F complex is hetero-

trimeric, consisting of a cap-binding protein, eIF4E (4E in Figure 4.2b), an RNA-dependent helicase, eIF4A (4A in Figure 4.2b), and a large protein serving as an adapter in the complex, eIF4G (hook-like structure with N- and –C-terminal domains termed 4G in Figure 4.2b)[168,221]. Concomitantly, a ternary complex with GTP and the initiator Met-tRNA forms that associates with the 40S ribosomal subunit and several initiation factors, such as eIF1, eIF1A, and eIF3 (triangle termed F2 in Figure 4.2b). The 43S preinitiation complex binds to the eIF4F complex to form the 48S preinitiation complex. After completion of initiation, the initiation complex scans the mRNA for the translation start codon AUG, and GTP hydrolysis occurs. Finally, the translational elongation by the 80S ribosome starts.

Synergistically with the cap structure circularization of the mRNA by protein–protein interactions between proteins attached to the 3' and 5' ends of the mRNAs acts as a rate-limiting step in initiation to promote the initiation process (Figure 4.2b). For this, the eIF4G adapter protein in the initiation complex associates with its N-terminal domain with the poly(A) tail of the 3'UTP of the mRNA by binding to PABP (gray boxes in Figure 4.2b). Concomitantly, eIF4G recruits eIF3 (termed F3 in Figure 4.2b) with its C-terminal domain to the 40S ribosomal complex. In combination with eIF5 it may serve as an adapter for proteins associated with the heterotrimeric eIF2 complex and the Met-t-RNA[224]. When all the factors for translational initiation have assembled they promote initiation of translation. In mouse, expression of embryonal poly(A) binding protein (ePAB), an ortholog of *Xenopus* embryonal PABP, appears to be particularly relevant. It is present during maturation and at metaphase II, as well as in the one-cell and two-cell embryo[225]. The protein becomes undetectable from the four-cell stage. The expression up to major zygotic gene activation argues for a role in translational activation of maternally derived mRNAs during mammalian oocyte and early preimplantation development[226].

According to the need for circularization, the presence of a poly(A) tail and interaction of PABP with the eIF4F complex on mRNAs decide on whether and when mRNAs can be translated. In effect, it is also the timing of polyadenylation and modifications of molecules in the protein–protein interactions that influence translation. For instance, modification of the cap structure in maturing oocytes contributes to efficient translational initiation. The cap of certain mRNAs may be modified by methylation of riboses in the trinucleotide at the 5'UTR[227]. Such ribose methylation occurs concomitantly with recruitment and translational activation of mRNAs like Mos in *Xenopus* oocytes[227]. The cap-binding factor also becomes phosphorylated at resumption of maturation, probably by the MAP kinase pathway (Figure 4.2c[228]). This enhances the affinity of the protein for the mRNA 5' cap in the initiation event[222]. The hypermethylated cap within the eIF4F complex may ensure that certain molecules become very efficiently associated with polyribosomes and translated, right after polyadenylation. When eIF4G, which mediates the binding of the 5' cap to PABP, is enzymatically cleaved, the recruitment of stage-specifically expressed mRNAs coding for c-mos, cyclin B1, and other proteins to polyribosomes is blocked[179,229].

Post-translational mechanisms in mRNA recruitment

According to their function, most cellular mRNAs encoding housekeeping proteins that are efficiently translated during oocyte growth attain the poly(A) tail already in the nucleus (about 450 residues) and, after nuclear export, can directly associate with ribosomes. Initiation of translation can proceed according to the mechanisms shown in Figures 4.1 and 4.2b. As demonstrated above, especially during gametogenesis/oogenesis, several types of mRNAs appear to become deadenylated and masked by proteins associating with the mRNA, preventing their expression. Translational repression may involve masking factors, which associate with RNA in the cytoplasm but also already in the nucleus. For instance, association of a masking protein FRGY2, a DEAD-box RNA-helicase, with mRNA species starts within the nucleus of the growing *Xenopus* oocyte[230]. The catalytic subunits of casein kinase II (CkII) and two other proteins, FRGY2a and FRGY2b, were found to be involved in the masking of mRNAs. FRGY2 is phosphorylated by CkII, which appears to be important for the masking/unmasking reaction[231]. MSY2, the mouse ortholog of *Xenopus* FRY2 and of human contrin[232], functions as a co-activator of transcription in male germ cells and plays an important role in the translational repression and storage of both paternal and maternal mRNAs in spermatocytes, spermatids, and oocytes (see reference 233). In the mouse, MSY2 is one of the most abundant proteins (2% of total protein) in fully grown oocytes. Deletion in transgenic msy2–/– mice causes infertility in both sexes, and early loss of oocytes, and defects in ovulation in females[234]. The reduction of MSY2 in GV-arrested oocytes by using Zp3-promoter-based transgenic RNAi methodology for knockdown of expression also leads to subfertility or infertility. This is consistent with the proposed function of MSY2 to stabilize mRNAs in oocytes and thereby facilitate mRNA accumulation during oocyte growth. Specificity of binding appears to be linked to transcripts derived from genes with a Y-box-containing promoter. MSY2 is inactivated by degradation at resumption of oocyte maturation, which may contribute to the recruitment of maternal mRNAs at this transition.

The recruitment of stored maternal mRNAs for polyadenylation in the cytoplasm is a complex process that mainly relies on post-translational mechanisms and sequential synthesis and activation of stimulatory kinases. The processes have been studied most extensively in *Xenopus* oocytes, but appear largely conserved. For instance, as in *Xenopus*, masking and inhibition of polyadenylation by exposure to polyadenylation inhibitor 3'-deoxyadenosine (3'-dA) up to metaphase I prevents meiosis progression in in-vitro maturing bovine oocytes, possibly by inhibiting the constant lengthening of cyclin B1 mRNA[151]. Such observations in experimental models underline the significance of timed polyadenylation and expression of meiotic genes from stored, timely recruited mRNAs. Release from repression of masked, dormant RNAs requires the CPE (also termed adenylation control element, ACE) and a hexanucleotide downstream in the 3′UTR of the mRNA or a related consensus sequence. In masked mRNA the CPE is associated with the CPEB protein that, in turn, appears bound to the Maskin protein in stored deadenylated mRNAs (Figure 4.2c). This prevents the elongation initation complex efficiently docking to the 3′UTR of the mRNA because the message is rendered with a short poly(A) tail and has no site for binding of PABP. As described above, PABP is involved in ring formation. CPSF associated with the hexamer in the 3′UTP is also prevented from tight interaction with CPEB by the presence of Maskin and therefore cannot position the PAP on the 3′UTR for polyadenylation (upper part of Figure 4.2C). The two proteins CPEB and CPSF are in contact with the protein symplekin[161]. The latter helps to attract and activate the meiotic poly(A) polymerase Gld2. Once maskin is released and CPEB phosphorylated this may induce conformational changes so that Gld2 can elongate the poly(A) tail (lower part of Figure 4.2c). Maskin also binds translation initiation factor 4E (eIF4E), an interaction that excludes eIF4G and in this way prevents formation of the eIF4F initiation complex (Figure 4.2c).

However, upon resumption of maturation and activation of MPF/cdk1, maskin is phosphorylated by MPF and this releases it from CPEB and from eIF4F[164] (detachment in Figure 4.2c). Mutation of residues for MPF phosphorylation alleviates the cdk1-induced dissociation of maskin from eIF4E and translation initiation. Downstream from cdk1 activation another kinase, Eg2/aurora A kinase, a member of the

aurora family of mitotic serine/threonine kinases, is activated during maturation, which, in turn, can phosphorylate CPEB[235]. The quantity of aurora A/Eg2 protein is already high in the GV of mouse oocytes and remains stable during maturation up to metaphase II[236]. Phosphorylation of CPEB by aurora A participates in the control of sequential protein synthesis by enhancing the affinity of binding between CPEB and CPSF, promoted by attachment to symplekin[161]. CPSF in turn may recruit/position PAP. CPEB/CPSF proteins complexed by symplekin can target poly(A) polymerase GLD2 to catalyze polyadenylation of the 3′UTR of the message[161]. The mechanisms are conserved since mouse GLD-2 (mGld2), a recently identified cytoplasmic PAP, is also expressed in the oocytes exclusively after GVBD at meiosis I and II and appears essential for the progression from metaphase I to metaphase II during oocyte maturation[237]. Upon elongation of the poly(A) tail, PABP can bind and recruit eIF4G of the eIF4E complex for ring formation and stimulation of expression. Maskin may have several functions as it can be phosphorylated by different kinases and at different sites. Before maturation, Maskin is already phosphorylated by protein kinase A. This does not influence initiation of translation but appears critical for the protein to localize on the spindle of somatic cells[161]. After resumption of maturation, phosphorylation of Maskin by E2/aurora A kinase (Figure 4.2c) may help to promote microtubule growth from asters and contribute to the determination of microtubule steady-state length[238].

Apart from these mechanisms of translational initiation involving differential phosphorylation of Maskin, the early cytoplasmic polyadenylation and translational activation of multiple maternal mRNAs can also occur in a CPE- and CPEB-independent manner. The sequential action of distinct 3′-UTR-directed translational control mechanisms and related RNA-binding proteins can possibly coordinate the complex temporal patterns and extent of protein synthesis during vertebrate meiotic cell cycle progression in such cases[155,172,239]. Generally, it appears to be the context, for instance, the number and distance between the CPEs and the hexanucleotide, the presence of RNA-binding and interacting proteins, and the activity of kinases, which controls the timing and extent of polyadenylation[155,240]. As an example, DAZL proteins like human DAZ and BOULE stimulate translation by promoting initiation. Collier et al. showed that DAZL proteins interact with PABPs and thus may contribute to the activation of specific translationally silent mRNAs during germ cell development[241]. DAZL protein is abundantly expressed in mature human oocytes and embryos, and expression in the embryo may relate to quality and developmental capacity[242].

CONCLUSIONS AND PERSPECTIVES

Currently we are at a time when qualitative analysis of gene expression in mammalian oocytes of different species is progressing towards quantitative assessments, in order to proceed from genomics and proteomics to metabolomics and systems biology. We are still far from understanding the complex regulatory processes that govern regulation of gene expression in oocyte growth and maturation, in para- and autocrine signaling cascades during folliculogenesis, and in ovulation and early development. Even less so, we do not comprehend the influences of environment, in-vitro conditions, and aging on gene expression. However, several recent studies analyzing global gene expression or expression of particular genes in unstimulated versus stimulated cycles provide evidence that the endocrine environment has a profound influence and may greatly impinge on gene expression, and oocyte quality and developmental competence (e.g. references 2, 21, 116, and 243). For instance, the expression of the transcription factor Oct-4 is increased in primordial follicles of mice primed with PMSG, and following the LH surge in preovulatory antral oocytes[116]. This suggests that Oct-4 may not only have a role in regulation of gene expression to initiate growth, but also in the selection of oocytes for ovulation in response to endocrine signaling. Expression patterns of preovulatory oocytes of the mouse were shown to differ between oocytes obtained from unstimulated cycles and stimulated cycles, and this was associated with a better developmental potential of oocytes from the stimulated compared to the unstimulated cycle[2]. Such approaches may reveal pivotal components that are needed for normal development. Currently, there is a hunt for predictive indicators of oocyte health, in particular with respect to optimize in-vitro maturation. For instance, the expression of insulin-like growth factor II (IGF-II) was not found in metaphase II in-vitro grown oocytes from preantral follicle culture compared to in-vivo controls, and this was associated with reduced developmental potential after fertilization[113]. Differential expression related to maternal age and/or depletion of the follicular reserve is also of high relevance, especially in ART, when patients of advanced age ask for help in conception. Thus, there are reports suggesting that aging may affect expression of components of the spindle assembly checkpoint[244] and chromosome cohesion[43] that may contribute to increase risks for meiotic non-disjunction (errors in chromosome segregation). Other genes that appear repressed with advanced maternal age are candidate maternal effect genes required for early embryogenesis[144]. The large increase in numbers of libraries of genes expressed at distinct stages of oogenesis, coupled with improvement in methodology for assessing gene expression in silico as well as through experimental approaches, the availability of animal models, and the improvement in culture methods, now greatly facilitates comparative/subtractive and quantitative approaches to identify key factors in regulation and test for their influence on developmental potential (e.g. reference 245). The present review just provides a glimpse at the complexity of differential expression and its temporal, stage-specific regulation in oocytes. Apart from assessing expression at the translational and protein level, it should however be kept in mind that the spatio-temporal regulation is crucial in the context of oocyte quality, the polar distribution of cellular components, and the functional integrity at the level of the cytoskeleton and the chromatin configuration. Therefore, it is essential to analyze gene expression in a global fashion as well as by functional approaches to improve IVM and oocyte quality in ART.

ACKNOWLEDGMENTS

I thank Rudolf Eichenlaub (University of Bielefeld) for critical reading of the manuscript and Helen Picton (University of Leeds) for helpful information. I apologize to all whose work could not be cited due to limited space.

REFERENCES

1. Paredes A, Garcia-Rudaz C, Kerr B et al. Loss of synaptonemal complex protein-1, a synaptonemal complex protein, contributes to the initiation of follicular assembly in the developing rat ovary. Endocrinology 2005; 146: 5267–77.

2. Pan H, O'Brien MJ, Wigglesworth K et al. Transcript profiling during mouse oocyte development and the effect of gonadotropin priming and development in vitro. Devel Biol 2005; 286: 493–506.

3. De La Fuente R, Eppig JJ. Transcriptional activity of the mouse oocyte genome: companion granulosa cells modulate transcription and chromatin remodeling. Devel Biol 2001; 229: 224–36.

4. De La Fuente R, Viveiros MM, Burns KH et al. Major chromatin remodeling in the germinal vesicle (GV) of mammalian oocytes is dispensable for global transcriptional silencing but required for centromeric heterochromatin function. Devel Biol 2004; 275: 447–58.

5. Cao Q, Richter JD. Dissolution of the maskin-eIF4E complex by cytoplasmic poly adenylation and poly (A)-binding protein controls cyclin B1

6. mRNA translation and oocyte maturation. EMBO J 2002; 21: 3852–62.

6. Wilkie GS, Dickson KS, Gray NK. Regulation of mRNA translation by 5'- and 3'-UTR-binding factors. Trends Biochem Sci 2003; 28: 182–8.

7. Amleh A, Dean J. Mouse genetics provides insight into folliculogenesis, fertilization and early embryonic development. Hum Reprod Update 2002; 8: 395–403.

8. Serafica MD, Goto T, Trounson AO. Transcripts from a human primordial follicle cDNA library. Hum Reprod 2005; 20: 2074–91.

9. Choi T, Aoki F, Mori M et al. Activation of p34cdc2 protein kinase activity in meiotic and mitotic cell cycles in mouse oocytes and embryos. Development 1991; 113: 789–95.

10. Sagata, N. What does Mos do in oocytes and somatic cells? Bioessays 1997; 19: 13–21.

11. Araki K, Naito K, Haraguchi S et al. Meiotic abnormalities of c-mos knockout mouse oocytes: activation after first meiosis or entrance into third meiotic metaphase. Biol Reprod 1996; 55: 1315–24.

12. Tunquist BJ, Maller JL. Under arrest: cytostatic factor (CSF)-mediated metaphase arrest in vertebrate eggs. Genes Dev 2003; 17: 683–710.

13. Brunet S, Maro B. Cytoskeleton and cell cycle control during meiotic maturation of the mouse oocyte: integrating time and space. Reproduction 2005; 130: 801–11.

14. Rieder CL, Schultz A, Cole R et al. Anaphase onset in vertebrate somatic cells is controlled by a checkpoint that monitors sister kinetochore attachment to the spindle. J Cell Biol 1994; 127: 1301–10.

15. Marangos P, Carroll J. Fertilization and InsP3-induced Ca2+ release stimulate a persistent increase in the rate of degradation of cyclin B1 specifically in mature mouse oocytes. Devel Biol 2004; 272: 26–38.

16. Tung JJ, Hansen DV, Ban KH et al. A role for the anaphase-promoting complex inhibitor Emi2/XErp1, a homolog of early mitotic inhibitor 1, in cytostatic factor arrest of *Xenopus* eggs. Proc Natl Acad Sci USA 2005; 102: 4318–23.

17. Shoji S, Yoshida N, Amanai M et al. Mammalian Emi2 mediates cytostatic arrest and transduces the signal for meiotic exit via Cdc20. EMBO J 2006; 25: 834–45.

18. Morgan HD, Santos F, Green K et al. Epigenetic reprogramming in mammals. Hum Mol Genet 2005; 14(Spec No 1): R47–58.

19. Xu Y, Zhang JJ, Grifo JA et al. DNA methylation patterns in human tripronucleate zygotes. Mol Hum Reprod 2005; 11: 167–71.

20. Lucifero D, Mann MR, Bartolomei MS et al. Gene-specific timing and epigenetic memory in oocyte imprinting. Hum Mol Genet 2004; 13: 839–49.

21. Borghol N, Lornage J, Blachere T et al. Epigenetic status of the H19 locus in human oocytes following in vitro maturation. Genomics 2006; 87: 417–26.

22. Davidson EH. Gene Activity in Early Development. Academic Press, New York, 1986.

23. Gosden RG. Oogenesis as a foundation for embryogenesis. Mol Cell Endocrinol 2002; 186: 149–53.

24. Zheng P, Patel B, McMenamin M et al. Effects of follicle size and oocyte maturation conditions on maternal messenger RNA regulation and gene expression in rhesus monkey oocytes and embryos. Biol Reprod 2005; 72: 890–7.

25. Watanabe Y. Sister chromatid cohesion along arms and at centromeres. Trends Genet 2005; 21: 405–12.

26. Eichenlaub-Ritter U. Mouse genetic models for aneuploidy induction in germ cells. Cytogenet Genome Res 2005; 111: 392–400.

27. Revenkova E, Jessberger R. Keeping sister chromatids together: cohesins in meiosis. Reproduction 2005; 130: 783–90.

28. Yuan L, Liu JG, Hoja MR et al. Female germ cell aneuploidy and embryo death in mice lacking the meiosis-specific protein SCP3. Science 2002; 296: 1115–18.

29. Bannister LA, Reinholdt LG, Munroe RJ et al. Positional cloning and characterization of mouse mei8, a disrupted allele of the meiotic cohesin, Rec8. Genesis 2004; 40: 184–94.

30. Revenkova E, Eijpe M, Heyting C et al. Cohesin SMC1 beta is required for meiotic chromosome dynamics, sister chromatid cohesion and DNA recombination. Nat Cell Biol 2004; 6: 555–62.

31. Xu Y, Ashley T, Brainerd EE et al. Targeted disruption of ATM leads to growth retardation, chromosomal fragmentation during meiosis, immune defects, and thymic lymphoma. Genes Dev 1996; 10: 2411–22.

32. Pittman DL, Cobb J, Schimenti KJ et al. Meiotic prophase arrest with failure of chromosome synapsis in mice deficient for Dmc1, a germline-specific RecA homolog. Mol Cell 1998; 1: 697–705.

33. de Vries SS, Baart EB, Dekker M et al. Mouse MutS-like protein Msh5 is required for proper chromosome synapsis in male and female meiosis. Genes Dev 1999; 13: 523–31.

34. Woods LM, Hodges CA, Baart E et al. Chromosomal influence on meiotic spindle assembly: abnormal meiosis I in female Mlh1 mutant mice. J Cell Biol 1999; 145: 1395–406.

35. Kneitz B, Cohen PE, Avdievich E et al. MutS homolog 4 localization to meiotic chromosomes is required for chromosome pairing during meiosis in male and female mice. Genes Dev 2000; 14: 1085–97.

36. Baudat F, Manova K, Yuen JP et al. Chromosome synapsis defects and sexually dimorphic meiotic progression in mice lacking spo11. Mol Cell 2000; 6: 989–98.

37. Kolas NK, Svetlanov A, Lenzi ML et al. Localization of MMR proteins on meiotic chromosomes in mice indicates distinct functions during prophase I. J Cell Biol 2005; 171: 447–58.

38. Bhalla N, Dernburg AF. A conserved checkpoint monitors meiotic chromosome synapsis in Caenorhabditis elegans. Science 2005; 310: 1683–6.

39. Guillon H, Baudat F, Grey C et al. Crossover and noncrossover pathways in mouse meiosis. Mol Cell 2005; 20: 563–73.

40. Hunt PA, Hassold TJ. Sex matters in meiosis. Science 2002; 296: 2181–3.

41. Tay J, Richter JD. Germ cell differentiation and synaptonemal complex formation are disrupted

in CPEB knockout mice. Devel Cell 2001; 1: 201–13.

42. Tay J, Hodgman R, Sarkissian M et al. Regulated CPEB phosphorylation during meiotic progression suggests a mechanism for temporal control of maternal mRNA translation. Genes Dev 2003; 17: 1457–62.

43. Hodges CA, Revenkova E, Jessberger R et al. SMC1beta-deficient female mice provide evidence that cohesins are a missing link in age-related nondisjunction. Nat Genet 2005; 37: 1351–5.

44. Watanabe Y. Sister chromatid cohesion along arms and at centromeres. Trends Genet 2005; 21: 405–12.

45. Herbert M, Levasseur M, Homer H et al. Homologue disjunction in mouse oocytes requires proteolysis of securin and cyclin B1. Nat Cell Biol 2003; 5: 1023–5.

46. Tateno H, Akutsu H, Kamiguchi Y et al. Inability of mature oocytes to create functional haploid genomes from somatic cell nuclei. Fertil Steril 2003; 79: 216–18.

47. Heindryckx B, Lierman S, Van der Elst J et al. Chromosome number and development of artificial mouse oocytes and zygotes. Hum Reprod 2004; 19: 1189–94.

48. Galat V, Ozen S, Rechitsky S et al. Cytogenetic analysis of human somatic cell haploidization. Reprod Biomed Online 2005; 10: 199–204.

49. Chen SU, Chang CY, Lu CC et al. Microtubular spindle dynamics and chromosome complements from somatic cell nuclei haploidization in mature mouse oocytes and developmental potential of the derived embryos. Hum Reprod 2004; 19: 1181–8.

50. Hubner K, Fuhrmann G, Christenson LK et al. Derivation of oocytes from mouse embryonic stem cells. Science 2003; 300: 1251–6.

51. Fortune JE, Cushman RA, Wahl CM et al. The primordial to primary follicle transition. Mol Cell Endocrinol 2000; 163: 53–60.

52. Skinner MK. Regulation of primordial follicle assembly and development. Hum Reprod Update 2005; 11: 461–71.

53. Peters H. The development of the mouse ovary from birth to maturity. Acta Endocrinol (Copenh) 1969; 62: 98–116.

54. Juneja SC, Barr KJ, Enders GC et al. Defects in the germ line and gonads of mice lacking connexin43. Biol Reprod 1999; 60: 1263–70.

55. Kezele PR, Ague JM, Nilsson E et al. Alterations in the ovarian transcriptome during primordial follicle assembly and development. Biol Reprod 2005; 72: 241–55.

56. Carabatsos MJ, Elvin J, Matzuk MM et al. Characterization of oocyte and follicle development in growth differentiation factor-9-deficient mice. Devel Biol 1998; 204: 373–84.

57. Gittens JE, Kidder GM. Differential contributions of connexin37 and connexin43 to oogenesis revealed in chimeric reaggregated mouse ovaries. J Cell Sci 2005; 118(Pt 21): 5071–8.

58. Uda M, Ottolenghi C, Crisponi L et al. Foxl2 disruption causes mouse ovarian failure by pervasive blockage of follicle development. Hum Mol Genet 2004; 13: 1171–81.

59. Schmidt D, Ovitt CE, Anlag K et al. The murine winged-helix transcription factor Foxl2 is required for granulosa cell differentiation and ovary maintenance. Development 2004; 131: 933–42.

60. Kol S, Adashi EY. Intraovarian factors regulating ovarian function. Curr Opin Obstet Gynecol 1995; 7: 209–13.

61. Kumar TR, Wang Y, Lu N et al. Follicle stimulating hormone is required for ovarian follicle maturation but not male fertility. Nat Genet 1997; 15: 201–4.

62. Soyal SM, Amleh A, Dean J. FIGalpha, a germ cell-specific transcription factor required for ovarian follicle formation. Development 2000; 127: 4645–54.

63. Bayne RA, Martins da Silva SJ, Anderson RA. Increased expression of the FIGLA transcription factor is associated with primordial follicle formation in the human fetal ovary. Mol Hum Reprod 2004; 10: 373–81.

64. Spears N, Molinek MD, Robinson LL et al. The role of neurotrophin receptors in female germ-

cell survival in mouse and human. Development 2003; 130: 5481–91.

65. Paredes A, Romero C, Dissen GA et al. TrkB receptors are required for follicular growth and oocyte survival in the mammalian ovary. Devel Biol 2004; 267: 430–49.

66. Durlinger AL, Gruijters MJ, Kramer P et al. Anti-Mullerian hormone inhibits initiation of primordial follicle growth in the mouse ovary. Endocrinology 2002; 143: 1076–84.

67. Salmon NA, Handyside AH, Joyce IM. Expression of Sox8, Sf1, Gata4, Wt1, Dax1, and Fog2 in the mouse ovarian follicle: implications for the regulation of Amh expression. Mol Reprod Dev 2005; 70: 271–7.

68. Schmidt KL, Kryger-Baggesen N, Byskov AG et al. Anti-Mullerian hormone initiates growth of human primordial follicles in vitro. Mol Cell Endocrinol 2005; 234: 87–93.

69. Visser JA, Themmen AP. Anti-Mullerian hormone and folliculogenesis. Mol Cell Endocrinol 2005; 234: 81–6.

70. Ficicioglu C, Kutlu T, Baglam E et al. Early follicular antimullerian hormone as an indicator of ovarian reserve. Fertil Steril 2006; 85: 592–6.

71. Gandolfi TA, Gandolfi F. The maternal legacy to the embryo: cytoplasmic components and their effects on early development. Theriogenology 2001; 55: 1255–76.

72. Sirard MA. Resumption of meiosis: mechanism involved in meiotic progression and its relation with developmental competence. Theriogenology 2001; 55: 1241–54.

73. Gougeon A. Regulation of ovarian follicular development in primates: facts and hypotheses. Endocr Rev 1996; 17: 121–55.

74. Gougeon A. Ovarian follicular growth in humans: ovarian ageing and population of growing follicles. Maturitas 1998; 30: 137–42.

75. Schultz RM, LaMarca MJ, Wassarman PM. Absolute rates of protein synthesis during meiotic maturation of mammalian oocytes in vitro. Proc Natl Acad Sci USA 1978; 75: 4160–4.

76. Wassarman PM, Kinloch RA. Gene expression during oogenesis in mice. Mutat Res 1992; 296: 3–15.

77. Tian Q, Kopf GS, Brown RS et al. Function of basonuclin in increasing transcription of the ribosomal RNA genes during mouse oogenesis. Development 2001; 128: 407–16.

78. Kaplan G, Abreu SL, Bachvarova R. rRNA accumulation and protein synthetic patterns in growing mouse oocytes. J Exp Zool 1982; 220: 361–70.

79. Roest HP, Baarends WM, de Wit J et al. The ubiquitin-conjugating DNA repair enzyme HR6A is a maternal factor essential for early embryonic development in mice. Mol Cell Biol 2004; 24: 5485–95.

80. Sorensen RA, Wassarman PM. Relationship between growth and meiotic maturation of the mouse oocyte. Devel Biol 1976; 50: 531–6.

81. Wickramasinghe D, Ebert KM, Albertini DF. Meiotic competence acquisition is associated with the appearance of M-phase characteristics in growing mouse oocytes. Devel Biol 1991; 143: 162–72.

82. Eppig JJ, Schroeder AC. Capacity of mouse oocytes from preantral follicles to undergo embryogenesis and development to live young after growth, maturation, and fertilization in vitro. Biol Reprod 1989; 41: 268–76.

83. Bouniol-Baly C, Hamraoui L, Guibert J et al. Differential transcriptional activity associated with chromatin configuration in fully grown mouse germinal vesicle oocytes. Biol Reprod 1999; 60: 580–7.

84. Zuccotti M, Boiani M, Garagna S et al. Analysis of aneuploidy rate in antral and ovulated mouse oocytes during female aging. Mol Reprod Dev 1998; 50: 305–12.

85. Bjerregaard B, Maddox-Hyttel P. Regulation of ribosomal RNA gene expression in porcine oocytes. Anim Reprod Sci 2004; 82–83: 605–16.

86. Rajkovic A, Matzuk MM. Functional analysis of oocyte-expressed genes using transgenic models. Mol Cell Endocrinol 2002; 187: 5–9.

87. Neilson L, Andalibi A, Kang D et al. Molecular phenotype of the human oocyte by PCR-SAGE. Genomics 2000; 63: 13–24.

88. Robert C, Barnes FL, Hue I et al. Subtractive hybridization used to identify mRNA associ-

ated with the maturation of bovine oocytes. Mol Reprod Dev 2000; 57: 167–75.

89. Tanaka M, Hennebold JD, Miyakoshi K et al. The generation and characterization of an ovary-selective cDNA library. Mol Cell Endocrinol 2003; 202: 67–9.

90. Rajkovic A, Yan MSC, Klysik M et al. Discovery of germ cell-specific transcripts by expressed sequence tag database analysis. Fertil Steril 2001; 76: 550–4.

91. Stanton JL, Bascand M, Fisher L et al. Gene expression profiling of human GV oocytes: an analysis of a profile obtained by Serial Analysis of Gene Expression (SAGE). J Reprod Immunol 2002; 53: 193–201.

92. Goto T, Jones GM, Lolatgis N et al. Identification and characterisation of known and novel transcripts expressed during the final stages of human oocyte maturation. Mol Reprod Dev 2002; 62: 13–28.

93. Vallee M, Gravel C, Palin MF et al. Identification of novel and known oocyte-specific genes using complementary DNA subtraction and microarray analysis in three different species. Biol Reprod 2005; 73: 63–71.

94. Arraztoa JA, Zhou J, Marcu D et al. Identification of genes expressed in primate primordial oocytes. Hum Reprod 2005; 20: 476–83.

95. Pennetier S, Uzbekova S, Guyader-Joly C et al. Genes preferentially expressed in bovine oocytes revealed by subtractive and suppressive hybridization. Biol Reprod 2005; 73: 713–20.

96. Bermudez MG, Wells D, Malter H et al. Expression profiles of individual human oocytes using microarray technology. Reprod Biomed Online 2004; 8: 325–37.

97. Herrera L, Ottolenghi C, Garcia-Ortiz JE et al. Mouse ovary developmental RNA and protein markers from gene expression profiling. Devel Biol 2005; 279: 271–90.

98. Doneda L, Klinger FG, Larizza L et al. KL/KIT co-expression in mouse fetal oocytes. Int J Devel Biol 2002; 46: 1015–21.

99. Thomas FH, Ethier JF, Shimasaki S et al. Follicle-stimulating hormone regulates oocyte growth by modulation of expression of oocyte and granulosa cell factors. Endocrinology 2005; 146: 941–9.

100. Nilsson EE, Kezele P, Skinner MK. Leukemia inhibitory factor (LIF) promotes the primordial to primary follicle transition in rat ovaries. Mol Cell Endocrinol 2002; 188: 65–73.

101. Nilsson E, Parrott JA, Skinner MK. Basic fibroblast growth factor induces primordial follicle development and initiates folliculogenesis. Mol Cell Endocrinol 2001; 175: 123–30.

102. Kezele P, Nilsson EE, Skinner MK. Keratinocyte growth factor acts as a mesenchymal factor that promotes ovarian primordial to primary follicle transition. Biol Reprod 2005; 73: 967–73.

103. Moore GP, Lintern-Moore S. Transcription of the mouse oocyte genome. Biol Reprod 1978; 18: 865–70.

104. Eppig JJ, Wigglesworth K, Pendola FL. The mammalian oocyte orchestrates the rate of ovarian follicular development. Proc Natl Acad Sci USA 2002; 99: 2890–4.

105. Matzuk MM, Burns KH, Viveiros MM et al. Intercellular communication in the mammalian ovary: oocytes carry the conversation. Science 2002; 296: 2178–80.

106. Eppig JJ, Pendola FL, Wigglesworth K et al. Mouse oocytes regulate metabolic cooperativity between granulosa cells and oocytes: amino acid transport. Biol Reprod 2005; 73: 351–7.

107. Pangas SA, Matzuk MM. The art and artifact of GDF9 activity: cumulus expansion and the cumulus expansion-enabling factor. Biol Reprod 2005; 73: 582–5.

108. Juengel JL, McNatty KP. The role of proteins of the transforming growth factor-beta superfamily in the intraovarian regulation of follicular development. Hum Reprod Update 2005; 11: 143–60.

109. Hussein TS, Froiland DA, Amato F et al. Oocytes prevent cumulus cell apoptosis by maintaining a morphogenic paracrine gradient of bone morphogenetic proteins. J Cell Sci 2005; 118(Pt 22): 5257–68.

110. Dong J, Albertini DF, Nishimori K et al. Growth differentiation factor–9 is required during early ovarian folliculogenesis. Nature 1996; 383: 531–5.

111. Moore RK, Shimasaki S. Molecular biology and physiological role of the oocyte factor, BMP-15. Mol Cell Endocrinol 2005; 234: 67–73.

112. Simon AM, Goodenough DA, Li E et al. Female infertility in mice lacking connexin 37. Nature 1997; 385: 525–9.

113. Yan W, Ma L, Stein P et al. Mice deficient in oocyte-specific oligoadenylate synthetase-like protein OAS1D display reduced fertility. Mol Cell Biol 2005; 25: 4615–24.

114. Rajkovic A, Pangas SA, Ballow D et al. NOBOX deficiency disrupts early folliculogenesis and oocyte-specific gene expression. Science 2004; 305: 1157–9.

115. Becker M, Becker A, Miyara F et al. Differential in vivo binding dynamics of somatic and oocyte-specific linker histones in oocytes and during ES cell nuclear transfer. Mol Biol Cell 2005; 16: 3887–95.

116. Monti M, Garagna S, Redi C et al. Gonadotropins affect Oct–4 gene expression during mouse oocyte growth. Mol Reprod Dev 2006; 73: 685–91.

117. Dade S, Callebaut I, Paillisson A et al. *In silico* identification and structural features of six new genes similar to MATER specifically expressed in the oocyte. Biochem Biophys Res Commun 2004; 324: 547–53.

118. Song JL, Wessel GM. How to make an egg: transcriptional regulation in oocytes. Differentiation 2005; 73: 1–17.

119. Cohen MM Jr. The hedgehog signaling network. Am J Med Genet 2003; 123: 5–28.

120. Villaescusa JC, Allard P, Carminati E et al. Clast4, the murine homologue of human eIF4E-Transporter, is highly expressed in developing oocytes and post-translationally modified at meiotic maturation. Gene 2006; 367: 101–9.

121. Kaygun H, Marzluff WF. Translation termination is involved in histone mRNA degradation when DNA replication is inhibited. Mol Cell Biol 2005; 25: 6879–88.

122. Allard P, Yang Q, Marzluff WF et al. The stem-loop binding protein regulates translation of histone mRNA during mammalian oogenesis. Devel Biol 2005; 286: 195–206.

123. Cheung P, Lau P. Epigenetic regulation by histone methylation and histone variants. Mol Endocrinol 2005; 19: 563–73.

124. Vignon X, Zhou Q, Renard JP. Chromatin as a regulative architecture of the early developmental functions of mammalian embryos after fertilization or nuclear transfer. Cloning Stem Cells 2002; 4: 363–77.

125. Marshall TW, Link KA, Petre-Draviam CE et al. Differential requirement of SWI/SNF for androgen receptor activity. J Biol Chem 2003; 278: 30605–13.

126. Kono T. Influence of epigenetic changes during oocyte growth on nuclear reprogramming after nuclear transfer. Reprod Fertil Dev 1998; 10: 593–8.

127. Obata Y, Kaneko-Ishino T, Koide T et al. Disruption of primary imprinting during oocyte growth leads to the modified expression of imprinted genes during embryogenesis. Development 1998; 125: 1553–60.

128. Gioia L, Barboni B, Turriani M et al. The capability of reprogramming the male chromatin after fertilization is dependent on the quality of oocyte maturation. Reproduction 2005; 130: 29–39.

129. Fedoriw AM, Stein P, Svoboda P et al. Transgenic RNAi reveals essential function for CTCF in H19 gene imprinting. Science 2004; 303: 238–40.

130. Okano M, Bell DW, Haber DA et al. DNA methyltransferases Dnmt3a and Dnmt3b are essential for de novo methylation and mammalian development. Cell 1999; 99: 247–57.

131. Kim DH, Ko DS, Lee HC et al. Comparison of maturation, fertilization, development, and gene expression of mouse oocytes grown *in vitro* and *in vivo*. J Assist Reprod Genet 2004; 21: 233–40.

132. Hu Y, Betzendahl I, Cortvrindt R et al. Effects of low O_2 and ageing on spindles and chromosomes in mouse oocytes from pre-antral follicle culture. Hum Reprod 2001; 16: 737–48.

133. Paillisson A, Dade S, Callebaut I et al. Identification, characterization and metagenome analysis of oocyte-specific genes organized in clusters in the mouse genome. BMC Genomics 2005; 6: 76.

134. Tung JJ, Jackson PK. Emi1 class of proteins regulates entry into meiosis and the meiosis I to mei-

osis II transition in *Xenopus* oocytes. Cell Cycle 2005; 4: 478–82.

135. Parfenov V, Potchukalina G, Dudina L et al. Human antral follicles: oocyte nucleus and the karyosphere formation (electron microscopic and autoradiographic data). Gamete Res 1989; 22: 219–31.

136. Zuccotti M, Garagna S, Merico V et al. Chromatin organisation and nuclear architecture in growing mouse oocytes. Mol Cell Endocrinol 2005; 234: 11–17.

137. Kageyama S, Liu H, Nagata M et al. Stage specific expression of histone deacetylase 4 (HDAC4) during oogenesis and early preimplantation development in mice. J Reprod Dev 2006; 52: 99–106.

138. Borsuk E, Milik E. Fully grown mouse oocyte contains transcription inhibiting activity which acts through histone deacetylation. Mol Reprod Dev 2005; 71: 509–15.

139. Burns KH, Viveiros MM, Ren Y et al. Roles of NPM2 in chromatin and nucleolar organization in oocytes and embryos. Science 2003; 300: 633–6.

140. Tamada H, Van Thuan N, Reed P et al. Chromatin decondensation and nuclear reprogramming by nucleoplasmin. Mol Cell Biol 2006; 26: 1259–71.

141. Wu X, Viveiros MM, Eppig JJ et al. Zygote arrest 1 (Zar1) is a novel maternal-effect gene critical for the oocyte-to-embryo transition. Nat Genet 2003; 33: 1871–91.

142. Tong ZB, Gold L, Pfeifer KE et al. Mater, a maternal effect gene required for early embryonic development in mice. Nat Genet 2000; 26: 267–8.

143. Tong ZB, Gold L, De Pol A et al. Developmental expression and subcellular localization of mouse MATER, an oocyte-specific protein essential for early development. Endocrinology 2004; 145: 1427–34.

144. Hamatani T, Falco G, Carter MG et al. Age-associated alteration of gene expression patterns in mouse oocytes. Hum Mol Genet 2004; 13: 2263–78.

145. Hinkins M, Huntriss J, Miller D et al. Expression of Polycomb-group genes in human ovarian fol-

licles, oocytes and preimplantation embryos. Reproduction 2005; 130: 883–8.

146. Richter JD. Cytoplasmic polyadenylation in development and beyond. Microbiol Mol Biol Rev 1999; 63: 446–56.

147. Liang L, Soyal SM, Amleh A, Dean J. FIGalpha, a germ cell-specific transcription factor involved in the coordinate expression of the zona pellucida genes. Development 2000; 124: 4939–47.

148. Picton H, Briggs D, Gosden R. The molecular basis of oocyte growth and development. Mol Cell Endocrinol 1998; 145: 27–37.

149. Roller RJ, Kinloch RA, Hiraoka BY et al. Gene expression during mammalian oogenesis and early embryogenesis: quantification of three messenger RNAs abundant in fully grown mouse oocytes. Development 1989; 106: 251–61.

150. Bachvarova RF. A maternal tail of poly (A): the long and the short of it. Cell 1992; 69: 895–7.

151. Tay J, Hodgman R, Richter JD. The control of cyclin B1 mRNA translation during mouse oocyte maturation. Devel Biol 2000; 221: 1–9.

152. Fuchimoto D, Mizukoshi A, Schultz RM et al. Posttranscriptional regulation of cyclin A1 and cyclin A2 during mouse oocyte meiotic maturation and preimplantation development. Biol Reprod 2001; 65: 986–93.

153. Traverso JM, Donnay I, Lequarre AS. Effects of polyadenylation inhibition on meiosis progression in relation to the polyadenylation status of cyclins A2 and B1 during in vitro maturation of bovine oocytes. Mol Reprod Dev 2005; 71: 107–14.

154. Mendez R, Hake LE, Andresson T et al. Phosphorylation of CPE binding factor by Eg2 regulates translation of c-mos mRNA. Nature 2000; 404: 302–7.

155. Dai Y, Newman B, Moor R. Translational regulation of MOS messenger RNA in pig oocytes. Biol Reprod 2005; 73: 997–1003.

156. Dai Y, Lee C, Hutchings A et al. Selective requirement for Cdc25C protein synthesis during meiotic progression in porcine oocytes. Biol Reprod 2000; 62: 519–32.

157. El Mouatassim S, Guerin P, Menezo Y. Expression of genes encoding antioxidant

enzymes in human and mouse oocytes during the final stages of maturation. Mol Hum Reprod 1999; 5: 720–5.

158. Stebbins-Boaz B, Hake LE, Richter JD. CPEB controls the cytoplasmic polyadenylation of cyclin, Cdk2 and c-mos mRNAs and is necessary for oocyte maturation in *Xenopus*. EMBO J 1996; 15: 2582–92.

159. Hodgman R, Tay J, Mendez R et al. CPEB phosphorylation and cytoplasmic polyadenylation are catalyzed by the kinase IAK1/Eg2 in maturing mouse oocytes. Development 2001; 128: 2815–22.

160. Dickson KS, Bilger A, Ballantyne S et al. The cleavage and polyadenylation specificity factor in *Xenopus laevis* oocytes is a cytoplasmic factor involved in regulated polyadenylation. Mol Cell Biol 1999; 19: 5707–17.

161. Barnard DC, Ryan K, Manley JL et al. Symplekin and xGLD-2 are required for CPEB-mediated cytoplasmic polyadenylation. Cell 2004; 119: 641–51.

162. Rouhana L, Wang L, Buter N et al. Vertebrate GLD2 poly(A) polymerases in the germline and the brain. RNA 2005; 11: 1117–30.

163. Stebbins-Boaz B, Cao Q, de Moor CH et al. Maskin is a CPEB-associated factor that transiently interacts with eIF–4E. Mol Cell 1999; 4: 1017–27.

164. Barnard DC, Cao Q, Richter JD. Differential phosphorylation controls Maskin association with eukaryotic translation initiation factor 4E and localization on the mitotic apparatus. Mol Cell Biol 2005; 25: 7605–15.

165. Gray NK; Wickens M. Control of translation initiation in animals. Annu Rev Cell Dev Biol 1998; 14: 399–458.

166. Mendez R, Richter JD. Translational control by CPEB: a means to the end. Nat Rev Mol Cell Biol 2001; 2: 521–9.

167. Richter JD, Sonenberg N. Regulation of cap-dependent translation by eIF4E inhibitory proteins. Nature 2005; 433: 477–80.

168. de Moor CH, Meijer H, Lissenden S. Mechanisms of translational control by the 3′ UTR in development and differentiation. Semin Cell Dev Biol 2005; 16: 49–58.

169. Graindorge A, Thuret R, Pollet N et al. Identification of post-transcriptionally regulated *Xenopus tropicalis* maternal mRNAs by microarray. Nucleic Acids Res 2006; 34: 986–95.

170. Wassarman PM, Liu C, Litscher ES. Constructing the mammalian zona pellucida: some new pieces of an old puzzle. J Cell Sci 1996; 109(Pt 8): 2001–4.

171. Audic Y, Omilli F, Osborne HB. Postfertilization deadenylation of mRNAs in *Xenopus laevis* embryos is sufficient to cause their degradation at the blastula stage. Mol Cell Biol 1997; 17: 209–18.

172. Charlesworth A, Cox LL, MacNicol AM. Cytoplasmic polyadenylation element (CPE)- and CPE-binding protein (CPEB)-independent mechanisms regulate early class maternal mRNA translational activation in *Xenopus* oocytes. J Biol Chem 2004; 279: 17650–9.

173. Huarte J, Stutz A, O'Connell ML et al. Transient translational silencing by reversible mRNA deadenylation. Cell 1992; 69: 1021–30.

174. Paynton BV. RNA-binding proteins in mouse oocytes and embryos: expression of genes encoding Ybox, DEAD box RNA helicase, and polyA binding proteins. Devel Genet 1998; 23: 285–98.

175. Korner CG, Wormington M, Muckenthaler M et al. The deadenylating nuclease (DAN) is involved in poly(A) tail removal during the meiotic maturation of *Xenopus* oocytes. EMBO J 1998; 17: 5427–37.

176. Brevini-Gandolfi TA, Favetta LA, Mauri L et al. Changes in poly(A) tail length of maternal transcripts during *in vitro* maturation of bovine oocytes and their relation with developmental competence. Mol Reprod Dev 1999; 52: 427–33.

177. Wormington M, Searfoss AM, Hurney CA. Overexpression of poly(A) binding protein prevents maturation-specific deadenylation and translational inactivation in *Xenopus* oocytes. EMBO J 1996; 15: 900–9.

178. Alizadeh Z, Kageyama S, Aoki F. Degradation of maternal mRNA in mouse embryos: selective degradation of specific mRNAs after fertilization. Mol Reprod Dev 2005; 72: 281–290.

179. Eichenlaub-Ritter U, Peschke M. Expression in in-vivo and in-vitro growing and maturing

oocytes: focus on regulation of expression at the translational level. Hum Reprod Update 2002; 8: 21–41.

180. Mehlmann LM. Oocyte-specific expression of Gpr3 is required for the maintenance of meiotic arrest in mouse oocytes. Devel Biol 2005; 288: 397–404.

181. Freudzon L, Norris RP, Hand AR et al. Regulation of meiotic prophase arrest in mouse oocytes by GPR3, a constitutive activator of the Gs G protein. J Cell Biol 2005; 171: 255–65.

182. Hinckley M, Vaccari S, Horner K et al. The G-protein-coupled receptors GPR3 and GPR12 are involved in cAMP signaling and maintenance of meiotic arrest in rodent oocytes. Devel Biol 2005; 287: 249–61.

183. Dekel N. Cellular, biochemical and molecular mechanisms regulating oocyte maturation. Mol Cell Endocrinol 2005; 234: 19–25.

184. Lincoln AJ, Wickramasinghe D, Stein P et al. Cdc25b phosphatase is required for resumption of meiosis during oocyte maturation. Nat Genet 2002; 30: 446–9.

185. Duckworth BC, Weaver JS, Ruderman JV. G2 arrest in *Xenopus* oocytes depends on phosphorylation of cdc25 by protein kinase A. Proc Natl Acad Sci USA 2002; 99: 16794–9.

186. Perdiguero E, Nebreda AR. Regulation of Cdc25C activity during the meiotic G2/M transition. Cell Cycle 2004; 3: 733–7.

187. Han SJ, Conti M. New pathways from PKA to the Cdc2/cyclin B complex in oocytes: Wee1B as a potential PKA substrate. Cell Cycle 2006; 5: 227–31.

188. Masciarelli S, Horner K, Liu C et al. Cyclic nucleotide phosphodiesterase 3A-deficient mice as a model of female infertility. J Clin Invest 2004; 114: 196–205.

189. Richard FJ, Tsafriri A, Conti M. Role of phosphodiesterase type 3A in rat oocyte maturation. Biol Reprod 2001; 65: 1444–51.

190. Kawamura K, Kumagai J, Sudo S et al. Paracrine regulation of mammalian oocyte maturation and male germ cell survival. Proc Natl Acad Sci USA 2004; 101: 7323–8.

191. Polanski Z, Ledan E, Brunet S et al. Cyclin synthesis controls the progression of meiotic maturation in mouse oocytes. Development 1998; 125: 4989–97.

192. Mitra J, Schultz RM. Regulation of the acquisition of meiotic competence in the mouse: changes in the subcellular localization of cdc2, cyclin B1, cdc25C and wee1, and in the concentration of these proteins and their transcripts. J Cell Sci 1996; 109(Pt 9): 2407–15.

193. Lazar S, Gershon E, Dekel N. Selective degradation of cyclin B1 mRNA in rat oocytes by RNA interference (RNAi). J Mol Endocrinol 2004; 33: 73–85.

194. Revenkova E, Jessberger R. Keeping sister chromatids together: cohesins in meiosis. Reproduction 2005; 130: 783–90.

195. Kubiak JZ, Weber M, de Pennart H et al. The metaphase II arrest in mouse oocytes is controlled through microtubule-dependent destruction of cyclin B in the presence of CSF. EMBO J 1993; 12: 3773–8.

196. Heikinheimo O, Lanzendorf SE, Baka SG et al. Cell cycle genes c-mos and cyclin-B1 are expressed in a specific pattern in human oocytes and preimplantation embryos. Hum Reprod 1995; 10: 699–707.

197. Suzumori N, Burns KH, Yan W et al. RFPL4 interacts with oocyte proteins of the ubiquitin-proteasome degradation pathway. Proc Natl Acad Sci USA 2003; 100: 550–5.

198. Gebauer F, Richter JD. Synthesis and function of Mos: the control switch of vertebrate oocyte meiosis. Bioessays 1997; 19: 23–8.

199. Sagata N. What does Mos do in oocytes and somatic cells? Bioessays 1997; 19: 13–21.

200. Araki K, Naito K, Haraguchi S et al. Meiotic abnormalities of c-mos knockout mouse oocytes: activation after first meiosis or entrance into third meiotic metaphase. Biol Reprod 1996; 55: 1315–24.

201. Irniger S. Preventing fatal destruction: inhibitors of the anaphase-promoting complex in meiosis. Cell Cycle 2006; 5: 405–15.

202. Pinsky BA, Biggins S. The spindle checkpoint: tension versus attachment. Trends Cell Biol 2005; 15: 486–93.

203. Homer HA, McDougall A, Levasseur M et al. Mad2 is required for inhibiting securin and cyclin B degradation following spindle depolymerisation in meiosis I mouse oocytes. Reproduction 2005; 130: 829–43.

204. Vogt E, Betzendahl I, Eichenlaub-Ritter U. Model for aging: knockdown of Mad2 expression predisposes to non-disjunction in mammalian oocytes possessing aberrant spindles. Hum Reprod 2005, 20(Suppl 1):i70.

205. Paronetto MP, Giorda E, Carsetti R et al. Functional interaction between p90Rsk2 and Emi1 contributes to the metaphase arrest of mouse oocytes. EMBO J 2004; 23: 4649–59.

206. Winston NJ, Maro B. Calmodulin-dependent protein kinase II is activated transiently in ethanol-stimulated mouse oocytes. Devel Biol 1995; 170: 350–2.

207. Hansen DV, Tung JJ, Jackson PK. CaMKII and polo-like kinase 1 sequentially phosphorylate the cytostatic factor Emi2/XErp1 to trigger its destruction and meiotic exit. Proc Natl Acad Sci USA 2006; 103: 608–13.

208. Liu J, Maller JL. Calcium elevation at fertilization coordinates phosphorylation of XErp1/Emi2 by Plx1 and CaMK II to release metaphase arrest by cytostatic factor. Curr Biol 2005; 15: 1458–68.

209. Wianny F, Tavares A, Evans MJ et al. Mouse polo-like kinase 1 associates with the acentriolar spindle poles, meiotic chromosomes and spindle midzone during oocyte maturation. Chromosoma 1998; 107: 430–9.

210. Pahlavan G, Polanski Z, Kalab P et al. Characterization of polo-like kinase 1 during meiotic maturation of the mouse oocyte. Devel Biol 2000; 220: 392–400.

211. Anger M, Klima J, Kubelka M et al. Timing of Plk1 and MPF activation during porcine oocyte maturation. Mol Reprod Dev 2004; 69: 11–16.

212. Terret ME, Lefebvre C, Djiane A et al. DOC1R: a MAP kinase substrate that control microtubule organization of metaphase II mouse oocytes. Development 2003; 130: 5169–77.

213. Lefebvre C, Terret ME, Djiane A et al. Meiotic spindle stability depends on MAPK-interacting and spindle-stabilizing protein (MISS), a new MAPK substrate. J Cell Biol 2002; 157: 603–13.

214. Vinot S, Le T, Maro B et al. Two PAR6 proteins become asymmetrically localized during establishment of polarity in mouse oocytes. Curr Biol 2004; 14: 520–5.

215. Leader B, Lim H, Carabatsos MJ et al. Formin-2, polyploidy, hypofertility and positioning of the meiotic spindle in mouse oocytes. Nat Cell Biol 2002; 4: 921–8.

216. Hewitson L, Dominko T, Takahashi D et al. Unique checkpoints during the first cell cycle of fertilization after intracytoplasmic sperm injection in rhesus monkeys. Nat Med 1999; 5: 431–3.

217. Oh B, Hwang SY, Solter D et al. Spindlin, a major maternal transcript expressed in the mouse during the transition from oocyte to embryo. Development 1997; 124: 493–503.

218. Oh B, Hwang S, McLaughlin J et al. Timely translation during the mouse oocyte-to-embryo transition. Development 2000; 127: 3795–803.

219. Yao YQ, Xu JS, Lee WM et al. Identification of mRNAs that are up-regulated after fertilization in the murine zygote by suppression subtractive hybridization. Biochem Biophys Res Commun 2003; 304: 60–6.

220. Simerly C, Dominko T, Navara C et al. Molecular correlates of primate nuclear transfer failures. Science 2003; 300: 297.

221. Antczak M, Van Blerkom J. Temporal and spatial aspects of fragmentation in early human embryos: possible effects on developmental competence and association with the differential elimination of regulatory proteins from polarized domains. Hum Reprod 1999; 14: 429–47.

222. Edwards RG. Genetics of polarity in mammalian embryos. Reprod Biomed Online 2005; 11: 104–14.

223. Deb K, Sivaguru M, Yong HY et al. Cdx2 gene expression and trophectoderm lineage specification in mouse embryos. Science 2006; 311: 992–6.

224. Preiss T, Hentze MW. Starting the protein synthesis machine: eukaryotic translation initiation. Bioessays 2003; 25: 1201–11.

225. Wilkie GS, Gautier P, Lawson D et al. Embryonic poly(A)-binding protein stimulates translation in germ cells. Mol Cell Biol 2005; 25: 2060–71.

226. Seli E, Lalioti MD, Flaherty SM et al. An embryonic poly(A)-binding protein (ePAB) is expressed in mouse oocytes and early preimplantation embryos. Proc Natl Acad Sci USA 2005; 102: 367–72.

227. Kuge H, Brownlee GG, Gershon PD et al. Cap ribose methylation of c-mos mRNA stimulates translation and oocyte maturation in *Xenopus laevis*. Nucleic Acids Res 1998; 26: 3208–14.

228. Pyronnet S, Imataka H, Gingras AC et al. Human eukaryotic translation initiation factor 4G (eIF4G) recruits mnk1 to phosphorylate eIF4E. EMBO J 1999; 18: 270–9.

229. Keiper BD, Rhoads RE. Translational recruitment of *Xenopus* maternal mRNAs in response to poly(A) elongation requires initiation factor eIF4G–1. Devel Biol 1999; 206: 1–14.

230. Sommerville J, Ladomery M. Transcription and masking of mRNA in germ cells: involvement of Y-box proteins. Chromosoma 1996; 10: 435–43.

231. Braddock M, Muckenthaler M, White MR et al. Intron-less RNA injected into the nucleus of *Xenopus* oocytes accesses a regulated translation control pathway. Nucleic Acids Res 1994; 22: 5255–64.

232. Tekur S, Pawlak A, Guellaen G et al. Contrin, the human homologue of a germ-cell Y-box-binding protein: cloning, expression, and chromosomal localization. J Androl 1999; 20: 135–44.

233. Yang J, Medvedev S, Reddi PP et al. The DNA/RNA-binding protein MSY2 marks specific transcripts for cytoplasmic storage in mouse male germ cells. Proc Natl Acad Sci USA 2005; 102: 1513–18.

234. Yang J, Medvedev S, Yu J et al. Absence of the DNA-/RNA-binding protein MSY2 results in male and female infertility. Proc Natl Acad Sci USA 2005; 102: 5755–60.

235. Sasayama T, Marumoto T, Kunitoku N et al. Over-expression of Aurora-A targets cytoplasmic polyadenylation element binding protein and promotes mRNA polyadenylation of Cdk1 and cyclin B1. Genes Cells 2005; 10: 627–38.

236. Yao LJ, Zhong ZS, Zhang LS et al. Aurora-A is a critical regulator of microtubule assembly and nuclear activity in mouse oocytes, fertilized eggs, and early embryos. Biol Reprod 2004; 70: 1392–9.

237. Nakanishi T, Kubota H, Ishibashi N et al. Possible role of mouse poly(A) polymerase mGLD-2 during oocyte maturation. Devel Biol 2006; 289: 115–26.

238. Peset I, Seiler J, Sardon T et al. Function and regulation of Maskin, a TACC family protein, in microtubule growth during mitosis. J Cell Biol 2005; 170: 1057–66.

239. Sakurai T, Sato M, Kimura M. Diverse patterns of poly(A) tail elongation and shortening of murine maternal mRNAs from fully grown oocyte to 2-cell embryo stages. Biochem Biophys Res Commun 2005; 336: 1181–9.

240. Stebbins-Boaz B, Richter JD. Translational control during early development. Crit Rev Eukaryot Gene Expr 1997; 7: 73–94.

241. Collier B, Gorgoni B, Loveridge C et al. The DAZL family proteins are PABP-binding proteins that regulate translation in germ cells. EMBO J 2005; 24: 2656–66.

242. Cauffman G, Van de Velde H, Liebaers I et al. DAZL expression in human oocytes, preimplantation embryos and embryonic stem cells. Mol Hum Reprod 2005; 11: 405–11.

243. Walters KA, Binnie JP, Campbell BK et al. The effects of IGF-I on bovine follicle development and IGFBP-2 expression are dose and stage dependent. Reproduction 2006; 131: 515–23.

244. Steuerwald N, Cohen J, Herrera RJ et al. Association between spindle assembly checkpoint expression and maternal age in human oocytes. Mol Hum Reprod 2001; 7: 49–55.

245. Stein P, Svoboda P, Schultz RM. Transgenic RNAi in mouse oocytes: a simple and fast approach to study gene function. Devel Biol 2003; 256: 187–93.

246. De Moor CH, Richter JD. Translational control in vertebrate development. Int Rev Cytol 2001; 203: 567–608.

CHAPTER 5

Mechanism of oocyte maturation

Jason E Swain and Gary D Smith

INTRODUCTION

The oocyte is a unique cell, not only in structure and function, but in that it is the only cell in the female body that undergoes meiosis, or a reductional division in chromosome number from a diploid to a haploid state. Meiotic progression in the oocyte is known as oocyte maturation and, simply defined, is the re-initiation of the first meiotic division, progression to metaphase II (MII), and the accompanying cytoplasmic processes necessary for successful fertilization and early embryo development[1]. This definition implies that oocyte maturation is, in fact, composed of two inter-related processes: nuclear and cytoplasmic maturation. This chapter will outline the process of oocyte maturation, as well as address the cellular and molecular mechanisms regulating the process with the understanding that, the better a system is understood, the better the chances of improving the manipulation of oocytes to support efficient in-vitro maturation (IVM) and/or preventing aberrations that occur in vivo. Such improvements hold great potential considering defects in oocyte meiosis are a leading cause of aneuploidy-derived infertility and birth defects[2,3], as well as the immense potential benefits in-vitro oocyte maturation holds in

respect to treatment of human infertility and fertility preservation (see Parts III and IV).

OOCYTE MATURATION

Nuclear maturation

Oocyte nuclear maturation refers to modifications of nuclear components during meiosis (Figure 5.1). At birth mammalian oocytes are arrested in the diplotene stage of prophase of meiosis I and remain arrested in this chromatin-remodeling state while completing their growth and acquiring developmental competence. This growth and acquisition of developmental competence occurs during follicular development, prior to ovulation (see Chapter 1). This stage is characterized by the presence of an intact nuclear envelope or germinal vesicle (GV). A surge of gonadotropins preceding ovulation releases the oocyte from its quiescent state and signals re-initiation of meiosis, characterized in part by dissolution of the GV in a process known as GV breakdown (GVBD). During completion of prophase of the first meiotic division, homologous chromosomes undergo a process of pairing and recombination. Homologs then condense in preparation for a reductional division. A bipolar

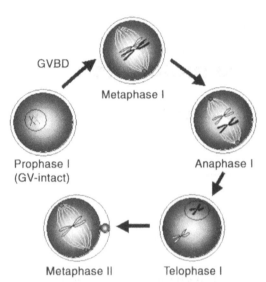

Figure 5.1 Schematic representation of oocyte nuclear maturation depicting an oocyte resuming meiosis and progressing from the GV-intact stage, undergoing dissolution of the nuclear envelope during germinal vesicle breakdown (GVBD), progressing through MI, anaphase, telophase, and finally re-arresting at MII until fertilization occurs. (Note that for visual purposes, proportions are not exact)

meiotic spindle forms and attaches to homologs at their centromeres. Subsequently, the physical contact between homologous pairs at chiasmata counteracts forces pulling apart the homologs, resulting in alignment of chromosomes along the metaphase plate, signaling completion of metaphase I (MI). The meiotic spindle then facilitates separation and segregation as homologs are pulled towards opposite poles at the beginning of anaphase. The oocyte progresses through telophase, resulting in disproportionate cytokinesis and extrusion of the first polar body. Finally, the oocyte proceeds directly to MII of meiosis II, forgoing interphase and DNA duplication, where it remains until fertilization occurs.

From this description of nuclear oocyte maturation, it is evident the process can be divided into six specific mechanistic events:

1. Meiotic resumption/GVBD

2. Chromatin condensation

3. Formation of the meiotic spindle apparatus

4. Separation and segregation of homologs

5. Disproportionate cytokinesis/polar body extrusion

6. Meiotic re-arrest.

Cytoplasmic maturation

Events comprising oocyte cytoplasmic maturation are less well defined than nuclear maturation, but equally important. For example, production of cortical granules from Golgi complexes and their subsequent proliferation and migration toward the oolemma is a critical step of oocyte maturation required for successful fertilization by helping prevent polyspermic penetration[4]. Redistribution of the endoplasmic reticulum and inositol-triphosphate (IP3) receptors corresponds to maturation of the oocyte as it develops the ability to produce sperm-induced Ca^{2+} oscillations[5,6]. Additionally, glutathione concentration increases during oocyte maturation, and inhibition of its synthesis suppresses sperm decondensation and formation of the male pronucleus[7]. Furthermore, cytoplasmic polyadenylation of maternal transcripts is an essential mechanism for temporal regulation of transcript stability and activation of protein translation, important to the developing embryo prior to the maternal–zygotic transition[8]. Regulation of energy substrate metabolism may be another indicator of successful oocyte cytoplasmic maturation, having implications for subsequent embryo development (see Chapter 2). Thus, cytoplasmic maturation includes relocation of organelles, synthesis and modification of proteins and mRNAs, as well as proper storage and timely reactivation of molecules and biochemical processes essential for supplying building materials required for successful fertilization, pronuclear formation, and preimplantation embryo development.

It is important to note that nuclear and cytoplasmic maturation are normally coordinated events, with GVBD releasing nuclear contents into the cytoplasm. This undoubtedly has some effect on cytoplasmic maturation. However, even though nuclear maturation can influence cytoplasmic maturation, at least some aspects of cytoplasmic maturation are independent of the nuclear event[9]. Therefore, although oocytes may appear 'meiotically mature' with respect to nuclear maturation and display extrusion of the first polar body, these oocytes may actually be lacking essential maternal factors required for subsequent fertilization, pronuclear formation, and embryonic development.

REGULATION OF OOCYTE MATURATION

Oocyte maturation is a complex process regulated through hormonal signals, interactions with surrounding somatic cells, and involvement of transcription factors regulating gene expression (see Chapters 3 and 4). Additionally, oocyte maturation is heavily regulated via reversible phosphorylation of proteins. Reversible phosphorylation is modulated through the actions of protein kinases and phosphatases, which phosphorylate and dephosphorylate phosphoproteins, respectively. This chapter discusses the roles of various protein kinases and phosphatases in relation to specific mechanistic events of oocyte maturation.

Meiotic resumption/GVBD

Meiotic resumption of oocytes in vivo is initiated in response to the preovulatory surge of luteinizing hormone (LH). However, pioneering work by Pincus and Enzmann[10] first described the process of spontaneous maturation of mammalian

oocytes, demonstrating that oocytes removed from antral follicles could complete maturation to MII in vitro. These oocytes were deemed 'meiotically competent'. Oocytes obtained from preantral follicles, however, were unable to complete the first meiosis, and were thus labeled 'meiotically incompetent'. Acquisition of meiotic competence is correlated with aspects of oocyte growth, such as oocyte size, follicular morphology, and chronologic age[11]. Thus, oocytes must complete their growth phase before being able to complete meiotic maturation (see Chapter 1).

It is apparent that surrounding somatic cells influence oocyte meiotic resumption. Physical separation of oocytes from granulosa within the antrum of intact follicles results in meiotic resumption, an effect prevented when oocytes regained contact with granulosa cells[12]. It is theorized that this breakdown in communication across gap junctions between somatic cells and the oocyte blocks delivery of an inhibitory somatic cell factor to the oocyte that maintains meiotic arrest. In the absence of this arresting factor, the oocyte resumes meiosis and progresses to MII, the developmental stage at which the oocyte is usually ovulated. However, evidence also exists to support the notion that somatic cell regulation of oocyte meiotic resumption is mediated via a positive factor[13]. Despite the fact that the identity of this inhibitory or stimulatory molecule remains to be determined, it is known that the resulting phosphorylation/dephosphorylation events are critical for resumption of meiosis and completion of oocyte maturation.

Germinal vesicle breakdown is the most visually apparent indicator of meiotic resumption in the oocyte and involves dissolution of the nuclear envelope (NE) (Figure 5.2). The NE consists of a network of filament-type proteins known as nuclear lamins[14]. Oocytes contain two lamins recognized by lamin B and lamin AC antibodies[15]. Phosphorylation of these nuclear lamins controls nuclear envelope integrity. Specifically, hypophosphorylation of nuclear lamins   maintains

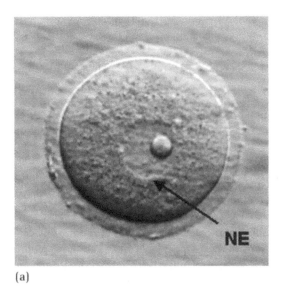
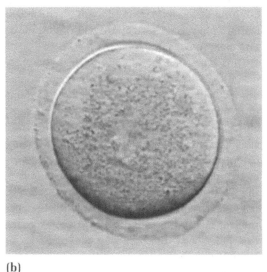

(a)   (b)

Figure 5.2 Micrographs of a (a) GV-intact oocyte (NE: nuclear envelope) and (b) an oocyte having undergone dissolution of the NE during GVBD

NE integrity, while hyperphosphorylation of lamins results in NE disassembly[14].

cAMP/protein kinase A (PKA)

Intraoocyte cyclic adenosine 5′-monophosphate (cAMP) levels, mediated by surrounding cumulus cells, are involved in maintaining meiotic arrest[16]. Culture of oocytes in the presence of cAMP analogs, cAMP elevating agents, and phosphodiesterase inhibitors prevents meiotic resumption, while cAMP antagonists allow maturation to proceed[13,17]. Furthermore, microinjection of the catalytic subunit of cAMP dependent kinase (PKA) inhibits spontaneous maturation[18]. This suggests the influence of cAMP on meiotic resumption is mediated through PKA. Recall that in the absence of cAMP, PKA exists as an inactive tetramer, comprised of two regulatory subunits and two catalytic subunits. Binding of cAMP to PKA regulatory subunits results in release and activation of catalytic subunits to phosphorylate target substrates (Figure 5.3a). Indeed, regulatory and catalytic subunits of PKA have been identified in oocytes[19,20]. Thus, uncoupling of gap junctions interrupts unidirectional flow of cAMP into the oocyte from surrounding cumulus cells, resulting in reduced PKA activity and resumption of meiosis (Figure 5.3b). Furthermore, A-kinase-anchoring-proteins (AKAPs) have been identified in oocytes and spatially regulate PKA activity by tethering the enzyme to specific subcellular regions[19,20], an extremely important regulatory mechanism in a cell as large as the oocyte.

Additionally, it should be mentioned that although elevated PKA activity within the oocyte inhibits meiotic resumption, increased PKA activity in surrounding cumulus cells actually stimulates oocyte meiosis[17]. This may be possible due to the existence of two PKA isozymes and two regulatory subunits with differential localization and affinities for cAMP[17]. In response to the preovulatory surge of LH, cAMP levels increase in cumulus cells[16], thus increasing PKA activity. This increase in PKA activity is partially responsible for phosphorylation of the gap junction protein connexin 43[21]. It is thought that phosphorylation of connexin 43 interrupts gap junction communication and prevents flow of cAMP into oocytes (Figure 5.3b).

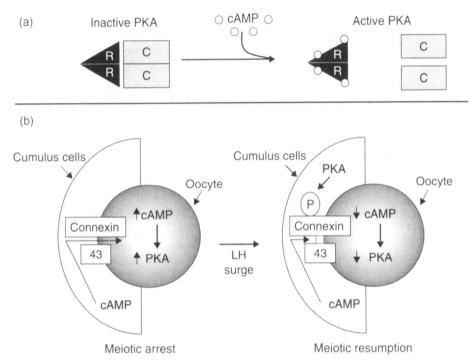

Figure 5.3 (a) In the absence of cAMP, PKA exists as an inactive tetramer, composed of two regulatory and two catalytic subunits. Binding of cAMP to regulatory subunits releases and activates catalytic subunits, allowing them to act on substrate proteins. (b) Representation of how increased cAMP levels flowing into the oocyte from surrounding cumulus cells through gap junctional protein, such as connexin 43, results in elevated intraoocyte PKA activity and meiotic block. In response to the preovulatory LH surge, connexin 43 is phosphorylated by PKA and gap junctional communication with the oocyte is blocked, resulting in decreased cAMP levels within the oocyte and decreased PKA activity, leading to meiotic resumption

Protein kinase C (PKC)

Similar to PKA, differential localization of various PKC isoforms also seems to dictate the effect of this kinase on oocyte meiotic resumption. Several isoforms of PKC have been identified in GV-intact oocytes, as well as in surrounding cumulus cells[22,23]. Direct activation of PKC in the mouse oocyte suppresses meiotic resumption, while stimulation of PKC in cumulus cells results in GVBD[22,24]. The role of PKC in oocyte meiotic maturation remains an interesting area of study due to the myriad of isoforms and conflicting reports of stimulatory and inhibitory effects on meiotic resumption in oocytes from various species[22].

Maturation promoting factor (MPF)

Another regulator of oocyte meiotic resumption and GVBD is MPF. Discovered by Masui and Markert in frog oocytes[25], MPF is actually a heterodimer consisting of p34[cdc2] kinase (CDK1) and cyclin B. Association of CDK1 with cyclin B is essential for MPF activity. Activation of MPF requires dephosphorylation of the kinase portion of the complex on tyrosine 15 and threonine 14 residue, as well as phosphorylation of cyclin

B[26]. However, protease control of cyclin B degradation has also been implicated in MPF regulation[11]. Maturation promoting factor's kinase activity fluctuates during oocyte meiotic progression, exhibiting undetectable activity in GV-intact oocytes, increasing around GVBD, peaking at MI, decreasing dramatically at anaphase I and telophase I, and peaking again when the oocyte re-arrests at MII[27]. With respect to regulation of meiotic resumption and GVBD, MPF moves into oocyte nuclei in conjunction with acquisition of meiotic competence[28] and is believed to regulate the phosphorylation and integrity of NE lamins[29] (Figure 5.4a).

Aurora A kinase

Aurora A kinase is one of three highly homologous aurora kinases found in mammals, shown in many somatic cell studies to regulate critical aspects of the cell cycle[30]. The serine/threonine aurora A kinase also plays a role in regulation of oocyte maturation[31,32]. Aurora A protein expression levels are highest in GV-intact oocytes where the kinase is concentrated within the germinal vesicle[32]. Furthermore, microinjection of anti-aurora A antibodies into the GV of mouse oocytes delays the onset of GVBD[32]. Upstream

regulators and downstream targets of aurora A involved in regulation of mammalian oocyte GVBD remain to be determined.

Protein phosphatase-1 (PP1)

Numerous kinases have been investigated and implicated in oocyte meiotic resumption and GVBD, while the role of specific protein phosphatases (PPs) has been less well studied. Classification of PPs is based on substrate specificity and sensitivity to defined inhibitors and results in four main types of PPs: PP1, PP2A, PP2B, and PP2C[33]. In addition, four isoforms of the PP1 catalytic subunit have been identified, varying at their carboxyl terminus: $PP1_\alpha$, $PP1_\delta$, $PP1_{\gamma1}$, and $PP1_{\gamma2}$[34–36]. An important discovery in phosphatase research was identification of the cell permeable inhibitor of PP1 and PP2A, okadaic acid (OA)[37]. Treatment of oocytes with OA results in premature meiotic resumption and GVBD[38,39]. Interestingly, PP1 translocates to the nucleus of oocytes following acquisition of meiotic competence[40] and specific inhibition of $PP1_\alpha$ pheno-mimics OA-stimulated GVBD, providing the first direct evidence that nuclear PP1 is involved in regulation of oocyte nuclear membrane integrity[41]. In addition, phosphorylation of

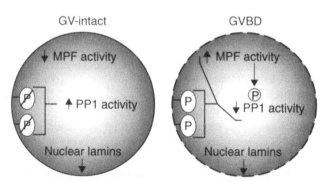

Figure 5.4 Proposed mechanism of regulation of nuclear lamin phosphorylation and nuclear envelope integrity during oocyte germinal vesicle breakdown (GVBD). Elevated PP1 activity in the nucleus results in lamin dephosphorylation and the presence of an intact GV. Upon meiotic resumption, MPF may directly phosphorylate lamins and/or phosphorylate and inactivate PP1, resulting in lamin phosphorylation and subsequent GVBD

PP1$_\alpha$ by MPF at Thr320 results in inactivation of PP1 in somatic cells[42]. Phosphorylation of PP1$_\alpha$ at Thr320 occurs during GVBD in oocytes[41], suggesting that inactivation of PP1 by MPF may be an important intracellular event in regulation of oocyte nuclear envelope dissolution (Figure 5.4).

cdc25 phosphatase

Another phosphatase involved in regulation of oocyte meiotic resumption is cdc25. cdc25 is a dual-specificity threonine/tyrosine phosphatase with three isoforms expressed in oocytes; cdc25a, cdc25b, and cdc25c[43,44]. Female mice deficient in cdc25b are sterile with oocytes arrested at prophase of meiosis I[45]. Injection of exogenous cdc25 into oocytes from these knockout animals allows oocytes to resume meiosis and progress to MII through activation of MPF[45]. Concentrations of transcripts encoding cdc25 are similar between meiotically competent and incompetent oocytes[28,46]; however, protein expression levels are greater in meiotically competent oocytes and are localized to the nucleus of GV-intact cells[28,46]. Activity of cdc25 is regulated by periodic changes in its phosphorylated state, with phosphorylation activating the enzyme[47]. During oocyte maturation, cdc25 becomes phosphorylated at or around GVBD and increases until reaching MII[46].

Chromatin condensation

Following meiotic resumption, chromatin begins condensing into individual metaphase chromosomes. Normal chromatin condensation is essential to ensure subsequent fidelity of chromosome segregation into daughter cells. Condensation permits the unencumbered movement of chromosomes by driving the resolution of chromosomes to reduce the likelihood of entrapment, tangling, or breakage of genetic material[48]. Thus, chromatin condensation is of great importance when considering causes of oocyte-derived embryonic aneuploidy.

Chromatin condensation is the result of long strands of DNA coiling around an octamer of two each of four regulatory proteins known as histones: H2A, H2B, H3, and H4[49]. These coiled structures of DNA and histones are referred to as nucleosomes. Additionally, a family of linker histones exists known as H1 histones, which function to fold DNA into a higher ordered structure. Phosphorylation of histone-H3 at ser10 and ser28 is tightly coupled to mitotic chromosome condensation[50,51], as well as during condensation events in pig[52] and mouse oocytes (unpublished data). It is thought phosphorylation of N-terminal tails of histone-H3 may act as a receptor or recruitment factor for condensation factors[53]. Alternatively, phosphorylation of the amino tail may reduce the affinity of histone-H3 for DNA and make the relatively compact chromatin fiber more readily accessible to condensation factors[53], like the condensin complex.

Condensin is an evolutionary conserved five-protein complex consisting of a heterodimeric SMC core (structural maintenance of chromosomes) and three non-SMC subunits, essential for proper mitotic chromosome condensation from yeast to mammals[53]. Condensin co-localizes with phosphorylated histone-H3[54]. In fact, direct binding of non-SMC condensin subunits to histone-H3 has been shown[55], an event potentially regulated by the phosphorylated state of the histone or the non-SMC components[53]. Although condensin subunits have not been identified in mammalian oocytes, the complex is present and necessary for proper meiotic chromosome condensation[48,56]. Thus, exploration of condensin's role in proper mammalian oocyte meiosis remains an exciting area of future study.

PP1

Treatment of oocytes with PP inhibitors, such as okadaic acid or calyculin-A, induces rapid chromatin condensation[39,57]. These treatments also result in increased phosphorylation of histone-H3 at Ser10[52]. Studies in our laboratory demonstrate the localization of $PP1_\delta$ and the endogenous PP1 regulator, inhibitor-2 (I2), to condensed chromatin in mouse oocytes (unpublished data, Figure 5.5a). In somatic cells, PP1 can directly dephosphorylate histone-H3, or regulate phosphorylation through regulation of aurora B kinase activity[58]. Interestingly, aurora B is also instrumental in condensin recruitment[59].

Thus, PP1 may be the OA sensitive PP regulating phosphorylation of histone-H3 and chromatin condensation during oocyte meiosis (Figure 5.5b).

MPF

In addition to meiotic resumption, MPF may also regulate chromatin condensation during oocyte

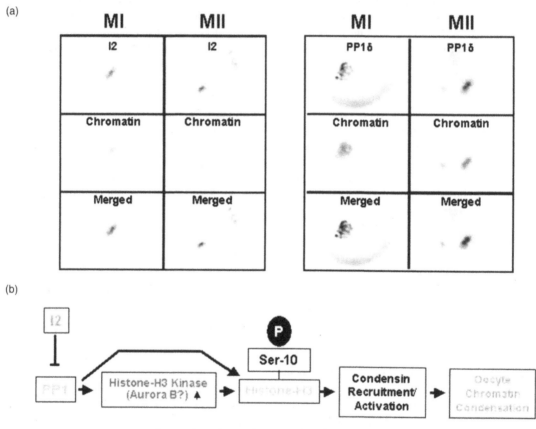

Figure 5.5 (a) Immunocytochemical analysis of $PP1_\delta$ and endogenous PP1 inhibitor I2 in mouse metaphase I and metaphase II oocytes. Both $PP1_\delta$ and I2 localize with condensed chromatin. (b) Proposed mechanism of how PP1 may regulate oocyte histone phosphorylation and chromatin condensation. During times of oocyte chromatin condensation, chromatin associated I2 may inhibit PP1 activity. This decrease in chromatin associated PP1 activity results in increased histone-H3 phosphorylation through direct effects, or via possible activation of a histone-H3 kinase (aurora B). This increased histone-H3 phosphorylation leads to chromatin condensation, possibly through recruitment and/or activation of condensation factors, such as the condensin complex (see color plate section)

maturation. Histone-H1 is a known substrate for MPF and is often used for the demonstration and quantification of MPF activity in mammalian oocytes[60]. Histone-H1 kinase activity has been demonstrated in oocyte extracts and its activity is greatest during chromatin condensation at MI and MII, with an oscillatory pattern mimicking that of MPF[61]. Recall histone-H1 is instrumental in obtaining higher ordered condensation of chromosomes. Therefore, MPF may regulate chromatin condensation, in part, due to regulation of histone-H1 phosphorylation. Maturation promoting factor may also directly regulate the phosphorylated state and activity of non-SMC components of the condensin complex[62]. It should be noted that oocyte chromatin condensation has been observed in the absence of cdc2 kinase activity[52] and histone-H1 phosphorylation may not be required for meiotic chromatin condensation[63]. However, normality of oocyte chromatin condensation under these circumstances may be compromised.

Meiotic spindle apparatus formation

Insight into regulation of meiotic spindle formation and function during oocyte maturation is extremely important, especially considering that in humans it is estimated that 10–25% of all human conceptions are chromosomally abnormal due to an error in chromosome segregation during meiosis[2,3]. Many of these abnormalities are lethal and result in spontaneous abortion within the first trimester. Furthermore, studies indicate greater than 95% of this human aneuploidy is attributable to defects within meiotic machinery of the oocyte[2]. Through understanding of regulatory components involved in oocyte spindle formation, it is hoped therapies can be developed to reduce the occurrence of these meiotic abnormalities and lower the incidence of resulting birth defects and aneuploidy derived infertility.

To ensure proper chromosome segregation, a dividing cell must form a functional spindle apparatus (Figure 5.6). The spindle apparatus is a conglomerate of microtubules comprised of α- and β-tubulin and associated structural proteins, acting to coordinate cyto- and karyokinetic events essential for normal chromosome segregation. These microtubule arrays are organized into a barrel-shaped bipolar structure and contain a blend of dense material at either pole known as microtubule organizing centers (MTOCs) or centrosomes[64]. The main structural proteins comprising oocyte centrosomes include γ-tubulin and pericentrin[65]. It is hypothesized that the phosphorylated state of centrosomal proteins regulates their function[66,67]. Indeed, studies indicate the phosphorylated state of oocyte centrosomes changes during meiotic maturation[68,69]. Similarly, microtubule associated proteins are also regulated by cell cycle-dependent reversible phosphorylation[70].

PP2A

Although inhibition of oocyte PPs with OA results in premature GVBD, oocytes fail to progress to MII due to severe meiotic spindle abnormalities[38,71]. Okadaic acid inhibition of PP1/PP2A in

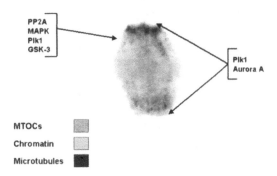

Figure 5.6 Micrograph of a mouse oocyte metaphase I meiotic spindle displaying microtubules (green/β-tubulin), condensed chromatin (blue/Hoescht), and centrosomes (red/γ-tubulin). Potential regulators of spindle component phosphorylation and activity are listed (see color plate section)

mouse oocytes results in malformation of the meiotic spindle, dispersion of centrosomal staining from spindle poles, and a disassociation of centrosomes from microtubules[72]. Thus, one or both of these PPs may regulate meiotic spindle formation and function. Immunocytochemical studies have shown PP2A[73] is localized to polymerized microtubules. Additionally, activity of PP2A increases at the time of first meiotic spindle formation[73]. Therefore, PP2A may regulate meiotic spindle formation though regulation of the phosphorylated state of some unidentified microtubule associated protein (Figure 5.6).

MAP kinase (MAPK)

The family of MAPKs (p44MAPK1 and p42MAPK2), also known as ERK1 and ERK2, respectively, are serine/threonine kinases that require phosphorylation to be activated[74]. Evidence suggests MAPKs are instrumental in regulation of microtubule dynamics and spindle formation in oocytes. Both ERK1 and ERK2 are activated after GVBD, and remain activated throughout the MI/MII transition[75], times when the meiotic spindle is formed and active. Additionally, active ERK1 and ERK2 are associated with oocyte centrosomes and spindles[73]. Lastly, inhibition of mouse oocyte MAPK activity results in compromised microtubule polymerization, no spindle formation, and aberrant condensation of chromosomes[73]. Specific protein targets of MAPK within the meiotic spindle and/or oocyte centrosome remain to be elucidated (Figure 5.6).

Polo-like kinase-1 (Plk1)

Another serine/threonine kinase that appears to regulate meiotic spindle and centrosome formation and function is Plk1. Much of the research focusing on Plk1 has focused on its role in regard to cancer. However, emerging data suggest Plk1 is also a regulator of oocyte meiosis. Levels of Plk1 protein increase following GVBD[76], a time at which the meiotic spindle is forming. Additionally, this kinase is localized to spindle poles in MI and MII oocytes and also localizes to the middle of the spindle during anaphase–telophase[76,77]. Neutralization of Plk1 activity in oocytes through antibody microinjection resulted in various MI spindle abnormalities and inability to progress to MII[78], possibly through alterations in MTOC activity (Figure 5.6).

Aurora A kinase

Aurora A is known to regulate oocyte GVBD[32]. Additionally, aurora A functions to regulate spindle formation and microtubule dynamics. Aurora A localizes to the spindle poles of MI and MII oocytes, and neutralization of kinase activity via antibody microinjection distorts MI spindle organization[32]. It is thought the activity and regulatory function of aurora A is dependent upon protein expression levels[32]. Specific protein targets for aurora A within the oocyte MTOCs remain to be elucidated. However, based on somatic cell studies, likely candidates include recruitment factors for γ-tubulin[79] (Figure 5.6).

Glycogen synthase kinase-3 (GSK-3)

A highly conserved serine/threonine protein kinase, GSK-3 was initially discovered as a kinase that phosphorylates and inactivates glycogen synthase[80]. The vast majority of research focusing on GSK-3 has been performed in neuronal and somatic cells, where it regulates phosphorylation of numerous microtubule associated proteins. In such a manner, GSK-3 influences microtubule polymerization, stability, spindle formation, and function[81–83]. Recently GSK-3 isoforms have been identified in oocytes[84]. Inhibition of GSK-3 activity results in modified organization of microtubules and altered spindle function, resulting in compromised segregation of homologs[84] (Figure 5.6).

Separation and segregation of homologs

As important as meiotic spindle formation in ensuring proper homolog distribution in the oocyte, is regulation of chromosome cohesion and separation. The majority of the understanding we have concerning mechanisms governing chromosome separation is derived from studies in somatic or non-mammalian cells. However, data are emerging regarding regulation of chromosome cohesion and separation during mammalian oocyte meiosis.

It has long been observed that there is a physical association between replicated copies of chromosomes and an abrupt release of this association as chromosomes segregate during cell division. This cytologic visible attachment is referred to as cohesion[85]. Cohesion must be sustained until anaphase because it is essential each copy of the chromosome be able to resist forces of microtubules while aligned on the metaphase plate and remain in a position to capture microtubules from opposite spindle poles to ensure each cell retains only one copy of the genetic material. At anaphase, chromosome cohesion is released.

In meiosis I, homologous chromosomes undergo a pairing and recombination prior to segregation. This process involves a sister chromatid from one homolog attaching to a sister chromatid of the other homolog at points called chiasmata. Consequently, in order for homologs to segregate at anaphase I, chiasmata between homologs must be resolved and cohesion along the arms of sister chromatids released[85]. Sister chromatid cohesion is regulated by a multi-subunit complex known as cohesin (Figure 5.7a)[85]. Indeed, components of the cohesin complex have been identified in oocytes during the first meiosis[86]. The cohesin complex holds homologous chromosomes together until separase activity results in their separation and allows homolog disjunction at anaphase (Figure 5.7b)[85,87]. Securin inhibits separase activity at metaphase

until it undergoes proteolysis, probably by the anaphase-promoting complex (APC) (Figure 5.7b)[88].

PP1/PP2A

It is evident that PP1 and/or PP2A regulate multiple aspects of oocyte maturation. Indeed, PPs may also regulate cohesion of sister chromatids and affect segregation of homologs. As mentioned, $PP1_\delta$ localizes to chromatin (unpublished data). Additionally, inhibition of PP1 and/or PP2A with OA during meiosis I results in MI oocytes with abnormal numbers of chromatids as well as MII oocytes with increased frequency of premature sister chromatid separation, single unpaired chromatids, and hyperploidy[89]. Thus PP1 and/or PP2A regulate the phosphorylated state and function of cohesin proteins on chromosomes (Figure 5.7b).

GSK-3

Recall that inhibition of oocyte GSK-3 results in abnormal segregation of homologs[84]. Recall also that $PP1_\delta$ and I2 localize to condensed oocyte chromatin (unpublished data). Residue Thr72 of I2 is a known substrate for GSK-3 phosphorylation[90]. Phosphorylation of Thr72 of I2, when complexed with PP1, results in PP activation. Therefore, inhibition of GSK-3 activity may result in reduced I2 phosphorylation and subsequent PP1 inactivation. Thus, errors in homolog segregation observed via inhibition of oocyte GSK-3 activity may not only be due to direct effects on microtubule associated proteins, but also on cohesins through regulation of PP1 (Figure 5.8).

MPF

It appears as if MPF also regulates separation of chromosomes during oocyte maturation. Homolog disjunction in mouse oocytes requires proteolysis of cyclin B1, a component of MPF (Figure 5.7b)[88]. Additionally, despite securin

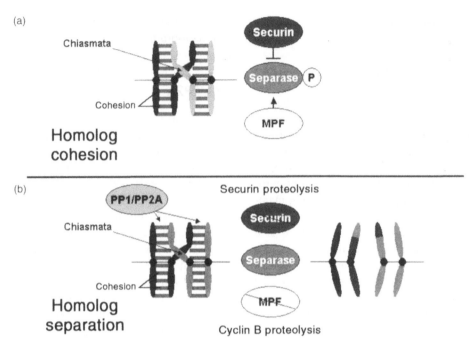

Figure 5.7 Proposed mechanism of control of homolog cohesion and separation during meiosis I of oocyte maturation. The cohesion complex (red) maintains cohesion between sister chromatids, while homologous chromosomes are connected at chiasmata. Separase activity is inhibited through the action of securin and phosphorylation of separase by MPF. Homologs separate when securin and the MPF component, cyclin B, undergo proteolysis, resulting in increased separase activity. Separase activity, along with desphosphorylation of cohesin complex components by PP1 and/or PP2A, allows for separation of sister chromatids, resolution of chiasmata, and separation of homologs (see color plate section)

degradation, sister chromatids do not separate during meiosis II in oocytes[91]. It is hypothesized that MPF regulates phosphorylation and activity of separase to control chromosome segregation during oocyte maturation (Figure 5.7b)[91].

Disproportionate cytokinesis/polar body extrusion

Normally, it is vitally important cell division results in two identical daughter cells with equal amounts of cytoplasm and organelles. However, asymmetric cell division is a fundamental mechanism for generating cell diversity during development by allowing unequal inheritance of cell fate determinants. Asymmetric cell division is readily apparent within the oocyte during meiosis with extrusion of a small polar body. Two major events are required to ensure asymmetric cell division during oocyte meiosis. The first involves the migration of the meiotic spindle toward the cell cortex, while the second event involves formation of a cortical domain over the spindle for formation of the cleavage furrow[92,93].

In oocytes, migration of the spindle appears to be regulated by interactions between chromosomes and the microfilament network[93]. A microfilament-binding protein, formin-2, appears to be essential for this process[94]. A network of microfilaments, nucleated by formin-2, may interact with actin binding proteins

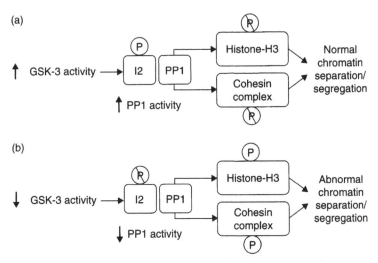

Figure 5.8 Proposed model for how intraoocyte GSK-3 regulates homolog separation and segregation during oocyte meiosis. (a) Active GSK-3 results in phosphorylation of I2 at Thr72, resulting in increased PP1 activity. This increased activity of PP1 results in a reduction of the phosphorylation of histone-H3 and/or the cohesin complex. This reduced phosphorylation is required for normal chromatin separation and/or segregation. (b) Inhibition of oocyte GSK-3 results in a lack of I2 phosphorylation, leading to inhibition of PP1 activity. This reduced PP1 activity results in hyperphosphorylation of histone-H3 and/or the cohesin complex, resulting in abnormal chromatin separation/segregation

associated with chromosomes to direct movement of the spindle along the shortest path to the cortex[93,95]. The direction of this migration results from the slight asymmetric position of the germinal vesicle[95]. Meanwhile, chromosomes located under the cortex appear to control formation of the cortical domain, the area to which the cleavage furrow is restricted. During spindle migration, an area devoid of microvilli and enriched in actin microfilaments forms in the area over the spindle to assist in formation of the cleavage furrow[93].

MAPK

The MAPK pathway may be involved in polar body formation and extrusion. Oocytes from mos⁻/mos⁻ mice, which lack a functional MAPK signaling pathway, form abnormally large polar bodies[95]. These oocytes maintain their ability to migrate their homologs, but the signaling distance instructing this movement is reduced. It is suggested MAPK may act as an 'amplifier' to increase the range of these signals by controlling phosphorylation and activity of the actin microfilament network, possibly through myosin IIA[95,96] or formin-2[93].

Meiotic re-arrest

After resuming meiosis, undergoing GVBD, and progressing through metaphase, anaphase, and telophase of meiosis I, oocytes forego interphase and DNA duplication and proceed directly to metaphase of meiosis II (MII). This is the stage at which the oocyte is ovulated in vivo. The oocyte will remain arrested at this stage until stimulated to resume the second meiotic division via activation by a spermatozoan. Historically, MII arrest was attributed to some unknown cytosolic factor activity (CSF)[25]. However, reversible phosphorylation, regulated via a balance of protein kinase and phosphatase activity, also plays a role in the re-arrest of oocytes at MII.

MPF

In addition to regulating meiotic resumption, MPF is involved in regulating MII arrest in oocytes. Levels of MPF activity peak during MII[27] and this high MPF activity is maintained through a continuous equilibrium between cyclin B synthesis and degradation[97]. A decrease in MPF activity is related to an enhanced ability of oocytes to release from MII arrest of meiosis I and proceed to meiosis II[98].

MAPK

Since initial experiments identified the importance of CSF in MII arrest, the components of CSF have been characterized and found to contain members of the MAPK signaling cascade[99]. MAPK activity remains elevated at MII[75]. Mos knockout mice, which have no functional MAPK, parthenogenetically activate without arrest at MII[100]. Subsequent studies demonstrated that inhibition of MAPK activity results in an inability of oocytes to re-arrest at MII[101,102]. It appears as if MAPK regulates this re-arrest by reactivation of MPF activity[101], possibly through decreasing the degradation of cyclin B[103].

CONCLUSIONS

The maturation of immature oocytes in vitro (IVM) is an extremely attractive avenue of research and offers numerous benefits over conventional in vitro fertilization (see subsequent chapters). However, although progress has been made in this field, there remains significant room for improvement. Oocyte meiotic non-disjunction, which results in embryonic aneuploidy, is a leading cause of congenital birth defects. With such high error rates occurring during natural oocyte meiosis, these problems may also be a concern when considering IVM. Therefore, through understanding of regulatory mechanisms involved in oocyte maturation, it is hoped strategies can be developed to refine and optimize conditions for IVM while circumventing potential problems such as chromosomal non-disjunction.

ACKNOWLEDGMENTS

The authors would like to express their appreciation to Dr Charles Bormann, Dr Carrie Smith, and Jordon Swain for the critical reading of this manuscript. We would like to thank Drs Tan, Chian, and Buckett for the invitation to participate in this collection of chapters. We apologize to those whose work we have not cited because of space limitations.

REFERENCES

1. Smith G. *In vitro* maturation of oocytes. Curr Womens Health Rep 2001; 1: 143–51.

2. Hassold T, Hunt P. To err (meiotically) is human: the genesis of human aneuploidy. Nat Rev Genet 2001; 2: 280–91.

3. Hunt PA. The control of mammalian female meiosis: factors that influence chromosome segregation. J Assist Reprod Genet 1998; 15: 246–52.

4. Sathananthan AH, Ng SC, Chia CM et al. The origin and distribution of cortical granules in human oocytes with reference to Golgi, nucleolar, and microfilament activity. Ann NY Acad Sci 1985; 442: 251–64.

5. Mehlmann LM, Terasaki M, Jaffe LA et al. Reorganization of the endoplasmic reticulum during meiotic maturation of the mouse oocyte. Devel Biol 1995; 170: 607–15.

6. Mehlmann LM, Mikoshiba K, Kline D. Redistribution and increase in cortical inositol 1,4,5-trisphosphate receptors after meiotic maturation of the mouse oocyte. Devel Biol 1996; 180: 489–98.

7. Perreault S, Barbee R, Slott V. Importance of glutathione in the acquisition and maintenance of sperm nuclear decondensing activity in maturing hamster oocytes. Devel Biol 1988; 125: 181–6.

8. Gandolfi TA, Gandolfi F. The maternal legacy to the embryo: cytoplasmic components and their effects on early development. Theriogenology 2001; 55: 1255–76.

9. Eppig JJ, Schultz RM, O'Brien M et al. Relationship between the developmental programs controlling nuclear and cytoplasmic maturation of mouse oocytes. Devel Biol 1994; 164: 1–9.

10. Pincus G, Enzmann E. The comparative behavior of mammalian eggs *in vivo* and *in vitro*. I. The activation of ovarian eggs. J Exp Med 1935; 62: 655–75.

11. Eppig J. Regulation of mammalian oocyte maturation. In: Adashi E, Leung P, eds. The Ovary. Raven Press Ltd, New York, 1993: 185–208.

12. Racowsky C, Baldwin K. In vitro and *in vivo* studies reveal that hamster oocyte meiotic arrest is maintained only transiently by follicular fluid, but persistently by membrana/cumulus granulosa cell contact. Devel Biol 1989; 134: 297–306.

13. Downs SM. The biochemistry of oocyte maturation. Ernst Schering Res Found Workshop 2002; 41: 81–99.

14. Stuurman N, Heins S, Aebi U. Nuclear lamins: their structure, assembly, and interactions. J Struct Biol 1998; 122: 42–66.

15. Maul G, Schatten G, Jimenez S et al. Detection of nuclear lamin B epitopes in oocyte nuclei from mice, sea urchins, and clams using a human autoimmune serum. Devel Biol 1987; 121: 368–75.

16. Dekel N. Regulation of oocyte maturation. The role of cAMP. Ann NY Acad Sci 1988; 541: 211–16.

17. Downs SM, Hunzicker-Dunn M. Differential regulation of oocyte maturation and cumulus expansion in the mouse oocyte–cumulus cell complex by site-selective analogs of cyclic adenosine monophosphate. Devel Biol 1995; 172: 72–85.

18. Bornslaeger E, Mattei P, Schultz R. Involvement of cAMP-dependent protein kinase and protein phosphorylation in regulation of mouse oocyte maturation. Devel Biol 1986; 114: 453–62.

19. Brown R, Ord T, Moss S et al. A-kinase anchor proteins as potential regulators of protein kinase A function in oocytes. Biol Reprod 2002; 67: 981–7.

20. Kovo M, Schillace R, Galiani D et al. Expression and modification of PKA and AKAPs during meiosis in rat oocytes. Mol Cell Endocrinol 2002; 192: 105–13.

21. Granot I, Dekel N. Phosphorylation and expression of connexin-43 ovarian gap junction protein are regulated by luteinizing hormone. J Biol Chem 1994; 269: 30502–9.

22. Downs SM, Cottom J, Hunzicker-Dunn M. Protein kinase C and meiotic regulation in isolated mouse oocytes. Mol Reprod Dev 2001; 58: 101–15.

23. Fan HY, Tong C, Li MY et al. Translocation of the classic protein kinase C isoforms in porcine oocytes: implications of protein kinase C involvement in the regulation of nuclear activity and cortical granule exocytosis. Exp Cell Res 2002; 277: 183–91.

24. Lu Q, Smith G, Chen D-Y et al. Activation of protein kinase C induces MAP kinase dephosphorylation and pronucleus formation in rat oocytes. Biol Reprod 2002; 67: 64–9.

25. Masui Y, Markert CL. Cytoplasmic control of nuclear behavior during meiotic maturation of frog oocytes. J Exp Zool 1971; 177: 129–45.

26. Gautier J, Maller JL. Cyclin B in *Xenopus* oocytes: implications for the mechanism of pre-MPF activation. Embo J 1991; 10: 177–82.

27. Naito K, Toyoda Y. Fluctuation of histone H1 kinase activity during meiotic maturation in porcine oocytes. J Reprod Fertil 1991; 93: 467–73.

28. Mitra J, Schultz R. Regulation of the acquisition of meiotic competence in the mouse: changes in the subcellular localization of cdc2, cyclin B1, cdc 25C and wee1, and in the concentration of these proteins and their transcripts. J Cell Sci 1996; 109: 2407–15.

29. Dessev G, Iovcheva-Dessev C, Bischoff J et al. A complex containing p34^{cdc2} and cyclin B phosphorylates the nuclear lamin and disassembles nuclei of clam oocytes in vitro. J Cell Biol 1991; 112: 523–33.

30. Nigg E. Mitotic kinases as regulators of cell division and its checkpoints. Nat Rev Mol Cell Biol 2001; 2: 21–32.

31. Yao LJ, Sun QY. Characterization of aurora-a in porcine oocytes and early embryos implies its functional roles in the regulation of meiotic maturation, fertilization and cleavage. Zygote 2005; 13: 23–30.

32. Yao LJ, Zhong ZS, Zhang LS et al. Aurora-A is a critical regulator of microtubule assembly and nuclear activity in mouse oocytes, fertilized eggs, and early embryos. Biol Reprod 2004; 70: 1392–9.

33. Cohen P. The structure and regulation of protein phosphatases. Annu Rev Biochem 1989; 58: 453–508.

34. Tognarini M, Villa-Moruzzi E. Analysis of the isoforms of protein phosphatase 1 (PP1) with polyclonal peptide antibodies. Methods Mol Biol 1998; 93: 169–83.

35. Zhang Z, Bai G, Shima M et al. Expression and characterization of rat protein phosphatases-1 alpha, -1 gamma 1, -1 gamma 2, and -1 delta. Arch Biochem Biophys 1993; 303: 402–6.

36. da Cruz e Silva EF, Fox CA, Ourmet CC et al. Differential expression of protein phosphatase 1 isoforms in mammalian brain. J Neurosci 1995; 15(5 Pt 1): 3375–89.

37. Bialojan C, Takai A. Inhibitory effect of a marine-sponge toxin, okadaic acid, on protein phosphatases. Specificity and kinetics. Biochem J 1988; 256: 283–90.

38. Rime H, Ozon R. Protein phosphatases are involved in the in vivo activation of histone H1 kinase in mouse oocyte. Devel Biol 1990; 141: 115–22.

39. Gavin AC, Tsukitani Y, Schorderet-Slatkine S. Induction of M-phase entry of prophase-blocked mouse oocytes through microinjection of oka-daic acid, a specific phosphatase inhibitor. Exp Cell Res 1991; 192: 75–81.

40. Smith G, Sadhu A, Mathies S et al. Characterization of protein phosphatases in mouse oocytes. Devel Biol 1998; 204: 537–49.

41. Swain JE, Wang X, Saunders TL et al. Specific inhibition of mouse oocyte nuclear protein phosphatase-1 stimulates germinal vesicle breakdown. Mol Reprod Dev 2003; 65: 96–103.

42. Dohadwala M, da Cruz e Silva E, Hall F et al. Phosphorylation and inactivation of protein phosphatase 1 by cyclin-dependent kinases. Proc Natl Acad Sci USA 1994; 91: 6408–12.

43. Wu S, Wolgemuth DJ. The distinct and developmentally regulated patterns of expression of members of the mouse Cdc25 gene family suggest differential functions during gametogenesis. Devel Biol 1995; 170: 195–206.

44. Wickramasinghe D, Becker S, Ernst MK et al. Two CDC25 homologues are differentially expressed during mouse development. Development 1995; 121: 2047–56.

45. Lincoln AJ, Wickramasinghe D, Stein P et al. Cdc25b phosphatase is required for resumption of meiosis during oocyte maturation. Nat Genet 2002; 30: 446–49.

46. Gall L, Ruffini S, Le Bourhis D et al. Cdc25C expression in meiotically competent and incompetent goat oocytes. Mol Reprod Dev 2002; 62: 4–12.

47. Izumi T, Walker DH, Maller JL. Periodic changes in phosphorylation of the Xenopus cdc25 phosphatase regulate its activity. Mol Biol Cell 1992; 3: 927–39.

48. Chan RC, Severson AF, Meyer BJ. Condensin restructures chromosomes in preparation for meiotic divisions. J Cell Biol 2004; 167: 613–25.

49. Alberts B. Molecular Biology of the Cell, 3rd edn. Garland, New York, 1994.

50. Wei Y, Mizzen CA, Cook RG et al. Phosphorylation of histone H3 at serine 10 is correlated with chromosome condensation during mitosis and meiosis in Tetrahymena. Proc Natl Acad Sci USA 1998; 95: 7480–4.

51. Goto H, Tomono Y, Ajiro K et al. Identification of a novel phosphorylation site on histone H3 coupled with mitotic chromosome condensation. J Biol Chem 1999; 274: 25543–9.

52. Bui HT, Yamaoka E, Miyano T. Involvement of histone H3 (Ser10) phosphorylation in chromosome condensation without CDC2 kinase and mitogen-activated protein kinase activation in pig oocytes. Biol Reprod 2004; 70: 1843–51.

53. Hirano T. Chromosome cohesion, condensation, and separation. Annu Rev Biochem 2000; 69: 115–44.

54. Schmiesing JA, Gregson HC, Zhou S et al. A human condensin complex containing hCAP-C-hCAP-E and CNAP1, a homolog of *Xenopus* XCAP-D2, colocalizes with phosphorylated histone H3 during the early stage of mitotic chromosome condensation. Mol Cell Biol 2000; 20: 6996–7006.

55. Ball AR, Jr, Schmiesing JA, Zhou C et al. Identification of a chromosome-targeting domain in the human condensin subunit CNAP1/hCAP-D2/Eg7. Mol Cell Biol 2002; 22: 5769–81.

56. Yu HG, Koshland DE. Meiotic condensin is required for proper chromosome compaction, SC assembly, and resolution of recombination-dependent chromosome linkages. J Cell Biol 2003; 163: 937–47.

57. Picard A, Capony J, Brautigan D et al. Involvement of protein phosphatases 1 and 2A in the control of M phase-promoting factor activity in starfish. J Cell Biol 1989; 109: 3347–54.

58. Murnion M, Adams R, Callister D et al. Chromatin-associated protein phosphatase 1 regulates aurora-B and histone H3 phosphorylation. J Biol Chem 2001; 276: 26656–65.

59. Giet R, Glover DM. Drosophila aurora B kinase is required for histone H3 phosphorylation and condensin recruitment during chromosome condensation and to organize the central spindle during cytokinesis. J Cell Biol 2001; 152: 669–82.

60. Dekel N. Protein phosphorylation/dephosphorylation in the meiotic cell cycle of mammalian oocytes. Rev Reprod 1996; 1: 82–8.

61. Jelinkova L, Kubelka M, Motlik J et al. Chromatin condensation and histone H1 kinase activity during growth and maturation of rabbit oocytes. Mol Reprod Dev 1994; 37: 210–15.

62. Kimura K, Hirano M, Kobayashi R et al. Phosphorylation and activation of 13S condensin by Cdc2 in vitro. Science 1998; 282: 487–90.

63. Shen X, Yu L, Weir JW et al. Linker histones are not essential and affect chromatin condensation *in vivo*. Cell 1995; 82: 47–56.

64. Schatten G. The centrosome and its mode of inheritance: the reduction of the centrosome during gametogenesis and its restoration during fertilization. Devel Biol 1994; 165: 299–335.

65. Combelles C, Albertini D. Microtubule patterning during meiotic maturation in mouse oocytes is determined by cell cycle-specific sorting and redistribution of gamma-tubulin. Devel Biol 2001; 239: 281–94.

66. Vandre D, Davis F, Rao P et al. Phosphoproteins are components of mitotic microtubule organizing centers. Proc Natl Acad Sci USA 1984; 81: 4439–43.

67. Centonze VE, Borisy GG. Nucleation of microtubules from mitotic centrosomes is modulated by a phosphorylated epitope. J Cell Sci 1990; 95(Pt 3): 405–11.

68. Messinger SM, Albertini DF. Centrosome and microtubule dynamics during meiotic progression in the mouse oocyte. J Cell Sci 1991; 100(Pt 2): 289–98.

69. Wickramasinghe D, Albertini D. Centrosome phosphorylation and the developmental expression of meiotic competence in mouse oocytes. Devel Biol 1992; 152: 62–74.

70. Cassimeris L. Accessory protein regulation of microtubule dynamics throughout the cell cycle. Curr Opin Cell Biol 1999; 11: 134–41.

71. Gavin A-C, Tsukitani Y, Schorderet-Slatkine S. Induction of M-phase entry of prophase-blocked mouse oocytes through microinjection of okadaic acid, a specific phosphatase inhibitor. Exp Cell Res 1991; 192: 75–81.

72. de Pennart H, Verlhac MH, Cibert C et al. Okadaic acid induces spindle lengthening and disrupts the interaction of microtubules with the kinetochores in metaphase II-arrested mouse oocytes. Devel Biol 1993; 157: 170–81.

73. Lu Q, Dunn RL, Angeles R et al. Regulation of spindle formation by active mitogen-activated protein kinase and protein phosphatase 2A during mouse oocyte meiosis. Biol Reprod 2002; 66: 29–37.

74. Cobb M, Boulton TG, Robbins DJ. Extracellular signal-regulated kinases: ERKs in progress. Cell Reg 1991; 2: 965–78.

75. Sobajima T, Aoki F, Kohmoto K. Activation of mitogen-activated protein kinase during meiotic maturation in mouse oocytes. J Reprod Fertil 1993; 97: 389–94.

76. Wianny F, Tavares A, Evans MJ et al. Mouse polo-like kinase 1 associates with the acentriolar spindle poles, meiotic chromosomes and spindle midzone during oocyte maturation. Chromosoma 1998; 107: 430–9.

77. Tong C, Fan H-Y, Lian L et al. Polo-like kinase-1 is a pivotal regulator of microtubule assembly during mouse oocyte meiotic maturation, fertilization, and early embryonic mitosis. Biol Reprod 2002; 67: 546–54.

78. Fan HY, Tong C, Teng CB et al. Characterization of Polo-like kinase-1 in rat oocytes and early embryos implies its functional roles in the regulation of meiotic maturation, fertilization, and cleavage. Mol Reprod Dev 2003; 65: 318–29.

79. Ducat D, Zheng Y. Aurora kinases in spindle assembly and chromosome segregation. Exp Cell Res 2004; 301: 60–7.

80. Embi N, Rylatt DB, Cohen P. Glycogen synthase kinase-3 from rabbit skeletal muscle. Separation from cyclic-AMP-dependent protein kinase and phosphorylase kinase. Eur J Biochem 1980; 107: 5195–227.

81. Ryves WJ, Harwood AJ. The interaction of glycogen synthase kinase-3 (GSK-3) with the cell cycle. Prog Cell Cycle Res 2003; 5: 489–95.

82. Doble BW, Woodgett JR. GSK-3: tricks of the trade for a multi-tasking kinase. J Cell Sci 2003; 116: 1175–86.

83. Jope RS, Johnson GV. The glamour and gloom of glycogen synthase kinase-3. Trends Biochem Sci 2004; 29: 95–102.

84. Wang X, Liu X, Dunn R et al. Glycogen synthase kinase-3 regulates mouse oocyte homologue segregation. Mol Reprod Devel 2003; 64: 96–105.

85. Lee JY, Orr-Weaver TL. The molecular basis of sister-chromatid cohesion. Annu Rev Cell Dev Biol 2001; 17: 753–77.

86. Prieto I, Tease C, Pezzi N et al. Cohesin component dynamics during meiotic prophase I in mammalian oocytes. Chromosome Res 2004; 12: 197–213.

87. Terret ME, Wassmann K, Waizenegger I et al. The meiosis I-to-meiosis II transition in mouse oocytes requires separase activity. Curr Biol 2003; 13: 1797–802.

88. Herbert M, Levasseur M, Homer H et al. Homologue disjunction in mouse oocytes requires proteolysis of securin and cyclin B1. Nat Cell Biol 2003; 5: 1023–5.

89. Mailhes JB, Hilliard C, Fuseler JW et al. Okadaic acid, an inhibitor of protein phosphatase 1 and 2A, induces premature separation of sister chromatids during meiosis I and aneuploidy in mouse oocytes in vitro. Chromosome Res 2003; 11: 619–31.

90. Sakashita G, Shima H, Komatsu M et al. Regulation of type 1 protein phosphatase/inhibitor-2 complex by glycogen synthase kinase-3β in intact cells. J Biochem 2003; 133: 165–71.

91. Madgwick S, Nixon VL, Chang HY et al. Maintenance of sister chromatid attachment in mouse eggs through maturation-promoting factor activity. Devel Biol 2004; 275: 68–81.

92. Maro B, Johnson M, Webb M et al. Mechanism of polar body formation in the mouse oocytes: an interaction between the chromosomes, the cytoskeleton and the plasma membrane. J Embry Exp Morphol 1986; 92: 11–32.

93. Maro B, Verlhac M. Polar body formation: new rules for asymetric divisions. Nat Cell Biol 2002; 4: E281–3.

94. Leader B, Lim H, Carabatsos MJ et al. Formin-2, polyploidy, hypofertility and positioning of the meiotic spindle in mouse oocytes. Nat Cell Biol 2002; 4: 921–8.

95. Verlhac M-H, Lefebvre C, Guillaud P et al. Asymmetric division in mouse oocytes: with or without Mos. Curr Biol 2000; 10: 1303–6.

96. Simerly C, Nowak G, de Lanerolle P et al. Differential expression and functions of cortical myosin IIA and IIB isotypes during meiotic maturation, fertilization, and mitosis in mouse oocytes and embryos. Mol Biol Cell 1998; 9: 2509–25.

97. Kubiak JZ, Weber M, de Pennart H et al. The metaphase II arrest in mouse oocytes is controlled through microtubule-dependent destruc-

tion of cyclin B in the presence of CSF. Embo J 1993; 12: 3773–8.

98. Kikuchi K, Izaike Y, Noguchi J et al. Decrease of histone H1 kinase activity in relation to parthenogenetic activation of pig follicular oocytes matured and aged *in vitro*. J Reprod Fertil 1995; 105: 325–30.

99. Sagata N. What does mos do in oocytes and somatic cells? Bioessays 1997; 19: 13–21.

100. Colledge WH, Carlton MB, Udy GB et al. Disruption of c-mos causes parthenogenetic development of unfertilized mouse eggs. Nature 1994; 370: 65–8.

101. Gordo AC, He CL, Smith S et al. Mitogen activated protein kinase plays a significant role in metaphase II arrest, spindle morphology, and maintenance of maturation promoting factor activity in bovine oocytes. Mol Reprod Dev 2001; 59: 106–14.

102. Tatemoto H, Muto N. Mitogen-activated protein kinase regulates normal transition from metaphase to interphase following parthenogenetic activation in porcine oocytes. Zygote 2001; 9: 15–23.

103. Minshull J, Sun H, Tonks NK et al. A MAP kinase-dependent spindle assembly checkpoint in *Xenopus* egg extracts. Cell 1994; 79: 475–86.

CHAPTER 6

Epigenetic modification during oocyte growth and maturation

Amanda L Fortier and Jacquetta M Trasler

INTRODUCTION

The growth and maturation of the oocyte is a complex and highly regulated process. An important aspect of oocyte maturation is the establishment of the correct epigenetic status. 'Epigenetics' refers to processes such as DNA methylation or histone modifications that regulate gene activity without affecting the actual DNA sequence, but are heritable through cell division. The epigenetic state of the male and female germ cells is not equivalent; this was first discovered as a result of ingenious nuclear transplantation experiments carried out in the mid 1980s demonstrating that uniparental embryos are not viable[1,2]. Subsequently, a subset of mammalian genes was found to be subject to genomic imprinting. Importantly, a number of imprinted genes are essential for fetal growth and development, including the functioning of the placenta. These genes are expressed in a parent-of-origin specific manner, as a result of the different epigenetic profiles acquired by imprinted genes during male and female gametogenesis. The best characterized epigenetic modification is the methylation of cytosine residues in DNA, which is involved in establishing genomic imprints in the germ line. This establishment occurs during the growth phase of oocyte development, and is beginning to be elucidated in greater detail. In recent years, increased concern has been focused on the potential for epigenetic dysregulation as a result of early embryo culture and assisted reproductive technologies[3,4].

Several recent reports have suggested that there might be an increased occurrence of the imprinting disorders Beckwith–Weidemann syndrome[5-8] and Angelman syndrome[9,10] in children conceived by in-vitro fertilization (IVF) or intracytoplasmic sperm injection (ICSI). Of particular interest is the fact that the described cases are almost all the result of maternal DNA methylation defects. These cases highlight the need for further study of the possible mechanisms of epigenetic dysregulation during assisted reproduction. In-vitro maturation and IVF raise concerns due to the prolonged exposure of the oocyte and early embryo to culture conditions and the use of exogenous gonadotropins. However, there may also be epigenetic causes for infertility in patients undergoing assisted reproductive technologies (ARTs). This chapter will review our current knowledge of the epigenetic modifications that occur in developing female germ cells including the erasure and establishment of methylation imprints, the aspects of current

ARTs, and the conditions they are designed to treat (i.e. infertility) that may perturb or reveal imprinting defects and suggest further studies that are required in this area.

DYNAMICS AND TIMING OF EPIGENETIC CHANGES IN THE OOCYTE

The oocyte undergoes many well-defined epigenetic changes during its growth and maturation. Levels of DNA methylation decrease in the primordial germ cells, which will give rise to the oocytes, as they migrate into the genital ridge. Following this period, methylation of a class of genes, referred to as imprinted genes, must be acquired in order to direct the expression of these genes from a single allele. The functional non-equivalence of the male and female germ lines was first discovered based on the results of nuclear transfer experiments in which uniparental embryos failed to develop normally[1,2]. Androgenetic mouse embryos created by the combination of two male pronuclei, hence lacking any maternal contribution, give rise to well-developed extraembryonic tissues with poor embryonic development. In contrast, gynogenetic embryos (containing two maternal pronuclei and no paternal contribution) or parthenogenetic mouse embryos derived by the activation of oocytes develop, at least for a short period, as relatively normal embryos, but have rather poor development of the extraembryonic tissues. Based on these studies, it was proposed that genes expressed from the paternal genome direct development of the extraembryonic tissues, in order to ensure optimal nutrient exchange in support of the developing embryo. In contrast, the maternal genome expresses genes that are involved in the development of the embryo proper. These observations led to the well-known 'conflict hypothesis' of genomic imprinting[11,12]. This hypothesis proposes that the paternal genome evolved in such a way that

genes are expressed to favor the optimal use of maternal resources in order to maximize fetal growth and development, while the maternal genome attempts to limit the investment in fetal growth to reserve resources for future pregnancies. Since the initial studies involving uniparental embryos, a subset of genes has been discovered that is expressed from a single allele only, depending on whether the gene is inherited on the maternally or paternally derived chromosome. The phenomenon leading to this uniparental expression is known as genomic imprinting.

Genomic imprinting is controlled by epigenetic means, as DNA sequence alone cannot distinguish between parental alleles or control allele-specific expression of genes. DNA methylation plays an important role in genomic imprinting, through the differential methylation of the parental alleles. Genomic imprinting is also associated with histone modifications, antisense transcripts, and non-coding RNAs, although the mechanisms are not well understood. As such, this chapter will concentrate on the role of DNA methylation in the oocyte.

Erasure of DNA methylation imprints in the mouse model system

The germ line arises from the migration of primordial germ cells into the genital ridge. The primordial germ cells appear to be marked by normal somatic DNA methylation patterns when they begin their migration, however these cells undergo widespread DNA demethylation around embryonic day (E) 10.5, as they migrate into the genital ridge. The earliest studies examining DNA methylation in the germ line used methylation-sensitive restriction enzymes together with Southern blotting or polymerase chain reaction (PCR). The results of these studies suggested that the primordial germ cell genome is completely demethylated by E13.5[13–16]. More recently, bisulfite sequencing has been used to further characterize the methylation status at various stages (Figure 6.1a). The methylation status of several imprinted genes has been examined, these include *H19*, *Snrpn*, *Peg3*, *Kcnq1ot1* (also named *Lit1*), *Igf2*, *Gtl2*, and *Rasgfr1*, as well as non-imprinted gene sequences such as α-*actin* and *my1C*[17,18]. These studies indicated that imprinted and non-imprinted single copy genes become completely demethylated between E10.5 and E13.5. Intriguingly, similar studies examining the methylation status of some repeat sequences, including long interspersed nuclear element 1 (LINE1), intracisternal A particle (IAP), and minor satellite sequences, found that these repetitive sequences are only partially demethylated in the primordial germ cell population[17,19–21] (Figure 6.2).

Analysis of gene expression has also been undertaken to examine the progress of epigenetic reprogramming in the germ line (Figure 6.1b). In primordial germ cells, monoallelic expression of imprinted genes would be expected prior to the erasure of methylation imprints. At E9.5, monoallelic expression of four imprinted genes was detected[19]. As development progressed, biallelic expression of *Snrpn* (E10.5) and of *H19* and *Igf2* (E11.5) was detected. Analysis of embryos generated by somatic cell nuclear transfer using nuclei from primordial germ cells isolated from mice at various gestational ages has also pointed to demethylation of the genome in primordial germ cells between E10.5 and E12.5[22,23].

Taken together, these results indicate that single copy genes, both imprinted and non-imprinted, undergo a rapid, and perhaps active, demethylation as the primordial germ cells migrate into the genital ridge. Repetitive sequences do not appear to be subject to the same complete demethylation process, but do undergo a partial demethylation during the same period. As a result of DNA demethylation, evidence to date suggests that the primordial germ cells of both sexes are epigenetically equivalent by E13.5[17,18,22,24].

Maternal imprint establishment

Initial studies in mice examining a few CpG sites in the endogenous imprinted gene *Igf2r*[25–27] and the imprinted transgenes *RSVIgmyc* and *MPA434*[14,28] first suggested that maternal imprints are acquired during oocyte growth. Further support for the functional importance of DNA methylation occurring during oocyte growth came from nuclear transplantation studies in which parthenogenetic embryos containing one genome from a neonate-derived non-growing oocyte and the other genome from a fully grown oocyte developed to E13.5, 3 days longer than normal parthenogenotes (in which both genomes were derived from fully grown oocytes,[27] Figure 6.3b). In these experiments, immature, non-growing oocytes were collected from mice at postnatal day 1, and these oocytes were fused to enucleated germinal vesicle (GV)-stage oocytes in order to provide the correct cytoplasmic environment for the fused oocytes to proceed to the metaphase (MII) stage. The chromosomes of the fused oocytes were then transferred to mature ovulated MII stage oocytes (whose nuclear material was removed) and the resulting parthenogenetic embryos were allowed to develop in pseudopregnant recipient mice[27,29] (Figure 6.3b). These embryos contained only one set of maternally imprinted chromosomes from the fully grown MII oocyte, and one set of chromosomes without any maternal imprint, from the non-growing oocyte. Expression studies in the resulting parthenogenetic embryos, made possible due to single nucleotide polymorphisms between the strains used (Figure 6.1b), confirmed that the paternally expressed genes *Snrpn*, *Peg1*, and *Peg3*, which are not normally expressed from the maternal genome, were expressed from the genome derived from the non-growing oocyte[29], whereas they were not expressed from the genome of the fully grown oocyte. This result suggests that primary maternal imprints are not yet established in immature non-growing oocytes.

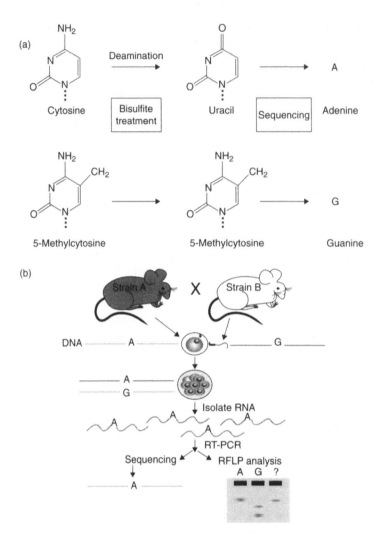

Figure 6.1 Schematic representation of techniques used to assess CpG methylation and allele-specific expression of imprinted genes in the mouse model. (a) Principle of bisulfite sequencing. DNA is treated with sodium bisulfite, resulting in a deamination of all non-methylated cytosine residues to uracil. 5-Methylcytosine residues are not modified in this reaction. Sequencing of the bisulfite-treated DNA allows for the identification of methylated and unmethylated cytosines within the region under study. (b) The presence of single nucleotide polymorphisms (SNPs) allows for identification of alleles that are transcribed. Two different strains are mated, with known sequence variants at imprinted genes. RNA is collected from the resulting embryo, and gene-specific RT-PCR is carried out. The resulting cDNA product can be sequenced to identify the relative proportion of the parental alleles present. Alternatively, if the SNP generates or abolishes a recognition site for a restriction enzyme, the relative contribution of parental alleles may be assessed using restriction enzyme digestion followed by electrophoretic separation. RT-PCR: reverse transcription–polymerase chain reaction; RFLP: restriction fragment length polymorphism; ?: test sample

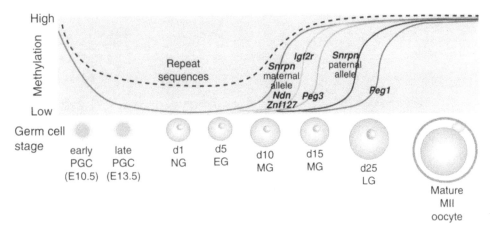

Figure 6.2 Methylation dynamics of imprinted genes and repeat sequences during female germ line development. The lower panel illustrates the stages of germ cell development shown in the top panel. The top panel illustrates the methylation dynamics of imprinted genes in the developing oocyte, beginning with the demethylation of imprinted and single copy genes in the primordial germ cells (red line). At this early stage, repeat sequences are not demethylated to the same extent as the single copy genes (dotted line). During oocyte growth, single copy genes become hypermethylated throughout the growth stages. Imprints are established asynchronously in the oocyte, with the latest imprints being established in the late growing stages. PGC: primordial germ cell; NG: non-growing oocyte; EG: early growing oocyte; MG: mid growth oocyte; LG: late growing oocyte; MII: metaphase II. Adapted from references 4 and 32 (see color plate section)

However, the resulting parthenogenotes could not develop to term, likely due to the absence of paternal imprints, since the nongrowing oocyte genome would, along with the genome from the fully grown oocyte, express those genes that are normally maternally expressed (paternally imprinted), resulting in a double dose of these genes. This possibility was supported by expression analysis that revealed expression of *H19* and coordinate repression of *Igf2*, which shares a differentially methylated domain with *H19*, from the non-growing oocyte genome[29]. The result would be biallelic expression of *H19* and loss of *Igf2* expression in the parthenogenotes. This led the authors to repeat this experiment with non-growing oocytes from mice carrying a large deletion of the *H19* gene as well as the differentially methylated domain between *H19* and *Igf2*, which were then used for nuclear transfer to mature MII oocytes. As a result, two live born parthenogenetic pups were obtained, with a marked normalization in expression of most imprinted genes examined[30]. One of these pups was allowed to develop to adulthood, and even went on to produce offspring. This experiment demonstrated that limited parthenogenetic development is possible in the mouse provided that imprinted gene expression is appropriately controlled. This was, however, only possible with large deletions of an imprinted gene region. It is important to note that this experiment had a very low success rate, as 371 morulae were transferred to pseudopregnant females, but only two pups survived to birth. Clearly, many questions remain to be answered about parthenogenesis and the relative importance of imprinted genes in normal development.

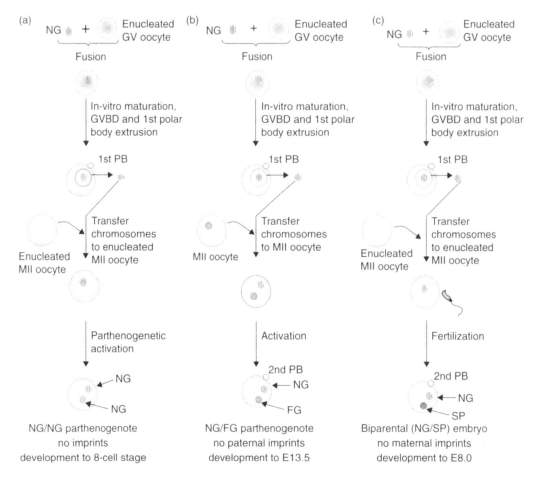

Figure 6.3 Schematic representation of nuclear transfer experiments revealing the developmental potential of oocytes at different stages of growth and maturation. Non-growing oocytes have not established maternal imprints (pink hatched nuclei). (a) When non-growing oocytes are used in nuclear transfer experiments followed by parthenogenetic activation of the oocyte, development stalls at the 8-cell stage. (b) When the nucleus of a non-growing oocyte is transferred to a mature MII oocyte which retains its nucleus (red nucleus) development proceeds to E13.5. (c) When the nucleus of a non-growing oocyte is transferred to an enucleated MII oocyte and fertilized with a normal spermatozoon (blue nucleus) development stalls at E8.0. NG: non-growing oocyte; GV: germinal vesicle stage oocyte; PB: polar body; MII: metaphase II; FG: fully grown (mature) oocyte; SP: sperm. Adapted from references 27 and 29 (see color plate section)

In other nuclear transplantation experiments, when the genomes from postnatal day 1 non-growing oocytes were transferred to enucleated MII oocytes, followed by parthenogenetic activation (ng/ng parthenogenetic embryos), devel-opment stalled at the eight-cell stage[27] (Figure 6.3a). In these parthenogenotes, no methylation imprints were present at all. In the absence of any methylation imprints, embryonic development cannot proceed to the blastocyst stage, possibly due to problems in early cell specification. When non-growing oocytes were transferred to enucleated MII oocytes and fertilized in vitro (ng/sp embryos), development proceeded to about E8.0 (Figure 6.3c). In this case, paternal methylation imprints would be present, whereas maternal imprints would not. These embryos are not equivalent to androgenotes, as they only have one paternally imprinted set of chromosomes. Development of these embryos to E8.0 suggests that maternal imprints are required for postimplantation development, and there is some evidence that cell type specification is disrupted as early as the blastocyst stage[27].

The nuclear transplantation experiments established that maternal methylation imprints are not present in early non-growing oocytes, but are present in mature MII oocytes. In order to determine the time period during which these methylation imprints are established, embryos were generated by nuclear transfer using the genomes from oocytes isolated at different days of postnatal development paired with genomes from fully grown oocytes. These embryos were used to examine maternal imprint establishment by detection of transcripts that are normally paternally expressed[31]. Loss of expression of the paternally expressed genes examined was interpreted as indicating the establishment of the maternal methylation imprint. Embryos constructed with the nuclei of the earliest non-growing oocytes, isolated from postnatal day 1 ovaries, expressed all of the genes that are normally only expressed from the paternal genome[31]. Embryos constructed with postnatal day 5 oocyte genomes were beginning to exhibit loss of expression of *Snrpn*, *Znf127*, and *Ndn*, whereas those constructed with genomes from oocytes from postnatal day 10 ovaries began to exhibit loss of *Peg3* expression, while *Snrpn*, *Znf127*, and *Ndn* expression was completely lost in most of the samples. When genomes isolated from oocytes in mid-growth (postnatal day 15) were used, loss of *Peg1* expression was observed in some embryos, and once oocytes that had

reached the fully grown stage in postnatal day 20 mice were used, imprints had been established at all paternally expressed genes in the resulting embryos[31] (Figure 6.2).

At the molecular level, bisulfite sequencing has been used to characterize the acquisition of DNA methylation imprints in oocytes at different stages of oocyte growth[32,33]. For these experiments, oocytes of increasingly larger sizes were isolated from ovaries collected at postnatal days 1, 5, 10, 15, and 25, similar to the experiments described above. Bisulfite sequencing (Figure 6.1a) was used to examine the methylation status of differentially methylated regions (DMRs) of four paternally expressed genes, *Snrpn*, *Igf2r*, *Peg1*, and *Peg3*. The results of this study indicated that imprint establishment occurred in a gene-specific manner, with *Snrpn* acquiring methylation first, followed by *Igf2r* and *Peg3*, while *Peg1* acquired the methylation imprint very rapidly in the latest stages of oocyte growth[32] (Figure 6.2). Importantly, this study also reports that the acquisition of the methylation imprint at the *Snrpn* DMR is related to oocyte diameter rather than specifically to the age of the female mouse. Oocytes isolated from postnatal day 15 ovaries were sized and the methylation status of the *Snrpn* DMR was assessed by bisulfite sequencing. In oocytes with diameters of 20–50 μm *Snrpn* was largely unmethylated, while in oocytes with diameters of 60–80 μm *Snrpn* was largely methylated[32].

Taken together, the nuclear transfer and bisulfite sequencing studies reveal that DNA methylation imprints are acquired progressively during the entire oocyte growth phase, as follicles progress from the primary to the antral stage. Interestingly, the methylation of specific genes is established at different stages in oocyte growth, with methylation of the genes examined being completed by the time oocytes arrest in MII (Figure 6.2). The difference in timing of imprint acquisition may be related to the different chromosomal locations of the imprinted gene clusters[32]. The relationship between oocyte size and methylation imprints could indicate that imprint establishment requires the accumulation of proteins involved in the enzymatic process; in support of this hypothesis, the expression of the DNA methyltransferase genes *Dnmt3a*, *Dnmt3b*, and *Dnmt3L* peaked in oocytes from postnatal day 15 ovaries[32].

Additionally, it was found that for at least one locus, the *Snrpn* gene, the methylation imprint is first established on the maternal allele, and is only acquired later on the paternal allele[32]. This indicates that the alleles are not equivalent following erasure (Figure 6.2). It is perhaps methylation at other sites that were not examined or differences in chromatin structure that mark the different parental alleles, and then direct the establishment of methylation imprints[32]. Further studies will be required to ascertain if all methylation imprints are established preferentially on one allele before the other, and if chromatin structure plays a role in maintaining the identity of the alleles in the absence of methylation.

Given that methylation imprints appear to be established asynchronously, with certain imprints not being established until late in oocyte growth, it is possible that certain methylation imprints are more susceptible to perturbation as a result of ARTs. The susceptibility of different loci to disruption will also require further study.

Studies in humans and other animals

Due to ethical limitations, little has been done to examine imprint establishment in human oocytes. It is known that parthenogenetic embryos do not develop in vivo, but are the cause of ovarian teratomas[34]. The establishment of a single maternal methylation imprint at the human *SNRPN* DMR has been examined using bisulfite sequencing. In an early study, using unfertilized oocytes from a fertility center, the *SNRPN* DMR was found to be largely unmethylated in aspirated oocytes[35], leading the authors to suggest that the *SNRPN* methylation imprint is established after fertilization. A later study

was conducted using GV-stage, metaphase I (MI) and MII oocytes that were unsuitable for transfer and were donated by patients for research purposes[36]. The *SNRPN* DMR was found to be highly methylated in GV stage oocytes, and the methylation was maintained in more mature oocytes. The results of this second study fit well with the data from the mouse, however more studies are required to clarify the timing of imprint establishment in human oocytes.

Hydatidiform moles are a common cause of gestational trophoblastic disease in women. Complete hydatidiform moles usually result from androgenetic pregnancies, and are marked by a complete lack of fetal tissue. An inherited form of complete hydatidiform molar pregnancy has been described, in which the resultant moles are phenotypically indistinguishable from the androgenetic complete hydatidiform moles, but on further genetic examination the moles are found to be biparental in origin[37]. Based on the recurrent, heritable incidence of biparental complete hydatidiform moles, as well as recurrence in women who have changed sexual partners, it was hypothesized that these biparental complete hydatidiform moles are the result of a defect in the maternal germ line[38]. Examination of the methylation status of several characterized imprinted gene DMRs was undertaken using bisulfite sequencing. Based on a limited number of clones, it appears that the maternal methylation imprint is absent in biparental complete hydatidiform moles[38]. These embryos are genomically equivalent to the ng/sp embryos generated by Kono et al.[27], where the genome of a non-growing oocyte lacking all methylation imprints was fertilized by a normal sperm nucleus. In the mouse, these embryos develop to approximately E8.0 with apparent developmental delay followed by embryonic loss[27]. Human biparental complete hydatidiform moles also fail to develop normally, with the human phenotype being much more severe than in the mouse, as there is an apparent lack of fetal tissue with expansive extraembryonic tissue[37].

The methylation status of four imprinted genes has been examined in tissues isolated from four different biparental complete hydatidiform moles, and the methylation patterns were found to be abnormal[39]. In particular, the genes that were normally maternally methylated showed a decrease in methylation and as a result were more like the paternal allele. Variability in the amount of hypomethylation was also observed between moles[39]. In contrast, the methylation status of imprinted genes was found to be normal in the somatic tissue of two women with recurrent biparental complete hydatidiform molar pregnancies[40], and thus the abnormal epigenotype of their molar pregnancies did not arise due to a general loss of methylation in all the mothers' cells. The studies conducted to date have not been able to identify whether the abnormal methylation pattern arose in the maternal germ line or after fertilization, as the moles studied were all from 6 weeks of gestation or later[40]. Judson et al.[38] have hypothesized that the underlying cause of familial recurrent biparental complete hydatidiform moles is a maternal germ line defect in which maternal imprints are not established. This is one possibility, although mutations in the known DNMT genes have been ruled out as causative in the familial biparental hydatidiform moles[41], implying that an as-of-yet unknown enzyme or protein is involved in the genesis of this disorder. El-Maarri et al.[40] proposed that the trophoblastic identity of the cells in complete hydatidiform moles may contribute to changes in methylation, as it has previously been shown that methylation is not strictly maintained in the placenta as it is in the embryonic compartment[42]. Clearly, more studies are required to determine the causation of familial recurrent biparental complete hydatidiform molar pregnancies.

The establishment of maternal imprints in oocytes has not been directly studied in other animal models. The majority of work has focused on techniques for parthenogenetic activation in vitro. Attempts have been made to generate parthenogenetic sheep, however these embryos die shortly after implantation and are growth retarded[43], while gynogenotes appear to develop normally at least to day 21 (implantation occurs between days 23 and 25 in sheep)[44]. However, later stages were not examined. Attempts have also been made to generate parthenogenetic marmoset monkeys[45]. These parthenogenotes developed to implantation but postimplantation development was limited.

THE DNA METHYLTRANSFERASES ARE INVOLVED IN ESTABLISHING METHYLATION IMPRINTS

As discussed above, methylation of important DNA sequences such as imprinted genes must be acquired during oogenesis to ensure proper gene expression in the embryo. The DNA methyltransferases (DNMTs) are currently the best-characterized enzymes involved in epigenetic reprogramming. The DNMTs catalyze a reaction in which a methyl group is transferred from the donor cofactor S-adenosylmethionine (SAM) to the 5′ carbon of a cytosine ring, resulting in 5-methylcytosine. In mammals, three families of DNMTs have been identified; these are grouped together based on sequence similarities in their C-terminal catalytic domains[46]. The DNMTs identified to date include DNMT1, which is the major DNMT in the mammalian system, as well as DNMT2[47], DNMT3a, DNMT3b[48], and DNMT3L[49,50]. The expression and activity of the DNMTs are summarized in Figure 6.4.

DNMT1

Mouse studies

DNMT1 has been assigned a role in maintenance methylation, based on early studies showing that this enzyme has a higher affinity for hemimethylated DNA than unmethylated DNA[51,52]. Three isoforms of *Dnmt1* transcripts have been

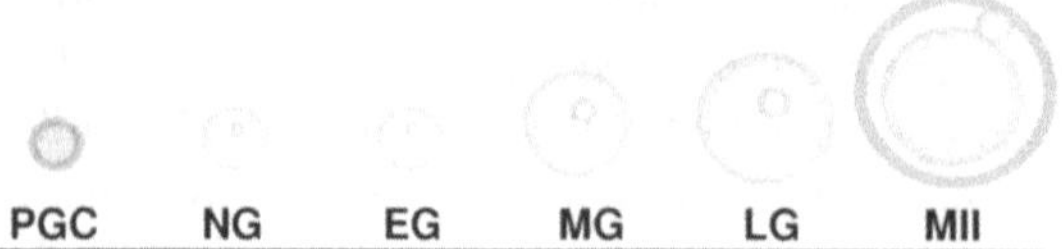

	PGC	NG	EG	MG	LG	MII
DNMT1	+	+	–	–	–	–
	maintenance methylation of repeat sequences					
DNMT1o	–	–	+	+	+	+
			cytoplasmic localization, no methylation activity			
DNMT3a	+	+	+	+	+	+
		de novo methylation – establishment of maternal imprints				
DNMT3b	+	+	+	+	+	+
		methylation of repeat sequences and chromosome stability				
DNMT3L	+	+	+	+	+	+
		de novo methylation – establishment of maternal imprints				

Figure 6.4 Summary of DNA methyltransferase (DNMT) expression and activity in the female germ line of the mouse. In the figure, (+) indicates that either transcript or protein expression has been detected at the stage indicated while (–) indicates that expression has not been detected to date. PGC: primordial germ cell; NG: non-growing oocyte; EG: early growing oocyte; MG: midgrowth oocyte; LG: late growing oocyte; MII: metaphase II oocyte

identified that use sex-specific first exons. *Dnmt1s* encodes the full-length protein that is expressed in somatic cells; *Dnmt1o* encodes an oocyte specific form of the protein, which lacks the first N-terminal 118 amino acids; while an untranslated isoform is generated in pachytene spermatocytes (*Dnmt1p*)[53,54]. During embryonic development, DNMT1 has been detected in primordial germ cells at E11.5 and remains strongly expressed until E13.5, at a time when methylation imprints are being erased, after which it decreases as cells enter meiotic prophase[17,55]. It has been suggested that during this stage of development, DNMT1 may be important for maintaining the methylation of repetitive elements, which do not undergo genome-wide demethylation to the same extent as imprinted genes. DNMT1o has been identified as the sole form of the protein that is present in the postnatal oocyte and the preimplantation embryo[54,56,57]. Detailed expression analysis revealed that DNMT1o is excluded from the oocyte nucleus after the early growing stage, and appears to be actively retained in the cortical region until the eight-cell stage postfertilization, when it enters the nucleus transiently, exiting by the 16-cell stage[54]. Based on this observation, it was postulated that oocytes must protect their meiotic chromosomes from inappropriate de novo methylation, raising the suggestion that DNMT1 may not act exclusively as a maintenance methyltransferase[54]. The ability of DNMT1 to act as a de novo methyltransferase in vivo remains to be determined.

To further examine the role of DNMT1o, the oocyte-specific isoform was deleted (knocked out) using gene targeting[56]. Male and female homozygous DNMT1o-deficient mice were obtained and appeared phenotypically normal, but the female mice were infertile. Characterization of this infertility revealed that the *Dnmt1o* knockout acts as a maternal effect lethal, where embryos derived from oocytes lacking DNMT1o rarely survive to birth[56]. Analysis of global methylation in embryos from homozygous null female mice revealed that the genome was normally methylated, including repeat regions and single copy sequences. Also, analysis of methylation of the 5′ region of *Snrpn* in oocytes collected from DNMT1o-null females demonstrated that imprints were properly acquired in the oocyte. In contrast, analysis of the embryos derived from such oocytes uncovered a non-stochastic loss of methylation on half of the normally imprinted alleles[56]. Intriguingly, this occurred for genes that received their imprints from the maternal as well as from the paternal germ line, implicating a defect in maintenance methylation at one stage of preimplantation development, the eight-cell stage. Thus, methylation imprints were properly established in the absence of DNMT1o, ruling it out as the primary de novo DNMT responsible for establishing maternal imprints in the oocyte.

Studies in humans and other animals

The *DNMT1* gene is conserved among chordates (reviewed in Goll and Bestor[46]). *DNMT1o* transcripts have been detected in human[41,58] and opposum oocytes[59], but have not been detected in bovine oocytes[60]. To date, mutations of the *DNMT1* gene have not been associated with any human disorders.

DNMT3a and DNMT3b

Two functional DNMTs have been identified in the DNMT3 family. These enzymes are more closely related to DNMTs across many species[46,61]. Members of the DNMT3 family appear to act primarily as de novo DNMTs[48]. Based on gene targeting experiments, DNMT3a and DNMT3b also appear to have discrete functions[62].

Mouse studies

As mentioned earlier, *Dnmt3a* expression peaks in growing oocytes and coincides with the time of acquisition of maternal methylation[32]. Two different splice variants of *Dnmt3a* have been identified, *Dnmt3a* and *Dnmt3a2*[63]. *Dnmt3a* encodes the full-length protein that was initially characterized and is known to have methyltransferase activity[48], while *Dnmt3a2* encodes a form of the protein that lacks 219 amino acids at the N-terminus while retaining similar methylation activity in vitro[63]. In vivo, *Dnmt3a* transcripts are ubiquitously expressed, while *Dnmt3a2* transcripts are detected in a tissue-restricted manner, specifically in cells known to undergo de novo methylation such as testis, ovary, spleen, and thymus[64]. *Dnmt3a2* transcripts are detected at slightly higher levels than *Dnmt3a* transcripts in whole ovaries at postnatal day 12, a time period when waves of oocyte growth and de novo methylation are occurring[64]. Interestingly, DNMT3a2 has been shown to localize specifically to euchromatin while DNMT3a localizes to heterochromatin[63]. Based on these pieces of information, DNMT3a2 may be involved in de novo methylation of single copy sequences. When *Dnmt3a* is knocked out in mice, the homozygous null animals develop to term and appear normal at birth, however they die at about 4 weeks of age[62]. Methylation in the homozygous null animals appears to be normal[62], indicating that another protein must compensate or cooperate with DNMT3A in vivo. To determine if loss of *Dnmt3a* specifically in the germ line resulted in a reproductive phenotype, a conditional allele was generated[65]. When *Dnmt3a* was removed from the germ line only, the mice were viable and reached adulthood, but when the germ line *Dnmt3a*-null female mice were crossed to wild-type males, no live pups were obtained[65]. Further examination revealed an embryonic lethal phenotype by E10.5, which must be due to a maternal effect as the males would contribute a normal *Dnmt3a* gene to the embryos[65]. In addition, maternal methylation imprints were not established, and gene expression of imprinted genes was dysregulated in the E10.5 embryos derived from mutant mothers[65]. Thus, DNMT3a is one of the key enzymes needed for the acquisition of maternal methylation imprints in oocytes.

One of the multiple isoforms of *Dnmt3b* likely can compensate for some of the functions of DNMT3a in its absence, as it has been shown that DNMT3a and DNMT3b have distinct functions in gene targeting experiments[62]. Six different isoforms of *Dnmt3b* have been identified to date, and all of the isoforms show different tissue-specific expression patterns[48,63,66,67]. *Dnmt3b1* and *Dnmt3b2* transcripts have been detected in the female germ line, however DNMT3b2 is the only functional isoform in the adult ovary and is therefore more likely to be important for de novo methylation in the oocyte[64]. *Dnmt3b2* and *Dnmt3b3* transcripts are both highly expressed in cells undergoing de novo methylation (testis, ovary, spleen, thymus, and liver), however DNMT3b3 appears to be unable to transfer methyl groups despite its ability to bind DNA[48,68,69]. As a result, it has been suggested that DNMT3b1 and DNMT3b2 may act as de novo methyltransferases while DNMT3b3 and possibly DNMT3b6 may be involved in regulating methylation[63]. *Dnmt3b* has been knocked out in mice, resulting in embryonic lethality[62]. Also, in homozygous null embryos recovered prior to E9.5, undermethylation of C-type retroviral sequences and IAP sequences was observed, suggesting that DNMT3b may be involved in the methylation of a subset of minor satellite repeats[62]. Again, to determine if loss of *Dnmt3b* specifically in the germ line caused a phenotype, a conditional allele was generated[65]. When *Dnmt3b* was removed from the germ line only, the mice were viable and reached adulthood, and live pups were obtained from matings of the DNMT3b-null females to wild-type males[65]. Methylation of the sequences examined was not affected in the offspring of mutant animals. These data suggest that DNMT3b is not essential for the establishment of maternal imprints, while the association of *DNMT3B* mutations with a human disease with severe chromosome instability (see below) suggests that DNMT3b is important for

maintaining chromosome stability by ensuring methylation of repeat sequences.

Studies in humans and other animals

The human *DNMT3* genes are highly homologous to the mouse *Dnmt3* genes[66]. In addition, the same genomic organization and use of transcript variants have also been observed for the human *DNMT3* genes[63,66,69]. *DNMT3A* appears to be ubiquitously expressed, while *DNMT3B* is detected at lower levels in the tissues examined, including testis and ovary[66]. In human oocytes, *DNMT3A* and at least two splice variants of *DNMT3B* are developmentally regulated[58]. Similarly, *DNMT3A* and *DNMT3B* have also been detected in fetal and adult ovaries in the bovine model[60].

Mutations in the human *DNMT3B* gene are associated with human disease, and to date this is the only DNMT known to be causative of human disease when mutated. Various mutations of the *DNMT3B* gene are associated with the genetic disorder known as immunodeficiency, centromeric instability, and facial anomalies (ICF) syndrome[67,70]. Among patients with ICF syndrome, cytogenetic abnormalities at centromeric regions of chromosomes 1, 9, and 16 occur due to a loss of methylation on the satellite DNA in these areas[71]. Interestingly, none of the patients are homozygous for null mutations of *DNMT3B*, suggesting that loss of DNMT3B function may be lethal in humans, as it is in mice[62]. These results also support the hypothesis that DNMT3B specifically methylates certain repeat sequences including satellite repeats.

DNMT3L

Mouse studies

Dnmt3L was identified based on sequence similarity to the *Dnmt3* family[49]. Characterization of the genomic organization of the gene revealed that it lacks the catalytic domain, thus it does not likely act as a cytosine methyltransferase[49]. An in-vitro assay confirmed that DNMT3L appears to lack the ability to methylate DNA[72]. Levels of *Dnmt3L* are low in the female embryonic gonad, and expression peaks in the postnatal ovary[55,64]. High levels of *Dnmt3L* coincide with oocyte growth which suggests a role in maternal imprint establishment[55]. In support of this hypothesis, when *Dnmt3L* was knocked out in mice, oogenesis appeared normal but the deficiency acted as a maternal effect lethal with embryos of homozygous null female mice dying by E9.5 with abnormalities in extraembryonic tissues[50,72]. Analysis of genome wide methylation revealed that global methylation levels appeared normal, but bisulfite sequencing revealed a loss of maternal, but not paternal methylation imprints[50,72]. Since DNMT3L lacks methyltransferase activity, it cannot be solely responsible for establishing the methylation imprints. Co-immunoprecipitation and co-immunolocalization experiments demonstrate that DNMT3L can form a complex with DNMT3a and DNMT3b in vivo[72], suggesting that DNMT3L may be involved in targeting active methyltransferases to imprinted genes in order to establish the methylation imprints in the oocyte.

Studies in humans and other animals

DNMT3L expression has been detected in human testis, ovary, and thymus[49], as well as in preimplantation embryos; however, DNMT3L has not been detected in isolated human oocytes[58]. These differences suggest that there may be differences in maternal imprint establishment between mouse and human oocytes; however, further studies are required.

EPIGENETICS IN ASSISTED REPRODUCTION: QUESTIONS AND CONCERNS

As the number of children born as a result of assisted reproduction increases, there are several aspects of these technologies which are a cause for concern with respect to epigenetic abnormalities. Among these, the association of epigenetic abnormalities with infertility, the impact of aging on epigenetics in the oocyte, the administration of exogenous gonadotropins, and the exposure of both immature oocytes and preimplantation embryos to in-vitro culture are beginning to be acknowledged as possible inducers of epigenetic dysregulation.

Aging oocytes as a cause of infertility

Fertility rates decline rapidly as women enter the fourth decade of life. This decrease in fertility has often been attributed to the loss of the ovarian reserve throughout the reproductive period. The effect of aging on oocyte quality has also been suggested as a reason for the decreasing fertility rates in older women. A single study has examined gene expression in aging oocytes of mice[73]. This study employed carefully designed microarray experiments to compare pooled oocytes from young mice (5–6 weeks) and from mice nearing the end of their reproductive span (42–45 weeks). Of note, this study found significant decreases in the levels of *Dnmt1o*, *Dnmt1s*, and *Dnmt3L*, and a significant increase in the expression of *Dnmt3b* in older oocytes collected from mice nearing the end of their reproductive lives. This result, while not providing direct evidence of epigenetic dysregulation, suggests that studies are required to examine the effect of aging on the epigenetics of oocytes.

Ovulation induction with gonadotropins

Gonadotropins are often used to stimulate the development and ovulation of multiple oocytes for assisted reproduction. The concern has been raised that this procedure may force oocytes to go through the final growth and maturation process too rapidly or rescue oocytes that might normally undergo atresia, and as a result oocytes may be of lower quality, or methylation imprints may not be properly established in all oocytes. Additionally, the administration of exogenous gonadotropins may affect the uterine environment due to disruption of the normal levels of endogenous hormones. A single study has examined the effect of superovulation on methylation status[74], however this group only examined the distribution of 5-methylcytosine by immunofluorescence, and not methylation status of specific genetic sequences. Comparison of two-cell embryos from superovulated or natural mating revealed an increase in the number of embryos with abnormal 5-methylcytosine staining patterns among the superovulated group[74].

To address the question of gonadotropin stimulation in humans, prospective or retrospective studies are required with experimental groups who have only undergone ovulation induction, as opposed to the more involved protocols of assisted reproduction. One such study has been reported, in which a large case-control prospective study was undertaken to compare obstetric outcomes of singleton pregnancies in women who had undergone ovulation induction to comparable unstimulated control females[75]. This study described an increased relative risk of gestational diabetes mellitus and pregnancy-induced hypertension. Neither of these illnesses can be attributed specifically to the hormonal stimulation, as the cause may be related to the underlying fertility or treatments[75]. Imprinted genes have yet to be examined.

Further studies are required to examine the effect of gonadotropin stimulation on methylation and expression of imprinted genes. These studies will require careful planning, as there is a decreased rate of implantation and embryonic development in the mouse model[76]. If similar studies are to be undertaken in humans, careful consideration of tissue collection from children conceived using ARTs would be required if the methylation and expression status of imprinted genes are to be examined.

Culture of preimplantation embryos

The effect of preimplantion culture on the methylation and expression of a few imprinted genes has been examined in the mouse[77–79]. Culture in Whitten's media resulted in biallelic expression of *H19*, with a concomitant loss of methylation at a single CpG site upstream of *H19*; however, *Snrpn* was unaffected[77]. Khosla et al.[78] examined relative expression levels of imprinted genes after preimplantation culture in media with or without serum. This group described a decrease in relative expression of *H19*, *Igf2*, and *Grb7*, and an increase in relative expression of *Grb10* in the serum treated group, however, these changes were not correlated to methylation changes[78]. Another recent study found that preimplantation culture resulted in a decrease in the expression of *H19*, *Igf2*, *Peg1*, and *Grb10*[79]. Differences in the results of these studies are likely due to the use of different culture media. Further studies are required to examine the effect of preimplantation culture on the methylation and expression of imprinted genes. These studies are complicated by the requirement to pool preimplantation embryos for expression or methylation studies; however, these problems could be partially averted by transferring cultured embryos to pseudopregnant female mice and allowing the embryos to develop to a stage at which the experiments would be possible on single embryos.

In-vitro growth and maturation of oocytes

In-vitro maturation of oocytes has certain advantages over standard protocols, such as the ability to avoid stimulation by gonadotropins prior to harvesting oocytes, as well as being both less expensive and involving a simpler treatment protocol[80]. The ability to grow and mature oocytes in vitro has important implications for individuals who lose ovarian function early in life, such as cancer patients. There are, however, concerns related to the epigenetics of the oocytes. The first studies using mouse models of in-vitro growth and maturation have shown that oocytes grown and matured in vitro can generate live offspring, albeit with a very low rate of success[81]. The in-vitro growth and maturation protocol in mouse models has been revised, including changes to media and supplements, and the introduction of a two-step protocol for the culture[82]. The revised protocol resulted in higher levels of live births, although the proportion of live births was still significantly lower than in the control group, derived from in-vivo grown and matured oocytes[82]. Importantly, mouse oocytes grown in vitro do not reach the same diameter as those grown *in vivo*[83,84]. This observation is important, as imprint establishment in mouse oocytes is related to the diameter of the oocyte as opposed to being related to time[32]. In support of this, a recent study described inappropriate methylation of several imprinted genes in oocytes grown and matured in an in-vitro follicular culture model[85]. Although this study was small, together with the other data it suggests that further studies into the effects of in-vitro culture on maternal imprint establishment are required. In pig oocytes, another possible example of epigenetic dysregulation has been described. Oocytes matured in vitro show a decreased rate of proper methylation reprogramming following fertilization in this model[86].

One of the primary advantages of the in-vitro maturation protocol is the avoidance of exogenous gonadotropin treatment[80], however pretreatment, or priming, with either follicle-stimulating hormone (FSH) or human chorionic gonadotropin (hCG) is being suggested by several groups (reviewed in Chian et al.[80]). The administration of exogenous gonadotropins raises the same concerns discussed previously. Additionally, the in-vitro maturation of oocytes requires these cells to be in a culture environment for longer periods of time versus that for IVF or ICSI alone. The extended culture times heighten the concern that epigenetic dysregulation may occur in the synthetic environment.

These additional concerns further support the need for detailed studies of the impact of ARTs on the epigenetics of the oocyte.

Assisted reproductive technologies or infertility: what is the cause of epigenetic dysregulation?

Further complicating the question of epigenetic dysregulation as a result of ARTs are two recent reports examining imprinting in subfertile individuals or couples. One group has examined methylation at two imprinted loci in sperm samples from normal fertile males and in oligozoospermic males with moderately or severely reduced sperm counts[87]. When the methylation of *H19*, which is normally hypermethylated in sperm, was examined by bisulfite sequencing, it was observed that both moderately and severely oligozoospermic sperm samples had lower levels of methylation than the normozoospermic controls. Of note, methylation was not completely lost at all sites examined, and the more severely oligozoospermic males exhibited more variability as well as an increased number of sites at which methylation was lost than their moderately affected counterparts. Examination of a maternally methylated gene, *MEST*, showed normal hypomethylation at all sites for all samples, indicating that maternal imprints were correctly erased in these samples[87]. The authors suggest that transmission of imprinting errors may be increased as a result of infertility treatment, although the imprinting errors may not strictly occur as a result of the treatment but may be associated with some forms of male factor infertility.

Further support for a role for epigenetic defects in infertility comes from a retrospective study involving children born with Angelman syndrome in Germany[88]. Parents were contacted and asked to complete a survey related to method of conception and time to pregnancy, as well as to submit tissue samples from parents and child in order to determine the genetic cause of the

Angelman syndrome. As a result, it was discovered that there was an increased incidence of imprinting defects in patients with Angelman syndrome born to subfertile couples, defined as couples with a time to pregnancy longer than two years. The authors further suggest that the imprinting disorder and subfertility may have a common cause, unrelated to ARTs.

These findings support a need for further studies into the effects of ARTs as well as the causes of and epigenetic states in subfertile males and females.

CONCLUSIONS

Important features of the dynamic epigenetic changes that occur during oocyte growth and maturation have been uncovered in recent years. The time of acquisition of maternal methylation imprints may be a stage that is vulnerable to the effects of the different types of ARTs. A growing amount of evidence suggesting an association of imprinting disorders with assisted reproduction highlights the need for further study of epigenetic defects associated with infertility as well as the different aspects of the techniques currently employed. Additionally, testing in animal models should precede the introduction of new treatments and technologies into the clinic setting. The reports linking human imprinting disorders and ARTs suggest that children conceived using these techniques should be followed closely after birth, and highlight the need for large, multi-center prospective studies to examine the incidence of imprinting disorders in this population.

ACKNOWLEDGMENTS

Jacquetta Trasler is a William Dawson Scholar of McGill University and a Scholar of the Fonds de la recherché en santé du Québec. Amanda Fortier is the recipient of a Studentship Award from the Montreal Children's Hospital Research Institute and a Canada Graduate Scholarship from the Canadian Institutes of Health Research (CIHR). This work was supported by the Program on Oocyte Health (www.ohri.ca/oocyte) funded under the Healthy Gametes and Great Embryos Strategic Initiative of the Canadian Institutes of Health Research (CIHR) Institute of Human Development, Child and Youth Health (IHDCYH), grant number HGG62293.

REFERENCES

1. McGrath J, Solter D. Completion of mouse embryogenesis requires both the maternal and paternal genomes. Cell 1984; 37: 179–83.

2. Surani MA, Barton SC, Norris ML. Development of reconstituted mouse eggs suggests imprinting of the genome during gametogenesis. Nature 1984; 308: 548–50.

3. Gosden R, Trasler J, Lucifero D et al. Rare congenital disorders, imprinted genes, and assisted reproductive technology. Lancet 2003; 361: 1975–7.

4. Lucifero D, Chaillet JR, Trasler JM. Potential significance of genomic imprinting defects for reproduction and assisted reproductive technology. Hum Reprod Update 2004; 10: 3–18.

5. DeBaun MR, Niemitz EL, Feinberg AP. Association of *in vitro* fertilization with Beckwith–Wiedemann Syndrome and epigenetic alterations in *LIT1* and *H19*. Am J Hum Genet 2003; 72: 156–60.

6. Maher ER, Brueton LA, Bowdin SC et al. Beckwith–Wiedemann syndrome and assisted reproduction technology (ART). J Med Genet 2003; 40: 62–4.

7. Gicquel C, Gaston V, Mandelbaum J et al. *In vitro* fertilization may increase the risk of Beckwith–Wiedemann syndrome related to the abnormal imprinting of the KCNQ1OT gene. Am J Hum Genet 2003; 72: 1338–41.

8. Halliday J, Oke K, Breheny S et al. Beckwith–Wiedemann syndrome and IVF: a case-control study. Am J Hum Genet 2004; 75: 526–8.

9. Cox GF, Burger J, Lip V et al. Intracytoplasmic sperm injection may increase the risk of imprinting defects. Am J Hum Genet 2002; 71: 162–4.

10. Orstavik KH, Eiklid K, van der Hagen CB et al. Another case of imprinting effect in a girl with Angelman syndrome who was conceived by intracytoplasmic semen injection. Am J Hum Genet 2003; 72: 218–19.

11. Moore T, Haig D. Genomic imprinting in mammalian development: a parental tug-of-war. Trends Genet 1991; 7: 45–9.

12. Moore T, Reik W. Genetic conflict in early development: parental imprinting in normal and abnormal growth. Rev Reprod 1996; 1: 73–7.

13. Monk M, Boubelik M, Lehnert S. Temporal and regional changes in DNA methylation in the embryonic, extraembryonic and germ cell lineages during mouse embryo development. Development 1987; 99: 371–82.

14. Chaillet JR, Vogt TF, Beier DR et al. Parental-specific methylation of an imprinted transgene is established during gametogenesis and progressively changes during embryogenesis. Cell 1991; 66: 77–83.

15. Kafri T, Ariel M, Brandeis M et al. Developmental pattern of gene-specific DNA methylation in the mouse embryo and germ line. Genes Dev 1992; 6: 705–14.

16. Brandeis M, Ariel M, Cedar H. Dynamics of DNA methylation during development. Bioessays 1993; 15: 709–13.

17. Hajkova P, Erhardt S, Lane N et al. Epigenetic reprogramming in mouse primordial germ cells. Mech Dev 2002; 117: 15–23.

18. Li JY, Lees-Murdock DJ, Xu GL et al. Timing of establishment of paternal methylation imprints in the mouse. Genomics 2004; 84: 952–60.

19. Szabo PE, Hubner K, Scholer H et al. Allele-specific expression of imprinted genes in mouse migratory primordial germ cells. Mech Dev 2002; 115: 157–60.

20. Lane N, Dean W, Erhardt S et al. Resistance of IAPs to methylation reprogramming may provide a mechanism for epigenetic inheritance in the mouse. Genesis 2003; 35: 88–93.

21. Lees-Murdock DJ, De Felici M, Walsh CP. Methylation dynamics of repetitive DNA elements in the mouse germ cell lineage. Genomics 2003; 82: 230–7.

22. Lee J, Inoue K, Ono R et al. Erasing genomic imprinting memory in mouse clone embryos produced from day 11.5 primordial germ cells. Development 2002; 129: 1807–17.

23. Yamazaki Y, Mann MR, Lee SS et al. Reprogramming of primordial germ cells begins before migration into the genital ridge, making these cells inadequate donors for reproductive cloning. Proc Natl Acad Sci USA 2003; 100: 12207–12.

24. Kato Y, Rideout WM, 3rd, Hilton K et al. Developmental potential of mouse primordial germ cells. Development 1999; 126: 1823–32.

25. Brandeis M, Kafri T, Ariel M et al. The ontogeny of allele-specific methylation associated with imprinted genes in the mouse. Embo J 1993; 12: 3669–77.

26. Stoger R, Kubicka P, Liu CG et al. Maternal-specific methylation of the imprinted mouse Igf2r locus identifies the expressed locus as carrying the imprinting signal. Cell 1993; 73: 61–71.

27. Kono T, Obata Y, Yoshimzu T et al. Epigenetic modifications during oocyte growth correlates with extended parthenogenetic development in the mouse. Nat Genet 1996; 13: 91–4.

28. Ueda T, Yamazaki K, Suzuki R et al. Parental methylation patterns of a transgenic locus in adult somatic tissues are imprinted during gametogenesis. Development 1992; 116: 831–9.

29. Obata Y, Kaneko-Ishino T, Koide T et al. Disruption of primary imprinting during oocyte growth leads to the modified expression of imprinted genes during embryogenesis. Development 1998; 125: 1553–60.

30. Kono T, Obata Y, Wu Q et al. Birth of parthenogenetic mice that can develop to adulthood. Nature 2004; 428: 860–4.

31. Obata Y, Kono T. Maternal primary imprinting is established at a specific time for each gene throughout oocyte growth. J Biol Chem 2002; 277: 5285–9.

32. Lucifero D, Mann MR, Bartolomei MS et al. Gene-specific timing and epigenetic memory in oocyte imprinting. Hum Mol Genet 2004; 13: 839–49.

33. Lucifero D, Mertineit C, Clarke HJ et al. Methylation dynamics of imprinted genes in mouse germ cells. Genomics 2002; 79: 530–8.

34. Mutter GL. Teratoma genetics and stem cells: a review. Obstet Gynecol Surv 1987; 42: 661–70.

35. El-Maarri O, Buiting K, Peery EG et al. Maternal methylation imprints on human chromosome 15 are established during or after fertilization. Nat Genet 2001; 27: 341–4.

36. Geuns E, De Rycke M, Van Steirteghem A et al. Methylation imprints of the imprint control region of the SNRPN-gene in human gametes and preimplantation embryos. Hum Mol Genet 2003; 12: 2873–9.

37. Helwani MN, Seoud M, Zahed L et al. A familial case of recurrent hydatidiform molar pregnancies with biparental genomic contribution. Hum Genet 1999; 105: 112–15.

38. Judson H, Hayward BE, Sheridan E et al. A global disorder of imprinting in the human female germ line. Nature 2002; 416: 539–42.

39. El-Maarri O, Seoud M, Coullin P et al. Maternal alleles acquiring paternal methylation patterns in biparental complete hydatidiform moles. Hum Mol Genet 2003; 12: 1405–13.

40. El-Maarri O, Seoud M, Riviere JB et al. Patients with familial biparental hydatidiform moles have normal methylation at imprinted genes. Eur J Hum Genet 2005; 13: 486–90.

41. Hayward BE, De Vos M, Judson H et al. Lack of involvement of known DNA methyltransferases in familial hydatidiform mole implies the involvement of other factors in establishment of imprinting in the human female germline. BMC Genet 2003; 4: 2.

42. Mann MR, Lee SS, Doherty AS et al. Selective loss of imprinting in the placenta following preimplantation development in culture. Development 2004; 131: 3727–35.

43. Feil R, Khosla S, Cappai P et al. Genomic imprinting in ruminants: allele-specific gene expression in parthenogenetic sheep. Mamm Genome 1998; 9: 831–4.

44. Hagemann LJ, Peterson AJ, Weilert LL et al. In vitro and early in vivo development of sheep gynogenones and putative androgenones. Mol Reprod Dev 1998; 50: 154–62.

45. Marshall VS, Wilton LJ, Moore HD. Parthenogenetic activation of marmoset (Callithrix jacchus) oocytes and the development of marmoset parthenogenones in vitro and in vivo. Biol Reprod 1998; 59: 1491–7.

46. Goll MG, Bestor TH. Eukaryotic cytosine methyltransferases. Annu Rev Biochem 2004.

47. Yoder JA, Bestor TH. A candidate mammalian DNA methyltransferase related to pmt1p of fission yeast. Hum Mol Genet 1998; 7: 279–84.

48. Okano M, Xie S, Li E. Cloning and characterization of a family of novel mammalian DNA (cytosine–5) methyltransferases. Nat Genet 1998; 19: 219–20.

49. Aapola U, Kawasaki K, Scott HS et al. Isolation and initial characterization of a novel zinc finger gene, DNMT3L, on 21q22.3, related to the cytosine–5-methyltransferase 3 gene family. Genomics 2000; 65: 293–8.

50. Bourc'his D, Xu GL, Lin CS et al. Dnmt3L and the establishment of maternal genomic imprints. Science 2001; 294: 2536–9.

51. Bestor TH. Activation of mammalian DNA methyltransferase by cleavage of a Zn binding regulatory domain. Embo J 1992; 11: 2611–17.

52. Yoder JA, Soman NS, Verdine GL et al. DNA (cytosine–5)-methyltransferases in mouse cells and tissues. Studies with a mechanism-based probe. J Mol Biol 1997; 270: 385–95.

53. Carlson LL, Page AW, Bestor TH. Properties and localization of DNA methyltransferase in preimplantation mouse embryos: implications for genomic imprinting. Genes Dev 1992; 6: 2536–41.

54. Mertineit C, Yoder JA, Taketo T et al. Sex-specific exons control DNA methyltransferase in mammalian germ cells. Development 1998; 125: 889–97.

55. La Salle S, Mertineit C, Taketo T et al. Windows for sex-specific methylation marked by DNA methyltransferase expression profiles in mouse germ cells. Devel Biol 2004; 268: 403–15.

56. Howell CY, Bestor TH, Ding F et al. Genomic imprinting disrupted by a maternal effect mutation in the Dnmt1 gene. Cell 2001; 104: 829–38.

57. Ratnam S, Mertineit C, Ding F et al. Dynamics of Dnmt1 methyltransferase expression and intracellular localization during oogenesis and preimplantation development. Devel Biol 2002; 245: 304–14.

58. Huntriss J, Hinkins M, Oliver B et al. Expression of mRNAs for DNA methyltransferases and methyl-CpG-binding proteins in the human female germ line, preimplantation embryos, and embryonic stem cells. Mol Reprod Dev 2004; 67: 323–36.

59. Ding F, Patel C, Ratnam S et al. Conservation of Dnmt1o cytosine methyltransferase in the marsupial *Monodelphis domestica*. Genesis 2003; 36: 209–13.

60. Golding MC, Westhusin ME. Analysis of DNA (cytosine 5) methyltransferase mRNA sequence and expression in bovine preimplantation embryos, fetal and adult tissues. Gene Expr Patterns 2003; 3: 551–8.

61. Bestor TH. The DNA methyltransferases of mammals. Hum Mol Genet 2000; 9: 2395–402.

62. Okano M, Takebayashi S, Okumura K et al. Assignment of cytosine-5 DNA methyltransferases Dnmt3a and Dnmt3b to mouse chromosome bands 12A2–A3 and 2H1 by in situ hybridization. Cytogenet Cell Genet 1999; 86: 333–4.

63. Chen T, Ueda Y, Xie S et al. A novel Dnmt3a isoform produced from an alternative promoter localizes to euchromatin and its expression correlates with active de novo methylation. J Biol Chem 2002; 277: 38746–54.

64. Lees-Murdock DJ, Shovlin TC, Gardiner T et al. DNA methyltransferase expression in the mouse germ line during periods of de novo methylation. Devel Dyn 2005; 232: 992–1002.

65. Kaneda M, Okano M, Hata K et al. Essential role for *de novo* DNA methyltransferase Dnmt3a in paternal and maternal imprinting. Nature 2004; 429: 900–3.

66. Xie S, Wang Z, Okano M et al. Cloning, expression and chromosome locations of the human DNMT3 gene family. Gene 1999; 236: 87–95.

67. Hansen RS, Wijmenga C, Luo P et al. The DNMT3B DNA methyltransferase gene is mutated in the ICF immunodeficiency syndrome. Proc Natl Acad Sci USA 1999; 96: 14412–17.

68. Aoki A, Suetake I, Miyagawa J et al. Enzymatic properties of de novo-type mouse DNA (cytosine-5) methyltransferases. Nucl Acids Res 2001; 29: 3506–12.

69. Weisenberger DJ, Velicescu M, Preciado-Lopez MA et al. Identification and characterization of alternatively spliced variants of DNA methyltransferase 3a in mammalian cells. Gene 2002; 298: 91–9.

70. Xu GL, Bestor TH, Bourc'his D et al. Chromosome instability and immunodeficiency syndrome caused by mutations in a DNA methyltransferase gene. Nature 1999; 402: 187–91.

71. Jeanpierre M, Turleau C, Aurias A et al. An embryonic-like methylation pattern of classical satellite DNA is observed in ICF syndrome. Hum Mol Genet 1993; 2: 731–5.

72. Hata K, Okano M, Lei H et al. Dnmt3L cooperates with the Dnmt3 family of de novo DNA methyltransferases to establish maternal imprints in mice. Development 2002; 129: 1983–93.

73. Hamatani T, Falco G, Carter MG et al. Age-associated alteration of gene expression patterns in mouse oocytes. Hum Mol Genet 2004; 13: 2263–78.

74. Shi W, Haaf T. Aberrant methylation patterns at the two-cell stage as an indicator of early developmental failure. Mol Reprod Dev 2002; 63: 329–34.

75. Maman E, Lunenfeld E, Levy A et al. Obstetric outcome of singleton pregnancies conceived by *in vitro* fertilization and ovulation induction compared with those conceived spontaneously. Fertil Steril 1998; 70: 240–5.

76. Ertzeid G, Storeng R. Adverse effects of gonadotrophin treatment on pre- and postimplantation development in mice. J Reprod Fertil 1992; 96: 649–55.

77. Doherty AS, Mann MR, Tremblay KD et al. Differential effects of culture on imprinted H19 expression in the preimplantation mouse embryo. Biol Reprod 2000; 62: 1526–35.

78. Khosla S, Dean W, Brown D et al. Culture of pre-implantation mouse embryos affects fetal development and the expression of imprinted genes. Biol Reprod 2001; 64: 918–26.

79. Fernandez-Gonzalez R, Moreira P, Bilbao A et al. Long-term effect of *in vitro* culture of mouse embryos with serum on mRNA expression of imprinting genes, development, and behavior. Proc Natl Acad Sci USA 2004; 101: 5880–5.

80. Chian RC, Lim JH, Tan SL. State of the art in in-vitro oocyte maturation. Curr Opin Obstet Gynecol 2004; 16: 211–19.

81. Eppig JJ, Schroeder AC. Capacity of mouse oocytes from preantral follicles to undergo embryogenesis and development to live young after growth, maturation, and fertilization *in vitro*. Biol Reprod 1989; 41: 268–76.

82. O'Brien MJ, Pendola JK, Eppig JJ. A revised protocol for *in vitro* development of mouse oocytes from primordial follicles dramatically improves their developmental competence. Biol Reprod 2003; 68: 1682–6.

83. Eppig JJ, O'Brien MJ. Development *in vitro* of mouse oocytes from primordial follicles. Biol Reprod 1996; 54: 197–207.

84. Kim DH, Ko DS, Lee HC et al. Comparison of maturation, fertilization, development, and gene expression of mouse oocytes grown *in vitro* and *in vivo*. J Assist Reprod Genet 2004; 21: 233–40.

85. Kerjean A, Couvert P, Heams T et al. *In vitro* follicular growth affects oocyte imprinting establishment in mice. Eur J Hum Genet 2003; 11: 493–6.

86. Gioia L, Barboni B, Turriani M et al. The capability of reprogramming the male chromatin after fertilization is dependent on the quality of oocyte maturation. Reproduction 2005; 130: 29–39.

87. Marques CJ, Carvalho F, Sousa M et al. Genomic imprinting in disruptive spermatogenesis. Lancet 2004; 363: 1700–2.

88. Ludwig M, Katalinic A, Gross S et al. Increased prevalence of imprinting defects in patients with Angelman syndrome born to subfertile couples. J Med Genet 2005; 42: 289–91.

CHAPTER 7

In-vitro development of small ovarian follicles

Ronit Abir, Shmuel Nitke, Avi Ben-Haroush, and Benjamin Fisch

RELEVANT ASPECTS OF EARLY IN-VIVO OOGENESIS AND FOLLICULOGENESIS WITH EMPHASIS ON HUMANS

The in-vivo development of germ cells and follicles from fetal to adult life will be discussed briefly, focusing on topics essential for the understanding of the later sections on the in-vitro processes. Despite the numerous studies performed on ovarian development, much is still unknown, especially regarding the early stages of oogenesis and folliculogenesis[1,2].

Human primordial germ cells (PGC) arrive from the yolk sac to the gonad from day 26 of pregnancy, and are then termed oogonia[2,3]. Recently, PGCs have also been identified in ovaries of adult mice[3,4] and women[3,5], but this issue needs to be further investigated.

Three events induce the development of human female fetal germ cells in the gonad (ovary): mitotic division cycles of the oogonia, meiotic division, and follicular assembly[2,3]. The number of female germ cells in the fetal ovary peaks at about 7 million in mid pregnancy and then drops drastically during the third trimester. Meiotic division usually commences gradually in the third month of gestation, and the diplothen stage is achieved within weeks of its initiation. At this point, the oogonia enlarge and acquire more intracellular organelles and are then termed oocytes. Just before birth, the oocytes are arrested in the diplothen stage of the prophase of the first meiotic division[2,3]. They have completed genetic recombination and do not undergo any additional nuclear maturation until puberty.

Follicular formation in humans begins during the fourth month of gestation. In rats and mice, this process occurs during the first postnatal days[3,6]. During follicular assembly there is a rapid proliferation of the nearby cells, and the oocytes become surrounded by a single layer of flattened somatic cells, termed granulosa cells (GC), enclosed by a basement membrane[1-3]. These cellular complexes are defined as *primordial follicles* (30–50 µm in diameter) and can be identified in the human from around 22 gestational weeks (GWs).

Most of the follicles in human ovaries of adults as well as fetuses remain primordial and reach ovulatory sizes (18–20 mm in diameter) within 6 to 9 months[1,3]. Primordial follicles are activated when their GC become cuboidal, and these are then termed *primary follicles* (50 µm–0.1 mm in diameter). Thereafter, the increased proliferation rate yields a multilaminar granulosa layer[1-3], *secondary follicles* (0.1–0.2 mm in diameter). In the human, a definitive theca layer is created from the surrounding stroma cells around the follicle when a secondary follicle contains three to six GC layers[1-3]. Steroid hormones are synthesized through complex interactions between the GC and theca cells. During the secondary follicular stage the oocyte starts to grow, while forming a glycoprotein coat, the *zona pellucida* (ZP), between itself and the innermost layer of the GC. The final follicular stage consists of the development of *antral follicles* (early antral follicle: 0.2–0.4 mm in diameter) containing fluid-filled cavities within several layers of cuboidal GC; the innermost layers surrounding the oocytes are termed *cumulus cells*. At ovulation, the first meiotic division is completed with the extrusion of the first polar body enclosed between the oocyte and the ZP, forming a mature oocyte.

The growth regulation of primordial follicles is not hormonal. Follicle-stimulating hormone (FSH) sustains follicular development and growth only from secondary stages. The exact factors that stimulate growth of primordial follicles are unknown and various growth factors have been suggested for this role[2,3] (see the section 'Factors that might be responsible for early oogenesis or folliculogenesis').

CLINICAL IMPORTANCE OF IN-VITRO MATURATION (IVM) OF PRIMORDIAL FOLLICLES

As cancer treatment improves, more young women of reproductive age are surviving[3]. However, many suffer from ovarian failure and premature menopause, as a consequence of the radiation and chemotherapy[3,7]. Ovarian failure has been recorded mostly after malignancies that affect younger patients: Hodgkin's and non-Hodgkin's lymphoma, leukemias, Ewing and bone sarcomas, brain and breast tumors. These patients have limited options for putative fertility restoration, as the cryopreservation of mature oocytes has shown limited success[3,8].

Currently, egg donation promises, in many cases, the only choice for pregnancy[2,3,9]. However, there is a shortage of donated oocytes worldwide. One possible solution to increase the pool of donated oocytes is to use immature oocytes from ovaries of aborted human fetuses. However, before this becomes clinically feasible, methods to mature fetal follicles in vitro need to be developed[3,10]. Moreover, the use of oocytes from aborted fetuses is highly controversial and is forbidden in many countries.

Be that as it may, most women prefer to use their own oocytes and, therefore, methods to preserve self-fertility are required. Human ovarian tissue containing immature primordial follicles has been successfully cryopreserved after retrieval by a simple laparoscopic operation[3,6,7]. This technique is aimed either at inducing ovarian function by re-plantation of ovarian tissue or, further into the future, by in-vitro maturation (IVM) of oocytes derived from the cryopreserved-thawed ovarian tissue, followed by routine in-vitro fertilization (IVF) and embryo transfer (ET). To date, three live births have been reported after transplantation of ovarian tissue[3,11-13]. However, some cancers, such as hematologic malignancies[3,14] and breast cancer[3,15], carry a possible risk of disease re-transmission by the ovarian grafts.[2,3] Although IVM of primordial follicles would avoid this possibility, because the in-vitro matured oocytes will not contain cancerous cells, this method has so far shown limited success (see the section 'IVM of primordial follicles from adults').

Ovarian cryopreservation could also perhaps benefit girls with Turner's syndrome (TS), especially those with mosaic karyotypes, whose ovaries often contain follicles, usually at early ages[3,9,16] (see also the section 'IVM of primordial follicles from adults'). In these cases, ovarian biopsies should be preferably cryopreserved even before the first signs of puberty, since most or all of the follicles might be lost once signs of puberty appear.

Indeed, once established, fertility restoration by cryopreserved-thawed ovaries may be preferred also by healthy women who choose to postpone childbearing until later in life[3]. IVM of primordial follicles for artificial reproduction technologies would obviate the complexity, cost, and emotional toll of the procedure, which requires superovulation and extensive monitoring during the follicular phase of the cycle. Furthermore, it would make oocyte donation simpler, because an ovarian biopsy could be retrieved by a simple operation without any hormonal stimulation with its attendant side-effects to the donor. Finally, IVM of primordial follicles would not only benefit human fertility programs but could also enhance efforts at conservation of endangered species.

ATTEMPTS AT IVM OF FETAL OOGONIA/OOCYTES

It is unknown whether oocytes from fetuses have the same developmental capacity as those from adults, and relatively few studies to date have investigated this possibility in mammals.[3] There are several reports on the in-vitro growth of oogonia from fetal mice to antral follicles[3,17] or mature oocytes[3,18]. Fetal bovine and baboon follicles have developed in vitro into primary and secondary follicles with GC proliferation, as demonstrated by their expression of proliferating cell nuclear antigen (PCNA)[3,19–21], which plays an essential role in cell cycle regulation[3,10,19–21]. However, although the diameters of both the fetal bovine follicles and their oocytes increased in culture, about 50% of the follicles were atretic[19].

In another study, human fetal ovaries (13–16 GWs) were cultured for 40 days and, after several weeks, the oogonia entered the initial stages of meiosis[3,22]. Fresh and frozen-thawed human fetal oogonia and primordial follicles (16–20 GWs) were also cultured for 2 months, and morphologically mature oocytes (with a first polar body) were obtained[3,23], although they were smaller than those developed in vivo. In a study

conducted in our laboratory[3,10], ovarian specimens obtained from second- and third-trimester human fetuses (22–33 GWs) were cultured for 4 weeks (Figure 7.1). The follicles survived in culture without any apparent increase in the number of primary and secondary follicles, in the expression of PCNA or bromodeoxyuridine (BrdU) incorporation (another marker for dividing cells) in the GC, or in the number of atretic follicles. However, a significant increase in the level of estradiol in the spent media samples was detected in the fourth week of culture, indicating steroidogenesis of secondary follicles.

IVM OF PRIMODIAL FOLLICLES FROM ADULTS

Experiments to mature human oocytes in vitro from primordial follicles have had limited

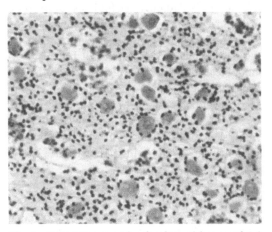

Figure 7.1 Micrograph of cultured human fetal follicles[10]. Section of human ovarian fetal follicles after 3 weeks in culture, stained for bromodeoxyuridine (BrdU) incorporation (DNA division). The tissue was taken from a 33 GWs fetus with achondroplasia. Note the normal primordial follicles, lack of brown BrdU staining in the GC indicating no proliferation, and brown staining only in the oocytes. Background blue staining is hematoxylin. Magnification × 400 (see color plate section)

success[2,3]. Researchers developing such maturation systems face two main problems: the signals involved in the transition of primordial follicles are unknown and there is a need to maintain the long-term survival and growth of the ovarian follicles under culture conditions.

Culture systems

There are two approaches to the culture of primary and primordial follicles[2,3]. The more popular one involves culturing whole slices of ovarian tissue (organ culture), such that the structural integrity of the ovarian tissue is maintained and, hence, the interactions between the surrounding stroma cells and the follicles are retained.

Using this method, primordial follicles from cows have been grown in organ culture to secondary stages[3,24]. Several studies also described the use of organ culture for human primordial follicles[3,25–31]. Although the follicles survived for up to 4 weeks, they did not develop beyond the secondary stages. There were no differences in the developmental capabilities of human ovarian follicles derived from fresh or frozen-thawed tissue[25]. Attempts to optimize the organ culture system yielded a reduced atresia rate[27,29] under serum-free conditions[27] and improved follicular survival in wells coated with diluted extracellular matrix[25,29] and with tissues cut in cubes rather than in long slices[3,29].

The second approach to follicular culture involves the use of isolated primordial and primary follicles[3,32,33] (Figures 7.2 and 7.3). Though whole tissue culturing is much easier than working with tiny follicles of 30–50 μm, the latter method enables researchers to directly monitor follicular growth during the culture period. This is of special importance considering the poorly populated human ovarian tissue in adults. For example, because of the low follicular content of ovaries from patients with TS, organ culture as well as ovarian transplantation could lead to the use of empty ovarian specimens, whereas the recruitment of isolated follicles would make it possible to determine the initial follicular content[2,3].

The first stage of isolation is incubation of the ovarian tissue with a cocktail of digesting enzymes (2 h for human tissue), usually of collagenase and DNase. This softens the stroma tissue and makes the isolation process easier[3,32,33]. The DNase breaks the sticky DNA ends, eliminating the risk of unprocessable digested ovarian tissue. The enzymatic treatment is followed by mechanical microdissection of the ovarian follicles in combination with repeated pipetting. Isolated mouse unilaminar follicles have been cultured to multi-laminar stages in collagen gels[34], and isolated rat follicles co-cultured with stroma cells on poly-L-lysine coated plates developed to preovulatory stages[35]. GC from isolated primary porcine follicles were found to proliferate in culture[36].

One group cultured bovine primary follicles isolated without enzymatic digestion[2,3,37]. The bovine ovarian tissue was cut into small fragments with a tissue chopper. The fragments were then transferred through nylon filters and morphologically normal primary follicles were isolated. These follicles were embedded in collagen gels and cultured. Follicular growth was slow and very limited (up to 24% in follicular diameter) and there was no oocyte growth; 43% of the oocytes were dead after 7 days of culture[37].

In another study, morphologically normal isolated primordial human follicles from fresh and frozen-thawed ovarian tissue survived for up to 5 days in culture, but without indications of actual growth[38]. Our group isolated human primordial and primary follicles from both fresh and frozen-thawed ovarian tissue[32,33] (Figures 7.2 and 7.3). Apart from an increase in lipid droplets in their GC, the isolated follicles appeared ultrastructurally normal compared with follicles in intact tissue blocks. After 24 h culture in collagen gels, 40% of the follicles showed an increase in the number of GC layers (to two or three) and in oocyte size (Figure 7.2). However, the follicles developed only within a supporting collagen gel matrix and not on collagen, poly-L-lysine, or extracellular matrix[33], or even within agar (Figure 7.3). Although others have demonstrated that human primordial follicles developed better in organ culture than as partially isolated follicles (with some stroma cells attached)[26], we found that only fully isolated follicles could grow in collagen gel culture. Partially isolated follicles only survived in culture, with no signs of GC proliferation or increase in oocyte diameter[33] (Figures 7.2 and 7.3).

The most promising studies of IVM of mammalian primordial follicles

Only in the mouse has the production of live young from cultured primordial follicles been successful[39,40]. This research group developed a two-stage culture system for murine primordial follicles. Primordial follicles were grown in organ culture to secondary follicles. The secondary follicles were then isolated enzymatically

and cultured further to mature oocytes, followed by routine IVF and ET. However, to date, only 59 live offspring (5.7% of embryos transferred) have been obtained[40]. The first mouse born was extremely obese and a postmortem examination revealed multiple malformations[39,40].

In some studies, ovarian tissue was grafted to hosts as an intermediate step in IVM of mammalian primordial follicles[41–43]. Specifically, fresh[41] and frozen-thawed[42] murine ovarian tissue was transplanted under the kidney capsule of immunodeficient mice[41,42]. The grafts were removed, and the secondary follicles were isolated and cultured until mature oocytes were obtained, and then further fertilized. Live born mice were reported after IVF and ET.

Similarly, porcine tissue containing primordial follicles was grafted[43], and when the grafts were removed, immature germinal vesicle (GV)-stage oocytes were aspirated from antral follicles. Seventeen percent underwent IVM, out of which 55% were fertilized successfully

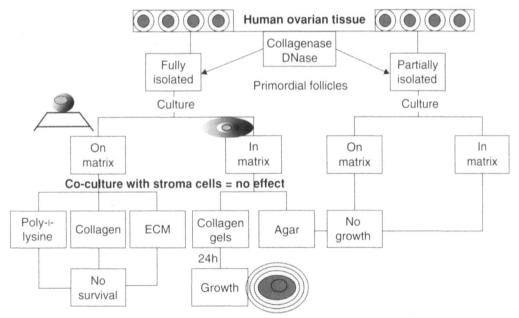

Figure 7.2 Strategies and results for culture of partially versus fully isolated human primordial follicles[32,33]. ECM: extracellular matrix

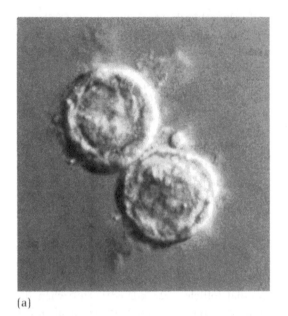
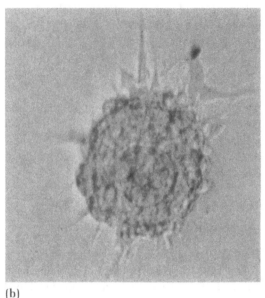

(a)   (b)

Figure 7.3   Micrograph of growing isolated human follicles[32,33]. (a) Two partially isolated human primordial follicles. Note the central oocytes surrounded by a single GC layer. Magnification × 400. (b) A secondary follicle developed in culture from a primordial follicle during 24 h in collagen gel. Note the central oocyte surrounded by several GC layers. Magnification × 400

in vitro to two-pronuclear-stage embryos. Despite these promising results[41–43], however, it is very unlikely that IVM of primordial follicles through animal hosts will ever be approved ethically for clinical purposes of production of human fertilizable oocytes.

FACTORS THAT MIGHT BE RESPONSIBLE FOR EARLY OOGENESIS OR FOLLICULOGENESIS

The stimulus that initiates the growth of primordial follicles into secondary, multilaminar follicles remains unknown[2,3]. Locally produced oocyte- and GC-derived paracrine factors have been found to mediate cell–cell interactions that are related to the initiation and progression of follicular development. Studies have localized to very small follicles certain cytokines, oncogenes, neurotropins, growth factors, or their receptors,

and have identified growth factors whose deficiency or that of their receptors in transgenic mice resulted in impaired PGC development or early folliculogenesis[2,3,44–48]. Therefore, these factors might possibly be candidates for initiation of early folliculogenesis. In the current chapter we will emphasize only on a portion of these factors: those that have actually affected mammalian PGC or follicular development in vitro or in vivo.

Growth factors that seem to promote growth of oogenia or primordial follicles

Table 7.1 summarizes the effects of various growth factors in activating primordial follicles in different mammalian species. *Insulin* or the *insulin like growth factor (IGF)* family probably activates mammalian primordial follicles in a species-specific manner[28,40,49]. The effects of

Table 7.1 Effects of growth factors on mammalian primordial follicles

GF	Species	Growth	FSH-R	Other	Effect Ab or Ab-R	References
BMP-4	Rat	To 1st follicles			Ab: *decrease* in oocytes, follicles, ovarian weight. *Increase*: apoptosis	51
BMP-7	Mouse	To 1st and 2nd follicles	Increase			54
bFGF	Rat	To 1st and 2nd follicles		*Increase*: stroma proliferation	Ab: *decrease* in growth	68
GDF-9	Rat	To 1st follicles		*Increase*: ovarian weight		52
	Human	To 1st and 2nd follicles		*Decrease*: atresia		53
Insulin	Human	To 1st follicles		*Decrease*: atresia		28
IGF-1	Human	To 1st follicles		(1) *Decrease*: atresia (2) PCNA expression in GC		28
IGF-2	Human	To 1st follicles		*Decrease*: atresia		28
LIF	Rat	To 1st and 2nd follicles		LIF + insulin >> LIF	Ab: *decrease* in growth	67
NGF	Rat	To 1st and 2nd follicles	Increase			56–58
SCF	Rat	To 1st and 2nd follicles			Ab-R: *decrease* in growth	63

GF: growth factor; FSH-R: follicle stimulating hormone receptor; 1st: primary; 2nd: secondary; Ab: antibody against the specific growth factor; Ab-R: antibody against the receptor for the specific growth factor; BMP-4: bone morphogenetic protein 4; BMP-7: bone morphogenetic protein 7; bFGF: basic fibroblast growth factor; GDF-9: growth differentiation factor 9; IGF-1: insulin like growth factor 1; IGF-2: insulin like growth factor 2; LIF: leukemia inhibiting factor; NGF: nerve growth factor; SCF: stem cell factor; PCNA: proliferating cell nuclear antigen; GC: granulosa cells

insulin on murine ovaries are unclear: one group described insulin inhibition of primordial follicles[40], whereas another showed that insulin, but not IGF-1, promoted the transition from the primordial to primary stages[49]. In humans, insulin, IGF-1, or IGF-2 reduced follicular atresia, and IGF-1 and IGF-2 induced follicular growth to primary stages[28]. However, PCNA expression in the GC was identified only with the addition of IGF-1.

Various members of the *transforming growth factor beta* (TGF-β) superfamily, such as *growth differentiation factor 9* (GDF–9), *bone-morphogenetic protein* (BMP)-4, 7, and 15, and *neurotropins* have been implicated in early folliculogenesis[2,3,47,50–54]. Treatment of neonatal rats with *GDF-9* increased ovarian weight and decreased the proportion of primordial follicles, with a concomitant increase in the proportions of primary and secondary follicles[52]. Treatment of cultured human primordial follicles with GDF-9 promoted their survival and progression to secondary stages with an increase in PCNA expression in the GC[53].

When rat primordial follicles were cultured with *BMP-4*, a significantly higher proportion of developing primary follicles and fewer arrested primordial follicles were observed[51]. By contrast, treatment with an anti-BMP-4 antibody resulted in a progressive loss of oocytes and primordial follicles, increased cellular apoptosis, and decreased ovarian size. Treatment of cultured murine primordial follicles with *BMP-7* stimulated the primordial–primary transition and the synthesis of the FSH receptor (FSH-R) mRNA[54]. Similarly, in-vivo injection of BMP-7 into the ovarian bursa of rats increased the number of primary, secondary, and antral follicles in parallel with a decrease in the number of primordial ovarian follicles[50]. Injecting *BMP-8b* into mice deficient in the BMP-8b gene rescued defective PGC[55].

Neurotropins are involved not only in ovarian innervation but also in follicular assembly and initiation of folliculogenesis[3,6,48]. Treatment of cultured rat primordial follicles with *nerve growth factor (NGF)* initiated the growth of primordial ovarian follicles, increased FSH-R mRNA expression, and increased the ovarian capacity to respond to FSH with cAMP formation and growth to secondary stages[56–58]. When fetal murine ovaries (containing oogonia), neonatal murine ovaries (containing primordial follicles), and human fetal ovaries (from fetuses aged 13–16 GWs) were cultured with a potent inhibitor of the neurotropins' receptors, the survival of oogonia and oocytes decreased[6,59].

Stem cell factor (SCF, kit ligand) regulates the survival and differentiation of migratory PGC and also of postmigratory PGC that are already settled in the murine gonad, primarily through its anti-apoptotic function[60–62]. The addition of SCF to the culture medium of isolated fetal murine oogonia co-cultured with GC resulted in meiotic resumption and fol-liculogenesis[18]. The addition of SCF to culture medium of postnatal rat ovaries containing primordial follicles induced follicular growth. By contrast, the addition of an anti-SCF-R antibody reduced growth and inhibited the activation of primordial follicles and the development to secondary follicles[62,63]. In pigs, SCF was found to be essential for the survival and proliferation of PGC[64].

Leukemia inhibiting factor (LIF) and *oncostatin M (OSM)* are members of the *interleukin 6 (IL-6)* family of cytokines[44,46], and are involved in the survival and proliferation of murine PGC. LIF has been found to regulate the growth, differentiation, and survival of the premigratory and postmigratory PGC in the developing murine[61,65] and porcine gonad[64,66], primarily through its anti-apoptotic function[60]. Antibodies against LIF receptor abolished PGC survival in culture[65]. Furthermore, LIF promoted the growth of rat primordial follicles in culture, whereas the addition of an anti-LIF antibody slightly decreased the number of developing follicles[67].

Basic fibroblast growth factor (bFGF, FGF-2) is a member of the *FGF* family[48]. It has been shown to promote the development of rat primordial follicles in vitro[68]. Specifically, the addition of bFGF to the culture medium induced a significant decrease in the number of primordial follicles with a corresponding increase in the number of primary and secondary follicles.

FSH and primordial follicles

The effect of *FSH* on mammalian primordial follicles is controversial and is probably species-dependent. In the mouse, FSH inhibited the activation of primordial follicles[40] and, in the cow, it had no effect on cultured primordial follicles[21]. Although FSH-R can be identified in human follicles only from the primary stages[69], in-vitro studies of isolated human primordial follicles[33] and primordial follicles in organ culture[27] suggested that FSH acts as a survival factor[27,33].

Nucleotide derivatives (secondary messengers) and primordial follicles

Nucleotide derivatives, such as *8-bromo guanosine 3',5'-cyclic monophosphate (8Br-cGMP)* and *cyclic adenosine monophosphate (cAMP)*, are important intracellular secondary messengers that might also be involved in the activation of primordial follicles[30,31,36]. GC from isolated porcine primary follicles proliferated in culture with the addition of 8Br-cAMP[36]. Slices of human ovaries cultured with 8Br-cGMP[30] or cAMP[31] showed increased growth to secondary stages; the proportion of viable follicles increased significantly in parallel with a decrease in atresia rates. 8Br-GMP also induced an increase in estradiol production in spent media samples, presumably because of the concurrent increase in the proportion of secondary follicles. However, these secondary follicles were smaller than those developed in vivo.

Possible involvement of multiple growth factors in early oogenesis or folliculogenesis

It is very unlikely that only a single growth factor is responsible for the development of PGC or primordial follicles in mammals.[3] Rather, various growth factors probably have similar effects on them, or stimulation from a combination of growth factors is required for their growth.

Indeed, studies have reported that growth promotion of murine migratory PGC was induced only by the combination of OSM, LIF, SCF, and bFGF[66,70]. Furthermore, OSM induction of the growth and survival of murine postmigratory PGCs was enhanced with the addition of LIF, SCF, and bFGF. Similarly, a combination of LIF, SCF, and IGF-1 promoted the survival in culture of murine oogonia[71,72] and led to a significant increase in the number of meiotic pachytene cells[72]. The addition of an antibody against glycoprotein 130, a receptor unit of various growth factors including LIF and OSM, blocked survival of the postmigratory colonizing murine PGC[70]. Likewise, in pigs, either LIF or SCF[64], or their combination[66], was essential for the survival and proliferation of PGC.

SCF or bFGF or insulin, or a combination of insulin with bFGF, or insulin with SCF and bFGF affected murine primordial follicles in a similar manner: a 25 to 30% increase in the level of primordial-to-primary follicle transition[49]. By contrast, treatment with insulin and SCF resulted in a 40% increase in the number of primary follicles. In the rat, the addition of LIF with insulin to cultured primordial follicles led to a greater number of developing follicles compared with LIF alone[67].

In mice, an inhibitor of the neurotropins' receptor decreased the survival of oocytes in newly formed primordial follicles, but this effect was rescued by the addition of bFGF to the culture medium[59]. In humans, there was a greater increase in the transition of primordial follicles to primary stages when insulin was added together with IGF-2 than when insulin and IGF-2 were each added alone[28].

Inhibitory factors on primordial follicles

Anti-Müllerian hormone (AMH), another member of the TGF-β superfamily, seems to inhibit the recruitment of primordial follicles for the growing phase[73]. Murine primordial follicles cultured with AMH showed a 40–50% reduction in the rate of growing follicles.

Some authors have suggested that *the oocyte* has an inhibitory action on the follicle, which can be overcome by the stimulation of factors arising from vesicular pericytes, such as Thy-differentiation protein[1,2].

Inhibitory effects on primordial follicle activation might also originate from *stroma cells*. Isolated human primordial follicles developed into secondary follicles already after 24 h of culture, only when they were fully isolated from the stroma layer[32,33]. Apparently, complete removal

DISCUSSION AND CONCLUSIONS

This review shows that the development of systems for the maturation of primordial as well as primary follicles is still in its infancy, and success so far is low.[3] Therefore, researchers need to continue their studies step-by-step using various follicular stages and culture systems (Figure 7.4). In humans and other species, follicular development from primordial stages onwards is complex and lengthy[1-3]. It is possible that the optimal culture medium for growth promotion needs to be very rich in supplements and species-specific. Growth factors should be added to the culture media of human primordial follicles to assess their in-vitro effect on folliculogenesis, alone and in combination. Various sequential media

of the stroma layer leads to a rapid release of inhibitory factors from the cells surrounding the follicles.

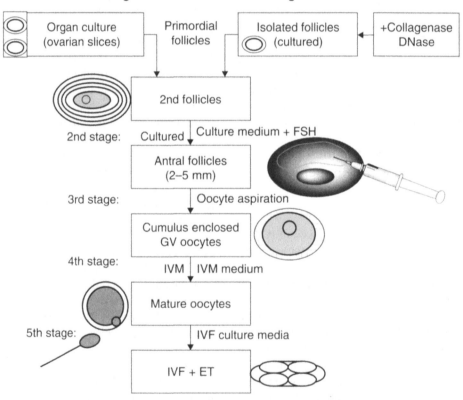

Figure 7.4 A possible strategy for the development of cultured human primordial follicles for an ultimate production of mature fertilizable oocytes. Note the five-stage strategy with sequential media: first stage – culture of primordial follicles (isolated or in organ culture) to secondary follicles with a medium rich in growth factors; second stage – culture of secondary follicles to small antral follicles with a medium containing FSH[1,2]; third stage – aspiration of cumulus enclosed GV-stage oocytes; fourth stage – culture of GV-stage oocytes to mature oocytes (with first polar body extrusion) using IVM medium[74]; fifth and final stage – standard IVF and ET

may also be necessary for every follicular stage, until a mature, healthy, and fertilizable human oocyte is obtained (Figure 7.4). It is very unlikely that human follicles could be brought in culture to an ovulatory size of 18–20 mm[1]; we expect that cumulus-enclosed GV-stage oocytes will be aspirated from small antral follicles obtained in culture and matured in vitro (Figure 7.4)[74].

The use of fetal follicles as a putative source of oocyte donations for IVF raises several ethical dilemmas[3,10]. So far, this possibility is remote, owing to the scarcity of in-vitro studies of fetal follicles and oogonia. In addition, most human abortions occur at early stages, and the respective oogonia from these ovaries develop very slightly in culture[22]. Studies conducted in our laboratory identified fewer receptors for various growth factors in GC of fetal primordial follicles that in those from adults[3,44–48], suggesting that it will be harder to develop a successful IVM system for fetal follicles than for primordial follicles from women. At the same time, a more in-depth understanding of the mechanisms involved in fetal folliculogenesis would assist researchers in improving the technology of IVM of small follicles from adults.[3] Therefore, studies on both mammalian fetal and adult follicles should be continued.

Currently, women who are about to receive anti-cancer treatment face limited options for fertility preservation[3,7]. Once the IVM technology of human primordial follicles is established, it will be possible to use oocytes that were matured and fertilized in vitro and thereby to avoid the dangers of malignancy re-transmission. The availability of such treatment will probably lead to its demand not only by cancer patients, but also by healthy women who choose to postpone childbearing until later in life. Moreover, taking into account the multiple malformations found in the first live mouse developed from a primordial follicle[2,3,40], after a successful acquisition of an IVM technology for primordial follicles, extensive research on their subsequent embryonic development will be necessary.

ACKNOWLEDGMENTS

Our original studies were partially sponsored by research grants from the Israel Cancer Association, the Israeli Ministry of Health, and Tel Aviv University. The authors are grateful to Ms G Ganzach from the Editorial Board of Rabin Medical Center for the English editing.

REFERENCES

1. Gougeon, A. Regulations of ovarian follicular development in primates: facts and hypotheses. Endocrinol Rev 1996; 17: 121–54.

2. Van den Hurk R, Abir R, Telfer EE et al. Preantral and antral follicles as possible source for fertilizable oocytes in human and bovine. Hum Reprod Update 2000; 6: 457–74.

3. Abir R, Nitke S, Ben-Haroush A et al. In vitro maturation of human primordial ovarian follicles – Clinical significance, process and methods for growth evaluation. Histol Histopathol 2006; 21: 887–98.

4. Johnson J, Canning J, Kaneko T et al. Germline stem cells and follicular renewal in the postnatal mammalian ovary. Nature 2004; 428: 145–50.

5. Bukovsky A, Caudle MR, Svetlikova M et al. Origin of germ cells and formation of new primary follicles in adult human ovaries. Reprod Biol Endocrinol 2004; 2: 20.

6. Ojeda SR, Romero C, Tapia V et al. Neurotrophic and cell–cell dependent control of early follicular development. Mol Cell Endocrinol 2000; 163: 67–71.

7. Abir R, Fisch B, Raz Ah et al. Preservation of fertility in women undergoing chemotherapy. Current approach and future prospects. J Assist Reprod Genet 1998; 15: 469–76.

8. Fabbri R, Porcu E, Marsella T et al. Human oocyte cryopreservation: new perspectives regarding oocyte survival. Hum Reprod 2001; 16: 411–16.

9. Abir R, Fisch B, Nahum R et al. Turner's syndrome and fertility: current status and possible future prospects. Hum Reprod Update 2001, 7: 603–10.

10. Biron-Shental T, Fisch B, Van Den Hurk R et al. Survival of frozen-thawed human ovarian fetal follicles in long-term organ culture. Fertil Steril 2004; 81: 716–19.

11. Donnez J, Dolmans MM, Demylle D et al. Livebirth after orthotopic transplantation of cryopreserved ovarian tissue. Lancet 2005; 364: 1405–10.

12. Meirow D, Levron J, Eldar-Geva T et al. Pregnancy after transplantation of cryopreserved ovarian tissue in a patient with ovarian failure after chemotherapy. N Engl J Med 2005; 353: 318–21.

13. Silber SJ, Lenahan KM, Levine DJ et al. Ovarian transplantation between monozygotic twins discordant for premature ovarian failure. N Engl J Med 2005; 353: 58–63.

14. Shaw J, Trounson A. Oncological implications in the replacement of ovarian tissue. Hum Reprod 1997; 12: 403–5.

15. Meirow D, Ben Yehuda D, Prus D et al. Ovarian tissue banking in patients with Hodgkin's disease: is it safe? Fertil Steril 1998; 69: 996–8.

16. Hreinsson JG, Otala M, Fridstrom M et al. Follicles are found in the ovaries of adolescent girls with Turner's syndrome. J Clin Endocrinol Metab 2002; 87: 3618–23.

17. Obata Y, Kono T, Hatada I. Maturation of mouse fetal germ cells *in vitro*. Nature 2002; 418: 497.

18. Klinger FG, De Felici M. *In vitro* development of growing oocytes from fetal mouse oocytes: stage-specific regulation by stem cell factor and granulosa cells. Devel Biol 2002; 244: 85–95.

19. Wandji SA, Srsen V, Voss AK et al. Initiation *in vitro* of growth of bovine primordial follicles. Biol Reprod 1996; 55: 942–8.

20. Wandji SA, Srsen, V, Nathanielsz, PW et al. Initiation of growth of baboon primordial follicles *in vitro*. Hum Reprod 1997; 12: 1993–2001.

21. Fortune JE, Kito S, Wandji SA et al. Activation of bovine and baboon primordial follicles *in vitro*. Theriogenology 1998; 49: 441–9.

22. Hartshorne GM, Barlow AL, Child TJ et al. Immunocytogenetic detection of normal and abnormal oocytes in human fetal ovarian tissue in culture. Hum Reprod 1999, 14: 172–82.

23. Zhang J, Liu J, Xu KP et al. Extracorporeal development and ultrarapid freezing of human fetal ova. J Assist Reprod Genet 1995; 12: 361–8.

24. Braw-Tal R, Yossefi, S. Studies *in vivo* and *in vitro* on the initiation of follicle growth in the bovine ovary. J Reprod Fertil 1997; 109: 165–71.

25. Hovatta O, Silye R, Abir R et al. Extracellular matrix improves the survival of human primordial and primary fresh and frozen-thawed ovarian follicles in long-term culture. Hum Reprod 1997; 12: 1032–6.

26. Hovatta O, Wright C, Krausz T et al. Human primordial, primary and secondary follicles in long-term culture: effect of partial isolation. Hum Reprod 1999; 14: 2519–24.

27. Wright CS, Hovatta O, Margara R et al. Effects of follicles stimulating hormone and serum substitution on the in-vitro growth of human ovarian follicles. Hum Reprod 1999; 14: 1555–62.

28. Louhio H, Hovatta O, Sjoberg J et al. The effects of insulin and insulin-like growth factor I and II on human ovarian follicles in long-term culture. Mol Hum Reprod 2000; 6: 694–8.

29. Scott JE, Carlsson IB, Bavister BD et al. Human ovarian tissue cultures: extracellular matrix composition, coating density and tissue dimensions. Reprod Biomed Online 2004; 9: 287–93.

30. Scott JE, Zhang P, Hovatta O. Benefits of 8-bromo-guanosine 3′,5′-cyclic monophosphate (8-br-cGMP) in human ovarian cortical tissue culture. Reprod Biomed Online 2004; 8: 319–24.

31. Zhang P, Louhio H, Tuuri T et al. *In vitro* effect of cyclic adenosine 3′, 5′-monophosphate (cAMP) on early human ovarian follicles. J Assist Reprod Genet 2004; 21: 301–6.

32. Abir R, Roizman P, Fisch B et al. Pilot study of isolated early human follicles cultured in collagen gels for 24 h. Hum Reprod 1999; 14: 1299–301.

33. Abir R, Fisch B, Nitke S et al. Morphological study of fully and partially isolated early human follicles. Fertil Steril 2001; 75: 141–6.

34. Torrance C, Telfer E, Gosden RG. Quantitative study of the development of isolated mouse preantral follicles in collagen gel culture. J Reprod Fertil 1989; 87: 367–74.

35. Cain L, Chatterjee S, Collins TJ. *In vitro* folliculogenesis of rat preantral follicles. Endocrinol 1995; 136: 3369–77.

36. Morbeck DE, Flowers WL, Britt JH. Response of granulosa cells isolated from primary and secondary follicles to FSH, 8-bromo-cAMP and epidermal growth factor *in vitro*. J Reprod Fertil 1993; 99: 577–84.

37. Schotanus K, Hage WJ, Van den Hurk R. Effects of conditioned media from murine granulosa cell lines on the growth of isolated bovine preantral follicles. Theriogenology 1997; 48: 471–83.

38. Oktay K, Nugent D, Newton H et al. Isolation and characterization of primordial follicles from fresh and cryopreserved human ovarian tissue. Fertil Steril 1997; 67: 481–6.

39. Eppig, JJ, O'Brien MJ. Development *in vitro* of mouse oocytes from primordial follicles. Biol Reprod 1996; 54: 197–207.

40. O'Brien MJ, Pendola JK, Eppig JJ. A revised protocol for *in vitro* development of mouse oocytes from primordial follicles dramatically improves their development competence. Biol Reprod 2003; 68: 1682–6.

41. Liu J, Van der Elst J, Van den Broecke R et al. Maturation of mouse primordial follicles by combination of grafting and *in vitro* culture. Biol Reprod 2000; 62: 1218–23.

42. Liu J, Van der Elst J, Van den Broecke R et al. Live offspring by in-vitro fertilization of oocytes from cryopreserved primordial mouse follicles after sequential *in vivo* transplantation and *in vitro* maturation. Biol Reprod 2001; 64: 171–8.

43. Kaneko H, Kikuchi K, Noguchi J et al. Maturation and fertilization of porcine oocytes from primordial follicles by a combination of xenografting and *in vitro* culture. Biol Reprod 2003; 69: 1488–93.

44. Abir R, Fisch B, Jin S et al. Immunocytochemical detection and RT-PCR expression of leukaemia inhibitory factor and its receptor in human fetal and adult ovaries. Mol Hum Reprod 2004; 10: 313–19.

45. Abir R, Fisch B, Jin S et al. Expression of stem cell factor and its receptor in human fetal and adult ovaries. Fertil Steril 2004; 82(Suppl 3): 1235–43.

46. Abir R, Ao A, Jin S et al. Immunocytochemical detection and reverse transcription polymerase chain reaction expression of oncostatin M (OSM) and its receptor (OSM-Rβ) in human fetal and adult ovaries. Fertil Steril 2005; 83(Suppl 1): 1188–96.

47. Abir R, Fisch B, Jin S et al. Presence of NGF and its receptors in ovaries from human fetuses and adults. Mol Hum Reprod 2005; 11: 229–36.

48. Ben-Haroush A, Abir R, Ao A et al. Expression of basic fibroblast growth factor (bFGF) and its receptors in human ovarian follicles from adults and fetuses. Fertil Steril 2005; 84: 1257–68.

49. Kezele PR, Nilsson EE, Skinner MK. Insulin but not insulin-like growth factor–1 promotes the primordial to primary follicle transition. Mol Cell Endocrinol 2002; 192: 37–43.

50. Lee WS, Otsuka F, Moore RK et al. Effect of bone morphogenetic protein–7 on folliculogenesis and ovulation in the rat. Biol Reprod 2001; 65: 994–9.

51. Nilsson EE, Skinner MK. Bone morphogenetic protein–4 acts as an ovarian follicle survival factor and promotes primordial follicle development. Biol Reprod 2003; 69: 1265–72.

52. Vitt UA, McGee EA, Hayashi M et al. *In vivo* treatment with GDF–9 stimulates primordial and primary follicle progression and theca cell marker CYP 17 in ovaries of immature rats. Endocrinology 2000; 141: 3814–20.

53. Hreinsson JG, Scott JE, Rasmussen C et al. Growth differentiation factor–9 promotes the growth, development, and survival of human ovarian follicles in organ culture. J Clin Endocrinol Metab 2002; 87: 316–21.

54. Lee W-S, Yoon S-J, Yoon T-K et al. Effects of bone morphogenetic protein–7 (BMP-7) on primordial follicular growth in the mouse ovary. Mol Reprod Dev 2004; 69: 159–63.

55. Ying Y, Qi X, Zhao GQ. Induction of primordial germ cells from murine epiblasts by synergistic action of BMP4 and BMP8B signalling pathways. Proc Natl Acad Sci USA 2001; 98: 7858–62.

56. Dissen GA, Hirshfield AN, Malamd S et al. Expression of neurotropins and their receptors in the mammalian ovary is developmentally

regulated: changes at the time of folliculogensis. Endocrinology 1995; 136: 4681–92.

57. Dissen GA, Romero C, Newman-Hirshfield A et al. Nerve growth factor is required for early follicular development in the mammalian ovary. Endocrinology 2001; 142: 2078–86.

58. Romero C, Parades A, Dissen GA. Nerve growth factor induces the expression of functional FSH receptors in newly formed follicles of the rat ovary. Endocrinology 2002; 143: 1485–94.

59. Spears N, Molinek MD, Robinson LLL et al. The role of neurotropin receptors in female germ-cell survival in mouse and human. Development 2003; 130: 5481–91.

60. Pesce M, Farrace MG, Piacentini M et al. Stem cell factor and leukemia germ cell survival by supporting programmed cell death (apoptosis). Development 1993; 118: 1089–94.

61. De Felici M. Regulation of primordial germ cell development in the mouse. Int Devel Biol 2000; 4: 575–80.

62. Driancourt M-A, Reynaud K, Cortvrindt R et al. Roles of KIT and KIT LIGAND in ovarian function. Rev Reprod 2000; 5: 143–52.

63. Parrot JA, Skinner MK. Kit-ligand/stem cell factor induces primordial follicle development and initiates folliculogenesis. Endocrinology 1999; 140: 4262–71.

64. Shim H, Anderson GB. *In vitro* proliferation of porcine primordial germ cells. Theriogenology 1998; 49: 521–8.

65. Cheng L, Gearing DP, White LS et al. Role of leukemia inhibitory factor and its receptor in mouse primordial cell growth. Development 1994; 120: 3145–53.

66. Durcova-Hills G, Prelle K, Muller S et al. Primary culture of porcine PGCs requires LIF and porcine membrane-bound stem cell factor. Zygote 1998; 6: 271–5.

67. Nilsson EE, Kezel P, Skinner MK. Leukemia inhibitory factor (LIF) promotes the primordial to primary follicle transition in rat ovaries. Mol Cell Endocrinol 2002; 188: 65–73.

68. Nilsson E, Parrot JA, Skinner MK. Basic fibroblast growth factor induces primordial follicle development and initiates folliculogenesis. Mol Cell Endocrinol 2001; 175: 123–30.

69. Oktay K, Briggs D, Gosden RG. Ontogeny of follicle-stimulating hormone receptor gene expression in isolated human ovarian follicles. J Clin Endocrinol Metab 1997; 82: 3748–51.

70. Koshimizu U, Taga T, Watanabe M et al. Functional requirement of gp130-mediated signalling of mouse primordial germ cells in vitro and derivation of embryonic germ (EG) cells. Development 1996; 122: 1235–42.

71. Morita Y, Manganaro TF, Tao XJ et al. Requirement for phosphatidylinositol–3′-kinase in cytokine-mediated germ cell survival during fetal oogenesis in the mouse. Endocrinology 1999; 140: 941–9.

72. Lyrakou S, Hulten MA, Hartshorne GM. Growth factors promote meiosis in mouse fetal ovaries *in vitro*. Mol Hum Reprod 2000; 8: 906–11.

73. Durlinger ALL, Visser JA, Themmen APN. Regulation of ovarian function: the role of anti-Müllerian hormone. Reproduction 2002; 124: 601–9.

74. Chian RC, Lim JH, Tan SL. State of the art in in-vitro oocyte maturation. Curr Opin Obstet Gynecol 2004; 16: 211–19.

CHAPTER 8

Maturation of primordial follicles – the next step

Julius Hreinsson, Inger Britt Carlsson, and Outi Hovatta

INTRODUCTION

The survival rates of patients after treatment against malignant disease have dramatically increased during the last few decades, primarily due to therapeutic improvements[1]. One of the possible side-effects of such treatments, however, is the loss of fertility, which can seriously affect the adult lives of survivors. Options for fertility preservation for men through cryopreservation and storage of sperm have been routinely available since the 1970s and are now considered an essential part of any comprehensive cancer care program[2]. The possibilities for women, however, have traditionally been more limited.

The gonadotoxic effect of chemotherapy and radiotherapy is well established; it is dose dependent and varies according to regimens used. A reduction in follicle numbers is seen[3] and the course of ovarian dysfunction is consistent with the destruction of a fixed number of follicles[4]. Temporary or permanent cessation of menstruation may follow therapy and a greatly elevated rate of premature menopause is found in women receiving treatment against malignancy[5]. Survivors of cancer in childhood have been shown to have a diminished ovarian reserve in spite of regular menstrual cycles and may have a shortened reproductive life span and early meno-

pause[6]. Radiotherapy causes destruction of the oocytes and reduction of the follicular reserve. Total body irradiation and high dose chemotherapy, for example before bone marrow transplantation, can be expected to destroy almost all of the oocytes in the ovaries of a female patient[7,8].

Strategies for preservation of fertility for women include cryopreservation of embryos, mature or immature oocytes, or follicles in ovarian cortical tissue. The first two options are not always possible, especially for young women and girls, since in-vitro fertilization (IVF) treatment is a prerequisite to obtain mature oocytes. The number of oocytes obtained at oocyte retrieval is limited at any age. Immature follicles are the largest proportion of the ovarian reserve and fertility preservation through cryopreservation of ovarian cortical biopsies is now offered in many of the larger university hospitals. This is a practical way for storing the large number of oocytes present in immature ovarian follicles. Patients with predicted premature menopause or Turner's syndrome may also benefit from these methods[9].

Good survival of human ovarian follicles in biopsied ovarian cortical tissue has been shown after cryopreservation and thawing using histologic evaluation, transmission electron microscopy, fluorescent viability markers, organ culture, and xenotransplantation to immunodeficient mice[10–16]. Live born individuals after cryopreservation and thawing of ovarian tissue followed by autotransplantation were first observed in experimental animals. This procedure has been successful in mice[17–21], sheep[22,23], and various other animals[24–27].

Developmental potential of the follicles and oocytes in thawed tissue has also been shown in humans by autotransplantation of thawed ovarian tissue. Evidence of follicular function following the procedure includes follicular development induced by follicle-stimulating hormone (FSH) stimulation, estradiol production, and ovulation[28]. Follicular and endometrial development have been observed[29] and hormonal analysis has shown a temporary decrease in FSH levels and estradiol production[30]. Oocyte collection and attempted IVF have also been reported after such a procedure[31].

Recently, two reports, one of a live born child and another of an ongoing pregnancy in human using this procedure, have been published[32,33], confirming the clinical motivation for cryopreservation of ovarian tissue. In survivors of cancer treatment there is a potential danger of re-introducing the original disease to the patient when autografting thawed tissue since malignant cells may reside in the tissue[34]. This depends on the type of cancer the patient had. This possible risk of re-transmission of cancer through autotransplantation of thawed tissue may be greatest in those patients who need fertility preservation most, for example patients with blood borne diseases such as leukemia. For these patients, culture from primordial to antral stages followed by oocyte maturation in vitro is probably the only safe alternative to obtain fertilizable oocytes.

FOLLICLE DEVELOPMENT

Ovarian follicles are formed as closed compartments consisting of an oocyte surrounded by a single layer of granulosa cells enclosed by a basal membrane. As follicles grow, the oocyte increases in size and the granulosa cells multiply in numbers. Formation of an antral cavity precedes ovulation and final oocyte maturation.

Culture of follicles in ovarian cortical tissue is a complex procedure. The whole process of in-vitro growth and maturation from the primordial stage has, until now, only been successful with live born pups in the mouse[35,36]. Using later stage follicles, also from mice, developmentally competent mature oocytes and live born young have been obtained[37–39]. In the human, the time for follicle growth from initiation until ovulation is a much longer process than in rodents. It has been estimated to take up to 200 days[40], although this may be an overestimation.

The early stages of follicle growth depend on a multitude of factors, including FSH for which human primary follicles already have receptors[41]. FSH acts as a survival factor and promotes the growth of the early follicles in vitro[42]. A number of growth factors which influence follicle growth and development have also been identified in recent years. Among these are the members of the TGF-β superfamily of growth factors, shown to be important at these early stages[43]. Of these, anti-Müllerian hormone (AMH, also known as Müllerian inhibiting substance or MIS) inhibits the initiation of growth of the primordial follicles both in human[44] and rat[45], although in 4-week cultures it has also been reported to promote the growth of the follicles[46]. Activins, inhibins, growth differentiation factor 9 (GDF-9), GDF-9B, and the bone morphogenetic proteins or BMPs have functions in follicle development have functions in various species, including humans[46–48]. Other factors, such as kit ligand and stem cell factor, have also been shown to affect early follicle growth in the human[49,50].

During growth the follicles migrate into the medullar region of the ovary. Gonadotropins, especially FSH, are of primary importance for follicular growth and they sustain follicular steroidogenesis. According to the 'two-cell, two-gonadotropins' theory, theca interstitial cells are stimulated by LH to produce aromatizable androgens that are transported to the granulosa cells where they are converted to estrogens by aromatizing enzymes which are induced by FSH[51]. When the follicles have reached a size of 2 mm, they become more dependent on FSH for growth and the steroid production increases. When the middle part of the menstrual cycle approaches, there is a dramatic increase in estrogen, followed by an LH and to a lesser extent an FSH surge. This triggers the dominant follicle to ovulate[52]. After ovulation, the follicle reorganizes to become the corpus luteum, responsible for progesterone production and early maintenance of pregnancy.

COLLECTION OF OVARIAN TISSUE

Human ovarian tissue for research purposes is difficult to obtain. Ovarian biopsies may be collected during laparoscopic surgery, such as sterilizations or other gynecological operations. We have also obtained small ovarian biopsies (2 × 2 × 5 mm) during cesarean sections with good results[53]. For cryostorage of primordial follicles, a biopsy specimen from one ovary, one-fifth of the ovary or less, contains large numbers of follicles, especially in younger patients with good ovarian reserve.

To minimize apoptosis in the tissue, the biopsy is collected in warm Hepes-buffered culture medium, transported immediately to the laboratory, and processed for culture without delay. Whether the biopsy should be kept on ice until processing, or kept at physiologic temperature, has been the subject of some research[54,55]. When preparation is performed after any length of time, a cold collection medium may be recommended[56].

CULTURE OF OVARIAN CORTICAL TISSUE

The high density of the stroma in human ovarian cortical tissue has contributed to the delay in developing a successful system for isolating follicles. Enzymatic isolation of preantral follicles has been successful using human ovarian cortical tissue, where culture was performed for up to 5 days. In these follicles FSH was seen to induce follicular DNA synthesis, antrum formation in larger follicles, and estradiol production[57]. Culture of isolated human primordial follicles for over 24 h, however, has not been successful[58]. In a comparative study of isolated and non-isolated follicles, significantly better survival was seen for follicles cultured within tissue slices than among partially isolated follicles[59].

In organ culture, extracellular matrix has been shown to be beneficial for the survival of the follicles[14]. An immediate activation of growth of the primordial follicles has been observed, with a majority of the follicles leaving the latent primordial stage after one week of culture[59]. Using this culture system, follicle growth up to the secondary stage regularly occurs, and antral follicles are occasionally observed[14,59]. Also follicles in frozen-thawed ovarian tissue grow in such cultures[14]. It is important to use carefully tested freezing protocols[60,61]. In our studies, the optimal size of the pieces in culture was 1–2 mm³. Cubes of tissue were better than thin slices 1 × 1 × 4 mm due to the increased surface area for nutrient and waste exchange[62].

Several factors have been identified that are important for growth of the follicles in vitro. FSH was seen to reduce atresia and to increase the mean diameter of healthy follicles in organ culture. HSA supplemented with insulin/transferrin/selenium mix was also beneficial compared with serum[42]. Insulin and insulin-like growth factors I (IGF-I) and IGF-II have also been seen to improve survival of follicles and to increase the proportion of primary follicles after 2 weeks of culture[63]. GDF-9 significantly promoted the growth and survival of follicles in culture[53]. Due to progressive atresia of the follicles during long-term culture, we have investigated whether apoptosis can be prevented by adding 8-bromo-cyclic adenosine monophosphate (AMP) or guanosine monophosphate (GMP)[64,65]. On the basis of these studies we now regularly add cGMP as an apoptosis inhibitor to the culture medium[64]. Table 8.1 shows the hormones and growth factors that we have studied in this culture model and their effects, while other media constituents are shown in Table 8.2. In Figure 8.1a, a primordial follicle before culture is shown, while Figure 8.1b shows a primary follicle after 1 week of culture. After 2 weeks in culture (Figure 8.1c) and 4 weeks in culture (Figure 8.1d) the follicles are mostly secondary.

We are now using a culture medium which is composed of α-minimal essential medium, with added human serum albumin (5 mg/ml), 1% ITS (insulin, transferrin, selenium mixture for culture supplements), FSH (0.5 IU/ml), GDF-9 (various concentrations have been tested), cGMP (1.1 mg/ml), and antibiotic/antimycotic solution. We have been successful in culturing viable follicles for up to 6 weeks, at which stage the majority of the follicles are at secondary stage (Carlsson et al., unpublished). As we proceed with our work, we are testing new compo-

Table 8.1 Hormones and growth factors which our group has studied using ovarian cortical tissue organ culture of slices/cubes in extracellular matrix and the effect(s) observed

Supplement	Dose(s)	Length of culture	Results	Reference
rrGDF-9	200 ng/ml	14 days	• Increase in follicle activation and development • Decrease in atresia	Hreinsson et al., 2002[53]
8-br-cGMP	5 mM	14 days	• Increase in secondary follicles • Increase in E_2 • Decrease in atresia	Scott et al., 2004[64]
8-br-cAMP	0.5 mM	21 days	• Increase in secondary follicles • Decrease in atresia	Zhang et al., 2004[65]
rhSCF	1, 10, 100 ng/ml	14 days	• No effect on follicle growth	Carlsson et al., 2005[50]
monoclonal anti-c-*kit* antibody	800 ng/ml	7–14 days	• Rapid atresia of primordial oocytes	Carlsson et al., 2005[50]
rrAMH	10, 30, 100, 300 ng/ml	7 days	• Decrease in follicle activation • Decrease in atresia (at 100 ng/ml)	Carlsson et al., 2005[44]

Table 8.2 Media supplements and concentrations

Supplement	Dose	Effect
α-Minimal essential medium	N/A	• Serum free base
Human serum albumin	5 mg/ml	• Protein component
Insulin/transferrin/selenium	1%	• Growth supplements
Antibiotic/antimycotic	1%	• Contamination preventative
rhFSH	0.5 IU/ml	• Growth and maturation promoter

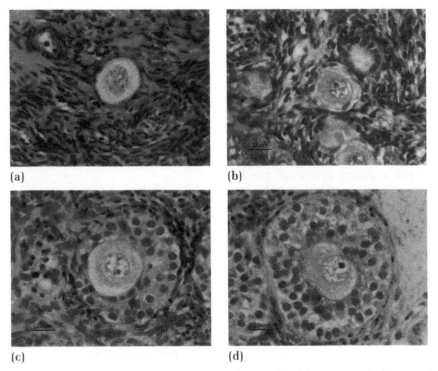

Figure 8.1 (a) Primordial follicle before culture; (b) primary follicle after 1 week of culture with GDF-9 at 200 ng/ml; (c) secondary follicle after 2 weeks of culture with GDF-9 at 200 ng/ml; (d) secondary follicle after 4 weeks of culture with GDF-9 at 200 ng/ml

sitions of the medium to improve antral follicle development. Antral follicles are a prerequisite for obtaining and removing the cumulus–oocyte complex for final maturation of the oocyte in vitro. The maturation of human primordial oocytes to metaphase II fertilizable oocytes is a long and complicated process, and much research is required before a reliable clinical procedure can be realized.

GOAL OF THESE TECHNIQUES – CURRENT PERSPECTIVES

The possibility of obtaining mature oocytes through in-vitro culture of follicles in ovarian tissue would benefit several patient groups. Women and girls having ovarian tissue cryopreserved to preserve their fertility prior to potentially sterilizing cancer treatment will need this technique to obtain fertilizable oocytes from the thawed tissue. Many of these survivors of cancer have been cured of blood borne malignancies precluding re-transplantation of the tissue for in-vivo development. Current techniques for re-transplantation of thawed ovarian tissue for other patients needing fertility preservation are not yet optimal. This includes patients with rheumatic diseases, premature menopause, Turner's syndrome, and localized malignancies. In-vitro culture allows closer observation of the follicles and potentially a better yield of oocytes from small follicles. With better understanding of follicle growth and oocyte maturation, these methods could also benefit women with certain gene defects, such as an inactivating mutation in the FSH receptor[66].

There is a great need to focus research on developing these techniques for human ovarian tissue due to a rapid accumulation of patients waiting to utilize cryopreserved ovarian cortical tissue. This follicle culture method offers us an excellent model for understanding the physiology of the oocyte, follicle recruitment, and development. The role of growth factors can also be critically examined using this method. If successful, this technique might also be beneficial for stem cell research as a source of oocytes for nuclear transfer. The ability to obtain large numbers of oocytes from ovarian tissue biopsies is a prerequisite for somatic cell nuclear transfer and stem cell derivation.

SUMMARY

Ovarian cortical tissue contains the vast majority of all oocytes. Culture of human ovarian cortical tissue to obtain mature fertilizable oocytes would be beneficial for young girls and women who have cryopreserved ovarian tissue and can be predicted to lose their oocytes due to chemotherapy, radiotherapy, or genetic causes. Further, it would be particularly important for women at risk of relapse of the malignancy after transplantation of frozen-thawed tissue, not to mention women with hematologic and ovarian malignancies. In the mouse, live offspring have been born after culture from primordial ovarian follicles, but in humans the process of follicular maturation is much longer and has not yet resulted in offspring. It has been shown that isolated human primordial follicles do not grow in culture. Within pieces of fresh and frozen-thawed human ovarian cortical tissue on extracellular matrix, follicles can be grown for many weeks. They regularly reach the secondary stage and occasionally the antral stage.

Several hormones have been shown to promote survival and growth of early follicles in vitro. We are currently adding FSH, insulin, GDF-9, and cGMP. Regular development to the antral follicle stage would be needed for cumulus-enclosed oocytes to be removed from the follicle for further in-vitro maturation (IVM) of the oocytes. The culture system has to be further developed before oocytes from primordial follicles can be used clinically.

REFERENCES

1. McVie JG. Cancer treatment: the last 25 years. Cancer Treat Rev 1999; 25: 323–31.

2. Kelleher S, Wishart SM, Liu PY et al. Long-term outcomes of elective human sperm cryostorage. Hum Reprod 2001; 16: 2632–9.

3. Nicosia SV, Matus-Ridley M, Meadows AT. Gonadal effects of cancer therapy in girls. Cancer 1985; 55: 2364–72.

4. Howell S, Shalet S. Gonadal damage from chemotherapy and radiotherapy. Endocrinol Metab Clin North Am 1998; 27: 927–43.

5. Byrne J, Fears TR, Gail MH et al. Early menopause in long-term survivors of cancer during adolescence. Am J Obstet Gynecol 1992; 166: 788–93.

6. Larsen EC, Muller J, Rechnitzer C et al. Diminished ovarian reserve in female childhood cancer survivors with regular menstrual cycles and basal FSH <10 IU/L. Hum Reprod 2003; 18: 417–22.

7. Wallace WH, Shalet SM, Crowne EC et al. Ovarian failure following abdominal irradiation in childhood: natural history and prognosis. Clin Oncol (R Coll Radiol) 1989; 1: 75–9.

8. Wallace WH, Thomson AB, Kelsey TW. The radiosensitivity of the human oocyte. Hum Reprod 2003; 18: 117–21.

9. Hreinsson JG, Otala M, Fridstrom M et al. Follicles are found in the ovaries of adolescent girls with Turner's syndrome. J Clin Endocrinol Metab 2002; 87: 3618–23.

10. Hovatta O, Silye R, Krausz T et al. Cryopreservation of human ovarian tissue using dimethylsulphoxide and propanediol-sucrose as cryoprotectants. Hum Reprod 1996; 11: 1268–72.

11. Gook DA, Edgar DH, Stern C. Effect of cooling rate and dehydration regimen on the histological appearance of human ovarian cortex following cryopreservation in 1, 2-propanediol. Hum Reprod 1999; 14: 2061–8.

12. Oktay K, Nugent D, Newton H et al. Isolation and characterization of primordial follicles from fresh and cryopreserved human ovarian tissue. Fertil Steril 1997; 67: 481–6.

13. Cortvrindt RG, Smitz JE. Fluorescent probes allow rapid and precise recording of follicle density and staging in human ovarian cortical biopsy samples. Fertil Steril 2001; 75: 588–93.

14. Hovatta O, Silye R, Abir R et al. Extracellular matrix improves survival of both stored and fresh human primordial and primary ovarian follicles in long-term culture. Hum Reprod 1997; 12: 1032–6.

15. Gook DA, Edgar DH, Borg J et al. Oocyte maturation, follicle rupture and luteinization in human cryopreserved ovarian tissue following xenografting. Hum Reprod 2003; 18: 1772–81.

16. Schmidt KL, Byskov AG, Nyboe Andersen A et al. Density and distribution of primordial follicles in single pieces of cortex from 21 patients and in individual pieces of cortex from three entire human ovaries. Hum Reprod 2003; 18: 1158–64.

17. Parrott DMV. The fertility of mice with orthotopic ovarian grafts derived from frozen tissue. J Reprod Fertil 1960; 1: 230–41.

18. Gunasena KT, Villines PM, Critser ES et al. Live births after autologous transplant of cryopreserved mouse ovaries. Hum Reprod 1997; 12: 101–6.

19. Sztein J, Sweet H, Farley J et al. Cryopreservation and orthotopic transplantation of mouse ovaries: new approach in gamete banking. Biol Reprod 1998; 58: 1071–4.

20. Liu J, Van der Elst J, Van den Broecke R et al. Live offspring by in vitro fertilization of oocytes from cryopreserved primordial mouse follicles after sequential in vivo transplantation and in vitro maturation. Biol Reprod 2001; 64: 171–8.

21. Snow M, Cox SL, Jenkin G et al. Generation of live young from xenografted mouse ovaries. Science 2002; 297: 2227.

22. Gosden RG, Baird DT, Wade JC et al. Restoration of fertility to oophorectomized sheep by ovarian autografts stored at –196 degrees C. Hum Reprod 1994; 9: 597–603.

23. Salle B, Demirci B, Franck M et al. Normal pregnancies and live births after autograft of frozen-thawed hemi-ovaries into ewes. Fertil Steril 2002; 77: 403–8.

24. Wang X, Chen H, Yin H et al. Fertility after intact ovary transplantation. Nature 2002; 415: 385.

25. Candy CJ, Wood MJ, Whittingham DG. Follicular development in cryopreserved marmoset ovarian tissue after transplantation. Hum Reprod 1995; 10: 2334–8.

26. Aubard Y, Newton H, Scheffer G et al. Conservation of the follicular population in irradiated rats by the cryopreservation and orthotopic autografting of ovarian tissue. Eur J Obstet Gynecol Reprod Biol 1998; 79: 83–7.

27. Gunasena KT, Lakey JR, Villines PM et al. Antral follicles develop in xenografted cryopreserved African elephant (Loxodonta africana) ovarian tissue. Anim Reprod Sci 1998; 53: 265–75.

28. Oktay K, Karlikaya G. Ovarian function after transplantation of frozen, banked autologous ovarian tissue. N Engl J Med 2000; 342: 1919.

29. Radford JA, Lieberman BA, Brison DR et al. Orthotopic reimplantation of cryopreserved ovarian cortical strips after high-dose chemotherapy for Hodgkin's lymphoma. Lancet 2001; 357: 1172–5.

30. Callejo J, Salvador C, Miralles A et al. Long-term ovarian function evaluation after autografting by implantation with fresh and frozen-thawed human ovarian tissue. J Clin Endocrinol Metab 2001; 86: 4489–94.

31. Tryde Schmidt KL, Yding Andersen C, Starup J et al. Orthotopic autotransplantation of cryopreserved ovarian tissue to a woman cured of cancer – follicular growth, steroid production and

oocyte retrieval. Reprod Biomed Online 2004; 8: 448–53.

32. Donnez J, Dolmans MM, Demylle D et al. Livebirth after orthotopic transplantation of cryopreserved ovarian tissue. Lancet 2004; 364: 1405–10.

33. Meirow D, Levron J, Eldar-Geva T et al. Pregnancy after transplantation of cryopreserved ovarian tissue in a patient with ovarian failure after chemotherapy. N Engl J Med 2005; 353: 318–21.

34. Shaw JM, Bowles J, Koopman P et al. Fresh and cryopreserved ovarian tissue samples from donors with lymphoma transmit the cancer to graft recipients. Hum Reprod 1996; 11: 1668–73.

35. Eppig JJ, O'Brien MJ. Development *in vitro* of mouse oocytes from primordial follicles. Biol Reprod 1996; 54: 197–207.

36. O'Brien MJ, Pendola JK, Eppig JJ. A revised protocol for *in vitro* development of mouse oocytes from primordial follicles dramatically improves their developmental competence. Biol Reprod 2003; 68: 1682–6.

37. Eppig JJ, Schroeder AC. Capacity of mouse oocytes from preantral follicles to undergo embryogenesis and development to live young after growth, maturation, and fertilization *in vitro*. Biol Reprod 1989; 41: 268–76.

38. Spears N, Boland NI, Murray AA et al. Mouse oocytes derived from *in vitro* grown primary ovarian follicles are fertile. Hum Reprod 1994; 9: 527–32.

39. Cortvrindt R, Smitz J, Van Steirteghem AC. A morphological and functional study of the effect of slow freezing followed by complete in-vitro maturation of primary mouse ovarian follicles. Hum Reprod 1996; 11: 2648–55.

40. Gougeon A. Dynamics of follicular growth in the human: a model from preliminary results. Hum Reprod 1986; 1: 81–7.

41. Oktay K, Briggs D, Gosden RG. Ontogeny of follicle-stimulating hormone receptor gene expression in isolated human ovarian follicles. J Clin Endocrinol Metab 1997; 82: 3748–51.

42. Wright CS, Hovatta O, Margara R et al. Effects of follicle-stimulating hormone and serum substi-tution on the in-vitro growth of human ovarian follicles. Hum Reprod 1999; 14: 1555–62.

43. Erickson GF, Shimasaki S. The role of the oocyte in folliculogenesis. Trends Endocrinol Metab 2000; 11: 193–8.

44. Carlsson IB, Scott JE, Visser JA et al. Anti-Müllerian hormone inhibits initiation of growth of human primordial ovarian follicles in vitro. Hum Reprod 2006; [Epub ahead of print].

45. Visser JA, Themmen AP. Anti-Mullerian hormone and folliculogenesis. Mol Cell Endocrinol 2005; 234: 81–6.

46. Schmidt KL, Kryger-Baggesen N, Byskov AG et al. Anti-Mullerian hormone initiates growth of human primordial follicles in vitro. Mol Cell Endocrinol 2005; 234: 87–93.

47. McGrath SA, Esquela AF, Lee SJ. Oocyte-specific expression of growth/differentiation factor-9. Mol Endocrinol 1995; 9: 131–6.

48. Juengel JL, McNatty KP. The role of proteins of the transforming growth factor-beta superfamily in the intraovarian regulation of follicular development. Hum Reprod Update 2005; 11: 143–60.

49. Driancourt MA, Reynaud K, Cortvrindt R et al. Roles of KIT and KIT LIGAND in ovarian function. Rev Reprod 2000; 5: 143–52.

50. Carlsson IB, M.P.E. L, Scott JE, Louhio H et al. Kit ligand and c-kit are expressed during early human ovarian follicular development and their interaction is required for the survival of follicles in long-term culture. *Reproduction* 2006; 131(4): 641–9.

51. Hillier SG, Whitelaw PF, Smyth CD. Follicular oestrogen synthesis: the 'two-cell, two-gonado-trophin' model revisited. Mol Cell Endocrinol 1994; 100: 51–4.

52. Yen SCC, Jaffe RB, Barbieri RL. Reproductive Endocrinology, 4th edn. WB Saunders Company, Philadelphia, Pennsylvania, 1999.

53. Hreinsson JG, Scott JE, Rasmussen C et al. Growth differentiation factor-9 promotes the growth, development, and survival of human ovarian follicles in organ culture. J Clin Endocrinol Metab 2002; 87: 316–21.

54. Weissman A, Gotlieb L, Colgan T et al. Preliminary experience with subcutaneous human ovarian cortex transplantation in the NOD-SCID mouse. Biol Reprod 1999; 60: 1462–7.

55. Lucci CM, Kacinskis MA, Rumpf R et al. Effects of lowered temperatures and media on short-term preservation of zebu (*Bos indicus*) preantral ovarian follicles. Theriogenology 2004; 61: 461–72.

56. Schmidt KL, Ernst E, Byskov AG et al. Survival of primordial follicles following prolonged transportation of ovarian tissue prior to cryopreservation. Hum Reprod 2003; 18: 2654–9.

57. Roy SK, Treacy BJ. Isolation and long-term culture of human preantral follicles. Fertil Steril 1993; 59: 783–90.

58. Abir R, Roizman P, Fisch B et al. Pilot study of isolated early human follicles cultured in collagen gels for 24 hours. Hum Reprod 1999; 14(5): 1299–301.

59. Hovatta O, Wright C, Krausz T et al. Human primordial, primary and secondary ovarian follicles in long-term culture: effect of partial isolation. Hum Reprod 1999; 14: 2519–24.

60. Hovatta O. Methods for cryopreservation of human ovarian tissue. Reprod Biomed Online 2005; 10: 729–34.

61. Hreinsson J, Zhang P, Swahn ML et al. Cryopreservation of follicles in human ovarian cortical tissue. Comparison of serum and human serum albumin in the cryoprotectant solutions. Hum Reprod 2003; 18: 2420–8.

62. Scott JE, Carlsson IB, Bavister BD et al. Human ovarian tissue cultures: extracellular matrix composition, coating density and tissue dimensions. Reprod Biomed Online 2004; 9: 287–93.

63. Louhio H, Hovatta O, Sjoberg J et al. The effects of insulin, and insulin-like growth factors I and II on human ovarian follicles in long-term culture. Mol Hum Reprod 2000; 6: 694–8.

64. Scott JE, Zhang P, Hovatta O. Benefits of 8-bromo-guanosine 3′,5′-cyclic monophosphate (8-br-cGMP) in human ovarian cortical tissue culture. Reprod Biomed Online 2004; 8: 319–24.

65. Zhang P, Louhio H, Tuuri T et al. In vitro effect of cyclic adenosine 3′, 5′-monophosphate (cAMP) on early human ovarian follicles. J Assist Reprod Genet 2004; 21: 301–6.

66. Aittomaki K, Herva R, Stenman UH et al. Clinical features of primary ovarian failure caused by a point mutation in the follicle-stimulating hormone receptor gene. J Clin Endocrinol Metab 1996; 81: 3722–6.

CHAPTER 9

Ovarian endocrinology

Frank J Broekmans and Bart CJM Fauser

INTRODUCTION

The ovary in the female adult has a cyclic function that is both autonomous as well as directed by the hypothalamic–pituitary axis. The development of primordial follicles towards the antral stages and the elimination of the vast majority of these developing follicles along the way are fully under control of local factors. It is from the small antral stage of follicular development onwards that pituitary gonadotropin hormones facilitate the menstrual cycle. Dominant follicle growth, ovulation of the oocyte, and corpus luteum formation represent the key processes of the ovarian cycle and much is dependent on the interplay between pituitary gonadotropins, ovarian steroids, and peptides. The ultimate goal of the menstrual cycle is the implantation of a vital embryo in the endometrium that has been prepared under the influence of ovarian steroids.

FUNCTIONAL OVARIAN ANATOMY

The human ovary is an ellipsoid organ with a clear white appearance. On full through-cut the medulla part should be distinguished from the cortex (Figure 9.1). The medulla is continuous with the mesovarium and contains mainly blood vessels and connective tissue. The cortical tissue comprises the largest part of the ovary and contains the stroma in which the follicles are embedded. At the periphery of the ovary the stroma tissue is very dense, giving the ovary its white appearance.

Histologically, the outer lining consists of a flat or cuboidal epithelial cell layer, often erroneously referred to as 'germinal epithelium'. It is capable of expressing the mucus gene MUC1 and the surface cells have cilia and apical microvilli. The surface epithelium plays a role in the transport of substances to and from the peritoneal cavity and in the repair of surface defects, for instance after ovulation. The ovarian stroma contains fibroblastic cells with limited steroidogenic properties and the capability of producing growth factors and growth factor binding proteins. As such, the stroma is involved in the functional separation of follicles and corpora lutea through both physical and biochemical measures[1]. Also, various inflammation cell types are found in the interstitial tissue that are involved in tissue repair after ovulation and the elimination of atretic follicles. The medullary part of the ovary contains the hilar vascular plexus and extrinsic innervation of both sympathetic as well as parasympathetic fibers, responsible for regulation of ovarian blood flow and steroid

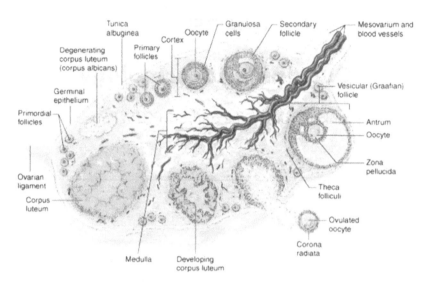

Figure 9.1 Section of the human ovary, showing the anatomic parts and the sequence of developmental stages of the follicles. Reprinted from Animal Reproduction Science, 78, Knight PG and Glister G: Local roles of TGF-β superfamily members in the control of ovarian follicle development, 165–183, 2003, with permission from Elsevier

synthesis of theca-interstitial cells. The cortex of the ovary contains large quantities of primordial follicles. This type of follicle consists of an oocyte surrounded by a single layer of flattened granulosa cells. Once the primordial follicle starts its development towards antral stages (primary follicle), the granulosa cells become cuboidal and an internal theca cell layer is acquired. These cells are elongated and separated from the granulosa cells by a basal membrane. With further expansion in follicle and oocyte size the outer thecal layer is developed by compressing the surrounding stroma, while the granulosa cells form several layers around the oocyte (secondary follicle, Figure 9.2), which by then becomes surrounded by the zona pellucida. The internal thecal layer is cell rich and highly vascularized and arterioles terminate in a network of capillaries at the basal membrane between the theca and granulosa layers.

As the secondary follicle is formed, FSH, androgen, and estrogen receptors develop in the granulosa and LH receptors in the thecal cells. Granulosa cells have no direct blood supply and

are dependent on the passage of nutritional and regulatory substances through the basal membrane between the granulosa cell layer and the blood supply of the internal theca. Granulosa cells are interconnected by gap junctions that ensure exchange and transport of small molecules and have cytoplasmic processes through the zona pellucida that contact the plasma mem-

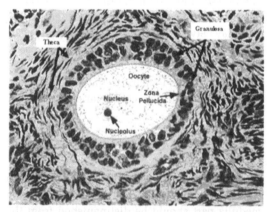

Figure 9.2 Histologic image of a primary human follicle

brane of the oocyte for exchange functions[2–4] The structural composition of the gap junctions is determined by proteins called connexins, that are encoded for by both the oocyte and granulosa cells.

In its development during the primary and secondary follicle stage the oocyte attains meiotic and developmental competence[5,6]. Meiotic competence refers to the ability to carry out the meiotic divisions with proper chromosome segregation and re-establishment of genomic imprinting. Developmental competence is the ability to support pre-embryo development by remodeling sperm DNA. Once fluid collection takes place between the multiple granulosa cell layers of the secondary follicle it eventually leads to the formation of an antrum. This process requires rapid influx of water, enabled by active ion transport by granulosa cells into the developing antrum, thereby increasing osmolarity. The antrum and its fluid are thought to enable the release of the cumulus–oocyte complex from the ruptured follicle at ovulation and to play a role in nutrient and waste exchange for the avascular granulosa layer. Granulosa cells from the antral wall are called mural cells and express the greatest steroidogenic activity and the highest level of LH receptors. The cells surrounding the oocyte are named cumulus cells and have low LH responding properties[7], while being active in producing the extracellular matrix that is necessary for the preovulatory expansion of the cumulus–oocyte complex (Figure 9.3).

The final stage of antral follicle development is the Graafian follicle, with a diameter of 15–25 mm, which rapidly increases its size through increased accumulation of fluid and granulosa cell proliferation. At ovulation the ovum is released from this follicle after having resumed meiosis and the granulosa and theca cells will differentiate into luteinized cells under the influence of the LH surge. Thereby follicular remnants remain endocrinally active as the corpus luteum, a highly vascularized structure which will regress into a corpus albicans some

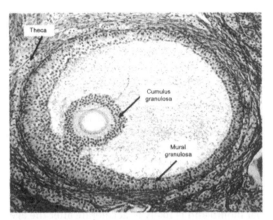

Figure 9.3 Histologic structure of the large antral follicle

9–11 days after ovulation, unless the exposure to human chorionic gonadotropin (hCG) released from an implanted blastocyst prevents this.

FOLLICLE DEVELOPMENT

Initial recruitment

In the third week of fetal development germ cells arise under the influence of transforming growth factor beta (TGF-β) superfamily members (bone morphogenetic proteins, BMPs)[8] in the yolk sac. From there the primordial germ cells migrate along the hindgut into the genital ridges, where they arrive at 6 weeks postfertilization[9] and start to proliferate. Migration and proliferation are under the control of kit ligand, integrin β, TIAR-1 and the Pog (proliferation of germ cells) gene, and leukemia inhibiting factor (LIF)[10–13]. At the fourth month of fetal development the ovaries contain some 6–7 million oogonia that develop into oocytes by entering the first meiotic division, after which they become arrested at the diplotene stage of the prophase[14,15]. Failure to enter meiosis will inevitably lead to apoptosis of the oogonium. Oocytes are then surrounded by a layer of flat granulosa cells to form primordial follicles. In humans, oocytes remain in this resting phase for many decades until resumption of meiosis is effected by exposure to the mid cycle LH peak. Through a steady flow of primordial follicles and non-meiotic oogonia into apoptosis or atresia, mediated by a deficiency in survival factors like kit ligand and LIF or cell death inducers like TGF-β and activin, at birth 1–2 million primordial follicles are left[16,17]. After birth the rate of loss of follicles slows down so that at menarche some 3 to 4 hundred thousands are left[18]. During the reproductive years the loss of primordial follicles remains steady at some thousand follicles per month and is likely to accelerate after the age of 37 until the ovaries have become devoid of any follicles around the menopause.

Of the 1–2 million follicles present at birth, only some 400 will eventually develop into an ovulating dominant follicle (Figure 9.4). The remaining follicles will undergo atresia in the course of postnatal life due to a process referred to as apoptosis (programmed cell death[20]). Atresia occurs at almost every stage of follicle

development, but not in postnatal primordial and dominant follicles. The development from the primordial follicle stage up till the moment of ovulation may take at least 6–8 months[21]. However, as in the fetal period, the vast majority of primordial follicles will never reach the stage of dominance and ovulation, but will undergo apoptosis or cell necrosis (Figure 9.5). It is proposed that follicle development before the antral stages is independent of FSH exposure and is regulated by intraovarian factors. As the normal fate of primordial follicles is programmed cell death, the 400 or so follicles that will reach full maturation and ovulation are rescued by processes that are principally dependent on gonadotropins.

Cyclic recruitment

From the size of 2 mm onwards, antral follicles gain FSH sensitivity as a result of increasing numbers of membrane receptors on their granulosa cells. Up to a follicle diameter of 5 mm only very

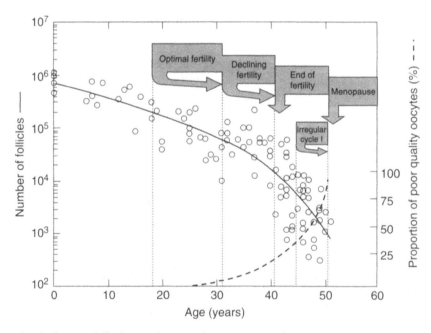

Figure 9.4 The decline in follicle number in relation to reproductive events with increasing female age. Reprinted with permission from Klinkert[19]

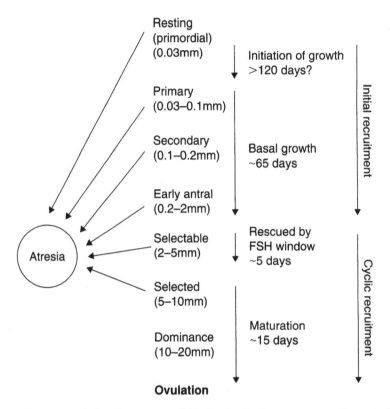

Figure 9.5 Classification and development of follicles in the human ovary. Reprinted and adapted with permission from te Velde and Pearson[22]

small amounts of gonadotropins are sufficient for follicle development[23,24]. For development into a dominant preovulatory follicle, exposure to higher levels of FSH is necessary. During that development, which will take about 2 weeks (Figure 9.6), the follicle will increase in size from 5 to about 20 to 25 mm just before ovulation[25]. Although the number of follicles that are present in the ovary in the small antral stage (2 to 5 mm) can amount to 20 to 25, only one follicle is selected to become the dominant follicle that will subsequently ovulate. The granulosa cells of this follicle have a high mitotic index and the follicular fluid contains FSH and estradiol. The mechanism underlying this single dominant follicle selection has become known as the threshold/window concept.

The demise of the corpus luteum at the end of the previous menstrual cycle and the resulting decrease in estradiol and inhibin A levels[26,27] cause FSH levels to rise at the end of the menstrual cycle[28]. By exceeding a certain threshold level[29,30], the cohort of FSH-sensitive antral follicles present at that time will start to grow and are thereby initially rescued from atresia. Rising FSH levels will, however, soon become depressed by negative feedback from estradiol[31] and inhibin B[32] produced by the cohort of developing antral follicles (Figure 9.7). Decreasing FSH levels provide the occurrence of a window or time period in which the FSH threshold of the individual follicles of the FSH sensitive cohort is exceeded[33,34]. The length of the time window and the hierarchy of FSH sensitivity of the various

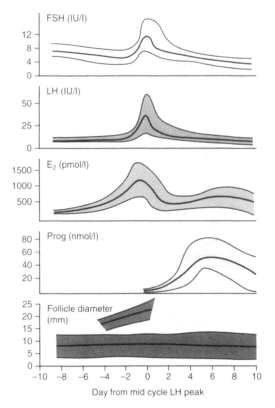

Figure 9.6 Endocrine fluctuations and follicle growth in the menstrual cycle. Reprinted with permission from Macklon and Fauser[39]

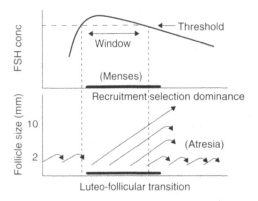

Figure 9.7 The FSH window/threshold concept for dominant follicle selection. Reprinted with permission from Macklon and Fauser[35]

follicles in the cohort will determine the number of follicles that are allowed to begin preovulatory development (dominant follicle growth). The single dominant follicle will gradually diminish its dependency on FSH and will start to produce rapidly increasing amounts of estradiol. The rising estradiol levels will subsequently further suppress the FSH plasma concentration, making dominant growth impossible for the other participants in the stimulated cohort[35,36]. Yet another mechanism whereby the dominant follicle escapes from becoming atretic is that the granulosa cells acquire LH receptors. Consequently, in addition to FSH, LH can support growth and differentiation of the dominant follicle and recent studies have shown that growth of the dominant follicle can be completed under the influence of LH alone[37,38].

The exponential rise in estradiol levels triggers the LH/FSH surge. As a result, resumption of meiosis in the oocyte, ovulation, and luteinization of the granulosa are established. The LH-induced synthesis of progesterone is believed to play an important role in the mechanism of follicle rupture. Enzymes that degrade the follicle wall, like plasminogen activators, the matrix metalloproteinase family members, and cadhepsin L, are expressed in granulosa cells under the influence of progesterone. Progesterone receptors induced in the granulosa cells by the LH surge are part of this autocrine loop phenomenon[40,41]. The end result of follicle wall degradation is the protrusion of the follicle through the ovarian capsule and the rupture and gentle release of the egg and follicular fluid. At this stage the expansion of the cumulus oophorus is a crucial process, enabling oocyte release from the follicle. LH-induced prostaglandin biosynthesis by COX/2 enzyme activity in granulosa cells is believed to play a role in the cumulus expansion[42]. Moreover, cumulus expansion results from LH-induced synthesis of hyaluronic acid[43].

Corpus luteum formation implies that a wide vascular network is formed which facilitates the delivery of precursors for steroid production and release of secretory products into the circulation. Vascularization is enabled by angiogenic factors like VEGF and FGF, produced by granulosa cells in response to the LH stimulus of the mid cycle surge. The luteinization of granulosa cells includes a loss of their mitotic potential and expression of genes that encode for enzymes involved in progesterone synthesis, like StAR, P450scc, and 3β-hydroxysteroid dehydrogenase. Granulosa-lutein cells therefore mainly deliver progesterone, but through continued expression of aromatase they also remain the source of estradiol production. Luteinized theca cells, through the 17α-hydroxylase/17–20 lyase enzyme, continue to produce androgen precursors, but also 17α-hydroxyprogesterone. Luteal function is principally maintained by exposure to LH pulses that coincide with fluctuations in progesterone levels[44], while the increasing presence of LH/hCG receptors in the course of the luteal phase enables a steady rise in progesterone levels. Progesterone itself is believed to support its own production in an autocrine fashion[45]. After the mid luteal progesterone peak the intrinsic life cycle of the corpus luteum inevitably results in its physical and functional demise. The mechanism of luteolysis, leading to the formation of a scarring tissue zone known as the corpus albicans, is poorly understood[46]. Reduced LH signaling efficiency, possibly related to the presence of prostaglandin F2α, results in a fall in the presence of steroidogenic enzymes with a drop in progesterone release. Also, apoptosis and autophagia triggered by cytokines of the TNF-α superfamily and interferon-γ will imply structural destruction of the steroidogenic cells. Luteolytic substances like TNF-α, endothelin-1, and MCP-1 are believed to alter endothelial function, with vascular damage and reduced perfusion of the corpus luteum as the consequence.

The emergence of hCG from an implanted embryo will stimulate steroidogenesis and prevent the programmed structural and functional demise of the corpus luteum. In contrast, under the influence of rising hCG, the corpus luteum will show hypertrophy of the luteinized granulosa and theca cells and further expansion of the vascular network. Rescue of the corpus luteum by hCG will lead to increased levels of progesterone, inhibin A, and relaxin at the end of the luteal phase and into the first weeks of pregnancy.

GONADOTROPIN CONTROL OF CYCLIC FOLLICULAR RECRUITMENT

FSH and LH are heterodimer glycoproteins composed of a common α subunit and a specific β subunit. Release of FSH and LH from the anterior pituitary cells is primarily directed by the secretion of gonadotropin-releasing hormone (GnRH) from autonomic nuclei located in the medial basal and ventral hypothalamus. The pulsatile release of GnRH into the pituitary stalk portal vein system ensures the synthesis and pulsatile release of LH and FSH from the pituitary. FSH release seems to have an additional autonomic component and has a relatively high plasma half life, resulting in the pulsatile pattern of FSH in the plasma being far less clear. Typically, the frequency of gonadotropin pulses is rather high in the follicular phase with relatively low amplitudes, while in the luteal phase pulse frequency slows down to every few hours with a clear increase in the amplitude.

Specificity of the interaction between hormone and receptor is regulated due to the presence of the β subunit. The human LH and FSH receptors are glycoproteins that belong to the family of G-protein-coupled transmembrane receptors and are encoded for by genes located on chromosome 2p21. Through the linkage to G proteins located in the inner part of the cell membrane, coupling to the intracellular effector system is ensured. In addition to the cyclic AMP pathway, calcium channels, protein kinase B and C, and mitogen activated kinase are believed to play a role in transforming the gonadotropin signal into specific cell function[47]. According to the two-cell two-gonadotropin theory, LH receptors are primarily present at the membranes of the internal theca cells, while the FSH receptor is expressed by granulosa cells (Figure 9.8). FSH receptor presence is attained in the early stage of antral follicle formation and FSH exposure in growing antral follicles will increase the number of FSH receptors, resulting in a feed forward system. In the course of an antral follicle obtaining dominance, FSH-induced LH receptors also

come to expression at the granulosa cell membrane, allowing LH to partially take over FSH actions and ensuring responsiveness of the pre-ovulatory follicle to the mid cycle LH surge[48].

The action of FSH at the level of the granulosa cell comprises enhancement of granulosa cell proliferation and differentiation, stimulation of the aromatase enzyme system that is responsible for the conversion of thecal

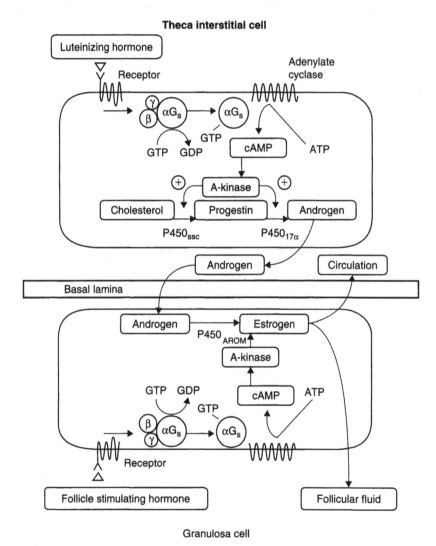

Figure 9.8 The two-cell two-gonadotropin concept [www.endotext.org/female/female1/figures1/figure19-gif]

androgens into estrogens, formation and development of the follicle antrum, maturation of the oocyte, presumably mediated through the function of the granulosa cells in the cumulus oophorus, as well as completion of the first meiotic division by the oocyte up to meiosis II metaphase stage.

The role of LH in the later stages of antral follicle development is mainly related to its effect on estradiol biosynthesis by regulating the production of androgens in the internal theca cells. LH also plays a role in supporting FSH in selection and regulation of the final growth of the dominant follicle[37,38]. In the course of dominant follicle growth only small amounts of LH are necessary for proper follicle function and high LH levels are believed to induce premature luteinization and atresia[49,50]. Finally, LH is uniquely essential for the process of ovulation of the dominant follicle and the resumption of meiotic division of the oocyte. Parallel to the process of ovulation, stimulation of the LH receptors at the granulosa level forces the granulosa cells to convert from an estradiol-producing unit into luteinized cells that produce both estradiol and progesterone. Corpus luteum function survival is dependent on the release of gonadotropins. However, in the absence of hCG release from an implanted blastocyst the corpus luteum will eventually regress in the late luteal phase. The subsequent fall in progesterone, estradiol, and inhibin A levels allows the levels of FSH to rise at the luteo-follicular transition, which induces the subsequent selection of a new cohort that delivers the dominant follicle for the upcoming cycle.

OVARIAN STEROID AND PROTEIN SYNTHESIS

Steroid hormone synthesis starts with the acquisition and storage of cholesterol by the steroid-producing theca cells. The enzyme complex cytochrome P450 side chain cleavage (P450-SSC) is responsible for the transformation of cholesterol into pregnenolone (Figure 9.9). For the rapid response to tropic hormones (especially LH) another enzyme, the steroid acute regulatory protein (StAR), is held responsible. Pregnenolone is further metabolized under the influence of two enzyme systems: the cytochrome P450-C17 and the 3β-hydroxy steroid dehydrogenase enzyme (3β-HSD). P450-C17 enables the transition of progestagens into androgens, first by allowing pregnenolone to change into 17OH-pregnenolone by hydroxylation (P450-17α-hydroxylase) and then by changing 17OH-pregnenolone into dehydroepiandrosterone (DHEA) through P450-17,20-lyase activity. The 3β-HSD enzyme converts the delta-5 steroids pregnenolone, 17OH-pregnenolone, and DHEA into the delta-4 steroids progesterone, 17OH-progesterone, and androstenedione, respectively. The 17β variant of HSD transforms androstenedione into testosterone. Finally, it is the CYP19 aromatase enzyme in the granulosa cells that converts C19 androgenic steroids into estradiol. This implies that granulosa cells are not capable of estradiol synthesis de novo, but fully rely upon androgen substrate production from the theca cells. The activity of the aromatase system is dependent on FSH exposure and, in the late proliferative phase, also on LH. Estradiol levels within the follicular fluid are extremely high. Through diffusion, estradiol reaches the blood circulation. Transport of steroids towards the effector organs is mainly through the blood system. In plasma they are bound to sex hormone binding globulin (SHBG) and albumin. Only in minor quantities do they circulate freely. Synthesis and release of SHBG from the liver is enhanced by estrogens and insulin, but decreases through the action of androgens. Steroid hormones will pass the cell membrane of the effector cell and bind to steroid receptors located at the cell nucleus. Steroid receptors are part of the superfamily of ligand-modified transcription factors that are responsible for growth, differentiation, and homeostasis.

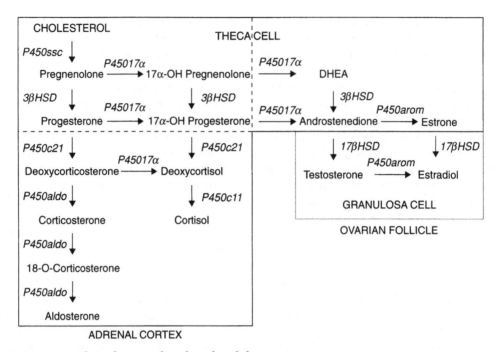

Figure 9.9 Steroid synthesis in the adrenal and the ovarian cortex

Apart from the classic target organs for steroid hormones like the endometrial tissue, cervix, fallopian tube, breast, bone, and brain, steroids also elicit effects in the ovary itself.

Progesterone synthesis from granulosa-lutein cells after ovulation is ensured by expression of the enzymes StAR, P450scc, and 3β-HSD (see Figure 9.9). Progesterone enhances corpus luteum function and induces development of the endometrium into the secretory stage.

Inhibins (A and B) are members of the TGF-β protein superfamily, with a common α-subunit but different β-subunits. The source of inhibin production is the granulosa cell. Inhibin B is secreted mainly from small antral follicles in the early follicular phase and levels fall to undetectable after the mid cycle gonadotropin surge. Inhibin A is low at the start of the cycle, but rises with dominant follicle growth into the preovulatory phase and will remain high until the mid luteal phase.

INTRAOVARIAN MODULATORS OF FOLLICLE DEVELOPMENT

The development of the primordial follicle up to the stage of ovulation and corpus luteum formation is, apart from extraovarian hormones like FSH and LH, regulated and controlled by a large number of para- and autocrine factors produced by granulosa cells, theca cells, and the oocyte itself. Most of these modulators are members of the superfamily of the TGF-β system[51], the insulin-like growth factor (IGF) system[52], and the epidermal growth factor (EGF) system[53,54], but ovarian steroid and protein hormones also play a role[55,56]. Intraovarian regulatory systems have not been elucidated to such an extent that there is full understanding of how primordial follicles eventually develop into the preovulatory follicle. Therefore in this section the role of intraovarian regulators will be discussed only briefly (Figure 9.10).

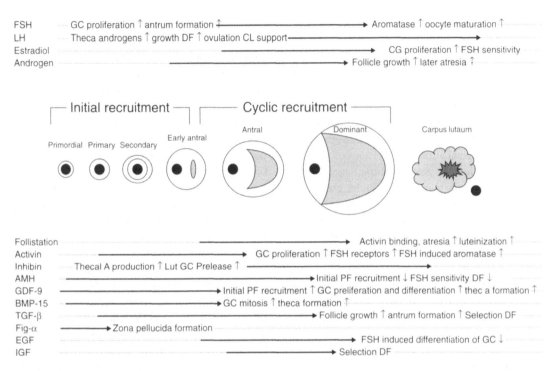

FSH — GC proliferation ↑ antrum formation → Aromatase ↑ oocyte maturation ↑
LH — Theca androgens ↑ growth DF ↑ ovulation CL support →
Estradiol → CG proliferation ↑ FSH sensitivity
Androgen → Follicle growth ↑ later atresia ↑

Initial recruitment — Cyclic recruitment

Antral — Dominant — Carpus lutaum

Primordial Primary Secondary — Early antral

Follistation → Activin binding, atresia ↑ luteinization ↑
Activin → GC proliferation ↑ FSH receptors ↑ FSH induced aromatase ↑
Inhibin — Thecal A production ↑ Lut GC Prelease ↑ →
AMH → Initial PF recruitment ↓ FSH sensitivity DF ↓
GDF-9 → Initial PF recruitment ↑ GC preliferation and differentiation ↑ thec a formation ↑
BMP-15 → GC mitosis ↑ theca formation ↑
TGF-β → Follicle growth ↑ antrum formation ↑ Selection DF
Fig-α → Zona pellucida formation
EGF → FSH induced differentiation of GC ↓
IGF → Selection DF

Figure 9.10 The role of intraovarian regulators in initial and cyclic recruitment of follicles. Bold arrows indicate the phase of development in which the modulator has (putative) action. Modified with permission from Knight and Glister[60] GC, Granulosa cell; DF, Dominant follicle; PF, Primordial follicle; Lut GC, Luteinized granulosa cells; CL, Corpus luteum

FSH is not necessary for the transition of primordial follicles into growing follicles as these follicles do not express FSH and LH receptors, and in FSH knockout mice the ovaries still contain growing follicles[57–59]. Still, LH and FSH regulation of early and late antral follicles may have indirect effects on the behavior of the primordial follicle pool, possibly through production by the antral follicles of one or more factors that affect the primordial pool. The transition of primordial follicles into growing follicles is a largely autonomous process in which growth differentiation factor-9 (GDF-9) and the bone morphogenetic protein 15 (BMP-15) are involved. GDF-9 is produced by the oocyte and considered an obligatory signal for further growth beyond the primordial stages[60,61]. It acts by promoting granulosa cell proliferation and differentiation

and by enabling the formation of a thecal cell layer in primary follicles[62,63]. The thecal cell layer develops from primary interstitial cells present in the fetal ovary under the influence of oocyte-derived GDF-9 and kit ligand produced by granulosa cells[64,65]. Recombinant GDF-9 has also been shown to stimulate initial follicle recruitment in vivo[66]. BMP-15 plays a comparably essential role in early follicular growth by stimulating granulosa cell mitosis and initiation of theca cell layer formation[67–70]. Zona pellucida (ZP) formation is regulated by oocyte-specific genes that encode for a number of ZP proteins. These genes are expressed under the control of Fig(factor in the germ line)-α. The zona protects the oocyte and is essential for normal fertilization[71,72]. During further stages of follicle development, oocytes continue to express GDF-9 and BMP-15. Anti-müllerian hormone (AMH), produced by the granulosa cells of the primary follicles, has been shown to have an inhibitory effect on the transition from primordial into developing follicles and as such has a functional counteraction to GDF-9. In the absence of AMH, as shown in the knockout model, the pool of primordial follicles is reduced at a much higher rate than in the normal situation[73].

After the follicle has developed into a primary and secondary growing follicle, granulosa cells initiate synthesis and release of inhibins, activin, and follistatin. In the early growing phase activins are predominantly produced that enhance granulosa cell proliferation and protect the follicle from becoming atretic[74–76]. In small antral follicles, activins promote the expression of FSH receptors, further assisting the growth of follicles in response to FSH, and support FSH-dependent aromatase activity, as well as reduce the LH-dependent androgen production by theca cells[74]. They also enhance oocyte maturation and as such activins seem to protect the growing follicle from demise and prepare it for its steroid producing functions, while stimulating FSH release from the pituitary. Much of their action becomes counteracted by follistatin, produced from small antral follicles, that selectively binds to activins and neutralizes the follicle development promoting actions of activins. Inhibins are involved in growing follicles from the antral stages onwards. They selectively suppress FSH release from the pituitary, thereby indirectly influencing FSH action on the follicle, and exert a paracrine action on theca cells where they enhance LH-induced androgen secretion[77–79]. As such inhibins play a role in both facilitating steroid synthesis and enabling dominant follicle selection. Activins and inhibins thus have opposing actions, where activins are dominant in the early stages of the growing follicle, while inhibins come into play much more when the follicle has become antral and attained sensitivity to gonadotropins.

TGF-β, produced by both theca and granulosa cells, is believed to play a role that is comparable to activin in promoting follicular growth and may also be involved in antrum formation by interfering with the role of connective tissue growth factor (CTGF) in extracellular matrix modeling and angiogenesis[80,81]. Epidermal growth factor and TGF-α have been shown to be potent inhibitors of FSH-dependent differentiation of granulosa cells.

When follicles have reached the antral stage of development the crucial factor for ongoing development is FSH. FSH action may, in part, become expressed through intermediary factors like steroids and proteins released from granulosa cells. Inhibins are capable of suppressing FSH release from the pituitary, but also enhance LH- and IGF-mediated androgen synthesis from theca cells. Follistatin is another factor that comes to expression in antral follicle stages and is known for its FSH-suppressing ability and binding of activins. The neutralization of activin action by follistatin is important to reduce the suppression of estrogen and progesterone production from granulosa cells in antral and dominant follicles. Estrogens produced from granulosa cells promote their proliferation and have anti-atretic effects, while augmenting intercellular gap junctions and formation of the follicular antrum. The role of androgens in antral follicles is believed to be mainly folliculotropic, as evidenced by the high quantities of androgen receptors in granulosa cells of preantral and antral follicles. In later stages of follicular growth androgens may exert atretogenic effects by interference with the aromatase system. AMH is capable of mitigating the FSH-induced follicular growth of antral follicles. Once the dominant follicle has been selected AMH expression becomes severely reduced, enabling an increase in the FSH effects on this dominant follicle. As such AMH may contribute to dominant follicle selection[82].

The process of dominant follicle selection and growth from the cohort of small antral follicles is believed to be regulated according to the threshold window concept, as explained earlier. Fine tuning of FSH levels seems to be the most important effector in this regulation. Still, the supposed changes in individual sensitivity for FSH within the cohort of follicles may be exerted by intraovarian paracrine and autocrine factors. Estradiol is believed to enhance the FSH response of the follicle and AMH exerts the opposite effect. In dominant follicles it is the production of these two substances that alters in such a way that the efficiency of the FSH stimulus is upgraded. Insulin-like growth factors and their binding proteins are believed to be the first factors that mark the attainment of dominance[83]. Members of the TGF-β family are known for their effects on steroid synthesis and induction of LH receptors in granulosa cells and growth inhibition of smaller subordinate antral follicles[61]. As such, the TGF and IGF systems may well be part of the integration of extraovarian signals and intrafollicular factors that determine whether a follicle will continue to develop into dominance or be diverted into atretic pathways.

REFERENCES

1. Jabara S, Christenson LK, Wang CY et al. Stromal cells of the human postmenopausal ovary display a distinctive biochemical and molecular phenotype. J Clin Endocrinol Metab 2003; 88: 484–92.

2. Matzuk MM, Burns KH, Viveiros MM, Eppig JJ. Intercellular communication in the mammalian ovary: oocytes carry the conversation. Science 2002; 296: 2178–80.

3. Albertini DF, Combelles CM, Benecchi E, Carabatsos MJ. Cellular basis for paracrine regulation of ovarian follicle development. Reproduction 2001; 121: 647–53.

4. Erickson GF, Shimasaki S. The physiology of folliculogenesis: the role of novel growth factors. Fertil Steril 2001; 76: 943–9.

5. Volarcik K, Sheean L, Goldfarb J et al. The meiotic competence of in-vitro matured human oocytes is influenced by donor age: evidence that folliculogenesis is compromised in the reproductively aged ovary. Hum Reprod 1998; 13: 154–60.

6. McLay DW, Carroll J, Clarke HJ. The ability to develop an activity that transfers histones onto sperm chromatin is acquired with meiotic competence during oocyte growth. Dev Biol 2002; 241: 195–206.

7. Lawrence TS, Dekel N, Beers WH. Binding of human chorionic gonadotropin by rat cumuli oophori and granulosa cells: a comparative study. Endocrinology 1980; 106: 1114–18.

8. Ying Y, Qi X, Zhao GQ. Induction of primordial germ cells from pluripotent epiblast. Sci World J 2002; 2: 801–10.

9. Motta PM, Makabe S, Nottola SA. The ultrastructure of human reproduction. I. The natural history of the female germ cell: origin, migration and differentiation inside the developing ovary. Hum Reprod Update 1997; 3: 281–95.

10. Anderson R, Fassler R, Georges-Labouesse E et al. Mouse primordial germ cells lacking beta1 integrins enter the germline but fail to migrate normally to the gonads. Development 1999; 126: 1655–64.

11. Cheng L, Gearing DP, White LS et al. Role of leukemia inhibitory factor and its receptor in mouse primordial germ cell growth. Development 1994; 120: 3145–53.

12. Beck AR, Miller IJ, Anderson P, Streuli M. RNA-binding protein TIAR is essential for primordial germ cell development. Proc Natl Acad Sci USA 1998; 95: 2331–6.

13. Agoulnik AI, Lu B, Zhu Q, Truong C, Ty MT, Arango N et al. A novel gene, Pog, is necessary for primordial germ cell proliferation in the mouse and underlies the germ cell deficient mutation, gcd. Hum Mol Genet 2002; 11: 3047–53.

14. Byskov AG. Differentiation of mammalian embryonic gonad. Physiol Rev 1986; 66: 71–117.

15. Baker TG. A quantitative and cytological study of germ cells in human ovaries. Proc R Soc Lond B Biol Sci 1963; 158: 417–33.

16. Peters H, Byskov AG, Grinsted J. Follicular growth in fetal and prepubertal ovaries of humans and other primates. Clin Endocrinol Metab 1978; 7: 469–85.

17. Peters H, Himelstein-Braw R, Faber M. The normal development of the ovary in childhood. Acta Endocrinol (Copenh) 1976; 82: 617–30.

18. Hillier SG. Regulation of follicular oestrogen biosynthesis: a survey of current concepts. J Endocrinol 1981; 89(Suppl): 3P–18P.

19. Klinkert ER. Clinical significance and management of poor response in IVF. Academic thesis, Utrecht, 2005.

20. Hsueh AJ, Billig H, Tsafriri A. Ovarian follicle atresia: a hormonally controlled apoptotic process. Endocr Rev 1994; 15: 707–24.

21. Gougeon A. Regulation of ovarian follicular development in primates: facts and hypotheses. Endocr Rev 1996; 17: 121–55.

22. te Velde ER, Pearson PL. The variability of female reproductive ageing. Hum Reprod Update 2002; 8: 141–54.

23. Hillier SG. Current concepts of the roles of follicle stimulating hormone and luteinizing hormone in folliculogenesis. Hum Reprod 1994; 9: 188–91.

24. Govan AD, Black WP. Ovarian morphology in oligomenorrhea. Eur J Obstet Gynecol Reprod Biol 1975; 5: 317–25.

25. Pache TD, Wladimiroff JW, de Jong FH, Hop WC, Fauser BCJM. Growth patterns of nondominant ovarian follicles during the normal menstrual cycle. Fertil Steril 1990; 54: 638–42.

26. Le Nestour E, Marraoui J, Lahlou N et al. Role of estradiol in the rise in follicle-stimulating hormone levels during the luteal–follicular transition. J Clin Endocrinol Metab 1993; 77: 439–42.

27. Roseff SJ, Bangah ML, Kettel LM et al. Dynamic changes in circulating inhibin levels during the luteal–follicular transition of the human menstrual cycle. J Clin Endocrinol Metab 1989; 69: 1033–9.

28. Hall JE, Schoenfeld DA, Martin KA, Crowley WFJ. Hypothalamic gonadotropin-releasing hormone secretion and follicle-stimulating hormone dynamics during the luteal–follicular transition. J Clin Endocrinol Metab 1992; 74: 600–7.

29. Brown JB. Pituitary control of ovarian function – concepts derived from gonadotrophin therapy. Aust NZJ Obstet Gynaecol 1978; 18: 47–54.

30. Schoemaker J, van Weissenbruch MM, Scheele F, van der Meer M. The FSH threshold concept in clinical ovulation induction. In: Evers JLH, ed. Ovulation Induction: The Difficult Patient. Bailliere Tindall, London, 1993: 297–308.

31. Zeleznik AJ, Hutchison JS, Schuler HM. Interference with the gonadotropin-suppressing actions of estradiol in macaques overrides the selection of a single preovulatory follicle. Endocrinology 1985; 117: 991–9.

32. Groome NP, Illingworth PJ, O'Brien M et al. Measurement of dimeric inhibin B throughout the human menstrual cycle. J Clin Endocrinol Metab 1996; 81: 1401–5.

33. Fauser BC, Van Heusden AM. Manipulation of human ovarian function: physiological concepts and clinical consequences. Endocr Rev 1997; 18: 71–106.

34. van Santbrink EJ, Hop WC, van Dessel TJ, de Jong FH, Fauser BC. Decremental follicle-stimulating hormone and dominant follicle development during the normal menstrual cycle. Fertil Steril 1995; 64: 37–43.

35. Macklon NS, Fauser BC. Follicle-stimulating hormone and advanced follicle development in the human. Arch Med Res 2001; 32: 595–600.

36. Schipper I, Hop WC, Fauser BC. The follicle-stimulating hormone (FSH) threshold/window concept examined by different interventions with exogenous FSH during the follicular phase of the normal menstrual cycle: duration, rather than magnitude, of FSH increase affects follicle development. J Clin Endocrinol Metab 1998; 83: 1292–8.

37. Zeleznik AJ. The physiology of follicle selection. Reprod Biol Endocrinol 2004; 2: 31.

38. Filicori M, Cognigni GE, Pocognoli P, Ciampaglia W, Bernardi S. Current concepts and novel applications of LH activity in ovarian stimulation. Trends Endocrinol Metab 2003; 14: 267–73.

39. Macklon N, Fauser BC. Regulation of follicle development and novel approaches to ovarian stimulation for IVF. Hum Reprod Update. 2000; 8: 141–154.

40. Borman SM, Chaffin CL, Schwinof KM, Stouffer RL, Zelinski-Wooten MB. Progesterone promotes

oocyte maturation, but not ovulation, in nonhuman primate follicles without a gonadotropin surge. Biol Reprod 2004; 71: 366–73.

41. Chaffin CL, Stouffer RL. Local role of progesterone in the ovary during the periovulatory interval. Rev Endocr Metab Disord 2002; 3: 65–72.

42. Norman RJ. Reproductive consequences of COX-2 inhibition. Lancet 2001; 358: 1287–88.

43. Zhuo L, Kimata K. Cumulus oophorus extracellular matrix: its construction and regulation. Cell Struct Funct 2001; 26: 189–96.

44. Filicori M, Butler JP, Crowley WF, Jr. Neuroendocrine regulation of the corpus luteum in the human. Evidence for pulsatile progesterone secretion. J Clin Invest 1984; 73: 1638–47.

45. Stouffer RL. Progesterone as a mediator of gonadotrophin action in the corpus luteum: beyond steroidogenesis. Hum Reprod Update 2003; 9: 99–117.

46. Davis JS, Rueda BR. The corpus luteum: an ovarian structure with maternal instincts and suicidal tendencies. Front Biosci 2002; 7: d1949–d1978.

47. Zeleznik AJ, Saxena D, Little-Ihrig L. Protein kinase B is obligatory for follicle-stimulating hormone-induced granulosa cell differentiation. Endocrinology 2003; 144: 3985–94.

48. Sullivan MW, Stewart-Akers A, Krasnow JS, Berga SL, Zeleznik AJ. Ovarian responses in women to recombinant follicle-stimulating hormone and luteinizing hormone (LH): a role for LH in the final stages of follicular maturation. J Clin Endocrinol Metab 1999; 84: 228–32.

49. Shoham Z, Jacobs HS, Insler V. Luteinizing hormone: its role, mechanism of action, and detrimental effects when hypersecreted during the follicular phase. Fertil Steril 1993; 59: 1153–61.

50. Shoham Z. The clinical therapeutic window for luteinizing hormone in controlled ovarian stimulation. Fertil Steril 2002; 77: 1170–7.

51. Findlay JK, Drummond AE, Dyson ML et al. Recruitment and development of the follicle; the roles of the transforming growth factor-beta superfamily. Mol Cell Endocrinol 2002; 191: 35–43.

52. Poretsky L, Cataldo NA, Rosenwaks Z, Giudice LC. The insulin-related ovarian regulatory system in health and disease. Endocr Rev 1999; 20: 535–82.

53. Ashkenazi H, Cao X, Motola S et al. Epidermal growth factor family members: endogenous mediators of the ovulatory response. Endocrinology 2005; 146: 77–84.

54. Park JY, Su YQ, Ariga M et al. EGF-like growth factors as mediators of LH action in the ovulatory follicle. Science 2004; 303: 682–4.

55. Findlay JK, Britt K, Kerr JB et al. The road to ovulation: the role of oestrogens. Reprod Fertil Dev 2001; 13: 543–7.

56. Findlay JK, Drummond AE, Britt KL et al. The roles of activins, inhibins and estrogen in early committed follicles. Mol Cell Endocrinol 2000; 163: 81–7.

57. Kumar TR, Wang Y, Lu N, Matzuk MM. Follicle stimulating hormone is required for ovarian follicle maturation but not male fertility. Nat Genet 1997; 15: 201–4.

58. Rannikki AS, Zhang FP, Huhtaniemi IT. Ontogeny of follicle-stimulating hormone receptor gene expression in the rat testis and ovary. Mol Cell Endocrinol 1995; 107: 199–208.

59. Oktay K, Briggs D, Gosden RG. Ontogeny of follicle-stimulating hormone receptor gene expression in isolated human ovarian follicles. J Clin Endocrinol Metab 1997; 82: 3748–51.

60. Aaltonen J, Laitinen MP, Vuojolainen K et al. Human growth differentiation factor 9 (GDF-9) and its novel homolog GDF-9B are expressed in oocytes during early folliculogenesis. J Clin Endocrinol Metab 1999; 84: 2744–50.

61. Knight PG, Glister C. Local roles of TGF-beta superfamily members in the control of ovarian follicle development. Anim Reprod Sci 2003; 78: 165–83.

62. Eppig JJ. Oocyte control of ovarian follicular development and function in mammals. Reproduction 2001; 122: 829–38.

63. Elvin JA, Yan C, Matzuk MM. Growth differentiation factor-9 stimulates progesterone synthesis in granulosa cells via a prostaglandin E2/EP2 receptor pathway. Proc Natl Acad Sci USA 2000; 97: 10288–93.

64. Erickson GF, Magoffin DA, Dyer CA, Hofeditz C. The ovarian androgen producing cells: a review of structure/function relationships. Endocr Rev 1985; 6: 371–99.

65. Nilsson EE, Skinner MK. Kit ligand and basic fibroblast growth factor interactions in the induction of ovarian primordial to primary follicle transition. Mol Cell Endocrinol 2004; 214: 19–25.

66. Vitt UA, McGee EA, Hayashi M, Hsueh AJ. In vivo treatment with GDF-9 stimulates primordial and primary follicle progression and theca cell marker CYP17 in ovaries of immature rats. Endocrinology 2000; 141: 3814–20.

67. Otsuka F, Yao Z, Lee T et al. Bone morphogenetic protein-15. Identification of target cells and biological functions. J Biol Chem 2000; 275: 39523–8.

68. Otsuka F, Shimasaki S. A novel function of bone morphogenetic protein-15 in the pituitary: selective synthesis and secretion of FSH by gonadotropes. Endocrinology 2002; 143: 4938–41.

69. Moore RK, Otsuka F, Shimasaki S. Molecular basis of bone morphogenetic protein-15 signaling in granulosa cells. J Biol Chem 2003; 278: 304–10.

70. Shimasaki S, Moore RK, Erickson GF, Otsuka F. The role of bone morphogenetic proteins in ovarian function. Reprod Suppl 2003; 61: 323–37.

71. Zhao M, Dean J. The zona pellucida in folliculogenesis, fertilization and early development. Rev Endocr Metab Disord 2002; 3: 19–26.

72. Soyal SM, Amleh A, Dean J. FIGalpha, a germ cell-specific transcription factor required for ovarian follicle formation. Development 2000; 127: 4645–54.

73. Durlinger AL, Kramer P, Karels B et al. Control of primordial follicle recruitment by anti-Mullerian hormone in the mouse ovary. Endocrinology 1999; 140: 5789–96.

74. Zhao J, Taverne MA, van der Weijden GC, Bevers MM, van den HR. Effect of activin A on in vitro development of rat preantral follicles and localization of activin A and activin receptor II. Biol Reprod 2001; 65: 967–77.

75. Phillips DJ. Activins, inhibins and follistatins in the large domestic species. Domest Anim Endocrinol 2005; 28: 1–16.

76. Muttukrishna S, Tannetta D, Groome N, Sargent I. Activin and follistatin in female reproduction. Mol Cell Endocrinol 2004; 225: 45–56.

77. Luisi S, Florio P, Reis FM, Petraglia F. Inhibins in female and male reproductive physiology: role in gametogenesis, conception, implantation and early pregnancy. Hum Reprod Update 2005; 11: 123–35.

78. Laven JS, Fauser BC. Inhibins and adult ovarian function. Mol Cell Endocrinol 2004; 225: 37–44.

79. Cook RW, Thompson TB, Jardetzky TS, Woodruff TK. Molecular biology of inhibin action. Semin Reprod Med 2004; 22: 269–76.

80. Harlow CR, Davidson L, Burns KH et al. FSH and TGF-beta superfamily members regulate granulosa cell connective tissue growth factor gene expression in-vitro and in vivo. Endocrinology 2002; 143: 3316–25.

81. Harlow CR, Hillier SG. Connective tissue growth factor in the ovarian paracrine system. Mol Cell Endocrinol 2002; 187: 23–7.

82. Weenen C, Laven JS, Von Bergh AR et al. Anti-Mullerian hormone expression pattern in the human ovary: potential implications for initial and cyclic follicle recruitment. Mol Hum Reprod 2004; 10: 77–83.

83. Fortune JE, Rivera GM, Yang MY. Follicular development: the role of the follicular microenvironment in selection of the dominant follicle. Anim Reprod Sci 2004; 82–83: 109–26.

CHAPTER 10

Clinical aspects of polycystic ovary syndrome

Jeffrey B Russell

HISTORICAL PERSPECTIVE

Sclerocystic disease of the ovaries was first described by Chereau[1]. He observed a thickened, pearly white, sclerotic capsule in those patients who had their ovaries removed that were thought to be diseased or damaged. In 1872, Robert Battey of Georgia described an operation for the removal of the ovaries through the vagina with the patient positioned on their side[2]. Battey suggested that ovarian extirpation of the ovary or 'ovarian ovariotomy' through the vagina be performed for severe dysmenorrhea, excessive menorrhagia, hysteroneurosis, a tendency toward epilepsy with menstruation, and pelvic pain due to pelvic engorgement where all other treatment options had failed. This became known as the Battey operation. In 1876, Battey published his first 10 cases. Six women had improved or complete resolution of their symptoms, whereas two had no relief. Two deaths occurred postoperatively from the procedure[2]. This became the widely accepted surgical procedure until it was challenged by a less radical, ovarian sparing approach recommended by Pozzi in 1884 and Waldo in 1895[3]. Their approach was to remove only the diseased portion of the ovary, which was later to be known as 'ovarian wedge resection'. Postoperatively, those patients who underwent partial ovarian resection were noted to initiate their menses.

In 1935, at the Michael Reese Hospital in Chicago, Irving Stein and Michael Leventhal correlated the symptoms of amenorrhea, hirsutism, infertility, and obesity with the large sclerotic ovaries in seven patients[4]. Expecting to find abnormal cells within the ovaries due to the severity of the clinical symptoms, they sent sections of the ovaries to pathology. The histologic appearance was the same as the previously reported 'polycystic' appearance of the ovary. They removed around 50–75% of the ovary. Their belief was that the thickened capsule inhibited ovulation. This became the only treatment for these patients to induce ovulation[5].

Many years later it would be shown that the effect of the ovarian wedge resection was to reduce the intraovarian testosterone level[6]. Resumption of menses was an unexpected finding following the surgery. Stein and Leventhal[4] then described a subgroup of patients with polycystic ovarian syndrome (PCOS) with symptoms of obesity, amenorrhea, hirsutism, the inability to conceive with bilateral ovarian engorgement as having Stein–Leventhal syndrome. Follow-up studies reported a reversal of amenorrhea to cyclic menses in 95% of patients and conception in 85% of patients in those treated with ovarian wedge resection[7].

HISTOLOGIC APPEARANCE

An early report of the histologic appearance of the ovary revealed numerous microfollicular cysts occupying the cortex of the ovaries[8]. These follicles were in various stages of maturation and atresia. The cyst walls were lined with a thin layer of granulosa cells and a thickened layer of theca interna. This was a clear difference from the histologic appearance of the normal ovary. The bilateral engorged ovaries observed on the histologic sections initiated the terminology 'polycystic ovaries'. The common feature that seems to bind the wide spectrum of the presenting disease is the multi-follicular histologic appearance found in the pathologic cross-section. Thus, the terminology of PCOS encompasses multiple clinical symptoms of menstrual dysfunction from oligo-ovulation to amenorrhea. Based on the microscopic appearance, the condition should actually be termed polyfollicular rather than polycystic.

DIAGNOSIS

It is estimated that 3 to 7% of women have PCOS. The varieties of clinical presenting symptoms are numerous. In a review of clinical symptoms, Goldzieher and Axelrod[9] documented that of patients who were surgically proven to have PCOS, 20% had no menstrual irregularity, 59% were not obese, and 31% were not hirsute. This report recognized the phenotypic heterogeneity of the disease.

The cardinal clinical feature of PCOS is the disruption of normal cyclic ovarian function. PCOS is associated with tonic or inappropriate luteinizing hormone (LH) secretion which independently increases androgen levels[10]. The common physiologic feature is the elevation in androgens and their precursors, resulting in menstrual irregularities, oligo-ovulation, signs of estrogen excess, and obesity[11,12]. The androgen excess contributes to the elevated level of the total estrogens from the peripheral conversion of androstendione to estrone. As a syndrome, PCOS does not have a single diagnostic criterion sufficient for the clinical diagnosis. Thus, PCOS remains a diagnosis of exclusion from other known menstrual dysfunction problems causing chronic anovulation disorders. Late onset congenital adrenal hyperplasia (LOCAH), premature ovarian failure, hyperandrogenism, ovarian hyperthecosis, Cushing's syndrome, pituitary tumors, and hypothalamic amenorrhea should be ruled out before the patient is given the diagnosis of PCOS. Unfortunately, many menstrual disorders routinely get categorized into the PCOS basket before these other conditions are ruled out.

WORKUP

The initial workup of women presenting with menstrual dysfunction or oligo-ovulation should include early follicular serum LH, follicle stimulating hormone (FSH), and estradiol (E_2) levels to exclude hypogonadotropic hypogonadism or premature ovarian failure. Patients with PCOS are part of a large spectrum where normal to slightly elevated gonadotropins and estrogenic environments are noted. Serum LH levels are frequently elevated in these patients. Serum 17OH-progesterone and a complete androgen profile will aid in the diagnosis of LOCAH and rule out the other disorders of androgen and chronic anovulation. In patients with centripetal obesity, fasting cortisol or 24 h urinary cortisol will eliminate inappropriate adrenocorticotropic hormone (ACTH) secretion. Routine measurements of serum prolactin levels are mildly elevated in hyperandrogenic patients. The free androgen level must be calculated secondary to the measurement of sex steroid binding globulin or total testosterone levels with the assistance of ammonia sulfate precipitation[13].

INAPPROPRIATE LH SECRETION

Due to the inappropriate secretion of LH, the serum levels were the mainstay of the laboratory diagnosis of PCOS. The relationship of circulating LH to FSH was found to be elevated or inverted in PCOS patients compared with controls[14]. Elevated LH serum concentrations appear to be secondary to increased amplitude and frequency of LH pulses from the hypothalamic–pituitary axis. The abnormal levels of LH have been shown to have detrimental effects on oocyte maturity and fertilization, as well as causing lower pregnancy and higher miscarriage rates[15]. Although this is controversial, the absolute LH value in relation to the FSH value may be clinically more important in assessing oocyte quality than the LH level alone.

ANDROGEN EXCESS

Patients with PCOS have excess androgens. Some patients manifest unwanted clinical features of these excess androgens with the appearance of hirsutism or male pattern hair growth[16,17]. It has been clearly shown that the hirsutism is caused by the local androgen stimulation by the conversion of testosterone to 5α-dihydrotestosterone (DHT) at the hair follicle by the enzyme 5α-reductase[18]. The wide disparity between those patients displaying androgen excess appears to be related to the local 5α-reductase activity. Studies have shown that increased levels of the metabolite 3α-androstanediol glucuronide (3α-diol G) have been associated with clitoromegaly, temporal balding, voice changes, and a full facial beard[19]. Overt clinical symptoms such as clitoromegaly, temporal balding, and voice changes should alert the clinician to rule out a virilizing tumor

before concluding the symptoms are from long-standing androgen excess[20].

Hyperandrogenism seems to be the most common clinical marker for PCOS patients. Patients with PCOS may still have the characteristic ultrasonographic appearance of the ovaries, but do not demonstrate an abnormality in any of the circulating androgen levels[21]. The limitations of this chemical marker of hyperandrogenism have come under considerable criticism due to the fact that:

(1) Age and body mass index (BMI) were not considered when normal values were established. There is also a wide variability of hair growth and patterns in the general population between different ethnic groups.

(2) Not all androgens may have been assessed in the patient's initial work-up.

(3) Normal ranges may not have been established in well characterized controlled populations from various geographic and ethnic backgrounds.

(4) The free testosterone or free androgens index (FAI) seem to be more sensitive in the assessment of hyperandrogenism. The level of free thyroid hormone must also be assessed, since improvement in insulin resistance seems to ameliorate a portion of these menstrual abnormalities[22].

OBESITY

Adipose tissue has long been known as the largest endocrine organ in the body as it provides the storage and metabolism of sex steroid hormones. Adipose tissue plays a critical role as it constitutes a dynamic portion of the endocrine–metabolic compartment. Obesity has long been associated as a clinical symptom for patients with PCOS. However, it is now known that obesity is not a universal clinical feature of PCOS, as a significant number of PCOS patients have a normal BMI[23]. There is also controversy about whether PCOS produces obesity or whether the high peripheral circulating estrogen level contributes to the etiology of obesity in this complex disorder.

The two types of obesity, upper vs. lower body, appear to have opposite endocrine environments. The upper body is associated with higher androgen production rates and elevated free testosterone levels, whereas lower body obesity is linked to increased levels of estrone from aromatization of androstenedione[24–26].

INSULIN RESISTANCE

Patients with PCOS have been clearly identified with insulin resistance[27–30]. PCOS is associated with peripheral insulin resistance, glucose intolerance, and hyperinsulinemia, regardless of the BMI. However, studies have shown that there appears to be a higher prevalence of insulin resistance in obese compared to non-obese PCOS patients. The endocrinologic biophysical profile of obese patients should be evaluated as they are at increased risk of developing type II diabetes[31,32]. Patients with several symptoms such as obesity, elevated blood pressure (BP) or hypertension, and cholesterolemia should be evaluated with an oral glucose tolerance test (OGTT) and further medical evaluation for the likelihood of developing full-blown type II diabetes as well as other significant medical problems[33]. Those patients with mild PCOS, by clinical assessment, may be evaluated with a fasting and a 2 h glucose tolerance test (GTT), along with fasting insulin level and biochemical indexes for hyperandrogenemia. In patients with severe insulin resistance, HAIR-AN (Hyper Androgenic Insulin Resistant Acanthosis Nigricans) syndrome must be ruled out[34,35].

The relationship between insulin resistance and PCOS appears to be directly correlated with a tissue defect impairing the insulin action sequence. Studies reveal that IGF-I and IGF-II in fat cells inhibit glycerol release and stimulate glucose transport and oxidation as effectively as insulin. IGF levels are found to be decreased in PCOS patients[36–38]. This may provide a key to the insulin hypersensitivity. A positive correlation has been reported between the degree of hyperinsulinemia and hyperandrogenemia[39]. Reduction of the hyperinsulinemia lowers hyperandrogenemia. However the converse does not apply and a reduction in the androgen levels does not correlate with a reduction in the insulin levels.

First degree relatives of PCOS patients with type II diabetes are known to be more insulin resistant than age and body matched indexed controls[40,41]. Insulin resistance was also seen even when compared to young and non-obese controls. The familial basis for this disorder was clearly demonstrated when the sisters of women with PCOS were found to be more insulin resistant than age and BMI matched controls[42]. The familial clustering has been confirmed, as well as the genetic association, with the identification of a single gene causing PCOS and male pattern baldness[43,44]. Other studies have also shown a genetic susceptibility to this disorder[45,46].

IMAGING

The introduction of ultrasound (u/s) has enabled the imaging of the ovaries to aid in the diagnosis of PCOS. The 'pearl-like' appearance of the ovary on u/s appears to be synonymous with PCOS. This clinical sign is a common feature in PCOS patients and is a common finding[45–47]. The ultrasound criteria used to define PCOS are as follows:

(1) The presence of 12 or more follicles in each ovary, measuring 2–9 mm in diameter;

(2) Ovarian volume greater than 10 mm;

(3) The ultrasound evaluation should be performed when there is no dominant follicle (> 12 mm) or a corpus luteum, present by u/s, or elevated progesterone (P_4) level[48].

Ovarian volume appears to be an even more quantitative measurement than stromal volume in the clinical practice setting[49]. Patients should not undergo u/s diagnostic information to confirm or exclude the u/s appearance of the polycystic ovary when an oral contraception or central access suppression has been initiated. The calculation of ovarian volume can be made from a simplified formula that multiplies together 0.5 times the length by the width by the thickness[50]. Ideally, ovarian measurements should be taken between cycle days 3 to 6. A progesterone withdrawal bleed should be considered in those patients without menses for three months before assessing both clinical and ultrasonographic information.

It is estimated that between 6 and 35% of women have the u/s appearance of PCOS, but of these women with u/s findings, not all have PCOS[51]. Women having the ultrasonographic appearance of polycystic ovaries on cursory u/s evaluation in the absence of the clinical symptoms of an anovulatory disorder with regular menstrual·cycles or the identification of any elevated androgen levels, should not be considered as having the diagnosis of PCOS. These patients are at risk for developing ovarian hyperstimulation syndrome (OHSS) with gonadotropins for controlled ovulation induction (OI). There are no long-term studies concerning the transition from the u/s appearance of the ovaries and the development of PCOS. However, these patients should be counseled and monitored at yearly intervals for any changes in the endocrine androgenic profile.

Several studies have looked at ovarian stromal blood flow, with high resolution two-dimensional (2D), three-dimensional (3D) u/s, Doppler imaging, and quantization of the Doppler signal, using the 3D power as a critical marker for the appearance of the ovary to further evaluate and assess the degree of PCOS[52]. The vascularized blood flow index (VFI) and vascularization index (VI) are all significantly higher in patients with PCOS than in those with normal ovaries[53].

TREATMENT

The treatment focus for patients with PCOS is to establish normal cyclic ovulatory function in those patients desiring to conceive. In those patients not desiring to conceive, treatment should be aimed at restoring menstrual cyclicity and suppression of hyperandrogenism. New oral contraceptive medications combine the suppression of hyperandrogenism and increase sex steroid binding globulins.

Ovulation induction

Patients seeking fertility who are anovulatory, oligo-anovulatory, or amenorrheic are treated with ovulation medications. Traditionally, OI can be initiated with clomiphine citrate and/or human menopausal gonadotropins (HMGs). Patients with elevated levels of androgens can be treated with a low dose of dexamethasone. Dexamethasone at bedtime reduces testosterone, androstenedione, and dehydroepiandrosterone sulfate in 21–46% of PCOS patients through the blunting of the ACTH peak[54]. Dexamethasone can reduce free testosterone by 50%.

Metformin, an insulin-sensitizing agent commonly used for type II diabetes, reduces the insulin response, decreasing hepatic gluconeogenesis and reducing androgens, and was found to restore normal menstrual cycles in chronic anovulatory patients[55].

Letrozole, a third generation aromatase inhibitor, is an agent which suppresses the biosynthesis of estrogen and reduces the negative feedback effect on the hypothalamic–pituitary system. This increases the secretion of FSH. Letrozole has been recently used for OI in anovulatory PCOS women resistant to clomiphene or with inadequate endometrial thickness during clomiphene treatment[56]. At a daily dose of 2.5 mg from days 3 to 7 of the menstrual cycle, ovulation was seen in 9 of 12 cycles (75%) treated with letrozole and only in 8 of 18 cycles (44.4%) treated with clomiphene, while the endometrium on the day of hCG administration was thicker in the letrozole group[56].

Insulin-sensitizing agents

Several insulin-sensitizing agents have been studied in the treatment of PCOS. They include metformin, thiazolidinediones, troglitazone, rofiglitazone, pioglitazone, and D-chiro-inositol[57]. The most extensively used insulin-sensitizing drug in the treatment of PCOS is metformin. Hyperinsulinemia is critical in the development of hyperandrogenemia and disrupts follicular genesis. Metformin is an orally administered agent used to lower the blood glucose level in non-insulin-dependent diabetics. It is antihyperglycemic in its action, but does not cause hypoglycemia, increased glucose uptake, or utilization in the muscle tissue.

Metformin enhances insulin sensitivity in the liver, where the peripheral tissue inhibits hepatic glucose production. Metformin has been studied and has been mostly shown to restore menstrual cycles and confirm ovulation in anywhere between 25 and 90% of cases[57]. A recent analysis of 13 randomized controlled trials showed that metformin increased the ovulation rate almost four times compared to placebo when it was administered in combination with clomiphene citrate[58]. In clomiphene resistant women, a significantly higher ovulation rate from metformin plus clomiphene citrate was seen when compared to clomiphene citrate plus placebo[59].

The benefits of metformin for OI are important as it does not confer the same risks of ovarian hyperstimulation or multiple pregnancies compared with clomiphene citrate or HMG. Although metformin has not yet been listed as one of the treatments for ovulation, several randomized controlled trials revealed that metformin plus clomiphene citrate is superior when compared to clomiphene citrate alone or with placebo[59].

Metformin has also been studied in women who continued the treatment during pregnancy.

One study has shown the clear benefit of reducing gestational diabetes in those women with PCOS who took metformin throughout their pregnancies[60]. The safety of metformin as a category B medication allows its use in patients who do conceive. One study has shown a reduction in first trimester spontaneous abortions.

In an excellent systematic review of metformin in patients with PCOS, Costello and Eden[58] did an analysis of the literature on metformin used as a single agent or in combination with other ovulatory inducing medications in restoring menses or establishing a pregnancy.

Their review indicated that for 3 to 6 months PCOS patients have a 60% chance of regular menses and ovulation. The addition of clomiphene citrate to metformin shows that for up to 9 months patients have approximately a 66% chance of regular menses and ovulation and 34% have a chance of pregnancy.

Surgical treatment

In 1984, an attempt to introduce a minimally invasive surgical treatment for PCOS and move away from the classical wedge resection, using laparoscopic surgical treatment of the polycystic ovary, was reported[61]. Gjonnaess studied 62 women with PCOS who were treated surgically with serial systematic electrocautery of the ovarian capsule. He reported that ovulation occurred within 3 months in 92% of the patients who underwent the surgical procedure, with regular menses established in 51 (86%) of the patients proven by an elevated progesterone level. Seven of nine women with a diagnosis of PCOS who had been previously treated with clomiphene citrate up to 150 mg for OI showed signs of ovulation with elevated progesterone levels after ovarian drilling. The remaining two patients, who did not spontaneously ovulate, did become responsive with use of clomiphene citrate. Gjonnaess reported a pregnancy rate of up to 80% of those treated with ovulation inducing medications. The proposed theory was that there were local factors within the ovary which were responsible for triggering ovulation.

Laparoscopic ovarian drilling (LOD) is a surgical treatment used to debulk the ovarian tissue either with monopolar, bipolar electrocautery, or with laser energy (Figures 10.1 and 10.2). There are different techniques to accomplish the task of volume reduction of the ovaries, all of which seem to have a beneficial effect in reducing the excess androgen levels, the hallmark of this condition. LOD was studied in preventing cancellation in patients undergoing controlled ovulation induction for IVF due to their risk of severe OHSS. Rimington et al.[62] studied 25 women who underwent ovarian electrocautery followed by gonadotropin therapy. This study found that, when compared to a control, the patients who underwent laparoscopic ovarian electrocautery after pituitary desensitization followed by gonadotropin therapy had a reduced risk of cancellation of their cycle due to impending or actual OHSS.

Parsanezhad et al.[63] studied ovarian stromal blood flow following LOD in 52 women and found serum concentrations of LH and testosterone were significantly decreased. Systolic velocity blood flow decreased significantly as well as pulsatile index and resistance index. The study showed a total of 73% of the women ovulated. This finding was inversely related to the pulsatile index and testosterone level. Those patients who did not have ovulatory cycles showed less of a change in their Doppler pulsatile index than those who ovulated. In an attempt to identify predictors of success for LOD Amer et al. looked at markers[64].

Obesity, hyperandrogenism, and long duration of infertility seemed to be the most profound clinical predictors of success from LOD. In addition, higher levels of LH often seemed to be a high predictor of success in those patients undergoing LOD.

Because of the invasive process of the surgical procedure, the risk of a general anesthetic does not justify LOD as a first line treatment in those patients with severe PCOS. The introduction of the insulin-sensitizing agents should be tried with or without clomiphene citrate as a first line treatment, depending on the results of the initial physiologic presentation. In those clomiphene citrate resistant patients, LOD is an excellent option. LOD may also help with patients who are at high risk for severe OHSS or who have been unable to achieve controlled ovarian stimulation without the significant risks associated with OHSS.

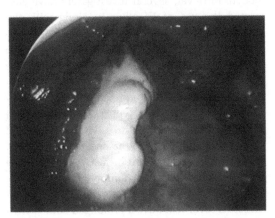

Figure 10.1 Engorged polycystic ovary before LOD

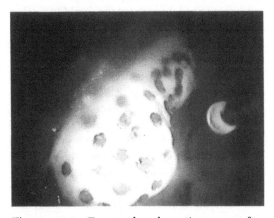

Figure 10.2 Engorged polycystic ovary after LOD with a Nd:YAG laser at 20 watts

Unstimulated IVF cycles

Immature oocyte retrieval is another treatment option recently presented for PCOS patients. Edwards[65], in 1965, leading up to the first in-vitro fertilization (IVF), studied in-vitro maturation (IVM) in mammalian species including human oocytes[65]. It was not until 1991, when Cha et al.[66] reported the use of immature oocytes excised from ovarian tissue, that the full clinical potential was actually realized. Cha established a triplet pregnancy with immature oocytes after they were matured, fertilized, and then transferred as frozen-thawed embryos to a recipient during a donor oocyte cycle. In 1994, Trounson et al.[67] brought the clinical feasibility of IVM with immature oocytes to PCOS patients when they were able to retrieve immature oocytes with u/s guidance transvaginally. They matured the immature oocytes, fertilized them, and then transferred embryos to the intrauterine cavity during the same cycle from which the oocytes were retrieved. This was a tremendous breakthrough for patients who had had a very difficult time with the use of gonadotropins and the high risk of ovarian hyperstimulation and the associated complications. Since that time, several other groups have reported successful transvaginal u/s guided oocyte retrieval, maturation, fertilization, transfer, and implantation[68–70]. IVM is now being used throughout the world in a select group of patients.

Due to the abundance of follicles in the ovary, PCOS patients present an excellent clinical opportunity for the retrieval of unstimulated immature eggs. Although Cha started the process of IVM through oophorectomized patients, it was really brought to clinical practise by Trounson. To enhance the success rate of IVM after retrieval of unstimulated oocytes, Chian et al.[71] reported utilizing human chorionic gonadotropin (hCG) priming, which seems to improve the maturation rate and 2PN fertilization rate for those patients undergoing immature oocyte retrieval (IOR).

OVARIAN HYPERSTIMULATION SYNDROME

One of the complications associated with the clinical treatment of PCOS with gonadotropins is the OHSS. OHSS is a serious, potentially life-threatening, iatrogenic complication of controlled ovarian stimulation. An excellent comprehensive review by Whelan and Vlahos[72] evaluated the risk factors, staging, pathophysiology, prevention, management, and treatment of OHSS. The triggering factor for OHSS is the exogenous hCG injection given to mimic the LH surge. The pathophysiology of the disease process appears to be related to the increased capillary permeability resulting in an intravascular fluid shift in the third space.

Risk factors include young age, low body weight, high estradiol levels, number of oocytes retrieved, and PCOS. The baseline antral follicle count appears to correlate well with the risk of developing OHSS. The risks vary widely and the only consistent clinical presentation appears to be the patient's androgen profile in the development of OHSS. Surgical puncture, for those patients undergoing in-vitro follicular aspiration with IVF, has been reported to interfere with corpus luteum progesterone production, increasing the severity of OHSS. At the time of oocyte retrieval, several investigators have suggested the use of IV albumin along with the oocyte retrieval to decrease the risk of developing OHSS. Although this has been reported to be successful, several conflicting studies have shown no benefit to the use of IV albumin.

OHSS has been determined to be a time limited phenomenon. The typical course with full recovery, even for severe cases, will run anywhere from 10 to 28 days from the onset of symptoms. A declining level of serum hCG is responsible for the self-limiting resolution of the disease. Conversely, patients who conceive with a rising hCG level will have a prolonged course with ascites, shortness of breath, pulmonary effusion, and possible deep vein thrombosis (DVT) due to loss of vascular capillary permeability. Mild to moderate ovarian hyperstimulation can be managed on an outpatient basis. Abdominal bloating, mild shortness of breath (SOB), and weight gain should be re-evaluated by the clinician to decide between hospital vs. outpatient management. Limited physical activity is essential as the disease progresses, with the worst symptoms occurring around early evening. Rapid weight gain with intravascular depletion, decreased urine output of <1000 ml/day, or fluid discrepancies between intake and output should alert the clinician to worsening conditions. Baseline electrolytes, hemodynamic concentration, ovarian u/s measurements, fluid volume, abdominal girth, and daily weight are critical to the ongoing assessment and should be evaluated.

Patients with severe OHSS should be admitted to hospital for close monitoring of vital signs, strict intake and output measurements, white blood cell count (WBC), hemoglobin and hematocrit, electrolyte panel, and liver function tests. The clinician should also run a full coagulopathy panel, and an X-ray to rule out pulmonary infiltrates with SOB. In addition, baseline pulse oximeter studies are essential to assess pulmonary reserve and function. Patients with severe OHSS are hypovolemic with an increase in third space fluid retention. Patients are typically hypernatremic with low urinary output and do not respond well to fluid restriction. On admission, patients should start protein supplementation or albumin infusions.

Paracentesis has become an integral part of the management of third spacing in these patients and the procedure can be performed with a transvaginal approach with a paracervical block using an oocyte retrieval needle[73]. The needle is connected through an adapter to a 1000 ml vacuum suction bottle. The patient should be monitored for hemodynamic stability during the procedure. Between 2 and 3 liters should be drawn off during this time. Less than 2 liters may put the patient at undue risk for such a small volume to be retrieved and more than 3 liters may put

too much of a shift on the patient's intravascular space. The procedure can be repeated typically every 48 to 72 h, or as the symptoms and clinical signs of worsening conditions avail themselves. If pulmonary ascites is present, the paracentesis may actually reduce the pulmonary ascites if the fluid is primarily located in the lower pleural space. Consideration of a thoracocentesis may be an option by a pulmonologist in those severe cases with a compromised pulmonary function.

Patients with PCOS have a major risk of OHSS with the controlled ovarian stimulation protocols. The side-effects include weight gain, bloating, nausea, vomiting, mood swings, and possible hospitalization. Numerous protocols have been suggested, including albumin treatments, paracenteses, and cryopreserving all embryos along with bed rest in an attempt to reduce the disadvantages of controlled OHSS in these patients.

REFERENCES

1. Jenks EW. Historical sketch. American System of Gynecology 1896; 1: 17–67.

2. Traite de Gynecologic Clinique et Operatoire, 2nd edn. Paris, 1890.

3. Graham H. Eternal Eve: The History of Gynecology and Obstetrics. Doubleday and Co, Garden City, NJ, 1951.

4. Stein IF, Leventhal ML. Amenorrhea associated with bilateral polycystic ovaries. Am J Obstet Gynecol 1935; 29: 181.

5. Stein IF. Bilateral polycystic ovaries. Am J Obstet Gynecol 1945; 50: 385.

6. Judd HL, Rigg LA, Anderson DC et al. The effect of ovarian wedge resection on circulating gonadotropins and ovarian steroid levels in patients with polycystic ovary syndrome. J Clin Endocrinol 1976; 43: 347.

7. Graf MA, Bielfeld P, Graf C et al. Patterns of gonadotropin secretion with hyperandrogenaemic amenorrhea before and after ovarian wedge resection. Hum Reprod 1994; 9: 1022–6.

8. Hughesdon PE. Morphology and morphogenesis of the Stein–Levanthal ovary and of so-called hyperthecosis. Obstet Gynec 1982; 37: 59–77.

9. Goldzieher JW, Axelrod LR. Clinical and biochemical features of polycystic ovarian disease. Fertil Steril 1963; 14: 631.

10. Lobo RA, Kletzky OA, Campeau JD et al. Elevated bioactive luteinizing hormone in women with the polycystic ovary syndrome. Fertil Steril 1983; 39: 674.

11. Rebar RW, Judd HL, Yen SSC et al. Characterization of the inappropriate gonadotropin secretion in polycystic ovary syndrome. J Clin Invest 1976; 57: 1320.

12. Chang RJ. Ovarian steroid secretion in polycystic ovarian disease. Semin Reprod Endocrinol 1984; 2: 244.

13. Tremblay RR, Dube JY. Plasma concentration of free and non-TeBG bound testosterone in women on oral contraceptives. Contraception 1974; 10: 599–605.

14. Quigley ME, Kakoff JS, Yen SSC. Increased luteinizing hormone sensitivity to dopamine inhibition in polycystic ovary syndrome. J Clin Endocrinol Metab 1981; 52: 231.

15. Tarlatizis BC, Grimbizis G, Pournaropoulos et al. The prognostic value of basal LH:FSH ratio in the treatment of patients with PCOS by assisted reproduction. Hum Reprod 1995; 10: 2545–9.

16. Ehrmann DA, Rosenfeld RL. Hirsutism – beyond the steroidogenic block. N Engl J Med 1990; 323: 909–11.

17. Bardin CW, Lipsett MB. Testosterone and androstenedione blood production rates in normal women and women with idiopathic hirsutism or polycystic ovaries. J Clin Invest 1967; 46: 891–902.

18. Lobo RA, Goebelsmann U, Horton R. Evidence for the importance of peripheral tissue events in the development of hirsutism in polycystic ovary syndrome. J Clin Endocrinol Metab 1983; 57: 393.

19. Lobo RA, Goebelsmann U. Evidence for reduced 3b-ol-hydroxysteroid dehydrogenase activity in some hirsute women thought to have polycystic ovary syndrome. J Clin Endocrinol Metab 1981; 53: 394.

20. Lobo RA. The role of the adrenal in polycystic ovary syndrome. Semin Reprod Endocrinol 1984; 2: 251.

21. Balen AH, Conway GS, Kaltsas G et al. Polycystic ovary syndrome: the spectrum of the disorder in 1741 patients. Hum Reprod 1995; 10: 2107–11.

22. Marca A, Morgante, DeLeo V. Evaluation of hypothalamic–pituitary–adrenal axis in amenorrheic women with insulin-dependent diabetes. Hum Reprod 1999; 14: 298–302.

23. Jialal I, Naiker P, Reddi K et al. Evidence for insulin resistance in nonobese patients with polycystic ovarian disease. J Clin Endocrinol Metab 1987; 64: 1066.

24. Pasquali R, Casimirri F, Balestra V et al. The relative contribution of androgens and insulin in determining abdominal fat distribution in premenopausal women. J Endocrinol Invest 1991; 14: 839.

25. Ostlund RE Jr, Staten M, Kohrt W et al. The ratio of waist to hip circumference, plasma insulin level, and glucose intolerance as independent predictors for the HDL2 cholesterol level in older adults. New Engl J Med 1990; (322): 229–234.

26. Kirschner MA, Samojlik E, Drejka M et al. Androgen–estrogen metabolism in women with upper body versus lower body obesity. J Clin Endocrinol Metab 1990; 70: 473.

27. Chang RJ, Nakamura RM, Judd HL et al. Insulin resistance in nonobese patients with polycystic ovarian disease. J Clin Endocrinol Metab 1983; 57: 356.

28. Burghen GA, Givens JR, Kitabchi AE. Correlation of hyperandrogenism with hyperinsulinism in polycystic ovarian disease. Fertil Steril 1980; 50: 113.

29. Dunaif A, Segal KR, Futterweit W et al. Profound peripheral insulin resistance, independent of obesity, in polycystic ovary syndrome. Diabetes 1989; 38: 1165.

30. Morales AJ, Laughlin GA, Butzow T et al. Insulin, somatotropic and luteinizing hormone axes in lean and obese women with polycystic ovary syndrome: common and distinct features. J Clin Endocrinol Metab 1996; 81: 2854.

31. Reavens GM. Role of insulin resistance in human disease. Diabetes 1988; 37: 1595.

32. O'Meara NM, Blackman JD, Ehrman DA et al. Defects in β-cell function in functional ovarian hyperandrogenism. J Clin Endocrinol Metab 1993; 76: 1241.

33. Deutsch MI, Mueller WH, Malina RM. Androgyny in fat patterning is associated with obesity in adolescents and young adults. Ann Hum Biol 1985; 12: 275.

34. Barbieri RL, Ryan KJ. Hyperandrogenism, insulin resistance and Acanthosis Nigricans: a common endocrinopathy with distinct pathophysiologic features. Am J Obstet Gynecol 1982; 147: 90.

35. Dunaif A, Green G, Phelps RG et al. Acanthosis Nigricans, insulin action, and hyperandrogenism: clinical, histological, and biochemical findings. J Clin Endocrinol Metab 1991; 73: 590.

36. Dunaif A, Scott D, Finegood D et al. The insulin-sensitizing agent roglitazon improves metabolic and reproductive abnormalities in the polycystic ovary syndrome. J Clin Endocrinol Met 1996; 81: 3299.

37. The Rotterdam ESHRE/ASRM-sponsored PCOS consensus workup group. Revised 2003 consensus on diagnostic criteria and long-term health risks related to polycystic ovary syndrome. Hum Reprod 2004; 19: 41–7.

38. Shoupe D, Kumar DD, Lobo RA. Insulin resistance in polycystic ovary syndrome. Am J Obstet Gynecol 1983; 147: 588.

39. Robinson S, Kiddy D, Gelding SV et al. The relationship of insulin insensitivity to menstrual pattern in women with hyperandrogenism and polycystic ovaries. Clin Endocrinol (Oxf) 1993; 39: 351–5.

40. Wolk A, Renn W, Overkamp D et al. Insulin action and secretion in healthy, glucose tolerant first degree relatives of patients with type 2 diabetes mellitus. Influence of body weight. Exp Clin Endocrinol Diabetes 1999; 107: 140–7.

41. Raskauskiene D. Reduced insulin sensitivity in healthy first degree relatives of patients with type 2 diabetes mellitus. The 22nd Joint Meeting of the British Endocrine Societies, Vol 5, Glasgow, United Kingdom, 2003, 93.

42. Norman RJ, Masters S, Hague W. Hyperinsulinaemia is common in family members with polycystic ovary syndrome. Fertil Steril 1996; 66: 942–7.

43. Yildiz BO, Yarali H, Oguz H et al. Glucose intolerance, insulin resistance, and hyperandrogenemia in first degree relatives of women with polycystic ovary syndrome. J Clin Endocrinol Metab 2003; 88: 2031–6.

44. Hague WM, Adams J, Reeders ST et al. Familial polycystic ovaries: a genetic disease? Clin Endocrinol (Oxf) 1988; 29: 593–605.

45. Carey AH, Chan KL, Short F et al. Evidence for a single gene effect causing polycystic ovaries and male pattern baldness. Clin Endocrinol (Oxf) 1993; 38: 653–8.

46. Franks S. Gharani N, Waterworth D et al. The genetic basis of polycystic ovary syndrome. Hum Reprod 1997; 12: 2641–8.

47. Orsini LF, Venturoli S, Lorusso R et al. Ultrasonic findings in polycystic ovarian disease. Fertil Steril 1985; 43: 709–14.

48. Adams J, Polson DW, Abdulwahid N. Multifollicular ovaries: clinical and endocrine features and response to gonadotropin releasing hormone. Lancet 1985; 2: 1375–8.

49. Fulghesu AM, Ciampelli M, Belosi C et al. A new ultrasound criterion for the diagnosis of polycystic ovary syndrome: the ovarian stroma/total area ratio. Fertil Steril 2001; 76: 326–31.

50. Swanson M, Sauerbrie EE, Cooperberg PL. Medical implications of ultrasonically detected polycystic ovaries. J Clin Ultrasound 1981; 9: 219–22.

51. Farquhar CM, Birdsall M, Manning P et al. The prevalence of polycystic ovaries on ultrasound scanning in a population of randomly selected women. Aust NZ J Obstet Gynaecol 1994; 34: 67–72.

52. Ng EHY, Chan CCW, Yeung WSB et al. Comparison of ovarian stromal blood flow between fertile women with normal ovaries and infertile women with polycystic ovary syndrome. Hum Reprod 2005; 20: 1881–6.

53. Pan HA, Wu MH, Cheng YC et al. Quantification of Doppler signal in polycystic ovary syndrome using three-dimensional power Doppler ultrasonography: a possible new marker for diagnosis. Hum Reprod 2002; 17: 201–6.

54. Vanky E, Salvesen KA, Carlsen SM. Six-month treatment with low-dose dexamethasone further reduces androgen levels in PCOS women treated with diet and lifestyle advice, and metformin. Hum Reprod 2004; 19: 529–33.

55. Haas DA, Carr BR, Attia GR. Effects of metformin on body mass index, menstrual cyclicity, and ovulation induction in women with polycystic ovary syndrome. Fertil Steril 2003; 79: 469–81.

56. Mitwally MFM, Casper RF. The aromatase inhibitor, letrozole: a promising alternative for clomiphene citrate for induction of ovulation. Fertil Steril 2000; 74: S35.

57. Kashyap S, Wells GA, Rozenwaks Z. Insulin-sensitizing agents for patients with polycystic ovarian syndrome. Hum Reprod 2004; 19: 2474–83.

58. Costello MF, Eden JA. A systematic review of the reproductive system effects of metformin in patients with polycystic ovary syndrome. Fertil Steril 2003; 79: 1–13.

59. Palomba S, Orio F, Falbo A et al. Prospective parallel randomized, double-blind, double-dummy controlled clinical trial comparing clomiphene citrate and metformin as the first-line treatment for ovulation induction in nonobese anovulatory women with polycystic ovary syndrome. J Clin Endocrinol Metab 2005; 90: 4068–74.

60. Checa MA, Requena A, Salvador C. Insulin-sensitizing agents: use in pregnancy and as therapy in polycystic ovary syndrome. Hum Reprod Update 2005; 11: 375–90.

61. Gjonnaess E. Polycystic ovarian syndrome treated by ovarian electrocautery through the laparoscope. Fertil Steril 1984; 41: 20–2.

62. Rimington MR, Walker SM, Shaw RW. The use of laparoscopic ovarian electrocautery in preventing cancellation of in vitro fertilization cycles due to risk of ovarian hyperstimulation syndrome in women with polycystic ovaries. Hum Reprod 1997; 12: 1443–7.

63. Parsanezhad ME, Bagheri MH, Alborzi S et al. Ovarian stromal blood flow changes after laparoscopic ovarian cauterization in women with polycystic ovary syndrome. Hum Reprod 2003; 18: 1432–7.

64. Amer SAK, LI, TC, Ledger WL. Ovulation induction using laparoscopic ovarian drilling in women with polycystic ovarian syndrome: predictors of success. Hum Reprod 2004; 19: 1719–24.

65. Edwards RG. Maturation in vitro of mouse, sheep, cow, pig, rhesus monkey and human ovarian oocytes. Nature 1965; 208: 349–51.

66. Cha KY, Koo JJ, Ko JJ et al. Pregnancy after in vitro fertilization of human follicular oocytes collected from nonstimulated cycles, their culture in vitro and their transfer in a donor oocyte program. Fertil Steril 1991; 55: 109–13.

67. Trounson A, Wood C, Kaunsche A. In vitro maturation and fertilization and developmental competence of oocytes recovered from untreated polycystic ovarian patients. Fertil Steril 1994; 62: 353–62.

68. Russell JB, Knezevich, KM, Fabian KF et al. Unstimulated immature oocyte retrieval: early versus midfollicular endometrial priming. Fertil Steril 1997; 67: 616–20.

69. Son WY, Lee SY, Lim JH. Fertilization, cleavage and blastocyst development according to the maturation timing of oocytes in in vitro maturation cycles. Hum Reprod 2005; 20: 3204–7.

70. Du LeA, Kadock IJ, Bourcigaux N et al. In vitro oocytes maturation for the treatment of infertility associated with polycystic ovarian syndrome: the French experience. Hum Reprod 2005; 20: 420–4.

71. Chian RC, Buckett WM, Tulandi T et al. Prospective randomized study of human chorionic gonadotropins priming before immature oocyte retrieval from unstimulated women with polycystic ovarian syndrome. Hum Reprod 2000; 15: 165–170.

72. Whelan JG, Vlahos NF. The ovarian hyperstimulation syndrome. Fertil Steril 2000; 73: 883–896.

73. Padilla SL, Zamaria S, Baramki TA et al. Abdominal paracentesis for the ovarian hyperstimulation syndrome with severe pulmonary compromise. Fertil Steril 1990; 53: 365–7.

CHAPTER 11

The ultrasound diagnosis of the polycystic ovary

Adam H Balen

INTRODUCTION

Historically the detection of the polycystic ovary required visualization of the ovaries at laparotomy and histologic confirmation following biopsy[1]. As further studies identified the association of certain endocrine abnormalities in women with histologic evidence of polycystic ovaries, biochemical criteria became the mainstay for diagnosis. Well recognized clinical presentations included menstrual cycle disturbances (oligo/amenorrhea), obesity, and hyperandrogenism manifesting as hirsutism, acne, or androgen-dependent alopecia. Clinical features, however, vary considerably between women, and indeed some women with polycystic ovaries do not appear to display any of the common symptoms[2,3]. Likewise, the biochemical features associated with PCOS are not consistent in all women[4,5]. There is considerable heterogeneity of symptoms and signs amongst women with PCOS and for an individual these may change over time[5,6].

It has been considered necessary to redefine the polycystic ovary syndrome (PCOS) and include within it an appropriate definition of the polycystic ovary[7,8]. At the joint ASRM/ESHRE consensus meeting on PCOS held in Rotterdam, 2003, a refined definition of the PCOS was agreed[9], which, for the first time, includes a description of the morphology of the polycystic ovary (Table 11.1). The new definition requires the presence of two out of the following three criteria:

(1) Oligo- and/or anovulation;

(2) Hyperandrogenism (clinical and/or biochemical);

(3) Polycystic ovaries, with the exclusion of other etiologies[9].

Transabdominal ultrasound

Transabdominal and/or transvaginal ultrasound have now become the most commonly used diagnostic methods for the identification of polycystic ovaries. The characteristic features are accepted as being an increase in the size (volume) of the ovary due to a greater number of follicles and volume of stroma as compared with normal ovaries. Swanson et al.[10] were the first to use high-resolution real-time ultrasound (static B-scanner 3.5 MHz, transabdominal) to describe polycystic ovaries. The follicles were noted to be 2–6 mm in diameter, but the number of follicles was neither recorded nor defined. Stromal characteristics were not described. The

Table 11.1   The Ultrasound Assessment of the Polycystic Ovary: International Consensus Definitions[21]

1. The polycystic ovary should have at least one of the following: either 12 or more follicles measuring 2–9 mm in diameter or increased ovarian volume (>10 cm^3). If there is evidence of a dominant follicle (>10 mm) or a corpus luteum, the scan should be repeated the next cycle.
2. The subjective appearance of polycystic ovaries should not be substituted for this definition. The follicle distribution should be omitted as well as the increase in stromal echogenicity and/or volume. Although the latter is specific to PCO, it has been shown that the measurement of the ovarian volume is a good surrogate for the quantification of the stroma in clinical practice.
3. Only one ovary fitting this definition or a single occurrence of one of the above criteria is sufficient to define the PCO. If there is evidence of a dominant follicle (>10 mm) or corpus luteum, the scan should be repeated next cycle. The presence of an abnormal cyst or ovarian asymmetry, which may suggest a homogeneous cyst, necessitates further investigation.
4. This definition does not apply to women taking the oral contraceptive pill, as ovarian size is reduced, even though the 'polycystic' appearance may persist.
5. A woman having PCO in the absence of an ovulation disorder or hyperandrogenism ('asymptomatic PCO') should not be considered as having PCOS, until more is known about this situation.
6. In addition to its role in the definition of PCO, ultrasound is helpful to predict fertility outcome in patients with PCOS (response to clomiphene citrate, risk for ovarian hyperstimulation syndrome (OHSS), decision for in-vitro maturation of oocytes). It is recognized that the appearance of polycystic ovaries may be seen in women undergoing ovarian stimulation for IVF in the absence of overt signs of the polycystic ovary syndrome. Ultrasound also provides the opportunity to screen for endometrial hyperplasia.
7. The following technical recommendations should be respected:
   • State-of-the-art equipment is required and should be operated by appropriately trained personnel.
   • Whenever possible, the transvaginal approach should be preferred, particularly in obese patients.
   • Regularly menstruating women should be scanned in the early follicular phase (days 3–5). Oligo/amenorrhoeic women should be scanned either at random or between days 3–5 after a progestogen-induced bleed.
   • If there is evidence of a dominant follicle (>10 mm) or a corpus luteum, the scan should be repeated the next cycle.
   • Calculation of ovarian volume is performed using the simplified formula for a prolate ellipsoid ($0.5 \times$ length $\times$ width $\times$ thickness).
   • Follicle number should be estimated both in longitudinal and antero-posterior cross-sections of the ovaries. Follicle size should be expressed as the mean of the diameters measured in the two sections.

The usefulness of 3D ultrasound, Doppler, or MRI for the definition of PCO has not been sufficiently ascertained to date and should be confined to research studies.

early studies were hampered by the limitations of static B-scanners, which were superseded by high-resolution real-time sector scanners in the early 1980s[11,12]. Ultrasound was used to describe the ovarian appearance in women classified as having PCOS (by symptoms and serum endocrinology) rather than to make the diagnosis.

The transabdominal ultrasound criteria of Adams et al.[13] attempted to define a polycystic ovary as one which contains, in one plane, at least 10 follicles (usually between 2 and 8 mm in diameter) arranged peripherally around a dense core of ovarian stroma or scattered throughout an increased amount of stroma. This was a seminal paper which has been most often quoted in the literature on the PCOS. The Adams' criteria have been adopted by many subsequent studies which have used ultrasound scanning to detect polycystic ovaries[2,5,14–19].

Transvaginal ultrasound

Transabdominal ultrasound has been largely superseded by transvaginal scanning because of greater resolution and in many cases patient preference – as the need for a full bladder is avoided which saves time and may be more comfortable[20]. Whilst this may be the case in the context of infertility clinics, where women are used to having repeated scans, it was found that 20% of women who were undergoing routine screening declined a transvaginal scan after having first had a transabdominal scan[19]. Furthermore, the transabdominal approach is required for adolescent girls who are yet to commence sexual activity. The transvaginal approach may not always be acceptable for research studies; for example, in a population-based survey, Michelmore et al.[3] detected polycystic ovaries by transabdominal ultrasound in 33% of a population of young women.

The transvaginal approach gives a more accurate view of the internal structure of the ovaries, avoiding apparently homogeneous ovaries as described with transabdominal scans, particularly in obese patients. With the transvaginal route, high frequency probes (> 6 MHz) having a better spatial resolution but less examination depth can be used because the ovaries are close to the vagina and/or the uterus and because the presence of fatty tissue is usually less disruptive (except when very abundant). The consensus definition of polycystic ovaries as visualized transvaginally has been recently proposed (Table 11.1)[3].

Three-dimensional ultrasound

The recent innovation of three-dimensional (3D) ultrasound and the use of color and pulsed Doppler ultrasound are techniques which may further enhance the detection of polycystic ovaries, and which may be more commonly employed in time[21,22]. Three-dimensional ultrasound requires longer time for storage and data analysis, increased training, and more expensive equipment. Nardo et al.[23] found good correlations between 2D and 3D ultrasound measurements of ovarian volume and polycystic ovary morphology.

FEATURES OF THE POLYCYSTIC OVARY

Surface area and volume

It is necessary to identify each ovary and measure the maximum diameter in each of three planes (longitudinal, antero-posterior, and transverse). It is recognized that, because of the irregular shape of the ovary, any calculation of the volume of a sphere, or prolate ellipse, is at best an estimate. Modern ultrasound machines can calculate volume once the callipers have been used to measure the ovary and an ellipse is drawn around the outline of the ovary. The ultrasound software for this calculation appears to be accurate.

Calculation of ovarian volume has been traditionally performed using the formula for a prolate ellipsoid ($\pi/6 \times$ maximal longitudinal, antero-posterior, and transverse diameters)[13,24,25]. As $\pi/6 = 0.5233$ a simplified formula for a prolate ellipse is ($0.5 \times$ length $\times$ width $\times$ thickness)[10,26–29]. In practice this formula is easy to use and of practical value.

A large number of different ultrasound formulae with different weightings for the different diameters were used to calculate ovarian volume and the prolate spheroid formula ($\pi/6 \times$

antero-posterior diameter[2] × transverse diameter) was found to correlate well with ovarian volume as assessed by 3D ultrasound[23]. A similar correlation was found with the spherical volume method ($\pi/6$ × [(transverse diameter + antero-posterior diameter + longitudinal diameter)/3])[3]. As polycystic ovaries appear to be more spherical than ovoid it was suggested that the formula should be modified[23].

In the first study to assess ovarian volume, the simplified formula for a prolate ellipse was used for the calculation and found on average to be 12.5 cm[3] (range 6–30 cm[3])[10]. This formula was also used by Hann et al.[26] who reported considerable variety in ultrasound characteristics in women with polycystic ovary syndrome. They took the upper limit of ovarian volume to be 5.7 cm[3] based on data from Sample et al.[24]. In that study ovarian volume was calculated using the more accurate formula for a prolate ellipsoid (0.5233 × maximal longitudinal, antero-posterior, and transverse diameters)[24]. Women with PCOS were compared with normal controls and were found to have significantly greater ovarian volume (14.04 ± 7.36 cm[3] vs. 7.94 ± 2.34 cm[3]) and smaller uterine volume. There was no record of timing of the scan in relation to the menstrual cycle in either PCOS or control subjects.

In the paper of Adams et al.[13] polycystic ovaries were found to have a higher volume (14.6 ± 1.1 cm[3]) than both multicystic (8.0 ± 0.8 cm[3]) and normal ovaries (6.4 ± 0.4 cm[3]). Uterine cross-sectional area was also greater in women with PCOS than in those with multicystic or normal ovaries (26.0 ± 1.4 vs. 13.1 ± 0.9 vs. 22.4 ± 1.0 cm[2]), which is a reflection of the degree of estrogenization.

A large study of 80 oligo/amenorrheic women with PCOS was compared with a control group of 30 using a 6.5 MHz transvaginal probe[29]. Based on mean ± 2 SD data from the control group, the cut-off values were calculated for ovarian volume (13.21 cm[3]), ovarian total area (7.00 cm[2]), ovarian stromal area (1.95 cm[2]), and stromal/area ratio (0.34). The sensitivity of these parameters

for the diagnosis of PCOS was 21%, 4%, 62%, and 100%, respectively, suggesting that a stromal/area ratio > 0.34 is diagnostic of PCOS[29]. Whilst these data may be useful in a research setting, the measurement of ovarian stromal area is not easily achieved in routine daily practice.

Thus the consensus definition for a polycystic ovary includes an ovarian volume of greater than 10 cm[3]. It is recognized that not all polycystic ovaries will be enlarged to this size or greater and that the consensus is based on the synthesis of evidence from many studies that have reported a greater mean ovarian volume for polycystic ovaries combined with a consistent finding of a smaller mean volume than 10 cm[3] for normal ovaries. The consensus view is that until more data are collected and validated the volume of the polycystic ovary should be calculated using the more widely accepted criterion of a prolate ellipsoid[30].

Uterine size and relationship to ovarian size

The size of the uterus is often enlarged in women with PCOS because of the increased degree of estrogenization[5,13]. It had been suggested that the ratio of ovarian:uterine volume is never higher than 1.0 in women with polycystic ovaries[31]. Orsini et al.[25], however, found a wide range of ovarian:uterine volumes and this diagnostic criterion was subsequently abandoned.

Follicles: size and number

We now know that it is oocyte-containing follicles that we are observing when describing the polycystic ovary, rather than pathologic or atretic cystic structures. The early literature often refers to 'cysts' rather than follicles and as the latter are indeed small cysts – that is a 'sac containing fluid' – the terminology poly*cystic* ovary syndrome has remained.

Sample et al.[24] described the follicles as < 8 mm whilst Swanson et al.[10] noted the follicles to be 2–6 mm in diameter, but a prerequisite number was neither recorded or defined. Orsini et al.[25] described ovaries as either being predominantly solid if fewer than four small (< 9 mm) cystic structures were detected in the ovary or predominantly cystic if multiple small (neither quantified) cystic structures or at least one large (> 10 mm) cyst were present. Patients with PCOS usually had follicles of between 4 and 10 mm, but occasionally follicles of 15 mm – presumably indicative of follicular recruitment. The seminal paper of Adams et al.[13] described the polycystic ovary as having, in one plane, at least 10 follicles (usually between 2 and 8 mm in diameter), usually arranged peripherally – although when scattered through the stroma it was suggested that the follicles were usually 2–4 mm in diameter[13]. Others claimed that the transvaginal definition of a polycystic ovary should require the presence of at least 15 follicles (2–10 mm in diameter) in a single plane[16].

Jonard et al.[32] studied 214 women with PCOS (oligo/amenorrhea, elevated serum LH and/or testosterone, and/or ovarian area > 5.5 cm^2) and 112 with normal ovaries to determine the importance of follicle number per ovary (FNPO). A 7 MHz transvaginal ultrasound scan was performed and three different categories of follicle size analyzed separately (2–5, 6–9, and 2–9 mm).

The size range of the follicles has been considered important by some, with polycystic ovaries tending to have smaller follicles than normal or multicystic ovaries[4,33]. The mean FNPO was similar between normal and polycystic ovaries in the 6–9 mm range, but significantly higher in the polycystic ovaries in both the 2–5 and 2–9 mm ranges. A FNPO of ≥ 12 follicles of 2–9 mm gave the best threshold for the diagnosis of PCOS (sensitivity 75%, specificity 99%)[32] (Table 11.2). The authors suggest that intraovarian hyperandrogenism promotes excessive early follicular growth up to 2–5 mm, with more follicles able to enter the growing cohort which then become arrested at the 6–9 mm size. Thus the consensus definition for a polycystic ovary is one that contains 12 or more follicles of 2–9 mm diameter[30].

Multi-cystic and polycystic ovaries

The multi-cystic ovary is one in which there are multiple (≥ 6) follicles, usually 4–10 mm in diameter with normal stromal echogenicity[13]. Again, the terminology might be better annotated as multi-follicular rather than multi-cystic. The multi-follicular appearance is characteristically seen during puberty and in women recovering from hypothalamic amenorrhea – both situations being associated with

Table 11.2 Receiver operating characteristic (ROC) curve data for the assessment of polycystic ovaries[32]

FNPO	Area under the ROC curve	Threshold	Sensitivity (%)	Specificity (%)
2–5 mm	0.924	10	65	97
		12	57	99
		15	42	100
6–9 mm	0.502	3	42	69
		4	32.5	80
		5	24	89
2–9 mm	0.937	10	86	90
		12	75	99
		15	58	100

follicular growth without consistent recruitment of a dominant follicle[34,35]. It is therefore necessary to make careful consideration of the clinical picture and endocrinology.

Stromal echogenicity

The increased echodensity of the polycystic ovary is a key histologic feature[33], but is a subjective assessment that may vary depending upon the setting of the ultrasound machine and the patient's body habitus. In a study by Ardaens et al.[36], subjectively increased stromal hyperechogenicity assessed transvaginally appeared exclusively to be associated with PCOS.

Normal stromal echogenicity is said to be less than that of the myometrium, which is a simple guide that will take into account the setting of the ultrasound machine. Stromal echogenicity has been described in a semi-quantitative manner with a score for normal (= 1), moderately increased (= 2), or frankly increased (= 3)[28]. In this study the total follicle number of both ovaries combined correlated significantly with stromal echogenicity. Follicle number also correlated significantly with free androgen index. A further study comparing women with PCOS with controls found that the sensitivity and specificity of ovarian stromal echogenicity in the diagnosis of polycystic ovaries were 94% and 90%, respectively[37].

Echogenicity has been quantified by Al-Took et al.[38] as the sum of the product of each intensity level (ranging from 0 to 63 on the scanner) and the number of pixels for that intensity level divided by the total number of pixels in the measured area: Mean = $(\Sigma x_i f_i)/n$, where n = total number of pixels in the measured area, x = intensity level (from 0 to 63), and f = number of pixels corresponding with the level. The stromal index was calculated by dividing the mean stromal echogenicity by the mean echogenicity of the entire ovary in order to correct for cases in which the gain was adjusted to optimize image definition[38]. Using these measurements the stromal index did not predict responsiveness to clomiphene citrate and neither did the stromal index differ after ovarian drilling[38].

Another approach used a 7.5 MHz transvaginal probe with histogram measurement of echogenicity[39]. The mean echogenicity was defined as the sum of the product of each intensity level (from 0 to 63) using the same formula as Al-Took et al.[38]. The ovaries from women with PCOS had greater total volume, stromal volume, and peak stromal blood flow compared with normal ovaries, yet mean stromal echogenicity was similar. The stromal index (mean stromal echogenicity: mean echogenicity of the entire ovary) was higher in PCOS, due to the finding of a reduced mean echogenicity of the entire ovary[39]. The conclusion is that the subjective impression of increased stromal echogenicity is due both to increased stromal volume alongside reduced echogenicity of the multiple follicles.

Stromal area or volume

Dewailly et al.[40] designed a computer-assisted method for standardizing the assessment of stromal hypertrophy. Patients with hyperandrogenism, of whom 68% had menstrual cycle disturbances, were compared with a control group and a group with hypothalamic amenorrhea. Transvaginal ultrasound (5 MHz) was used and polycystic ovaries defined as the presence of 'abnormal ovarian stroma and/or the presence of at least 10 round areas of reduced echogenicity < 8 mm in size on a single ovarian section and/or an increased cross-sectional ovarian area (>10 cm²)'[36,40]. The computerized technique for reading the scans involved a longitudinal section in the middle part of the ovary and calculation of the stromal area and the area of the follicles. Of 57 women with hyperandrogenism, 65% had polycystic ovaries visualized on ultrasound and elevated serum testosterone and LH concentrations were found in 50% and 45%, respectively. There was no correlation between LH and androstenedione concentrations. Stromal area, however, correlated significantly with androstenedione and 17 hydroxyprogesterone (17OHP), but not testosterone, LH, or insulin concentrations; follicle area did not correlate with endocrine parameters[40]. Thus it was suggested that the analysis of ovarian stromal area is better than quantification of the follicles in polycystic ovaries.

Three-dimensional ultrasound has been shown to be a good tool for the accurate measurement of ovarian volume, and more precise than 2D ultrasound[21]. Three groups of patients were defined:

(1)   Those with normal ovaries,

(2)   Those with asymptomatic polycystic ovaries, and

(3)   Those with polycystic ovary syndrome[41].

The ovarian and stromal volumes were similar in groups 2 and 3, and both were greater than group 1. Stromal volume was positively correlated with serum androstenedione concentrations in group 3 only[41]. The mean total volume of the follicles was similar in all groups, indicating that increased stromal volume is the main cause of ovarian enlargement in polycystic ovaries.

In summary, ovarian volume correlates well with ovarian function and is both more easily and reliably measured in routine practice than ovarian stroma. Thus in order to define the polycystic ovary neither qualitative nor quantitative assessment of the ovarian stroma is required.

Blood flow

The combination of transvaginal ultrasound with color Doppler measurements is beginning to provide a detailed picture of follicular events around the time of ovulation and also allows assessment of the uterine blood flow to predict endometrial receptivity[42,43]. Blood flow through the uterine and ovarian arteries has been extensively investigated in spontaneous and stimulated cycles[44]. Color (or 'power') Doppler also allows assessment of the vascular network within the ovarian stroma. Intraovarian stromal blood flow is significantly higher in polycystic ovaries than normal ovaries and its measurement, either in the early follicular phase or following pituitary suppression, has been found to be predictive of follicular response to ovarian stimulation for IVF[45,46].

A number of studies of color Doppler measurement of uterine and ovarian vessel blood flow have demonstrated a low resistance index in the stroma of polycystic ovaries (i.e. increased flow) and correlations with endocrine changes[47–49]. Battaglia et al.[50] reported a good correlation between serum androstenedione concentrations and the LH:FSH ratio with the number of small follicles, and the LH:FSH ratio also correlated well with the stromal artery pulsatility index. In another study, the blood flow was more frequently visualized in PCOS (88%) than in normal patients (50%) in the early follicular phase and seemed to be increased[51].

The resistance index (RI) and pulsatility index (PI) have been found to be significantly lower in PCOS than in normal patients and the peak systolic velocity (PVS) greater[52]. No correlation was found with the number of follicles and the ovarian volume, but there was a positive correlation between LH levels and increased PVS. Zaidi et al.[22] found no significant difference in PI values between the normal and PCOS groups, while the ovarian flow, as reflected by the PVS, was increased in the former.

The assessment of Doppler blood flow may have some value in predicting the risk for ovarian hyperstimulation during gonadotropin therapy[53]. Increased stromal blood flow has also been suggested as a more relevant predictor of ovarian response to hormonal stimulation[39,46] than parameters such as ovarian or stromal volume. The measurement of Doppler blood flow requires specific expertise and machinery and at the present time is not necessary as part of the diagnostic criteria for the polycystic ovary.

DEFINING THE POLYCYSTIC OVARY

With all imaging systems, the ovarian size (i.e. volume) together with the number of preantral follicles are the key and consistent features of polycystic ovaries. Pache and colleagues performed a series of studies to distinguish between normal and polycystic ovaries and to determine the key features of the polycystic ovary[4,28,37]. First PCOS was defined (on the basis of elevated testosterone or LH) and transvaginal ultrasound (5 MHz) was used to compare those with the syndrome to a control group[37]. Women with amenorrhea had similar ultrasound features to those with oligomenorrhea. Control ovaries never had a volume of more than 8.0 cm³ or more than 11 follicles. The mean number of follicles was 10 in polycystic ovaries and 5 in normal ovaries. Median values for mean ovarian volume were 5.9 cm³ in controls and 9.8 cm³ in PCOS ($p < 0.001$); mean follicular size and number were 5.1 vs. 3.8 and 5.0 vs. 9.8 for controls and PCOS, respectively. Stromal echogenicity was also significantly increased in the PCOS patients, based on a semi-quantitative assessment[37]. The greatest power of discrimination between normal and polycystic ovaries was provided by a combined measurement of follicular size and ovarian volume (sensitivity 92%, specificity 97%).

A later study from the same group defined normal ovarian morphology in a control group of 48 normally cycling women and compared both ultrasound and endocrine parameters with those in patients with normogonadotropic oligomenorrhea or amenorrhea[54]. In the normal ovaries the mean number of follicles per ovary was 7.0 ± 1.7 and none had more than 9 follicles or an ovarian volume of greater than 10.7 ml. Polycystic ovaries were therefore considered to have ≥ 10 follicles and a volume of ≥ 10.8 ml.

From their data, Jonard et al.[32] proposed a new definition of the polycystic ovary: increased ovarian area (> 5.5 cm²) or volume (> 11 cm³) and/or the presence of ≥ 12 follicles of 2–9 mm diameter (as a mean of both ovaries). According to the literature review and to the discussion at the joint ASRM/ESHRE consensus meeting on PCOS held in Rotterdam in 2003 a consensus definition was decided (Table 11.1)[30]. There are circumstances where the above definition does not fit, until more data are collected:

- In women taking the combined oral contraceptive pill, the ovarian volume is suppressed but the appearance may still be polycystic[55].

- Polycystic ovaries can also be detected in postmenopausal women and whilst, not surprisingly, smaller than in premenopausal women with polycystic ovaries, they are still larger (6.4 cm³ vs. 3.7 cm³) with more follicles (9.0 vs 1.7) than normal postmenopausal ovaries[56]. However, no threshold is available.

- Criteria to discriminate polycystic ovaries in adolescent girls from multi-cystic ovaries have not been established[57]. Indeed it appears that PCOS manifests for the first time during the adolescent years, which are critical for future ovarian and metabolic function[58].

The incidental discovery of polycystic ovaries at ultrasound is common in women undergoing investigation for any gynecological complaint, such as pelvic pain, unexplained bleeding, or infertility. If polycystic ovaries are observed in ovulatory infertile women (in whom PCOS is not the cause of infertility), the information is very important when designing a 'superovulation' protocol because there is an increased risk of OHSS. Also, it may be useful to look for a family history of PCOS, as some siblings may have symptomatic, yet undiagnosed, PCOS. In addition, metabolic features of hyperinsulinism may be present and deserve careful evaluation since they could indicate risks for long-term health.

ACKNOWLEDGMENTS

The contents of this chapter are drawn from the ESHRE/ASRM Consensus Meeting on PCOS, Rotterdam 2003, from which the following paper was published on ovarian morphology: Balen AH, Laven JSE, Tan SL, Dewailly D. Ultrasound assessment of the polycystic ovary: international consensus definitions. Hum Reprod Update 2003; 9: 505–14.

I wish to acknowledge my co-authors from the consensus workshop on the definitions of the polycystic ovary, Professor Didier Dewailly (Lille, France), Dr Joop Laven (Rotterdam, The Netherlands), and Professor SL Tan (Montreal, Canada).

REFERENCES

1. Stein IF, Leventhal ML. Amenorrhea associated with bilateral polycystic ovaries. Am J Obstet Gynaecol 1935; 29: 181–91.

2. Polson DW, Adams J, Wadsworth J et al. Polycystic ovaries – a common finding in normal women. Lancet 1988; 1: 870–2.

3. Michelmore KF, Balen AH, Dunger DB et al. Polycystic ovaries and associated clinical and biochemical features in young women. Clin Endocrinol Oxf 1999; 51: 779–86.

4. Pache TD, de Jong FH, Hop WC et al. Association between ovarian changes assessed by transvaginal sonogrophy and clinical and endocrine signs of the polycystic ovary syndrome. Fertil Steril 1993; 59: 544–9.

5. Balen AH, Conway GS, Kaltsas G et al. Polycystic ovary syndrome: the spectrum of the disorder in 1741 patients. Hum Reprod 1995; 10: 2107–11.

6. Elting MW, Korsen TJM, Rekers-Mombarg LTM et al. Women with polycystic ovary syndrome gain regular menstrual cycles when ageing. Hum Reprod 2000; 15: 24–8.

7. Balen AH, Michelmore K. What is polycystic ovary syndrome? Are national views important? Hum Reprod 2002; 17: 2219–27.

8. Homburg R. What is polycystic ovary syndrome? A proposal for a consensus on the definition and diagnosis of polycystic ovary syndrome. Hum Reprod 2002; 17: 2495–9.

9. Fauser B, Tarlatzis B, Chang J et al. The Rotterdam ESHRE/ASRM-sponsored PCOS consensus workshop group. Revised 2003 consensus on diagnostic criteria and long-term health risks related to polycystic ovary syndrome (PCOS). Hum Reprod 2004; 19: 41–7; and The Rotterdam ESHRE/ASRM-sponsored PCOS consensus workshop group. Revised 2003 consensus on diagnostic criteria and long-term health risks related to polycystic ovary syndrome (PCOS). Fertil Steril 2004; 81: 19–25.

10. Swanson M, Sauerbrei EE, Cooperberg PL. Medical implications of ultrasonically detected polycystic ovaries. J Clin Ultrasound 1981; 9: 219–22.

11. Campbell S, Goessens L, Goswamy R et al. Real-time ultrasonography for determination of ovarian morphology and volume. Lancet 1982; 1: 425–8.

12. Orsini LF, Rizzo N, Calderoni P et al. Ultrasound monitoring of ovarian follicular development: a comparison of real-time and static scanning techniques. J Clin Ultrasound 1983; 11: 207–11.

13. Adams J, Polson DW, Abdulwahid N et al. Multifollicular ovaries: clinical and endocrine features and response to pulsatile gonadotropin releasing hormone. Lancet 1985; 2: 1375–9.

14. Conway GS, Honour JW, Jacobs HS. Heterogeneity of the polycystic ovary syndrome: clinical, endocrine and ultrasound features in 556 patients. Clin Endocrinol Oxf 1989; 30: 459–70.

15. Kiddy DS, Sharp PS, White DM et al. Differences in clinical and endocrine features between obese and non-obese subjects with polycystic ovary syndrome: an analysis of 263 consecutive cases. Clin Endocrinol Oxf 1990; 32: 213–20.

16. Fox R, Corrigan E, Thomas PA et al. The diagnosis of polycystic ovaries in women with oligo-amenorrhoea: predictive power of endocrine tests. Clin Endocrinol Oxf 1991; 34: 127–31.

17. Abdel Gadir A, Khatim MS, Mowafi RS et al. Implications of ultrasonically diagnosed polycystic ovaries. I. Correlations with basal hormonal profiles. Hum Reprod 1992; 7: 453–7.

18. Clayton RN, Ogden V, Hodgkinson J et al. How common are polycystic ovaries in normal women and what is their significance for the fertility of the population? Clin Endocrinol Oxf 1992; 37: 127–34.

19. Farquhar CM, Birdsall M, Manning P et al. The prevalence of polycystic ovaries on ultrasound scanning in a population of randomly selected women. Aust NZ J Obstet Gynaecol 1994; 34: 67–72.

20. Goldstein G. Incorporating endovaginal ultrasonography into the overall gynaecologic examination. Am J Obstet Gynecol 1990; 160: 625–32.

21. Kyei-Mensah A, Maconochie N, Zaidi J et al. Transvaginal three-dimensional ultrasound: reproducibility of ovarian and endometrial volume measurements. Fertil Steril 1996; 66: 718–22.

22. Zaidi J, Campbell S, Pittrof R et al. Ovarian stromal blood flow in women with polycystic ovaries – a possible new marker for diagnosis? Hum Reprod 1995; 10: 1992–6.

23. Nardo LG, Buckett WM, Khullar V. Determination of the best-fitting ultrasound formulaic method for ovarian volume measurement in women with polycystic ovary syndrome. Fertil Steril 2003; 79: 632–3.

24. Sample WF, Lippe BM, Gyepes MT. Grey-scale ultrasonography of the normal female pelvis. Radiology 1977; 125: 477–83.

25. Orsini LF, Venturoli S, Lorusso R et al. Ultrasonic findings in polycystic ovarian disease. Fertil Steril 1985; 43: 709–14.

26. Hann LE, Hall DA, McArdle CR et al. Polycystic ovarian disease: sonographic spectrum. Radiology 1984; 150: 531–4.

27. Saxton DW, Farquhar CM, Rae T et al. Accuracy of ultrasound measurements of female pelvic organs. Br J Obstet Gynaecol 1990; 97: 695–9.

28. Pache TD, Hop WC, Wladimiroff JW et al. Transvaginal sonography and abnormal ovarian appearance in menstrual cycle disturbances. Ultrasound Med Biol 1991; 17: 589–93.

29. Fulghesu AM, Ciampelli M, Belosi C et al. A new ultrasound criterion for the diagnosis of polycystic ovary syndrome: the ovarian stroma:total area ratio. Fertil Steril 2001; 76: 326–31.

30. Balen AH, Laven JSE, Tan SL et al. Ultrasound Assessment of the Polycystic Ovary: International Consensus Definitions. Hum Reprod Update 2003; 9: 505–14.

31. Parisi L, Tramonti M, Casciano S et al. The role of ultrasound in the study of polycystic ovarian disease. J Clin Ultrasound 1982; 10: 167–72.

32. Jonard S, Robert Y, Cortet-Rudelli C et al. Ultrasound examination of polycystic ovaries: is it worth counting the follicles? Hum Reprod 2003; 18: 598–603.

33. Hughesdon PE. Morphology and morphogenesis of the Stein–Leventhal Ovary and of so-called 'hyperthecosis'. Obstet Gynecol Surv 1982; 37: 59–77.

34. Venturoli S, Porcu E, Fabbri R et al. Ovaries and menstrual cycles in adolescence. Gynecol Obstet Invest 1983; 17: 219–23.

35. Stanhope R, Adams J, Jacobs HS et al. Ovarian ultrasound assessment in normal children, idiopathic precocious puberty, and during low dose pulsatile gonadotrophin releasing hormone treatment of hypogonadotrophic hypogonadism. Arch Dis Child 1985; 60: 116–9.

36. Ardaens Y, Robert Y, Lemaitre L et al. Polycystic ovarian disease: contribution of vaginal endosonography and reassessment of ultrasonic diagnosis. Fertil Steril 1991; 55: 1062–8.

37. Pache TD, Wladimiroff JW, Hop WC et al. How to discriminate between normal and polycystic ovaries: transvaginal ultrasound study. Radiology 1992; 83: 421–3.

38. Al-Took S, Watkin K, Tulandi T et al. Ovarian stromal echogenicity in women with clomiphene citrate-sensitive and clomiphene citrate-resistant polycystic ovary syndrome. Fertil Steril 1999; 71: 952–4.

39. Buckett WM, Bouzayen R, Watkin KL et al. Ovarian stromal echogenicity in women with normal and polycystic ovaries. Hum Reprod 1999; 14: 618–21.

40. Dewailly D, Robert Y, Helin I et al. Ovarian stromal hypertrophy in hyperandrogenic women. Clin Endocrinol 1994; 41: 557–62.

41. Kyei-Mensah A, Tan SL, Zaidi J et al. Relationship of ovarian stromal volume to serum androgen concentrations in patients with polycystic ovary syndrome. Hum Reprod 1998; 13: 1437–41.

42. Zaidi J, Jurkovic D, Campbell S et al. Circadian variation in uterine artery blood flow indices during the follicular phase of the menstrual cycle. Ultrasound Obstet Gynecol 1995; 5: 406–10.

43. Zaidi J, Tan SL, Pitroff R et al. Blood flow changes in the intra-ovarian arteries during the peri-ovulatory period – relationship to the time of day. Ultrasound Obstet Gynecol 1996; 7: 135–40.

44. Tan SL, Zaidi J, Campbell S et al. Blood flow changes in the ovarian and uterine arteries during the normal menstrual cycle. Am J Obstet Gynecol 1996; 175: 625–31.

45. Zaidi J, Barber J, Kyei-Mensah A et al. Relationship of ovarian stromal blood flow at the baseline ultrasound scan to subsequent follicular response in an in vitro fertilization program. Obstet Gynecol 1996; 88: 779–84.

46. Engmann L, Sladkevicius P, Agrawal LR et al. Value of ovarian stromal blood flow velocity measurement after pituitary suppression in the prediction of ovarian responsiveness and outcome of in vitro fertilization treatment. Fertil Steril 1999; 71: 22–9.

47. Battaglia C, Artini PG, D'Ambrogio G et al. The role of colour Doppler imaging in the diagnosis of polycystic ovary syndrome. Am J Obstet Gynecol 1995; 172: 108–13.

48. Loverro G, Vicino M, Lorusso F et al. Polycystic ovary syndrome: relationship between insulin sensitivity, sex hormone levels and ovarian stromal blood flow. Gynecol Endocrinol 2001; 15: 142–9.

49. Pan H-A, Wu M-H, Cheng Y-C et al. Quantification of Doppler signal in polycystic ovary syndrome using 3-D power Doppler ultrasonography: a possible new marker for diagnosis. Hum Reprod 2002; 17: 201–6.

50. Battaglia C, Genazzani AD, Salvatori M et al. Doppler, ultrasonographic and endocrinological environment with regard to the number of small subcapsular follicles in polycystic ovary syndrome. Gynecol Endocrinol 1999; 13: 123–9.

51. Battaglia C, Artini PG, Genazzani AD et al. Color Doppler analysis in lean and obese women with polycystic ovaries. Ultrasound Gynaecol Obstet 1996; 7: 342–6.

52. Aleem FA, Predanic MP. Transvaginal color Doppler determination of the ovarian and uterine blood flow characteristics in polycystic ovary disease. Fertil Steril 1996; 65: 510–16.

53. Agrawal R, Conway G, Sladkevicius P et al. Serum vascular endothelial growth factor and Doppler blood flow velocities in in vitro fertilization: relevance to ovarian hyperstimulation syndrome and polycystic ovaries. Fertil Steril 1998; 70: 651–8.

54. Van Santbrink EJP, Hop WC, Fauser BCJM. Classification of normogonadotropic infertility: polycystic ovaries diagnosed by ultrasound versus endocrine characteristics of polycystic ovary syndrome. Fertil Steril 1997; 67: 452–8.

55. Franks S, Adams J, Mason HD et al. Ovulatory disorders in women with polycystic ovary syndrome. Clin Obstet Gynecol 1985; 12: 605–32.

56. Birdsall MA, Farquhar CM. Polycystic ovaries in pre and post-menopausal women. Clin Endocrinol 1996; 44: 269–76.

57. Herter LD, Magalhaes JA, Spritzer PM. Relevance of the determination of ovarian volume in adolescent girls with menstrual disorders. J Clin Ultrasound 1996; 24: 243–8.

58. Balen AH, Danger D. Pubertal maturation of the internal genitalia. Ultrasound Obstet Gynaecol 1995; 6: 164–5.

CHAPTER 12

Prediction and prevention of ovarian hyperstimulation syndrome

Aykut Bayrak and Richard J Paulson

INTRODUCTION

Ovarian hyperstimulation syndrome (OHSS) is an iatrogenic condition encountered in patients undergoing ovulation induction. The incidence of moderate to severe forms of OHSS occurs in 1–2% of assisted reproductive technology (ART) cycles. The clinical symptom complex of ovarian enlargement, abdominal distension, nausea/vomiting, ascites, and oliguria characterizes the syndrome. Although OHSS is almost exclusively observed in controlled ovarian hyperstimulation (COH) cycles using exogenous gonadotropins, rarely clomiphene citrate administration can cause similar clinical features. The existence of this syndrome was first reported in 1961[1]. Whereas transvaginal ultrasound and serum estradiol (E_2) determinations have made monitoring of the clinical response to gonadotropins far more precise, the incidence of OHSS per treatment cycle has not lessened in the past 30 years.

Although most cases of OHSS are considered mild and limited to tolerable gastrointestinal side-effects, serious complications such as ischemic stroke[2], acute myocardial infarction[3,4], forearm amputation[5], and death have been reported[6]. OHSS is a self-limiting entity in most cases over the course of a few days in non-conceptional cycles. However, worsening OHSS can be observed in conceptional cycles in which endogenous human chorionic gonadotropin (hCG) production continues and resolution of the syndrome is delayed. Since 1967, various investigators using both clinical and laboratory data have classified OHSS as mild, moderate, or severe, with various subgrades[1,7–10]. Although useful for study purposes, these schemes are unnecessarily complex. Firstly, comprehensive monitoring has revealed that many features found in 'mild' and 'moderate' OHSS are common in most patients with average response to gonadotropins and could probably be considered the upper limits of a normal spectrum of response[11]. Secondly, some criteria for severe OHSS, such as hydrothorax or hypercoagulability, can exist without other stigmata of the syndrome[12,13]. Lastly, for the purpose of management, only two categories of cases are important: cases that require hospitalization (severe) and cases that don't (mild) (Table 12.1).

PATHOPHYSIOLOGY

The underlying physiologic derangement primarily responsible for OHSS is increased vascular permeability. Capillary leakage leads to commonly observed ascites and pleural or

Table 12.1 Criteria for hospitalization

Abdominal pain requiring narcotic analgesics

Coagulopathy

Electrolyte imbalance

Hematocrit >45%

Hemorrhage

Oliguria/anuria

Respiratory distress (dyspnea, tachypnea)

Severe nausea and vomiting that prevents oral intake

Hemodynamic instability (hypotension, dizziness, syncope)

---

pericardial effusion. Simultaneously, decreased circulating blood volume gives rise to oliguria, which may result in electrolyte abnormalities and renal failure. Hyperviscosity of circulating blood, a result of low plasma volume, may predispose to thrombosis and embolization. However, there is evidence that hypercoagulability may be an independent process related to high estrogen levels[14].

The precise physiologic factor that mediates increased vascular permeability was initially unknown. Estrogens were initially thought to be the cause since estrone (E_1) and E_2 levels during ovarian stimulation were elevated and E_2 was known to have effects on vascular permeability in the uterus. However, Polishuk and Schenker were unable to induce OHSS in rabbits by administering high doses of E_1[15].

Histamine received considerable attention as a putative mediator after Knox was able to prevent ovarian enlargement and ascites by administering antihistamines to hyperstimulated rabbits[16]. However, subsequent research failed to reveal elevated plasma histamine levels or an increased number of ovarian mast cells in OHSS[17].

Serotonin, another vasomotor amine, was also studied in rabbits by using two antiserotonin drugs, both of which failed to prevent OHSS[18]. Because prostaglandins (PGs), specifically PGI_2, have been implicated in ovulation and increased follicle wall permeability, one may hypothesize that they cause or contribute to OHSS. However, no increases in levels of PGI_2 metabolites were noted in stimulated cycles compared with the normal luteal phase[19]. Furthermore, PG inhibition with indometacin was ineffective in decreasing ovarian size or ascites in rabbits[20].

Prolactin levels are elevated in OHSS[21]. Additionally, exogenous prolactin has been shown to increase ascites formation[22]. Elevated levels of testosterone, progesterone, interleukin-6 and interleukin-18, and inflammatory cytokines associated with increased vascular permeability, have also been described[21,23–25]. However, their putative role as a causative agent has not been substantiated.

Recent data have pointed to angiogenic factors in the ovary as potential agents responsible for the clinical syndrome of OHSS. These substances appear to be associated with neovascularization of the corpus luteum. In a hyperstimulated ovary, their levels are greatly increased and their normal physiologic role is magnified into the syndrome of OHSS. These substances include angiotensin II and vascular endothelial growth factor (VEGF), but there may be others.

Evidence supporting the role of angiotensin II is indirect but suggestive. Firstly, a complete prorenin–renin–angiotensin cascade exists within the ovary, and production of several components of this system appears to be enhanced by gonadotropins[26,27]. High levels of prorenin, renin, and angiotensin II have been found in follicular fluid, blood, and ascites of patients with the syndrome[26–30]. Secondly, angiotensin II has been found to increase vascular permeability in rabbits – probably by contraction of vascular endothelial cells[31].

If this hypothesis is substantiated by clinical data in humans, it may be possible to treat or prevent OHSS by inhibiting production or action of angiotensin II. Angiotensin converting enzyme (ACE) inhibitors are currently used to treat hypertension and congestive heart failure. Moreover, recent evidence has suggested that ACE inhibitors help reduce vascular permeability in rabbit OHSS, as well as other abnormal vascular permeability syndromes.

In glomerular nephropathy (nephron protein leakage) and diabetic retinopathy (also a high prorenin state), ACE inhibition has been successfully used to reduce or prevent vascular leakage[32,33]. Moreover, in a controlled trial of the ACE inhibitor enalapril (Vasotec) in gonadotropin-stimulated rabbits, we were able to prevent OHSS completely in nearly half the treated animals[34]. In the remainder, weight gain was small or absent, and there was no hemoconcentration compared with controls.

However, while encouraging, these data need to be confirmed in humans before this form of therapy can be recommended. A recent report suggested for the first time in humans that the combination of an ACE inhibitor (alacepril) and an angiotensin II receptor blocker (candesartan cilexetil), in addition to cryopreservation, may prevent OHSS in patients at very high risk (E_2 levels $\geq$ 8000 pg/ml) for this syndrome[35]. It should be noted that ACE inhibitors have been associated with oligohydramnios and renal failure when used in later pregnancy.

VEGF is the other ovarian angiogenic factor thought to be involved in the pathogenesis of OHSS. VEGF stimulates endothelial cell proliferation and angiogenesis[36], and increases capillary permeability, which causes extravasation of protein-rich fluids, and these effects result in OHSS. VEGF levels are increased in serum, follicular, and peritoneal fluid of women who develop OHSS[37,38], and its levels correlate with the severity of the syndrome[39]. It has been reported that anti-VEGF antibodies can reverse the increased vascular permeability activity of the follicular fluid recovered from patients with OHSS[36]. These findings suggest that VEGF has a significant contribution to the pathogenesis of OHSS.

Leptin levels are elevated in patients with polycystic ovary syndrome, who are at a greater risk for OHSS during ART cycles. Whether leptin plays a role in OHSS is unclear, but levels of leptin were reported to be lower in patients with OHSS in one study[40] and were not associated in another[41].

More recently, spontaneous development of familial gestational OHSS has been described resulting from a mutation in the follicle-stimulating hormone (FSH) receptor. The mutation in the FSH receptor decreases the sensitivity of the receptor, thus allowing hCG and thyroid-stimulating hormone to stimulate it. Inappropriate stimulation of the FSH receptor results in clinical signs and symptoms of OHSS during gestation without a history of gonadotropin use for ovulation induction or in-vitro fertilization (IVF)[42–44]. Additionally, OHSS has been reported in women with FSH-secreting pituitary adenomas[45–47].

PREVENTION

Until adequate treatment is devised, prevention of OHSS remains the most effective way of avoiding serious sequelae. The most important prevention technique is identification of patients at high risk for severe disease, although even in this group such a development is relatively uncommon (Table 12.2).

Foremost among risk factors is luteal phase stimulation. The incidence of severe OHSS is significantly higher in patients who have either endogenous or exogenous hCG stimulation. It has been advocated that the ovulatory dose of hCG be withheld in 'high-risk' patients. While this measure is usually effective, it may not be necessary in patients receiving ovarian hyperstimulation for one of the ARTs. These women may undergo follicle aspiration followed by IVF and elective cryopreservation of all embryos, thus precluding the possibility of pregnancy and substantially reducing risk.

Table 12.2 Risk factors for severe ovarian hyperstimulation syndrome

---

Young age

Low body mass index

Known 'high responder'

High dose gonadotropins

High estradiol levels

Luteal phase stimulation with human chorionic gonadotropin

Polycystic appearance of ovaries on ultrasound

Polycystic ovary syndrome

Pregnancy

By contrast, in patients receiving gonadotropins for ovulation induction, withholding ovulatory hCG may be prudent. However, cases of OHSS have occurred both in spontaneous cycles and in stimulated cycles where hCG was withheld but in which the patient had a spontaneous luteinizing hormone surge and became pregnant[48,49]. Cancellation of a cycle may be avoided by conversion to an IVF cycle with cryopreservation[50]. A prospective randomized trial concluded that elective cryopreservation of zygotes in patients at risk for OHSS reduced the risk of the syndrome[51]. However, a recent Cochrane review suggested that there may be insufficient evidence to support routine cryopreservation of embryos[52].

Even though hCG may play a role in the development of OHSS, lowering the dose of hCG to trigger ovulation does not seem to reduce the risk of OHSS[53]. Reviews and studies suggesting such an improvement with the use of lower doses of hCG may be biased by other treatment modalities co-administered to prevent OHSS[54-56]. Additionally, when different recombinant hCG doses were compared with urinary hCG to trigger ovulation, the risk of OHSS was not reduced with lower doses[57].

It has been suggested previously that the number of gestational sacs could be predictive of OHSS 4 weeks after embryo transfer[58]. However, a recent report suggested that OHSS did not occur more frequently in twin than singleton pregnancies[59].

We retrospectively compared 133 cycles of COH consisting of 68 patients undergoing IVF and 67 oocyte donors, all of whom had extremely high degrees of ovarian response to COH (E_2 > 4000 pg/ml and more than 25 eggs collected)[60]. Donors, who received no luteal support and did not become pregnant, had no cases of severe OHSS. By contrast, among the IVF patients, there were six women with severe OHSS, four of whom later demonstrated clinical pregnancies. It is possible that pregnancy, even if subclinical, is a necessary condition for the development of severe OHSS.

Intravenous administration of albumin at the time of follicle aspiration has been advocated as a prophylactic measure for high-risk patients undergoing IVF[61]. Four prospective randomized trials supported this practice[62-65] and one study did not[66]. A meta-analysis of these five trials concluded that administration of intravenous albumin at the time of oocyte retrieval would be beneficial in patients at high risk for OHSS[67]. Based on the meta-analysis, in order to prevent one case of OHSS, 18 patients need to be treated with intravenous albumin. It should also be noted that the use of albumin was compared against similar volumes of crystalloid. It is possible that larger volumes of crystalloid, which would have a similar magnitude of effect on intravenous volume, may have matched the potential benefit of albumin. One conclusion from these data may be that volume expansion at the time of follicle aspiration is useful.

Repeated[68] and selective[69] follicle aspiration has been advocated as a possible means to reduce the number of preovulatory follicles and, thus, the risk of OHSS. Others have advocated a 'controlled drift', in which hyperresponding patients are maintained on gonadotropin-releasing hormone (GnRH) agonist therapy without gonadotropin stimulation for several days before hCG administration[70,71]. This approach results in diminished E_2 levels, but ascites has been noted[71]. In a prospective randomized study, early unilateral follicle aspiration was compared with coasting for prevention of OHSS. There was no difference in the incidence of OHSS between the two groups[72]. Because the incidence of severe OHSS may be low even in so-called 'high-risk' patients, it is not valid to conclude that the absence of OHSS in a small group of patients receiving a particular treatment proves the efficacy of that treatment. A recent Cochrane review concluded that, as yet, there is lack of evidence to support the routine use of coasting to prevent OHSS[73].

Administration of methylprednisolone was reported to reduce the risk of OHSS in a retrospective study[74]. Prospective randomized trials have shown that glucocorticoids, GnRH agonists, or administration of ketoconazole do not prevent OHSS[75–77]. Additionally, a recent review of randomized controlled trials failed to demonstrate a reduction in the incidence of severe OHSS with the use of GnRH antagonists compared to GnRH agonists in IVF-embryo transfer cycles[78]. Low dose hCG alone or in combination with low dose FSH can stimulate the growth of antral follicles in the mid/late follicular phase and result in the demise of the smaller follicles[79]. Although not yet tested for the prevention of OHSS, selective growth of larger antral follicles and the failure of growth of smaller preovulatory follicles might have a beneficial effect against the development of OHSS.

TREATMENT

Once OHSS is diagnosed, a clinical decision should be made as to whether the patient needs to be treated as an inpatient or outpatient. Women with mild OHSS are generally managed as outpatients with oral analgesics and close clinical monitoring. Patients should be advised to refrain from intercourse and impacting exer-

cise because this may worsen abdominal pain and possibly result in ovarian cyst rupture or even ovarian torsion. Although bed rest is commonly recommended as a part of the treatment algorithm, strict bed rest may actually increase the risk of thromboembolism and therefore light activity should be encouraged. Close surveillance with physical examinations (not pelvic), testing for complete blood count and electrolytes, monitoring urine output, ultrasound monitoring of ascites, measurement of weight, and frequent communication with the patient regarding the signs and symptoms of worsening OHSS are essential components of outpatient management. Early diagnosis of pregnancy is essential because the increasing hCG levels may worsen the clinical picture rapidly.

Severe OHSS requires hospitalization (Table 12.1) and careful hemodynamic and fluid monitoring. The goal of management is to maintain urine output and electrolyte homeostasis until spontaneous resolution (as indicated by diuresis) occurs. Close clinical assessment and laboratory testing allow monitoring of progression and response to the treatment modalities[80].

A recent report suggested that Dextran 40 infusion to inpatients with severe OHSS when compared to albumin infusion may result in a faster recovery from hemoconcentration and leukocytosis[81]. In a preliminary study, inpatients who initially had a poor response to albumin had improvement in clinical symptoms associated with ascites when treated with the oral dopamine prodrug docarpamine[82].

Prophylaxis against thrombosis is necessary because numerous cases of thromboembolic phenomena and their sequelae have been reported. Subcutaneous heparin (5000 IU twice a day) is typically used in severe OHSS cases to prevent thromboembolic phenomena. However, it is unclear at what point anticoagulation measures should be discontinued since thrombosis has been reported several weeks after resolution of other stigmata of severe OHSS[13]. Although relatively rare, signs and symptoms of acute thrombus or embolism should prompt the clinician to obtain diagnostic testing immediately, initiate therapeutic anticoagulation, and provide appropriate supportive care.

Paracentesis, achieved by the abdominal[83] or transvaginal[84] route, offers substantial symptomatic relief of symptoms, especially if respiratory compromise is present. It is not clear if OHSS resolves more quickly after paracentesis than with conservative treatment, although one study[84] suggested that hospital stay might be shortened. Since the ascites fluid contains elevated levels of prorenin and angiotensin II[28,29] it is tempting to speculate that drainage of this fluid may provide symptomatic relief by more than just mechanical means. Paracentesis may also be beneficial in improving urine output by lowering the intra-abdominal pressure and decreasing renal arterial resistance[85]. One report[86] suggested that chest tube drainage of pleural effusion could reduce abdominal ascites.

SUMMARY

Severe OHSS is a rare but dangerous complication of gonadotropin therapy. Its stigmata are the result of fluid derangements caused by increased vascular permeability. Current evidence points to angiotensin II and VEGF as the most likely mediators. Prevention of the syndrome in IVF cycles for high-risk patients may include administration of intravenous albumin, avoidance of luteal stimulation by hCG, and, in selected cases, elective cryopreservation of all embryos. Lowering the hCG dose to trigger ovulation does not have a protective effect against OHSS in IVF cycles. However, in ovulation-induction cycles, consider withholding hCG in high-risk cycles or converting to an IVF cycle.

Since OHSS is self-limiting, treatment should be conservative. Hospitalization is necessary only in severe cases. Treatment goals should include maintenance of circulating volume, electrolyte balance, and urine output, and pro-

phylaxis against thromboembolism. Abdominal paracentesis may provide substantial symptomatic relief in cases of OHSS and may be combined with drainage of pleural effusions in cases of respiratory distress. Patients who become pregnant are at an additional risk for developing severe illness and therefore should be more closely monitored.

REFERENCES

1. Esteban-Altirriba J. Le syndrome d'hyperstimulation massive des ovaires. Rev Fr Gynecol Obstet 1961; 56: 555–64.

2. Togay-Isikay C, Celik T, Ustuner I et al. Ischaemic stroke associated with ovarian hyperstimulation syndrome and factor V Leiden mutation. Aust NZ J Obstet Gynaecol 2004; 44: 264–6.

3. Akdemir R, Uyan C, Emiroglu Y. Acute myocardial infarction secondary thrombosis associated with ovarian hyperstimulation syndrome. Int J Cardiol 2002; 83: 187–9.

4. Ludwig M, Tolg R, Richardt G et al. Myocardial infarction associated with ovarian hyperstimulation syndrome. JAMA 1999; 282: 632–3.

5. Mancini A, Milardi D, Di Pietro ML et al. A case of forearm amputation after ovarian stimulation for in vitro fertilization-embryo transfer. Fertil Steril 2001; 76: 198–200.

6. Cluroe AD, Synek BJ. A fatal case of ovarian hyperstimulation syndrome with cerebral infarction. Pathol 1995; 27: 344–6.

7. Rabau E, David A, Serr DM et al. Human menopausal gonadotropins for anovulation and sterility. Results of 7 years of treatment. Am J Obstet Gynecol 1967; 98: 92–8.

8. Schenker JG, Weinstein D. Ovarian hyperstimulation syndrome: a current survey. Fertil Steril 1978; 30: 255–68.

9. Golan A, Ron-el R, Herman H et al. Ovarian hyperstimulation syndrome: an update review. Obstet Gynecol Surv 1989; 44: 430–40.

10. Navot D, Bergh PA, Laufer N. Ovarian hyperstimulation syndrome in novel reproductive

technologies: prevention and treatment. Fertil Steril 1992; 58: 249–61.

11. Blankstein J, Shalev J, Saadon T et al. Ovarian hyperstimulation syndrome: prediction by number and size of preovulatory ovarian follicles. Fertil Steril 1987; 47: 597–602.

12. Jewelewicz R, Vande Wiele RL. Acute hydrothorax as the only symptom of ovarian hyperstimulation syndrome. Am J Obstet Gynecol 1975; 121: 1121.

13. Mills MS, Eddowes HA, Fox R et al. Subclavian vein thrombosis: a late complication of ovarian hyperstimulation syndrome. Hum Reprod 1992; 7: 370–1.

14. Kaaja R, Siegberg R, Tiitinen A et al. Severe ovarian hyperstimulation syndrome and deep venous thrombosis. Lancet 1989; 2: 1043.

15. Polishuk WZ, Schenker JG. Ovarian overstimulation syndrome. Fertil Steril 1969; 20: 443–50.

16. Knox GE. Antihistamine blockade of the ovarian hyperstimulation syndrome. Am J Obstet Gynecol 1974; 118: 992–4.

17. Erlik Y, Naot Y, Friedman M et al. Histamine levels in ovarian hyperstimulation syndrome. Obstet Gynecol 1979; 53: 580–2.

18. Zaidise I, Friedman M, Lindenbaum ES et al. Serotonin and the ovarian hyperstimulation syndrome. Eur J Obstet Gynecol Reprod Biol 1983; 15: 55–60.

19. Hurwitz A, Krausz M, Eldar-Geva T et al. Production of 6-keto-PGF1α in hyperstimulated cycles: in vivo and in vitro studies. Int J Fertil 1991; 36: 252–6.

20. Pride SM, Yuen BH, Moon YS et al. Relationship of gonadotropin-releasing hormone, danazol, and prostaglandin blockade to ovarian enlargement and ascites formation of the ovarian hyperstimulation syndrome in the rabbit. Am J Obstet Gynecol 1986; 154: 1155–60.

21. Yuen BH, McComb P, Sy L et al. Plasma prolactin, human chorionic gonadotropin, estradiol, testosterone, and progesterone in the ovarian hyperstimulation syndrome. Am J Obstet Gynecol 1979; 133: 316–20.

22. Leung P, Yuen BH, Moon YS. Effect of prolactin in an experimental model of the ovarian hyper-stimulation syndrome. Am J Obstet Gynecol 1983; 145: 847–9.

23. Schumbert Z, Spitz I, Diamant Y et al. Elevation of serum testosterone in ovarian hyperstimulation syndrome. J Clin Endocrinol Metab 1975; 40: 889–92.

24. Friedlander MA, Loret de Mola JR, Goldfarb JM. Elevated levels of interleukin-6 in ascites and serum from women with ovarian hyperstimulation syndrome. Fertil Steril 1993; 60: 826–33.

25. Barak V, Elchalal U, Edelstein M et al. Interleukin-18 levels correlate with severe ovarian hyperstimulation syndrome. Fertil Steril 2004; 82: 415–20.

26. Morris RS, Paulson RJ. The ovarian renin angiotensin system: recent advances and their relationship to assisted reproductive technologies. Assist Reprod Rev 1993; 3: 88–94.

27. Morris RS, Paulson RJ. Ovarian derived prorenin–angiotensin cascade in human reproduction. Fertil Steril 1994; 62: 1105–14.

28. Delbaere A, Bergmann PJ, Gervy-Decoster C et al. Angiotensin II immunoreactivity is elevated in ascites during severe ovarian hyperstimulation syndrome: implications for pathophysiology and clinical management. Fertil Steril 1994; 62: 731–7.

29. Delbaere A, Bergmann PJ, Englert Y. Features of the renin–angiotensin system in ascites and pleural effusion during severe ovarian hyperstimulation syndrome. J Assist Reprod Genet 1997; 14: 241–4.

30. Itskovitz-Eldor J, Kol S, Lewit N et al. Ovarian origin of plasma and peritoneal fluid prorenin in early pregnancy and in patients with ovarian hyperstimulation syndrome. J Clin Endocrinol Metab 1997; 82: 461–4.

31. Robertson AL, Khairallah PA. Effects of angiotensin II and some analogues on vascular permeability in the rabbit. Circ Res 1972; 31: 923–31.

32. Stornello M, Valvo EV, Puglia N et al. Angiotensin converting enzyme inhibition with a low dose of enalapril in normotensive diabetics with persistent proteinuria. J Hypertens 1988; 6: S464–6.

33. Larsen M, Hommel E, Parving HH et al. Protective effect of captopril on the blood–retina barrier

in normotensive insulin-dependent diabetic patients with nephropathy and background retinopathy. Graefes Arch Clin Exp Ophthalmol 1990; 228: 505–9.

34. Morris RS, Wong IL, Kirkman E et al. Inhibition of ovarian-derived prorenin to angiotensin cascade in the treatment of ovarian hyperstimulation syndrome. Hum Reprod 1995; 10: 1355–8.

35. Ando H, Furugori K, Shibata D et al. Dual renin–angiotensin blockade therapy in patients at high risk of early ovarian hyperstimulation syndrome receiving IVF and elective embryo cryopreservation: a case series. Hum Reprod 2003; 18: 1219–22.

36. Levin ER, Rosen GF, Cassidenti DL et al. Role of vascular endothelial cell growth factor in ovarian hyperstimulation syndrome. J Clin Invest 1998; 102: 1978–85.

37. Lee A, Christenson LK, Stouffer RL et al. Vascular endothelial growth factor levels in serum and follicular fluid of patients undergoing in vitro fertilization. Fertil Steril 1997; 68: 305–11.

38. Agrawal R, Tan SL, Wild S et al. Serum vascular endothelial growth factor concentrations in in vitro fertilization cycles predict the risk of ovarian hyperstimulation syndrome. Fertil Steril 1999; 71: 287–93.

39. Abramov Y, Barak V, Nisman B et al. Vascular endothelial growth factor plasma levels correlate to the clinical picture in severe ovarian hyperstimulation syndrome. Fertil Steril 1997; 67: 261–5.

40. Ayustawati, Shibahara H, Hirano Y et al. Serum leptin concentrations in patients with severe ovarian hyperstimulation syndrome during in vitro fertilization-embryo transfer treatment. Fertil Steril 2004; 82: 579–85.

41. Salamalekis E, Makrakis E, Vitoratos N et al. Insulin levels, insulin resistance, and leptin levels are not associated with the development of ovarian hyperstimulation syndrome. Fertil Steril 2004; 82: 244–6.

42. Vasseur C, Rodien P, Beau I et al. A chorionic gonadotropin-sensitive mutation in the follicle-stimulating hormone receptor as a cause of familial gestational spontaneous ovarian hyper-

stimulation syndrome. N Engl J Med 2003; 349: 753–9.

43. Smits G, Olatunbosun O, Delbaere A et al. Ovarian hyperstimulation syndrome due to a mutation in the follicle-stimulating hormone receptor. N Engl J Med 2003; 349: 760–6.

44. Montanelli L, Delbaere A, Di Carlo C et al. A mutation in the follicle-stimulating hormone receptor as a cause of familial spontaneous ovarian hyperstimulation syndrome. J Clin Endocrinol Metab 2004; 89: 1255–8.

45. Mor E, Rodi IA, Bayrak A et al. Diagnosis of pituitary gonadotroph adenomas in reproductive aged women. Fertil Steril 2005; 84: 757.

46. Valimaki MJ, Tiitinen A, Alfthan H et al. Ovarian hyperstimulation caused by gonadotroph adenoma secreting follicle-stimulating hormone in 28-year-old woman. J Clin Endocrinol Metab 1999; 84: 4204–8.

47. Shimon I, Rubinek T, Bar-Hava I et al. Ovarian hyperstimulation without elevated serum estradiol associated with pure follicle-stimulating hormone-secreting pituitary adenoma. J Clin Endocrinol Metab 2001; 86: 3635–40.

48. Rosen GF, Lew MW. Severe ovarian hyperstimulation in a spontaneous singleton pregnancy. Am J Obstet Gynecol 1991; 165: 1312–13.

49. Lipitz S, Ben-Rafael Z, Bider D et al. Quintuplet pregnancy and third-degree ovarian hyperstimulation despite withholding human chorionic gonadotropin. Hum Reprod 1991; 6: 1478–9.

50. Lessing JB, Amit A, Libal Y et al. Avoidance of cancellation of potential hyperstimulation cycles by conversion to in vitro fertilization-embryo transfer. Fertil Steril 1991; 56: 75–8.

51. Ferraretti AP, Gianaroli L, Magli C et al. Elective cryopreservation of all pronucleate embryos in women at risk of ovarian hyperstimulation syndrome: efficiency and safety. Hum Reprod 1999; 14: 1457–60.

52. D'Angelo A, Amso N. Embryo freezing for preventing ovarian hyperstimulation syndrome. Cochrane Database Syst Rev 2002; 2: CD002806.

53. Schmidt DW, Maier DB, Nulsen JC et al. Reducing the dose of human chorionic gonadotropin in high responders does not affect the outcomes

of *in vitro* fertilization. Fertil Steril 2004; 82: 841–6.

54. Orvieto R, Ben-Rafael Z. Role of intravenous albumin in the prevention of severe ovarian hyperstimulation syndrome. Hum Reprod 1998; 13: 3306–9.

55. Hillensjo T, Wikland M, Wood M. Albumin in the prevention of severe OHSS. Hum Reprod 1999; 14: 1664–5.

56. Isik AZ, Vicdan K. Combined approach as an effective method in the prevention of severe ovarian hyperstimulation syndrome. Eur J Obstet Gynecol Reprod Biol 2001; 97: 208–12.

57. Chang P, Kenley S, Burns T et al. Recombinant human chorionic gonadotropin (rhCG) in assisted reproductive technology: results of a clinical trial comparing two doses of rhCG (Ovidrel^R) to urinary hCG (Profasi^R) for induction of final follicular maturation in *in vitro* fertilization-embryo transfer. Fertil Steril 2001; 76: 67–74.

58. Lyons CA, Wheeler CA, Frishman GN et al. Early and late presentation of the ovarian hyperstimulation syndrome: two distinct entities with different risk factors. Hum Reprod 1994; 9: 792–9.

59. De Neubourg D, Mangelschots K, Van Royen E et al. Singleton pregnancies are as affected by ovarian hyperstimulation syndrome as twin pregnancies. Fertil Steril 2004; 82: 1691–3.

60. Morris RS, Paulson RJ, Sauer MV et al. Predictive value of serum oestradiol concentrations and oocyte number in severe ovarian hyperstimulation syndrome. Hum Reprod 1995; 10: 811–14.

61. Asch RH, Ivery G, Goldsman M et al. The use of intravenous albumin in patients at high risk for severe ovarian hyperstimulation syndrome. Hum Reprod 1993; 8: 1015–20.

62. Shoham Z, Weissman A, Barash A et al. Intravenous albumin for the prevention of severe ovarian hyperstimulation syndrome in an in vitro fertilization program: a prospective, randomized, placebo-controlled study. Fertil Steril 1994; 62: 137–42.

63. Gokmen O, Ugur M, Ekin M et al. Intravenous albumin versus hydroxyethyl starch for the prevention of ovarian hyperstimulation in an in-vitro fertilization programme: a prospective randomized placebo controlled study. Eur J Obstet Gynecol Reprod Biol 2001; 96: 187–92.

64. Isik AZ, Gokmen O, Zeyneloglu HB et al. Intravenous albumin prevents moderate-severe ovarian hyperstimulation in in vitro fertilization patients: a prospective, randomized and controlled study. Eur J Obstet Gynecol Reprod Biol 1996; 70: 179–83.

65. Shalev E, Giladi Y, Matilsky M et al. Decreased incidence of severe ovarian hyperstimulation syndrome in high risk in vitro fertilization patients receiving intravenous albumin: a prospective study. Hum Reprod 1995; 10: 1373–6.

66. Ben-Chetrit A, Eldar-Geva T, Gal M et al. The questionable use of albumin for the prevention of ovarian hyperstimulation syndrome in an IVF programme: a randomized placebo-controlled trial. Hum Reprod 2001; 16: 1880–4.

67. Aboulghar M, Evers JH, Al-Inany H. Intra-venous albumin for preventing severe ovarian hyperstimulation syndrome. Cochrane Database Syst Rev 2002; 2: CD001302.

68. Amit A, Yaron Y, Yovel I et al. Repeated aspiration of ovarian follicles and early corpus luteum cysts in an in-vitro fertilization programme reduces the risk of ovarian hyperstimulation syndrome in high responders. Hum Reprod 1993; 8: 1184–6.

69. Ingerslev HJ. Selective follicular reduction following ovulation induction by exogenous gonadotrophins in polycystic ovarian disease. A new approach to treatment. Hum Reprod 1991; 6: 682–4.

70. Urman B, Pride SM, Yuen BH. Management of overstimulated gonadotrophin cycles with a controlled drift period. Hum Reprod 1992; 7: 213–17.

71. Sher G, Zouves C, Feinman M et al. 'Prolonged coasting': an effective method for preventing severe ovarian hyperstimulation syndrome in patients undergoing in-vitro fertilization. Hum Reprod 1995; 10: 3107–9.

72. Egbase PE, Sharhan MA, Grudzinskas JG. Early unilateral follicular aspiration compared with coasting for the prevention of severe ovarian

hyperstimulation syndrome: a prospective randomized study. Hum Reprod 1999; 14: 1421–5.

73. D'Angelo A, Amso N. Coasting (withholding gonadotrophins) for preventing ovarian hyperstimulation syndrome. Cochrane Database Syst Rev 2002; 3: CD002811.

74. Lainas T, Petsas G, Stavropoulou G et al. Administration of methylprednisolone to prevent severe ovarian hyperstimulation syndrome in patients undergoing *in vitro* fertilization. Fertil Steril 2002; 78: 529–33.

75. Tan SL, Balen A, el Hussein E et al. The administration of glucocorticoids for the prevention of ovarian hyperstimulation syndrome in in vitro fertilization: a prospective randomized study. Fertil Steril 1992; 58: 378–83.

76. Hughes EG, Fedorkow DM, Daya S et al. The routine use of gonadotropin-releasing hormone agonists prior to in vitro fertilization and gamete intrafallopian transfer: a meta-analysis of randomized controlled trials. Fertil Steril 1992; 58: 888–96.

77. Parsanezhad ME, Alborzi S, Pakniat M et al. A double-blind, randomized, placebo-controlled study to assess the efficacy of ketoconazole for reducing the risk of ovarian hyperstimulation syndrome. Fertil Steril 2003; 80: 1151–5.

78. Al-Inany H, Aboulghar M. Gonadotrophin-releasing hormone antagonists for assisted conception. Cochrane Database Syst Rev 2001; 4: CD001750.

79. Filicori M, Cognigni GE, Tabarelli C et al. Stimulation and growth of antral ovarian follicles by selective LH activity administration in women. J Clin Endocrinol Metab 2002; 87: 1156–61.

80. The Practice Committee of the American Society for Reproductive Medicine. Ovarian hyperstimulation syndrome. Fertil Steril 2003; 80: 1309–14.

81. Endo T, Kitajima Y, Hayashi T et al. Low-molecular-weight dextran infusion is more effective for the treatment of hemoconcentration due to severe ovarian hyperstimulation syndrome than human albumin infusion. Fertil Steril 2004; 82: 1449–51.

82. Tsunoda T, Shibahara H, Hirano Y et al. Treatment for ovarian hyperstimulation syndrome using an oral dopamine prodrug, docarpamine. Gynecol Endocrinol 2003; 17: 281–6.

83. Padilla SL, Zamaria S, Baramki TA et al. Abdominal paracentesis for the ovarian hyperstimulation syndrome with severe pulmonary compromise. Fertil Steril 1990; 53: 365–7.

84. Aboulghar MA, Mansour RT, Serour GI et al. Ultrasonically guided vaginal aspiration of ascites in the treatment of severe ovarian hyperstimulation syndrome. Fertil Steril 1990; 53: 933–5.

85. Maslovitz S, Jaffa A, Eytan O et al. Renal blood flow alteration after paracentesis in women with ovarian hyperstimulation. Obstet Gynecol 2004; 104: 321–6.

86. Rinaldi ML, Spirtos NJ. Chest tube drainage of pleural effusion correcting abdominal ascites in a patient with severe ovarian hyperstimulation syndrome: a case report. Fertil Steril 1995; 63: 1114–17.

CHAPTER 13

Clinical problems associated with ovarian stimulation for conventional IVF (excluding OHSS)

Gabor Kovacs

INTRODUCTION

Although the world's first IVF baby Louise Brown was conceived within a natural menstrual cycle[1], it soon became obvious that if IVF was to progress from a research tool to a clinical treatment, the use of controlled ovarian hyperstimulation was necessary. Initially it was the use of clomiphene citrate[2] that was utilized to produce multiple follicles, soon to be followed by injections of gonadotropins[3]. Soon the use of the natural cycle was virtually abandoned and various regimens utilizing follicle-stimulating hormone (FSH) were introduced.

The next breakthrough was the utilization of gonadotropin releasing hormone agonists (GnRH-A)[4], which suppressed luteinizing hormone (LH) release, preventing spontaneous ovulation and allowing hormonal monitoring to be significantly decreased, thus making treatment much easier. More recently, GnRH antagonists have been utilized[5] and allow the suppression of LH with a shorter administration, which is preferred by many patients[6].

There have been many modifications of controlled ovarian hyperstimulation (COH) for IVF but the basic principles remain – the utilization of FSH to recruit more of the developing primary oocytes to progress to maturation rather than atresia, thus giving the clinician more follicles to aspirate, resulting in several oocytes to be inseminated, hopefully resulting in a choice of embryos for transfer, and some for freezing. These protocols of COH are responsible for IVF reaching a success rate which has enabled it to be a readily available clinical treatment for subfertility, the world over.

However, as with most things in life, new procedures and treatments will also have associated with them new problems. The most serious complication of COH is ovarian hyperstimulation syndrome (OHSS), which is a potentially life-threatening complication. This complication is discussed in detail in Chapter 14. In this chapter we will confine ourselves to the discussion of other clinical problems associated with COH for IVF.

CHOOSING THE CORRECT DOSE OF FSH (UNDERDOSING/OVERDOSING)

Choosing the correct starting dose for a COH cycle is important. Administering too low a dose of FSH will result in insufficient follicles maturing, and the cycle may then have to be abandoned with the wasted time, effort, and hormones. Various starting doses for COH have been developed. Overdosing may result in OHSS, a potentially serious complication. Table 13.1 lists starting dose according to patient's age, basal FSH level, and PCO status, as devised at Monash IVF.

Administering the medication

With the daily use of injectable forms of FSH, administered by healthy patients who are not in hospital, it soon became generalized practice that women should be taught to self-administer. When this responsibility is transferred from the medical/nursing staff, potential new problems of administration arise. Protocols to teach patients and their partners about preparing the medication and administering injections had to be developed, and the techniques had to be taught to the users. Any deviations from dosage or method of administration could have an adverse outcome.

Medication preparation

During the use of the urinary product human menopausal gonadotropin (HMG), the FSH had to be reconstituted from a powder form.

Inadequate technique of dissolving the powder or incompletely aspirating the contents of the ampule would result in underdosing. With the recombinant product, rFSH [Gonal-F (Serono, Geneva) and Puregon® (Organon, Oss, The Netherlands)], the hormone comes as a solution ready to use, thus avoiding preparation errors. With the recently developed pens, administration has become even easier, and mistakes in dosing should be far fewer.

The triggering of follicular maturation is still mostly by human chorionic gonadotropin (hCG), which is supplied in a powder form, and the possible consequences described above still apply. However, recombinant LH is now available as Luveris (Serono, Geneva), which comes in a solution form thus avoiding the problems of preparation.

Hormone storage

With gonadotropins being supplied in a solution rather than powder form, in order to maintain efficacy, stricter conditions with regard to temperature for storage apply. Both Puregon and Gonal F need to be stored in a refrigerator, between 2 and 8°C.

Table 13.1 Starting dose of follicle-stimulating hormone for IVF as used at Monash IVF

			RECOMMENDED DAILY DOSE OF FSH	
Patient criteria				*FSH dose*
Female age	*day 3 FSH*	*PCO/ PCOS*	*Recombinant FSH Puregon®*	*Recombinant FSH Gonal-F® with metformin*
<38	≤10	No	200	225
<38	>10	No	450	450
<38	≤10	Yes	150	150
≥38	≤10	No	200	225
≥38	>10	No	450	450
≥38	≤10	Yes	200	225

For subsequent cycles, the dose may be adjusted when previous response to FSH is reviewed

Injecting technique

When gonadotropins were first utilized it was standard practice to administer them by intramuscular injection, However, it was shown that subcutaneous administration of FSH was just as effective. Of course subcutaneous injections were much easier and could be self-administered. FSH pens are even more user friendly.

ADMINISTERING THE RIGHT MEDICATION – NEED FOR hCG

One of the commonest reasons for failing to recover oocytes from preovulatory follicles is the failure to administer hCG at the appropriate time prior to oocyte collection. Usually hCG is administered 34 to 38 h prior to planned oocyte collection.

What to do if there is doubt about hCG administration?

If several preovulatory follicles have been drained and no oocyte has been recovered, it is recommended that follicular fluid be tested on an hCG dipstick to ensure the presence of hCG within the follicles[7], confirming that the appropriate dose of hCG has been administered. If the test is negative, re-administration of hCG and postponing the oocyte collection until 36 hours after the administration of hCG should be considered.

LUTEAL SUPPORT

It is generally accepted that in cycles where the GnRH agonist has been used there is a need for luteal support. Because of the increased risk of OHSS with booster doses of hCG, it is now routine practice to administer progesterone (P_4) supplementation during the luteal phase in the form of progestogen, either as progesterone pessaries,

vaginal cream progesterone 8%, 90 mg/1.125 g gel, prolonged release (Crinonone, Serono, Geneva), or by injection.

Side-effects of P_4 administration

Some women complain of both local and generalized side-effects from the use of vaginal progesterone, as characterized by premenstrual symptoms. Both vaginal preparations can cause local vaginal irritation.

MONITORING

Ultrasound

The main method of monitoring the ovarian response to COH is to follow the growth and development of ovarian follicles. Ultrasound gives a physical measurement of the number and size of follicles that are developing. It is therefore imperative to have a reliable transvaginal ultrasound monitoring service available, in order to make decisions about the timing of hCG administration and subsequent oocyte recovery. Any limitations of such a monitoring service will impact on the efficacy of the whole IVF treatment cycle.

Hormonal

With the reliance on ultrasound, the assessment of hormone levels has become less important, although some units still depend on estradiol (E_2) levels to help with decision making. With the use of GnRH agonists and antagonists, the measurement of LH is no longer relevant.

OOCYTE COLLECTION

Anesthesia/analgesia

The analgesia/anesthesia used varies from unit to unit. If general anesthesia is used there are risks of anesthetic complications, the most common being the risk of vomiting and inhaling. With intravenous sedation, the cough reflex is maintained and the risk of inhalation is far less likely. There have been no anesthetic complications at Monash IVF Clayton in 18 000 oocyte collections during the last 15 years.

Surgical trauma

When the technique of transvaginal oocyte collection under ultrasound control was first utilized, there was concern about possible complications of blind transvaginal puncture of the ovary. Fortunately time has shown that complications are very rare. With the hyperstimulated ovary resting next to the upper vagina, the aspiration needle can enter the ovary without damage to the bowel or other organs. Sometimes the ovary is behind the uterus, and oocyte collection is only possible by passing the needle through the myometrium. This does not seem to lead to complications in most instances.

The stimulated ovary lies adjacent to the iliac vessel, and on transverse ultrasonic view they may appear like follicles, but damage to the vessels is also rare. Initially, to reduce the risk of introducing the needle too deeply, an injection gun was developed. The operator measured the distance of the follicle from the end of the needle guide, and this distance was preset. The needle was spring loaded, and a trigger was released which then fired the needle into the follicle. As operators became more comfortable with ultrasound guided follicle puncture, freehand needling has become universally used.

Bruising/discomfort

It is fair to say that most women experience some degree of postoperative discomfort. This can be due to 'bruising' of the ovary due to the multiple punctures, to distension of the follicles with blood postoperatively, or the oozing of blood

from the drained follicles causing some degree of peritoneal irritation. The degree of discomfort is usually moderate, and whilst some women require some parenteral analgesia (usually a narcotic) immediately postoperatively, subsequently women can manage with oral analgesics. If severe pain persists, or especially if it develops some time after the oocyte collection, a complication should be suspected.

Bleeding

When oocyte collections were performed laparoscopically, it became apparent that the aspirated follicle filled with blood, and there was subsequent intraperitoneal bleeding. This bleeding was self-limiting, and the need for any surgical intervention was very rare. It was hoped that transvaginal oocyte collection was going to be just as safe, although the inability to inspect the pelvis postoperatively did cause some concern. With 20 years of experience behind us, we are now confident that postoperative bleeding is rare, and is usually self-limiting.

Bleeding can occur either from the ovary intraperitoneally, or from the vaginal skin, vaginally. It is our practice, that, if vaginal bleeding is excessive at the end of the procedure, an intravaginal pack is inserted to apply local pressure for about one hour. The pack is then removed and bleeding is almost always controlled. I personally have never used suturing of the vaginal vault to control bleeding, although this is occasionally performed at Monash IVF. With intraperitoneal bleeding a pelvic hematoma may result, which is then the basis for pelvic infection. This is discussed below under 'infection'.

Organ damage

With transvaginal scanning an excellent view of the ovaries is obtained, and with manipulation of the probe, the vaginal vault can be brought adjacent to the ovary. Bowel shadows can be identified and differentiated from the ovary. With some experience, freehand puncture can be safely carried out with little risk to other organs. There is some danger of perforating the ovary and damaging organs behind, and this was the reason for developing the 'aspiration gun'. However, it soon became apparent that freehand control was good, and rarely resulted in organ damage.

Infection

Because of the sensitivity of oocytes to antiseptics, the vagina is not sterilized prior to oocyte collection. Consequently, a sterile needle is inserted through the vagina, potentially pushing organisms from the vaginal flora intraperitoneally. Initially it was thought advisable to cleanse the vagina with saline or sterile water, but subsequent advice was that this just activated the vaginal organisms. Most clinicians use no preparation of the vagina, and fortunately we have learnt with time that the infection rate is low, although it does occur in 1 in 300 oocyte collections. Although usually not serious, and responsive to a course of antibiotics, the infection can sometimes be more severe and pelvic abscess may result, requiring drainage.

Ovarian torsion

This is a very rare complication of oocyte collection from a hyperstimulated ovary, where torsion resulting in gangrenous necrosis of the ovary may result. Suspicion of ovarian torsion should be aroused if the woman experiences a disproportionate amount of vomiting associated with localized pain. Clinical signs are that of an acute abdomen, and laparotomy is urgently required. If the blood supply appears intact after untwisting, conservative surgery can be undertaken, but if there is irreversible avascular necrosis, then oophorectomy needs to be carried out.

CONCLUSIONS

In a publication on in-vitro maturation (IVM) of oocytes, it is necessary to conclude with a comparison of what advantages this new technique has to offer over conventional COH. Of course in the absence of the use of significant doses of FSH, OHSS will not occur. Underdosing also is not relevant as it is the ovaries 'decision' how many primordial follicles it has available. As less medication has to be administered, the possibility of administering the wrong medication is decreased. Monitoring is less frequent than for stimulated cycles.

The clinical problems after oocyte collection are also somewhat different. The method of anesthesia is probably no different for IVM compared to COH, so the risks would be no different. Whilst the stimulated ovary after COH is bigger and maybe more vascular, the risk of the relative difficulty of aspirating small follicles probably balances the risk of trauma. Bruising and discomfort is less with IVM, as the ovaries are less vascular and do not fill up with blood, thus avoiding the discomfort caused by distended cysts. Bleeding is less common, as the unstimulated ovary is far less vascular. With respect to the risk of infection, there are no data yet available to compare postoocyte collection infection rates, but from first principles, as the blood filled ovarian follicles act as excellent culture media, their absence after IVM should result in a lower infection rate. As ovarian torsion is principally caused by distended blood cysts making the ovary uneven in consistency, this should not occur after unstimulated IVM.

In summary, as the lack of stimulation results in less disruption of the ovary, the consequences and complications of oocyte collection should be less severe and less common than after oocyte collection for IVF. We will have to wait until larger series of IVM are reported before we can confirm these advantages. The most significant advantage of IVM with respect to complications is the absence of OHSS, which is the most common significant, occasionally life threatening complication of COH.

REFERENCES

1. Steptoe PC, Edwards RG. Birth after reimplantation of a human embryo. Lancet 1978; 312: 366.

2. Trounson AO, Leeton JF, Wood EC et al. Pregnancies in humans by fertilization *in vitro* and embryo transfer in controlled ovulatory cycles. Science 1981; 212: 681–2.

3. Jones HW, Jones GS, Andrews MC et al. The program for *in vitro* fertilization at Norfolk. Fertil Steril 1982; 38: 14–21.

4. Porter RN, Smith W, Craft IL et al. Induction of ovulation for in-vitro fertilisation using buserelin and gonadotrophins. Lancet 1984; 324: 1284–5.

5. Olivennes F, Fanchin R, Bouchard P et al. Scheduled administration of a gonadotrophin-releasing hormone antagonist (Cetrorelix) on day 8 of in-vitro fertilization cycles: a pilot study. Hum Reprod 1995; 10: 1382–6.

6. Shapiro DB, Mitchell-Leef D. GnRH antagonist in *in vitro* fertilization: where we are now. Minerva Ginecol 2003; 55: 373–88.

7. Stankiewic M, Warnes G, Gilmore A et al. Unanticipated failure of oocyte recovery: a diagnostic and recovery algorhythm. Aust NZ J Obstet Gynecol 2005; 45(Suppl): A12.

CHAPTER 14

Management of ovarian hyperstimulation syndrome

Mark Sedler and Adam H Balen

INTRODUCTION

Consequences of stimulation of the ovaries include the serious and potentially life-threatening condition of ovarian hyperstimulation syndrome (OHSS). This can occur with any type of ovulation induction or superovulation therapy for assisted conception procedures. The development of OHSS can be reduced by the cautious use of preparations, careful monitoring of stimulation cycles, and prediction of 'at risk' patients. This overview will describe the syndrome and its pathophysiology in order to understand appropriate preventative strategies and management options.

The pathophysiologic hallmark of OHSS is a sudden increase in vascular permeability which results in the development of a massive extravascular exudate. This exudate accumulates primarily in the peritoneal cavity, causing protein-rich ascites. Loss of fluid into the third space causes a profound fall in intravascular volume, hemoconcentration, and suppression of urine formation. Loss of protein into the third space causes a fall in plasma oncotic pressure, which results in further loss of intravascular fluid. Secondary hyperaldosteronism occurs and causes salt retention. Eventually peripheral edema develops.

OHSS occurs after overstimulated ovaries have been exposed to hCG. The condition therefore results most commonly when sensitive (usually polycystic) ovaries are exposed to excessive quantities of FSH and then to hCG. That severe OHSS is often associated with pregnancy is probably related to the persistence of hCG in this situation. Even when the ovaries have been severely overstimulated, OHSS can be prevented by avoiding exposure of the ovaries to LH and/or hCG.

PREVALENCE

Most methods of ovarian stimulation can cause OHSS and it can even result from the use of oral anti-estrogens. In programs of ovulation induction the risk is related to the dose of gonadotropins and is rarer with low dose protocols. The overall risk is estimated to be about 4% and that of the severe form about 0.25%. In in-vitro fertilization (IVF) the prevalence varies in published series from 1 to 10%, being highest in those combining gonadotropin stimulation with treatment with a GnRH analog. Severe cases occur in 0.25–2% of IVF cycles[1].

There are no good data on the overall incidence of severe OHSS, as the severity of OHSS is often not standardized, although severe cases are those most likely to be reported. There have been case reports of thromboembolism and other severe sequelae of ovarian hyperstimulation, but good data are not kept centrally. The latest European database of all reported IVF cycles performed in 2000 presents the incidence of OHSS from registers of 17 of the 22 countries that submitted data[2]. There were 1586 cases of OHSS out of 146 342 cycles, equivalent to 1.1% of all stimulated cycles[2]. There were 376 cases reported from the UK to this database out of a total of 28 474 stimulated cycles, equivalent to 1.3%[2]. The North American databases do not report rates of OHSS[3].

A WHO report in 2002 estimated the overall incidence of severe OHSS as 0.2–1% of all assisted reproduction cycles[4] and the mortality has been estimated at 1:450 000–1:500 000 women undergoing superovulation[5]. There were no deaths in the European registry of 146 342 cycles in 2000[2]. A detailed assessment of mortality in a cohort of 29 700 Australian patients who had in the past undergone IVF failed to identify OHSS as a contributing cause to any of the 72 deaths from any cause[2]. Thus the mortality rate from OHSS would appear to be extremely low and difficult to quantify. It goes without saying that there is no acceptable rate of mortality as a result of fertility treatment. Furthermore there is no doubt that OHSS is a condition that should be taken extremely seriously because of the physical and emotional distress that it can cause and the thromboembolic risks.

CLASSIFICATION OF OHSS

Currently there is no unanimity in the classification of OHSS. The syndrome is graded according to its severity, with the 1989 classification by Golan et al.[6] having several clinical and practical advantages. Mild ovarian hyperstimu-

lation is divided into grades 1 and 2, moderate into grade 3, and grades 4 and 5 hyperstimulation equate to severe OHSS. Grade 1 is defined as abdominal distension and discomfort, progressing to grade 2 if additional clinical features of nausea, vomiting, ± diarrhea occur with additional ultrasonographic features of ovarian enlargement at 5–12 cm in diameter. Grade 3 includes the features of mild OHSS with the additional evidence of ascites by ultrasound scan. Grade 4 includes the features of moderate OHSS, with the addition of clinical evidence of ascites and/or hydrothorax and breathing difficulties. Grade 5 includes all the above features and a change in the blood volume with increased blood viscosity, hemoconcentration, coagulation abnormalities, and diminished renal perfusion and function.

The severest form of OHSS is a critical and life-threatening stage of the illness, with clinical evidence of intravascular volume depletion and hemoconcentration (reduced CVP, reduced cardiac output, hematocrit level >55%), severe expansion of the third space (tense ascites, pleural and pericardial effusions), and the development of hepatorenal failure (serum creatinine >1.6 g/dl, creatinine clearance <50 ml/min).

Additional risks include thromboembolic phenomenon, cerebrovascular and subclavian vein thrombosis, renal failure, adult respiratory distress syndrome, and cardiac tamponade secondary to pericardial effusion. Deaths have been recorded in women with the most severe form of OHSS. The advantages of Golan's classification are not needing to include cases of biochemical hyperstimulation (almost always present in assisted conception), abdominal distension/discomfort are the minimal presenting symptoms, and the incorporation of ultrasonographic findings (as OHSS is more frequently diagnosed by USS).

A more recent classification[7] subdivides the severe form of OHSS into three grades (Table 14.1). Here, the mild form of the disease is omitted from classification, as this can occur

Table 14.1 Clinical grading of ovarian hyperstimulation syndrome

---

Mild
Weight gain, thirst, abdominal discomfort
Mild distension
Ovaries >5 cm diameter

Moderate
Nausea and vomiting, distension, and pain
Dyspnea
Abdomen distended but not tense
Ascites detected by ultrasound

Severe
Evidence of intravascular fluid loss
Third space fluid accumulation (tense ascites, hydrothorax)
Hemoconcentration, hypovolemia, oliguria, hepatorenal failure

---

in most patients with ovarian stimulation and, moreover, the condition has no complications and does not require special treatment. The moderate condition includes symptoms of abdominal pain, distension and discomfort, nausea, and ultrasonic evidence of enlarged ovaries and ascites, but with normal hematologic and biochemical profiles. The severe form is subdivided into A, B, and C. Grade A includes symptoms of nausea, vomiting, diarrhea, oliguria, abdominal pain, and dyspnea, with clinical evidence of marked distension of the abdomen, ascites, and/or hydrothorax. Ultrasound scan shows evidence of large ovaries and marked ascites, but again the biochemical profile is normal. Grade B includes features of grade A with the addition of massive tension ascites, markedly enlarged ovaries, marked oliguria, and severe dyspnea, with the addition of a raised hematocrit, elevated serum creatinine, and abnormal liver function. Grade C includes further complications such as respiratory distress syndrome, renal shutdown, or venous thromboembolism.

CLINICAL PRESENTATION

The mild form includes weight gain, thirst, abdominal discomfort with bloating, and mild nausea. There are no clinical signs of dehydration or significant abdominal findings apart from some distension. Moderate OHSS is associated with more pronounced symptoms of nausea, vomiting, abdominal distension with pain, and dyspnea. The abdomen is distended but not tense and the ovaries may be palpable per abdomen with associated tenderness. Ascites may not be clinically demonstrable. No clinical evidence of fluid or electrolyte depletion is demonstrated.

Severe cases present with pronounced features of the moderate disease with clinical evidence of intravascular fluid loss (tachycardia, hypotension) and third-space fluid accumulation such as ascites and hydrothorax. Hypovolemia, hemoconcentration, oliguria, and electrolyte imbalance occur. The ovaries are usually grossly enlarged and can reach the level of the umbilicus. They are tender to palpation. In extreme cases acute respiratory distress from gross ascites and pleural effusion can occur. Other complications include pericardial effusion, hepato-renal failure, and thromboembolic phenomena[7].

A distinction has been made between early and late OHSS[8], with those presenting early (that is 3–7 days after hCG administration) having significantly higher serum estradiol concentrations than those presenting late (12–17 days after hCG), whilst there is no difference in the number of oocytes collected. Those presenting late are more likely to be pregnant and have a severe form of the syndrome, due to persistent hCG stimulation of the ovaries.

PATHOPHYSIOLOGY OF OHSS

The exact pathogenesis is unknown. The main pathophysiologic features are increased capillary permeability, new capillary formation (angiogenesis), and the existence of a vasoactive ovarian biochemical factor. All these factors are most prominent in the ovarian vasculature. While it has been known for many years that high circulating concentrations of estradiol are an immediate predictor of the syndrome, estrogen itself is not the cause of the sudden increase in vascular permeability. Such a change is not after all a feature of treatment with estrogen itself, even when the levels rise very abruptly, such as after an implant. While numerous compounds, such as prostaglandins, kallikreins, histamine, serotonin, and prolactin, etc., have been considered to mediate the process, the two prime movers in the development of OHSS are activation of the ovarian prorenin–renin–angiotensin system[9] and release of vascular endothelial growth factor (VEGF) from the ovary.

The follicle contains renin in an inactive form which is activated at mid cycle by LH (and by exposure of the ovary to hCG) and which then causes conversion of angiotensinogen to inactive angiotensin I and subsequent conversion to the active angiotensin II. This ovarian prorenin–renin–angiotensin system is thought to be involved in the neovascularization, which is so central a feature of the conversion of the avascular preovulatory follicle into the richly vascularized corpus luteum. Some years ago we reported excessive levels of renin activity in the plasma of a woman with severe, grade 3 OHSS at a stage of her illness when, as a consequence of treatment, the central venous pressure was several centimeters higher than normal (i.e. when secretion of renal renin would have been suppressed). Subsequent studies have shown that ascitic fluid in this syndrome contains very large amounts of angiotensin II compared with ascitic fluid obtained from women with liver failure. In rabbits angiotensin II increases peritoneal permeability and neovascularization. Moreover, in that species, treatment with an angiotensin-converting enzyme (ACE) inhibitor blocks the increase in peritoneal permeability that occurs in response to superovulation. Parallel studies have not, however, been performed in humans

because of concerns over the use of ACE inhibitors in pregnancy. There is no doubt of the involvement of the renin–angiotensin system in the pathogenesis of OHSS, with severity of OHSS and hematocrit being directly related to plasma renin activity (PRA) and also aldosterone concentration (the increased aldosterone production in OHSS is associated with increased PRA)[10].

VASCULAR ENDOTHELIAL GROWTH FACTOR

Vascular endothelial growth factor, also known as vascular permeability factor or vasculotropin, is a dimeric glycoprotein, which promotes growth and cell division of vascular endothelial cells. It increases capillary permeability. VEGF is expressed in steroidogenic and steroid-responsive cells, such as those involved in repair of endometrial vessels and in implantation[11]. In primates, production of VEGF increases after the LH surge and is reduced by suppression of LH secretion during the luteal phase. VEGF production by human luteinized granulosa cells is increased by incubation in vitro with hCG, as detected by measuring messenger RNA (indicating synthesis by the luteal cells), and VEGF itself, as detected by an immunofluorescent assay. Using a bioassay, which measured extravasation into the skin of an injected dye, McClure and colleagues[12] found increased amounts of VEGF in ascitic fluid obtained from patients with OHSS but not in ascitic fluid obtained from patients with liver failure. Most of the activity could be neutralized by incubation with an antiserum to recombinant human VEGF, indicating that VEGF is the major capillary permeability agent in OHSS. One might speculate that the activity that was not neutralized by the antiserum to VEGF was attributable to angiotensin II. Further studies have correlated follicular fluid concentrations of VEGF with OHSS and also with ovarian blood flow, as assessed by Doppler ultrasound flow studies[13]. Indeed serum VEGF concentrations have been proposed as a predictor for the development of the syndrome[14]. In hyperstimulated rats, vascular endothelial growth factor receptor-2 activation induces vascular permeability; this effect can be prevented by receptor blockade. A specific VEGF receptor-2 inhibitor, SU5416, has been shown to reverse increased vascular permeability[15].

The angiogenic response to LH or hCG is normally confined to a single dominant follicle. OHSS may be seen as an exaggeration of this response. Because of gonadotropin-stimulated overgrowth of follicles, VEGF, the major angiogenic mediator of vascularization of the corpus luteum, can no longer be confined to the ovary but spills over, first into the peritoneal cavity and then into the general circulation. Interestingly, a case report of OHSS in a spontaneous pregnancy, with fetal and placental triploidy (partial hydatidiform mole), has been reported[16], suggestive of the theory that VEGF is a causative factor of OHSS, but has no impact on the course of the disease.

Two other important factors for the genesis of OHSS are the use of luteal phase hCG support, potentially augmenting the already prevailing condition, and the risk associated with conception cycles. It has been found that OHSS is four times as frequent in conception cycles than in non-pregnant cycles. An increased incidence is also seen in multiple pregnancies, possibly the higher the multiple order, the increased risk and severity of the disease. This is certainly due to the continuing stimulation of the ovaries by the increasing levels of hCG produced by the conception cycle, causing longer duration and a more severe expression of the disease. Simply put, the addition of hCG to the situation is like adding 'fuel to the fire'.

RISK FACTORS FOR THE DEVELOPMENT OF OHSS (TABLE 14.2)

Two important risk factors can be identified before treatment starts, namely the presence of polycystic ovaries and young age.

Table 14.2 Prevention of ovarian hyperstimulation syndrome

- Pretreatment ultrasound assessment of ovaries: PCO?
- Care with gonadotropin administration: use low doses in women with PCO
- Care with GnRH analogs:
  emphasize use of ultrasound rather than estradiol concentrations
  note whether an LH-depleted gonadotropin preparation is being used
- Reduce use and dose of hCG:
  consider withholding ovulatory dose of hCG
  substitute progesterone for hCG in luteal phase
- Meticulous aspiration of all follicles
- Consider cryopreservation with deferred embryo transfer

Polycystic ovaries

Several studies have confirmed that patients most at risk are women with the characteristic appearance on ultrasound of polycystic ovaries. The essential point is the presence of polycystic ovaries, as detected by ultrasound, not the polycystic ovary syndrome. The polycystic ovary appearance (presence of >12 follicles of <9 mm diameter)[17] occurs in approximately 33% of normal women[18], but in 40% of patients undergoing IVF, irrespective of the indication for treatment[19]. The polycystic ovary is highly sensitive to gonadotropic stimulation.

Young age

Most cases of OHSS occur in younger women, usually less than 30 years, consistent with the greater ovarian responsiveness in this group compared with older women.

Factors as ovarian stimulation proceeds

Use of GnRH agonists

GnRH agonists protect the ovary from an endogenous LH surge, so facilitating more convenient scheduling of ovum pick-up. The protection so afforded renders the ovary more amenable to stimulation of multi-follicular development by high-dose gonadotropin treatment. Not surprisingly, this very advantage makes OHSS more common in treatment programs utilizing pituitary desensitization.

Development of multiple immature and intermediate sized follicles during treatment

The development of large numbers of immature and intermediate follicles during treatment indicates an exuberant response to gonadotropic stimulation, caused either by very sensitive, i.e. polycystic ovaries (the usual situation), or too high a dose of gonadotropin in women with normal ovaries. A large number of medium sized follicles (<14 mm in diameter) is an important risk factor, rather than a large number of mature follicles.

Exposure to LH/hCG and dose involved

The clinical observation that exposure of the ovaries to LH, and usually to hCG, is a sine qua non of its development and that pregnancy is frequently associated with the OHSS is consistent with the role of LH and hCG in stimulating the processes that mediate neovascularization and vascular permeability. An endogenous LH surge rarely provokes the development of OHSS unless pregnancy ensues. This may be due to the fact that the half-life of hCG preparations is longer than of natural hCG and possibly that the large doses of hCG given lead to a greater activity than

natural LH produces. It is possible that the higher the doses of exogenous LH/hCG used, the worse the potential for OHSS. These observations add plausibility to the clinical practice of attempting aspiration of all follicles in patients considered at risk because it is luteinized granulosa cells that are the source of the permeability factors.

PREDICTION AND PREVENTION OF OHSS

OHSS is an iatrogenic condition. The most effective management of OHSS is the accurate prediction and prevention of the disease. Ultrasound scanning and endocrine monitoring of follicular development are the main ways of prediction of the development of OHSS during ovarian stimulation. All patients undergoing ovarian stimulation, whether to correct anovulation or for assisted fertility techniques, should have a pretreatment ultrasound scan and if polycystic ovaries are detected, the dose of gonadotropin should be lowered, titrated gradually and slowly, and ultrasonographic follicular assessment and serum estradiol levels measured on day 5 of stimulation of IVF cycles, so that the dose can be adjusted accordingly, if needs be, for prevention of overstimulation. If pituitary desensitization has been used one should be sensitive to the loss of the normal 'protection' of the ovary caused by the block to estrogen-mediated positive feedback of LH release. If a long protocol of GnRH analog treatment is followed by treatment with one of the pure FSH preparations, one must also be aware that the lack of LH changes the usual relationship of follicle maturation and number to circulating estradiol levels. In this situation measurement of serum estradiol concentrations underestimates follicle development. It is therefore essential that endocrine monitoring is supported by high-quality ultrasound, otherwise low circulating estradiol concentrations may encourage further and inappropriate gonadotropic stimulation despite adequate follicular development. Meta-analyses of the different gonadotropin preparations have indicated no significant difference in risk of developing OHSS[20–24].

STRATEGIES FOR PREVENTING/ REDUCING OHSS RISK

For the patient with overstimulated ovaries who is approaching the time of hCG administration, several strategies to make treatment safer may be considered. The first is to administer a low dose of hCG to initiate oocyte maturation and/or ovulation (i.e. not more than a single injection of 5000 IU) and, in patients receiving GnRH analog treatment and who therefore require luteal support, to give progesterone (400 mg per vaginum for 14 days or gestone injections im) rather than hCG. It is current practice now to use progesterone routinely for luteal support. Recombinant LH has a shorter half-life than hCG and so may reduce the risk of short-term OHSS, although it will not influence OHSS resulting from hCG produced from the trophoblast of a developing pregnancy. In protocols where GnRH antagonists are used, the preovulatory trigger can be with a single dose of a GnRH agonist, instead of hCG – again a shorter-acting preparation, which should reduce the short-term risk of OHSS.

Consider the treatment of anovulatory infertility and the prevention of OHSS. Here the issue is the development of multiple *small* follicles. Thus, if there are more than six follicles with a diameter of 12 mm or more we advise discontinuing treatment or converting it to IVF. In the latter situation, having meticulously aspirated as many follicles as possible, one may cryopreserve the embryos and defer their transfer to another cycle. Alternatively, one may withhold hCG, continue treatment with the GnRH analog, and restart gonadotropin stimulation at a lower dose.

Follicular aspiration

Multiple follicular aspiration in IVF cycles (emptying most of the follicles of their follicular fluid and granulosa cells) has been suggested as a way of protecting against the development of OHSS[25]. Some studies show a confirmed benefit of using this technique, and others have shown no protective effect against OHSS development. However, a 20% incidence of severe OHSS occurred with repeated aspirations, against 70% in matched historic trials. It is also possible to aspirate most of the ovarian follicles 35 hours after the administration of hCG. The remaining intact follicles can still result in a singleton or twin pregnancy, whilst minimizing the risk of OHSS developing. Follicular aspiration induces intrafollicular hemorrhage, which has a negative impact on corpus luteum function[26]. Withdrawal of the follicular contents may significantly interfere with follicular maturation, potentially modifying the intraovarian mechanism responsible for the development of OHSS.

Early unilateral ovarian follicular aspiration (EUFA) has been performed in a prospective randomized study, versus no intervention[27]. Here, unilateral ovarian aspiration occurred 6–8 h prior to hCG administration. Fewer oocytes were recovered in the EUFA group, as expected, however fertilization, embryonic cleavage, and pregnancy rates were similar between the two groups. Although the development of OHSS was recorded in 25% of the EUFA group and 33.3% of the control group, severe OHSS developed in 12.5% and 6.6% of patients, respectively. The authors of this study concluded that early unilateral follicular aspiration, prior to hCG administration, failed to prevent or diminish the occurrence of severe OHSS.

Two years later, the same group performed a prospective, randomized study comparing EUFA 10–12 h after hCG administration versus coasting, for high-risk patients. Oocyte retrieval was then carried out in the contralateral ovary, 35–36 h after hCG administration. Interestingly, fewer oocytes were retrieved in the coasted group, but fertilization, embryonic cleavage, and pregnancy rates were similar in both groups. Severe OHSS occurred in 26.6% of the EUFA group, against 20% in the 'coasted' group. In conclusion, it was suspected that intraovarian bleeding induced by the aspiration of granulosa cells from one ovary may limit the production of ovarian mediators implicated in the pathogenesis of OHSS, thus reducing the risk of developing the severe condition. However the data on this are somewhat contradictory, and the number of cases insufficient to establish the efficacy of this method[28].

The coasting approach

Coasting, or delaying hCG, uses a controlled 'drift' period as an alternative to cancellation of the cycle, yielding favorable pregnancy rates (25% per cycle) with low severe OHSS complications (2.5%). In one study by Sher et al.[29], gonadotropins were withheld in 17 patients whose serum estradiol levels were >6000 pg/ml and daily administration of the GnRH analog was continued until estradiol levels had fallen to <3000 pg/ml. At this point, 10 000 IU hCG were administered to trigger ovulation. During the first 48 h of initial coasting, the estradiol levels continued to rise, but the follicular diameter reduced by approximately 2.3 mm/day. The estradiol levels plateaued and fell after 96 h. No follicular increase in diameter was seen after 72 h of coasting. The coasting period lasted 4–9 days; hCG administration was reduced on days 12–16. Interestingly, 35% of the cycles led to viable pregnancies and all 17 patients developed signs of grade 2–3 OHSS, however none led to severe OHSS. An update review abstract from the Cochrane Library[30], however, identified 13 studies (of which only one met the strict inclusion criteria), showing no difference in the incidence of moderate or severe OHSS, or pregnancy rates, between the groups.

Abandoning the treatment cycle

In patients having IVF and using gonadotropin containing LH activity (i.e. HMG preparations), the following are conservative criteria for ovarian responses, above which there is a significant risk of OHSS: a serum estradiol of greater than 10 000 pmol/l (3000 pg/ml) together with 20 or more follicles of 12 mm diameter or more. In the interpretation of estradiol concentrations one needs to recognize the aforementioned effects of using LH-depleted gonadotropin preparations in women receiving GnRH analogs in a 'long' protocol (less estrogen than usual is made so estradiol concentrations underestimate the intensity of the ovarian response). For patients with a serum estradiol greater than 17 000 pmol/l (5500 pg/ml) with more than 40 follicles, hCG should be withheld and treatment abandoned. Treatment with the GnRH analog is, however, continued and when the ovaries regain their normal size, ovarian stimulation is resumed at a lower dose.

Cryopreservation of all developed embryos

When serum estradiol concentrations are 10 000–17 000 pmol/l with 20–40 follicles hCG may be given, but the embryos are cryopreserved and transferred at a later date. The obvious advantages of this strategy are reduction in the incidence and severity of OHSS, in addition to preserving the potential benefits of the original cycle. Continuing a GnRH analog during the luteal phase can help to keep the ovaries quiescent. However, this may not eliminate the risk completely.

Prevention of OHSS using intravenous albumin

It has been suggested that administration of intravenous albumin to patients at high risk of developing OHSS may prevent the onset of the condition[31]. Albumin potentially increases serum oncotic pressure, reverses leakage of fluids from the intravascular spaces, and prevents to some degree the shift of fluid into the third space. However, the role of albumin in OHSS prevention is multi-factorial. First, it sequesters the vasoactive substance released from the corpora lutea. Interestingly, OHSS symptoms usually develop 3–10 days after hCG administration, regardless of embryo transfer. As albumin has a half-life of 10–15 days, its timely infusion during oocyte retrieval and immediately afterwards may serve to bind and inactivate this factor. Second, it sequesters any additional substance, which may have been synthesized as a result of OHSS. Third, its oncotic properties serve to maintain the intravascular volume and prevent the ensuing effects of hypovolemia, ascites, and hemoconcentration.

A prospective, randomized, placebo-controlled trial of albumin versus normal saline administration, in patients at high risk of developing OHSS, has been described. Four out of 15 cases in the control group developed OHSS, whereas there were no cases in the 16 patients treated with albumin (p <0.05)[32]. In contrast, however, Ng et al. reported that 2 cases out of 49, treated with albumin, developed severe OHSS. This was similar to a prior incidence of a 6% OHSS rate in 158 historic, matched controls, who received an equal volume of lactated ringers solution[33].

Despite the literature, the efficacy of albumin in preventing OHSS still requires further validation. It is unclear whether albumin administration, at the time of oocyte retrieval, would be effective in preventing the manifestations of late OHSS, which tend to be more severe than the early form of the disease, and also more likely to be associated with pregnancy. Also the dosage and optimal timing of administration of the albumin need to be established.

The use of gonadotropin releasing hormone antagonists

It has been suggested that the use of GnRH antagonist cycles might reduce the risk of OHSS[34] combined also with administration of a GnRH agonist to trigger oocyte maturation[35], although there are as yet insufficient data. In one trial involving 701 patients, the use of the GnRH antagonist Ganirelix versus GnRH agonists (e.g. Buserelin) resulted in fewer cases of OHSS (3.5% vs. 5.9%), however the ongoing pregnancy rate was 20.3%, compared to 25.7% in the GnRH agonist group[36].

Glucocorticoids

Studies comparing the effectiveness of glucocorticoid administration versus no steroid administration in preventing OHSS concluded that there was a similar incidence of the disease in both groups, irrespective of whether all degrees or only moderate and severe OHSS were considered[37].

In-vitro maturation

In-vitro maturation (IVM) of human oocytes is a scientific and clinical challenge, which has potential benefits for certain patient groups undergoing assisted reproductive treatments. These include patients who have a tendency to undergo a vigorous ovarian response to ovarian stimulation and are at risk of OHSS. Patients who have polycystic ovaries with a previous history of excessive ovarian stimulatory response, or who developed severe OHSS, or needed cycles canceling due to the risk of continuing the stimulatory regimen, could benefit from IVM technology in the future. IVM technology could well reduce the risk of OHSS.

Metformin

The association between insulin resistance and PCOS has resulted in the use of metformin to enhance insulin sensitivity and improve ovarian function. Furthermore, metformin has been shown to improve the response of polycystic ovaries to stimulation, with the suggestion of a more co-ordinated follicular response together with a reduced likelihood of hyperstimulation[38]. Indeed in patients with polycystic ovaries we have found in a prospective randomized trial, in which all patients were given a low dose of stimulation (100 IU FSH) that the use of metformin reduced the incidence of severe OHSS from 20.4% to 3.8% ($p < 0.023$)[39].

COMPLICATIONS OF OHSS

Thromboembolism

The most serious complication of OHSS is cerebrovascular accident. Hemoconcentration, high levels of factor V, platelets, fibrinogen, profibrinogen, fibrinolytic inhibitors, and thromboplastins are all found in patients with OHSS. The cytokine interleukin-6 was also found to be elevated in patients with OHSS[40], as compared to controls. Whether this is directly responsible for or contributes to the clinical manifestations of OHSS is unclear. However, unquestionably, all the above factors will contribute to the vascular complications described.

When considering the pathophysiology of the OHSS it is easy to appreciate the potential risk of deep venous thrombosis (DVT) and thromboembolic events. Indeed there has been an expanding literature on this association in recent years. Not only is there a hypercoagulable state but also the combination of enlarged ovaries and ascites leads to reduced venous return (increased venous pressure) from the lower limbs, which, combined with immobility, places the patient at risk of DVT. Furthermore, the thrombotic event need not only be in the lower limbs. A review of the world literature found that 75% of cases reported were in venous sites, with 60% in the upper limb, head, and neck veins (including internal jugular and subclavian veins), with an associated risk of pulmonary embolism of 4–12%, whilst the remaining 25% were arterial thromboses and were mostly intracerebral[41]. It is difficult to give an explanation for these more unusual

sites of thrombosis in young women, unless there is relative overreporting because of their rarity. The hypercoagulable state of OHSS may, in addition to the general vascular changes described in the previous section, relate to a change in clotting factors, which may be due to the recognized hematologic changes of pregnancy:

- Increased concentrations of factors VII, VIII, IX, X, XII, and fibrinogen;

- Reduced concentrations of protein S, antithrombin III, and fibrinolysis.

Whether this thrombophilic state is secondary to high circulating estrogen concentrations is less clear, as the thrombophilic state of pregnancy tends to occur closer to term and postpartum. It is possible that women who develop OHSS have a tendency to thrombophilias (e.g. deficiency of protein C, S, or antithrombin III or factor V Leiden expression), although the majority of women appear to screen negative after the event. An alternative theory is a leakage of factors such as antithrombin III into the ascitic fluid, thus resulting in a relative plasma deficiency[42]. Venous thrombosis in the lower limb most often resolves without long-term sequelae, unless pulmonary embolism occurs, which may be fatal. Upper limb venous thrombosis may lead to disabling long-term disability, with persistent discomfort, cramp, weakness, and cold hands. Cerebral thrombosis may resolve completely but it can also lead to various forms of long-term disability.

Liver dysfunction

Markedly abnormal liver function tests and significant morphologic abnormality at the ultrastructural level can occur. These changes may be due to the increased estrogen levels (also seen after combined oral contraceptive and anabolic steroid use) and may be compensatory in response to increased demand on the liver enzymes, rather than a true pathologic alteration.

Respiratory complications

Respiratory distress, including adult respiratory distress syndrome, secondary to ascitic fluid accumulation and pleural effusion, has been described. Aspiration of ascitic and pleural fluid usually relieves symptoms – as well as the other management strategies for treating OHSS (see later). An actual case of acute hydrothorax, presenting as the only manifestation of the OHSS, after IVF treatment, has been reported[43].

Renal complications

Prerenal failure (a complication of the hypovolemia secondary to fluid transudation into the third space compartments) and hydro-ureter are associated with OHSS. Pressure on the kidneys by tense ascites may also impair renal output, which can then improve dramatically after paracentesis.

Adnexal torsion

Torsion occurs, mainly due to enlargement with multiple follicular or luteal cysts, which can worsen in pregnancy due to increasing ovarian size. Cohen et al.[44], in one study, reported a 16% torsion rate in pregnant patients, compared with 2.3% in non-pregnant women. Patients with severe OHSS complicated by adnexal torsion have successfully undergone laparoscopic untwisting of ischemic and hemorrhagic adnexum.

MANAGEMENT OF OHSS

In general, all patients receiving gonadotropin therapy should be warned about the risks of OHSS and its symptoms. Information booklets and advice sheets with details about OHSS should be given to these patients. This should include the telephone number and contact name of the liaison person in the treating clinic. If OHSS is suspected, a full clinical examination and assessment of the patient is required. An assessment of the general condition, including vital signs, daily abdominal girth and weight, strict fluid balance, especially urinary output, is undertaken. The degree of hypovolemia and any secondary complications are determined.

Investigations include full blood count, serum urea and electrolytes, liver function, serum proteins, renal function tests, full coagulation profile, weight of the patient, and ultrasonography (transabdominally will give more accurate dimensions of the ovarian enlargement, but estimation of pelvic/pouch of Douglas fluid accumulation will be difficult) of the pelvis and abdomen/liver. If respiratory and/or renal compromise is suspected, then regular blood gases and acid–base balance are also needed. The frequency of these investigations depends on the patient's clinical condition. In patients with OHSS, a raised white cell count, hemoconcentration, hyponatremia, and hypoalbuminemia can occur.

As mentioned above, ultrasonography can visualize the extent of ovarian enlargement, the size and number of corpora lutea cysts, and the degree of pelvic (transvaginal scanning) and/or abdominal fluid accumulation (transabdominal scan). Pleural and pericardial effusions can be visualized by chest X-ray assessment. Invasive hemodynamic monitoring, for example CVP and PAP lines, may be needed under certain circumstances, in which volume expanders are employed in the management of the condition.

Mild OHSS

Mild ovarian hyperstimulation is very common and is managed expectantly, its importance being that it should alert both patient and doctor to the risk of a more severe condition developing. As mentioned above, the patient should be encouraged to weigh herself daily and have a high fluid and protein intake. Full observations with outpatient follow-up and reassurance are all that is needed. Most cases of the mild condition resolve within 1 to 3 weeks. Women suspected to be at risk of developing moderate/severe OHSS need an appointment for review prior to potential embryo transfer (to decide if clinically well enough for transfer of embryos and potential conception) and/or 4–6 days after oocyte retrieval.

Moderate OHSS

A marked increase in weight (more than 5 kg) with the development of abdominal distension, nausea, and vomiting indicates the onset of moderate hyperstimulation and the need for hospitalization. Patients are often admitted to their nearest hospital and not the specialist unit providing ovarian stimulation, so good liaison is essential. We recommend patients be issued with an advice sheet concerning the symptoms of OHSS and what to do if they suspect it may be happening to them. In non-conception cycles, moderate ovarian hyperstimulation can be expected to resolve with the development of menstruation, although the ovarian cysts may persist for a month or more.

Patients with moderate hyperstimulation need reassurance and explanation, together with hospitalization. Oral fluids are encouraged, although vomiting may make an intravenous infusion necessary. Analgesics may be required for abdominal pain/discomfort. Preferred drugs are paracetamol, with or without codeine and pethidine for very severe pain. Non-steroidal anti-inflammatory drugs such as diclofenac should be avoided, although indometacin has been used experimentally with good results. Anti-emetics such as metoclopramide or stemetil are given as needed. Table 14.3 indicates the surveillance that should be undertaken.

If luteal support is required progesterone should be used. Full-length thromboembolic prevention stockings and heparin 5000 IU twice daily are advised to reduce the risk of DVT. The possibility of pregnancy must always be thought

Table 14.3 Surveillance of moderate and severe ovarian hyperstimulation

Circulation
- Intravascular contraction:
  monitor CVP (consider administration of colloids)
  look for pleural and pericardial effusion
- Hemoconcentration:
  measure hematocrit, white blood cell count, coagulation profile

Hepatic function
Measure ascites (girth, ultrasound) and consider paracentesis
Monitor liver function tests, in particular serum albumin

Renal function
Monitor urine output (consider administration of crystalloids)
Paracentesis, dialysis

of, unless gametes/embryos have not been transferred. Most patients have relief of symptoms by the end of the first week after oocyte retrieval/artificial insemination. The presence of symptoms beyond this period may well reflect the increased corpora lutea activity, secondary to their stimulation by trophoblastic derived hCG, if pregnancy ensues.

Severe OHSS

The development of clinically detectable and usually painful ascites together with a deterioration in respiratory, circulatory, and renal function indicates the development of severe hyperstimulation and, in most cases, the need for admission to an intensive care unit. The intravascular volume should be monitored by measurements of central venous pressure, renal function by meticulous attention to input and urine output, and hemoconcentration by measurement of hematocrit (or packed cell volume – PCV), whose level reflects intravascular volume depletion and blood viscosity. A hematocrit of over 45% is a serious warning sign and a measurement greater than 55% signals a life-threatening situation. There may be a striking leukocytosis, the white cell count rising up to 40 000/ml. Measurement of body weight, serum urea, creatinine, and electrolytes, together with serum albumin and liver function tests and periodic assessments of the coagulation profile, are mandatory. A chest X-ray is needed if pleural or pericardial effusions are suspected.

The main treatment policy is the correction of circulating volume and electrolyte imbalance. Infusion of colloid is required to maintain intravascular volume, correct hypovolemia, as indicated by restoration of normal central venous pressure, and to obtain adequate renal function. The choice lies between human albumin (50–100 ml of 20% solution, repeated as required) or intravenous dextran or hydroxyethyl starch, although the latter compounds carry the risk of anaphylactic reaction and dextran has been implicated in severe adult respiratory distress syndrome (ARDS). Crystalloid (usually normal saline) is administered for rehydration.

A CVP line is recommended for gauging fluid balance and IV requirements and daily measurements of abdominal girth and body weight are needed. If urine flow remains suppressed despite restoration of central venous pressure and rehydration, abdominal paracentesis, under direct vision, using ultrasound guidance, should be undertaken. Other indications for this procedure are the need for symptomatic relief from abdominal distension and discomfort, breathing difficulties from a tense ascites, oliguria, rising serum creatinine, falling creatinine clearance, and hemoconcentration unresponsive to medical therapy. Drainage of ascitic fluid can be performed transabdominally or, better still, transvaginally. This must always be performed under direct vision using ultrasound scanning to avoid damage to the enlarged ovaries and bowel[45]. Severe oliguria or renal failure persisting despite these measures usually necessitates dialysis.

A pleural tap of a hydrothorax should be considered for relief of dyspnea or acute respiratory distress[46]. Cardiac tamponade from pericardial effusion is rare but may prove fatal if not rapidly relieved. Careful cardiologic assessment together with cardiac ultrasound should therefore feature in the management of these patients. Urgent drainage of the pericardial fluid by suitable specialists is needed in this situation. One must be aware of the possibility of re-accumulation of fluid in any of these cavities. Anticoagulation is used prophylactically (heparin 5000 IU, twice daily) against the coagulopathy/thromboembolic phenomenon, due to hemoconcentration, and is also indicated for treatment if there is clinical evidence of thromboembolism or a deteriorating coagulation profile (increasing hypercoagulability).

OTHER MEDICAL TREATMENTS FOR OHSS

Prostaglandin synthetase inhibitors

There is no evidence that drugs such as indometacin are protective against OHSS. In fact, they may reduce the renal prostaglandin that maintains renal function, thus reducing the renal perfusion, in an already compromised patient.

Danazol

Rabbit studies have shown no protective effect for this drug against OHSS development.

Antihistamines

These may stabilize membrane permeability, thus reducing the ascites/pleural effusions caused by OHSS. However, the course of the OHSS is not appreciably altered.

Diuretics

The only place for the use of diuretics is where pulmonary congestion or edema is present. Prior volume expansion must be used as, if it is not, further reduction of the intravascular space may occur, worsening the already existing hypovolemia. Otherwise diuretics are contraindicated in these patients.

Dopamine

This is used in oliguric patients with severe OHSS to improve renal function[47]. Dopamine increases renal blood flow and glomerular filtration via stimulation of the dopaminergic receptors present in the kidney vasculature. This will avoid fluid and salt restriction, and prevent acute renal failure.

THE SURGICAL TREATMENT OF OHSS

Surgery should generally be avoided in patients with the OHSS. However, indications for surgical intervention include evidence of ovarian torsion, rupture or marked hemorrhage of the ovarian cysts, intraperitoneal bleeding, and the presence of an ectopic pregnancy associated with OHSS. A laparotomy should be avoided if at all possible and, if necessary, should only be performed by experienced gynecologists. The ovarian tissue is very friable in this situation and so a great deal of care is needed at surgery.

It has been suggested that torsion of ovaries in patients who conceive after gonadotropin therapy represents a special entity, requiring special attention and early diagnosis. The first case of unwinding of a cystic ovary via the laparoscope, in which torsion had occurred in a patient with OHSS, has been reported[48]. Even a dark, hemorrhagic and ischemic looking adnexum, on visualization via laparoscopy, may be saved by simply unwinding it through the laparoscope.

ASPIRATION OF ASCITIC FLUID AND PLEURAL EFFUSION IN SEVERE OHSS

Abdominal paracentesis was first proposed for the treatment of OHSS in patients with respiratory distress secondary to massive ascites accumulation[49]. The increased intra-abdominal hydrostatic pressure in patients with tense ascites acts via the diaphragm to increase the intrathoracic pressure and hence decrease the transmural filling of the heart. As the mean right atrial pressure increases, the venous return is thus impeded. Abdominal paracentesis relieves intra-abdominal pressure, which reduces IVC and hepatic wedge pressure, thus increasing venous return and the filling of the heart. This in turn increases cardiac output and stroke volume.

Paracentesis has been shown to be followed by an increase in urinary output and improvement in renal function (increased creatinine clearance of 50%), and a decrease in the patient's weight, leg edema, and abdominal circumference[50]. The use of an ultrasound scan guided procedure reduces the risk of puncturing or damaging the enlarged cystic ovaries and, in general, the risks of paracentesis seem negligible. Repeated procedures may be needed as the fluid recurs in the third spaces, and as the fluid is rich in protein, removal of this fluid in an already hypoproteinemic patient can be disadvantageous.

Nonetheless, early paracentesis may result in a swift resolution of symptoms. Aspiration of ascitic fluid is important in relieving symptoms and improving the general condition of patients, as well as improving urinary output. The average hospital stay, duration of severe symptoms, and disturbed electrolyte balance were found to be much shorter in patients who underwent aspiration of ascitic fluid than in patients who were managed conservatively. No adverse hemodynamic effects were seen as a result of aspiration of a large amount of ascitic fluid, however replacement of plasma proteins is needed due to the high protein content of the aspirated fluid. Repeated aspirations are required in approximately 30% of patients. It takes on average 3–5 days for a large amount of ascitic fluid to re-accumulate. Transvaginal ultrasound scan guided aspiration of the ascitic fluid is an effective and safe procedure, giving easy access to the most dependent fluid in the pouch of Douglas. As mentioned previously, suitable specialists can perform drainage of pleural and pericardial fluid, if clinically indicated.

SUMMARY

The OHSS is a severe and potentially fatal complication of ovarian hyperstimulation for assisted conception, and may also occur after ovulation induction for anovulatory infertility. The overall incidence of moderate/severe OHSS ranges from 1 to 10% of IVF cycles, however only 0.5–2% of cases will be severe in nature. Those at greatest risk are young women with sensitive, usually polycystic ovaries on ultrasound scan, with at least 50% of PCOS patients developing some degree of OHSS with ovarian gonadotropin stimulation. Patients with anovulatory infertility with menstrual disorders are more likely to develop OHSS than amenorrheic patients. Other risk factors for developing OHSS include a greater ovarian reserve to superovulation therapy, the use of hCG to trigger ovarian response or for luteal phase support and endogenous hCG by early pregnancy in conception cycles. The use of gonadotropin releasing hormone agonist (GnRH-a) and HMG cycles also increases the risk.

OHSS is four times more frequent in pregnant than in non-conception cycles and the pregnancy rate in hyperstimulated cycles is three times that of non-hyperstimulated cycles. The pathogenesis is unknown, but a predominant chemical mediator, possibly a prorenin–renin–angiotensin system, has been implicated.

The most effective management is the accurate prediction of the patients most at risk and prevention. This can be achieved by using cautious, slow, and gradual low doses of gonado-tropins and reducing regimens in women with polycystic ovaries. Combined sonography and endocrine monitoring should improve prediction rates. The presence of 20 or more small and intermediate sized follicles and/or a serum estradiol level of >3000 pg/ml should alert the clinician. If an exuberant ovarian response is observed and the patient has clinical symptoms of overstimulation, then the dose of hCG can be reduced, delayed (coasting), or omitted (thus canceling the cycle). Another alternative, if the patient is clinically well, and more than 30 oocytes are collected, is to perform the oocyte retrieval and to cryopreserve all the generated embryos. Although this will avoid a pregnancy in this cycle, preventing any trophoblastic hCG worsening the condition, at least the cycle is not 'wasted'. The embryos can be replaced in subsequent HRT cycles, however this regimen does not eliminate totally the possibility of OHSS developing in the fresh cycle.

In patients deemed at risk, a lower dosage of exogenous hCG, e.g. 5000 IU (instead of 10 000 IU), should be used to trigger ovulation, and progesterone, not hCG, used for luteal phase support. Administration of albumin at the time of oocyte retrieval may reduce the risk of developing severe OHSS.

Mild OHSS is treated conservatively, with outpatient surveillance to detect the minority of patients who will go on to develop the more severe condition. All patients should be advised as regards adequate fluid and protein intake. Patients with moderate or severe OHSS should be hospitalized. Strict fluid balance, regular serum biochemistry, and prophylaxis against thromboembolism are needed in these patients. Fluid and electrolyte imbalance, as well as hypovolemia, should always be corrected. Adequate analgesia is needed for abdominal pain and discomfort. Both transvaginal aspiration and abdominal paracentesis of ascitic fluid, under ultrasonographic guidance (avoiding damage to enlarged ovaries), are used to relieve symptoms of abdominal distension and respiratory distress, caused by massive ascites accumulation. This improves venous return, cardiac output, renal function, and urinary output. In cases of pleural effusion, a pleural tap can help relieve symptoms.

Such an approach demands close contact with the patient and good liaison with colleagues in other centers who may be providing emergency care. Early referral to an intensive care unit will help to correct hemodynamic disturbances but the reproductive specialist must continue to play an active role in management. Secondary complications of OHSS include venous thromboembolism, respiratory distress, and hepato-renal failure. Although isolated reports of death due to complications of OHSS have been reported[51], death is very rare following ovarian stimulation, occurring in approximately 1 in 400–500 000 stimulation cycles.

REFERENCES

1. Navot D, Bergh PA, Laufer N. Ovarian hyperstimulation syndrome in novel reproductive techniques: prevention and treatment. Fertil Steril 1992; 58: 249–61.

2. European IVF-monitoring programme for ESHRE. Assisted reproductive technology in Europe, 2000. Results generated from European registers by ESHRE. Hum Reprod 2004; 19: 490–503.

3. Society for Assisted Reproductive Technology, The American Society for Reproductive Medicine. Assisted reproductive technology in the United States: 2000 results. Fertil Steril 2004; 81: 1207–2000.

4. Hugues JN. Ovarian stimulation for assisted reproductive technologies. In Vayena E, Rowe PJ, Griffin PD, eds. Current Practices and Controversies in Assisted Reproduction. World Health Organisation, Geneva, Switzerland, 2002: 102–25.

5. Brinsden PR, Wada I, Tan SL et al. Diagnosis, prevention and management of ovarian hyperstimulation syndrome. Br J Obstet Gynaecol 1995; 102: 767–72.

6. Golan A, Ron-El R, Herman A et al. Ovarian hyperstimulation syndrome: an update review. Obstet Gynaecol Surv 1989; 44: 430–40.

7. Aboulghar MA, Mansour RT. Ovarian hyperstimulation syndrome: classifications and critical analysis of preventive measures. Hum Reprod Update 2003; 9: 275–89.

8. Mathur R, Akande AV, Keay SD et al. Distinction between early and late ovarian hyperstimulation syndrome. Fertil Steril 2000; 73: 901–7.

9. Ong A, Eisen V, Rennie DP et al. The pathogenesis of ovarian hyperstimulation syndrome. Clin Endocrinol 1991; 34: 43–8.

10. Fabregues F, Balasch J, Manau D et al. Haematocrit, leukocyte and platelet counts and the severity of ovarian hyperstimulation syndrome. Hum Reprod 1998; 13: 2406–10.

11. Shweiki D, Itin A, Neufeld G et al. Patterns of expression of vascular endothelial growth factor (VEGF) and VEGF receptors in mice suggest a role in hormonally regulated angiogenesis. J Clin Invest 1993; 91: 2235–43.

12. McClure N, Healy DL, Rogers PAW et al. Vascular endothelial growth factor as capillary permeability agent in ovarian hyperstimulation syndrome. Lancet 1994; 34: 235–6.

13. Agrawal R, Conway G, Sladkevicius P et al. Serum vascular endothelial growth factor and Doppler flow velocities in in vitro fertilization: relevance to ovarian hyperstimulation syndrome and polycystic ovaries. Fertil Steril 1998; 70: 651–8.

14. Agrawal R, Tan SL, Wild S et al. Serum vascular endothelial growth factor concentrations in in vitro fertilization cycles predict the risk of ovarian hyperstimulation syndrome. Fertil Steril 1999; 71: 287–93.

15. Gomez R, Simon C, Ramohi J et al. Vascular endothelial growth factor receptor-2 activation induces vascular permeability in hyperstimulated rats, and this effect is prevented by receptor blockade. Endocrinology 2002; 143: 4339–48.

16. Ludwig M, Gembruch U, Bauer O et al. Ovarian hyperstimulation syndrome (OHSS) in a spontaneous pregnancy with fetal and placental triploidy: information about the general patho-

physiology of OHSS. Hum Reprod 1998; 8: 2082–7.

17. Balen AH, Laven JSE, Tan SL et al. Ultrasound Assessment of the Polycystic Ovary : International Consensus Definitions. Hum Reprod Update 2003; 9: 505–14.

18. Michelmore KF, Balen AH, Dunger DB et al. Polycystic ovaries and associated clinical and biochemical features in young women. Clin Endocrinol 1999; 51: 779–86.

19. MacDougall MJ, Tan SL, Balen AH et al. A controlled study comparing patients with and without polycystic ovaries undergoing in-vitro fertilisation. Hum Reprod 1993; 8: 233–7.

20. Daya S, Gunby J, Hughes EG et al. FSH versus hMG for IVF cycles: a meta-analysis. Fertil Steril 1995; 64: 347–54.

21. Agrawal R, Holmes J, Jacobs HS. Follicle-stimulating hormone or hMG for ovarian stimulation in *in vitro* fertilization cycles: a meta-analysis. Fertil Steril 2000; 73: 338–43.

22. Daya S, Gunby J. Recombinant versus urinary FSH for ovarian stimulation in assisted reproduction cycles. Cochrane Database Syst Rev 2000; 4: CD002810.

23. Al-Inany H, Aboulghar M, Mansour R et al. Meta-analysis of recombinant versus urinary-derived FSH: an update. Hum Reprod 2003; 18: 305–13.

24. Van Wely M, Westergaard LG, Bossuyt PM et al. HMG versus recombinant follicle stimulation hormone for ovarian stimulation in assisted reproductive cycles. Cochrane Database Syst Rev 2003; 1: CD003973.

25. Egbase PE, Makhseed M, Al Sharhan M et al. Timed unilateral ovarian follicular aspiration prior to the administration of human chorionic gonadotrophin for the prevention of severe OHSS in IVF; a prospective randomized study. Hum Reprod 1997; 12: 2603–6.

26. Gonen Y, Powell WA, Casper RF. Effects of follicular aspiration on hormonal parameters in patients undergoing ovarian stimulation. Hum Reprod 1991; 6: 356–8.

27. Egbase PE, Al Sharhan M, Grudzinskas JG. Early unilateral follicular aspiration compared to coasting for the prevention of severe OHSS;

28. Delvigne A, Rozenberg S. Epidemiology and prevention of ovarian hyperstimulation syndrome (OHSS): a review. Hum Reprod Update 2002; 8: 559–77.

29. Sher G, Zouves C, Feinman M, Maassarani G. 'Prolonged coasting': an effective method for preventing severe ovarian hyperstimulation syndrome in patients undergoing in-vitro fertilization. Hum Reprod 1995; 10(12): 3107–9.

30. D'Angelo A, Amso N. 'Coasting' (withholding gonadotrophins) for preventing ovarian hyperstimulation syndrome (cochrane review). Cochrane Database Syst Rev 2003; (3): CD002811.

31. Asch RH, Shoham Z. Comparison of intravenous albumin and transfer of fresh embryos, with cryopreservation of all embryos for subsequent transfer, in prevention of ovarian hyperstimulation syndrome. Fertil Steril 1996; 65: 992–6.

32. Shoham Z, Weissman A, Barash A et al. Intravenous albumin for the prevention of severe ovarian hyperstimulation syndrome, in an in-vitro fertilisation program: a prospective, randomised, placebo controlled study. Fertil Steril 1994; 62:137–42.

33. Ng E, Leader A, Claman P. Intravenous albumen does not prevent the development of severe OHSS in an IVF programme. Hum Reprod 1995; 10: 107–10.

34. Orvietto R. Can we eliminate severe ovarian hyperstimulation syndrome? Hum Reprod 2005; 2: 320–2.

35. Kol S. Luteolysis induced by a GnRH agonist is the key to prevention of ovarian hyperstimulation syndrome. Fertil Steril 2004; 81: 1–5.

36. Drug Information Service; The University of Utah Health Sciences Center. New Drugs Bulletins; Ganirelix Acetate (Antagon) 27 August 2004.

37. Tan SL, Balen A, Hussein EL et al. The administration of glucocorticoids for the prevention of ovarian hyperstimulation in IVF. A prospective randomized study. Fertil Steril 1992; 57: 378–83.

38. Lord JM, Flight IHK, Norman RJ. Insulin-sensitising drugs (metformin, troglitazone,

rosiglitazone, pioglitazone, D-chiro-inositol) for polycystic ovary syndrome. Cochrane Database Syst Rev 2003; 2: CD003053.

39. Tang T, Glanville J, Barth J, Balen AH. Metformin in patients with polycystic ovary syndrome (PCOS) undergoing IVF. A randomised, placebo-controlled, double-blind study. Hum Reprod 2006; 6: 1416–25.

40. Loret De Mora RJ, Pablo Flores J, Baumgardner GP et al. Elevated interleukin-6 levels in the ovarian hyperstimulation syndrome: ovarian immunohistochemical localization of interleukin-6 signal. Obstet Gynaecol 1996; 87: 581–7.

41. Stewart JA, Hamilton PJ, Murdoch AP. Thromboembolic disease associated with ovarian stimulation and assisted conception techniques. Hum Reprod 1997; 12: 2167–73.

42. Ryo E, Hagino D, Yano N et al. A case of ovarian hyperstimulation syndrome in which antithrombin III deficiency occurred because of its loss into ascites. Fertil Steril 1999; 71: 860–2.

43. Seow KM, Hwang JL, Tsai YL et al. Acute hydrothorax as the only manifestation of ovarian hyperstimulation syndrome after in vitro fertilization: case report and literature review. J Gynaecol Surg 2001; 17: 19–23.

44. Cohen SB, Weisz B, Seidman DS, Mashiach S, Lidor AL, Goldenberg M. Accuracy of the preoperative diagnosis in 100 emergency laparoscopies performed due to acute abdomen in nonpregnant women. J Am Assoc Gynecol Laparosc 2001; 8(1): 92–4.

45. Aboulgar MA, Mansour RT, Serour GI et al. Autotransfer of the ascitic fluid in the treatment of severe ovarian hyperstimulation syndrome. Fertil Steril 1993; 58: 1056–9.

46. Zosmer A, Katz Z, Lancet M et al. Adult respiratory distress syndrome complicating ovarian hyperstimulation. Fertil Steril 1987; 47: 524–6.

47. Ferraretti A P, Gianaroli L, Diotallevi L et al. A dopamine treatment for severe hyperstimulation syndrome. Hum Reprod 1992; 7:180–3.

48. Hurwitz A, Milwidsky A, Yagel S et al. Early unwinding of a torsion of an ovarian cyst as a result of hyperstimulation syndrome. Fertil Steril 1983; 40: 393.

49. Rabau E, Serr DM, David A et al. Human menopausal gonadotrophins for anovulation and sterility. Am J Obstet Gynaecol 1967; 98: 92–8.

50. Thaler I, Yoffe N, Kaftory J et al. Treatment of ovarian hyperstimulation syndrome: the physiological basis for a modified approach. Fertil Steril 1981; 36: 110–13.

51. Shenker JG, Weinstein D. Ovarian hyperstimulation syndrome: a current survey. Fertil Steril 1978; 30: 255–68.

CHAPTER 15

In-vitro maturation for the treatment of infertility with polycystic ovary syndrome

Hanadi Ba-Akdah, Hananel EG Holzer, Julie Lukic, and Seang Lin Tan

INTRODUCTION

The first live birth resulting from in-vitro fertilization (IVF) occurred in 1978[1] and, since then, over 2 million IVF babies have been born worldwide. IVF success rates have steadily improved over the years[2] and nowadays exceed spontaneous conception rates in fertile couples[3]. However, ovarian stimulation protocols are associated with high costs, daily injections of gonadotropins, and close monitoring, and carry a significant risk of causing ovarian hyperstimulation syndrome (OHSS)[4,5]. Papanikolaou et al.[6] found that the incidence of patients undergoing IVF requiring hospitalization for OHSS was 2%; in exceptional cases, where OHSS appropriate care is not given, it may even be fatal[7].

In-vitro maturation (IVM) is the maturation of immature oocytes in vitro from the germinal vesicle (GV) stage to the metaphase II (MII) stage of development, at which time they can be fertilized and subsequently undergo normal embryonic development. Clinical IVM is without ovarian stimulation. Therefore, IVM avoids OHSS, is clinically simple, and has a lower cost. As a result, it is a potentially useful treatment for infertility.

As GV oocytes will be successfully aspirated from about 60% of the tiny follicles during fol-

licular collection, the number of antral follicles is the major predictor clinically for the success of IVM[8]. Since the high number of antral follicles found in patients with polycystic ovary syndrome (PCOS) makes them more likely to develop OHSS, they are also prime candidates for IVM treatment. This applies even if the appearance of PCOS on ultrasound scan is not associated with an ovulatory disorder; that is, if patients have ultrasound-only polycystic ovaries (PCO)[9,10].

IN-VIVO AND IN-VITRO MATURATION OF OOCYTES

Oocytes are formed in the ovaries of a human female during fetal development but are arrested at the prophase I stage of meiosis. At birth, there are approximately 1 million primordial follicles in the ovaries[11]. Although large numbers of follicles can leave the primordial pool and begin to grow, very few will be selected to mature and to ovulate for potential fertilization. In response to rising levels of gonadotropins, the follicles will grow and become fully mature, but only after the onset of puberty will they be released into the fallopian tube by ovulation. During a woman's reproductive life, only about 400 to 500 mature oocytes will be released from the ovaries for potential fertilization. The process of follicular development within the ovary is directly influenced by gonadotropins, namely follicle stimulating hormone (FSH) and luteinizing hormone (LH). Gonadotropins (FSH and LH) are necessary for follicular development in vivo. The first meiotic division will occur in preovulatory follicles following the preovulatory LH surge, where the chromosomes progress from the metaphase I (MI) to the telophase I stage. After the first meiotic division and first polar body extrusion, the second meiotic division begins and a secondary metaphase plate (metaphase II) is formed at which time the oocyte is mature, enabling fertilization and early embryonic development to occur.

Hreinsson et al.[12] showed that the use of recombinant human chorionic gonadotropins (hCG) or recombinant LH is equally effective in promoting oocyte maturation in vitro. In addition, it is known that culture medium supplemented with a physiologic concentration of FSH or LH stimulates steroid secretions (estradiol and progesterone) from cultured granulosa and cumulus cells[13]. Therefore, it is likely that one of the actions of gonadotropins is mediated by either estradiol or progesterone, which may control oocyte maturation in vitro.

POLYCYSTIC OVARY SYNDROME (PCOS)

PCOS is a very heterogeneous syndrome and is the most common cause of anovulatory infertility. In the past, diagnosis of PCOS was made according to the National Institutes of Health (NIH) Consensus Criteria. However, more recently, the Rotterdam Consensus has revised the prerequisites whereby the diagnosis of PCOS now requires the presence of two out of the following three criteria: (1) oligo- or anovulation, (2) clinical and/or (3) biochemical signs of hyperandrogenism and polycystic ovaries at ultrasound scan[14].

Patients with PCOS might present with hirsutism, obesity, or frequently with cycle abnormalities (oligomenorrhea) and infertility (Figure 15.1). PCOS is the most widespread endocrinologic disorder among women of reproductive age as well as the most common cause of anovulatory infertility[15] and has been shown to exist in from 4% to 10% of the general population. Fertility treatments for women with PCOS include lifestyle management, administration of insulin-sensitizing agents, ovulation induction, ovarian stimulation, and IVF.

POLYCYSTIC OVARIES (PCO)

The definition of ultrasound-only polycystic ovaries (PCO) is the presence of 12 or more follicles in each ovary measuring 2–9 mm in diameter and increased ovarian volume (>10 ml) without any other manifestation of PCOS (Figure 15.2)[10]. Isolated PCO morphology without a full picture of PCOS has an incidence of 16–23%[16–18]. On ultrasound examination, women with ultrasound-only PCO were found to produce more follicles, oocytes, and embryos than women who had normal ovarian morphology[9,19].

The high number of antral follicles in patients with PCO makes them prime candidates for IVM

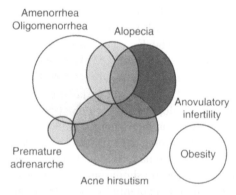

Figure 15.1 The spectrum of presentation in polycystic ovary syndrome (see color plate section)

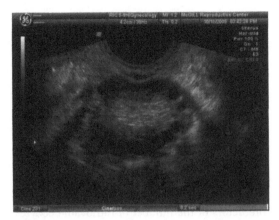

Figure 15.2 Ultrasound appearance of polycystic ovary

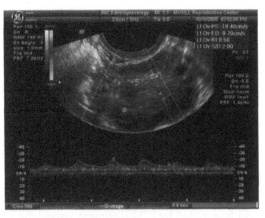

Figure 15.3 Stromal blood flow in polycystic ovary (see color plate section)

(treatment, even if the appearance of PCO in the scan is not associated with an ovulatory disorder. Indeed, the main clinical determinant of the success rates of IVM treatment is antral follicle count[8,20].

RISKS ASSOCIATED WITH IVF IN PCO/PCOS WOMEN

As previously mentioned, patients with PCO/PCOS have a greater risk of developing severe OHSS from gonadotropin stimulation than those who have normal ovaries[9]. Patients with PCO or PCOS are particularly more prone to develop OHSS, with an incidence of up to 6%[9]. The most severe manifestation of OHSS involves massive ovarian enlargement, multiple cysts, hemoconcentration, and third-space accumulation of fluid. The syndrome may be complicated by renal failure and oliguria, hypovolemic shock, thromboembolic episodes, and adult respiratory distress syndrome (ARDS), which, in extreme cases, may even be fatal, if appropriate care is not given. Ovarian volume, stromal volume, and stromal peak blood flow velocity are all significantly higher in the ovaries of women with PCO and PCOS (Figure 15.3). The reason for increased blood flow is probably because of the increased

vascular endothelial growth factor (VEGF) levels in PCO/PCOS patients. Serum VEGF seems to be a major capillary permeability factor in the development of OHSS ascites[21–24].

Several methods have been used to reduce the risk of OHSS, including starting stimulation with a lower dose of FSH, close monitoring by ultrasound scans and serum estradiol (E_2) level measurements, coasting, withholding or decreasing the hCG dose for final follicular maturation, administration of intravascular volume expanders, use of glucocorticoids[25], and decreasing the number of embryos transferred or freezing all the embryos and transferring in a later frozen embryo replacement cycle[26]. Despite many years of clinical experience, no method has been developed that will completely prevent severe OHSS after ovarian stimulation[27].

In assisted reproduction, the risk of multiple-follicle ovulation and subsequent multiple pregnancies in PCO/PCOS women is also of crucial importance[9,28]. When the outcome of in-vitro fertilization and embryo transfer (IVF-ET) in 76 patients with PCO diagnosed on pretreatment ultrasound scan was compared with that of 76 control patients who had normal ovaries, it was found that there was a 10.8% risk of OHSS in the PCO group compared with none (0%) in those with normal ovaries[9].

ADVANTAGES OF IVM

Because no expensive gonadotropin stimulation and no extensive monitoring scans are required, the cost of IVM treatment is lower than that of IVF. Furthermore, the side-effects of medications used in IVF, although mild, may be unpleasant.

The IVM treatment schedule is shorter, causing less stress, and it is not necessary to wait for 2 to 3 months between treatment cycles because no stimulation is involved. The risk of OHSS can be avoided by IVM treatment, especially in women with PCO/PCOS[5].

OUTLINE OF AN IVM TREATMENT CYCLE FOR WOMEN WITH PCO AND PCOS

The first pregnancy and delivery of a healthy baby after IVM of immature oocytes in a patient with PCOS was described by Trounson et al.[29]. In the following year, Barnes *et al.*[30] reported another pregnancy in a patient with PCOS treated with IVM combined with intracytoplasmic sperm injection (ICSI) and assisted hatching. In these early studies, the rates of maturation, fertilization, and cleavage were initially found to be higher in regularly ovulating women compared with irregularly ovulatory or anovulatory women with PCO; however, later studies have shown comparable maturation and fertilization rates[31,32]. When IVF was compared with IVM cycles in PCO women, the rates of fertilization and embryo cleavage were found to be similar[5].

Previous studies indicated that although immature oocytes recovered from unstimulated PCOS patients could be matured, fertilized, and developed in vitro, the implantation rate was still disappointingly low[5,33–35]. To compensate for this, endogenous priming with FSH or hCG has been suggested before oocyte retrieval and IVM.

Ultrasound

A baseline scan is performed between days 2 and 5 of the menstrual cycle to measure ovarian volume, ovarian stromal blood flow velocity, antral follicle count (AFC), size of the follicles, and endometrial thickness, and to detect whether any ovarian or uterine abnormalities are present. If the patient is amenorrheic, a withdrawal bleed with progestogens is induced. Although AFC, ovarian volume, and ovarian stromal maximal blood velocity are all predictors of the number of retrievable oocytes, we have found that when the other factors are controlled by multiple regression analysis, the antral follicle count is the only reliable predictor[8]. Between days 6 and 8 of the cycle, a second scan is performed to measure AFC and endometrial thickness. We and others have recently reported that atresia does not occur in the non-dominant follicles, even when a dominant follicle is present[36–38]. For this reason, we no longer cancel the procedure for patients who are found to have a dominant follicle. hCG is administered (see below) when the endometrial thickness is greater than 8 mm.

hCG priming and pretreatment with FSH

While the results of some studies indicate that pretreatment with FSH during the early follicular phase enhances both the number of oocytes retrieved and their rate of maturation[39], others have found that pretreatment with FSH produces no tangible benefits[40,41]. Based on the results of the latter studies, at our center we do not stimulate the ovaries with FSH prior to IVM oocyte collection.

Interest in the effects of hCG priming arose when morphologic and molecular differences were found between immature oocytes collected from stimulated cycles and those collected by cesarean section[42]. In 1999[43,44], we reported that the maturation rate of immature oocytes collected from women with PCOS was improved by administering 10 000 IU hCG 36 h prior to retrieval. Results of a randomized prospective study indicated that besides improving the maturation rate, priming with hCG also shortened the maturation process[44]. We determined that oocytes that had been matured for 24 h following collection produced better quality embryos than those that had been matured for 48 h[44]. Furthermore, our findings seem to indicate that hCG priming could increase the number of MII stage oocytes retrieved, resulting in a clinical pregnancy rate of >35% per cycle in young women up to 35 years of age[12,45–49]. Moreover, induced luteinization with hCG might enhance endometrial preparation, resulting in improved synchronization of embryonic development within the endometrium[50].

Retrieval of immature oocytes

Oocyte retrieval is performed under spinal anesthesia or intravenous sedation using 1 to 2 mg of fentanyl and midazolam. Intravenous fentanyl is administered at intervals of 15 to 20 minutes to a maximum dosage of 150 to 200 mg. In order to reduce the discomfort of the multiple needle punctures that are required by this procedure, 0.5% bupivacaine is infiltrated locally into the vagina. Oocyte retrieval is then performed under ultrasound guidance using a 19G, single-lumen aspiration needle. Because the aspiration pressure is reduced to 7.5 kPa and such a small gauge needle is used, bloodstained aspirate can frequently block the needle. Therefore, the needle is withdrawn from the vagina after aspirating a few follicles and is flushed to clear any obstruction. The procedure is repeated until all follicles seen are aspirated. Follicular fluid is collected in culture tubes containing a solution of 0.9% saline supplemented with 2 U/ml of heparin. Because immature oocytes are enclosed in tightly packed cumulus cells, curettage of the follicular wall is performed in order to dislodge the cumulus–oocyte complex.

Over the past 5 years, we have increased the average number of GV oocytes we collect per cycle from 10 to 15.

IVM and fertilization

Immature oocytes are incubated in a culture dish containing maturation medium supplemented with 75 mIU/ml of FSH and LH at 37°C in an atmosphere of 5% carbon dioxide and 95% air with high humidity and are checked for maturity 24 and 48 hours following culture. The oocytes are denuded of granulosa cells following retrieval, and mature oocytes (detected by the presence of an extruded polar body) are fertilized using intracytoplasmic sperm injection (ICSI). However, it has been demonstrated that when the sperm parameters are normal, ICSI may not always be required for the fertilization of oocytes collected through IVM[51]. Nevertheless, ICSI is generally performed on in-vitro matured oocytes because it reduces the risk of unexpected poor fertilization as compared with IVF. After ICSI, the oocytes are transferred into 1 ml of IVF medium in a tissue culture dish. Fertilization is determined 18 hours later by examining the oocytes for the appearance of two distinct pronuclei and two polar bodies.

Embryo transfer

The fertilized oocytes are further cultured up to day 2 or 3, following which an embryo transfer is performed. Prior to transfer, assisted hatching is performed to avoid reduced implantation due to a hardened zona pellucida. When a large number of embryos have formed, two alternatives are possible: a double transfer or a blastocyst transfer[52]. The former is performed on day 3 and repeated on day 5–6, while the latter involves extending the culture to the blastocyst stage at day 5 or 6 and transferring at that stage only. The embryo transfer technique is the same as that used for conventional IVF.

Endometrial preparation and luteal support

To achieve optimal endometrial growth, exogenous 17β-estradiol (micronized) is administered, starting on the day of oocyte retrieval. The dosage used depends on the endometrial thickness on the day of oocyte retrieval. When endometrial thickness is less than 6 mm, 12 mg a day is started; if the thickness is between 6 and 8 mm, then 10 mg a day is started; and if the thickness is more than 8 mm, then 6 mg is used – all in three divided doses. When an extremely thin endometrium (i.e. <4 mm) is recorded on ultrasound scan prior to collection, we have recently begun to administer estradiol treatment before oocyte collection. We are currently investigating an alternative approach whereby in-vitro matured oocytes are vitrified when the endometrial lining is very thin[53]. The endometrium is then prepared in an artificial cycle and, once it reaches a thickness of 8 mm, the oocytes are thawed, fertilized, and transferred. In an IVM treatment cycle, luteal support with daily intramuscular injections of progesterone in oil or Prometrium 200 mg (Schering Canada) three times per day, is started on the day that oocyte maturation is achieved and ICSI is performed. Estradiol and progesterone supplementation is continued until the twelfth week of pregnancy.

IVM OUTCOME

IVM pregnancy rates are correlated with the number of immature oocytes retrieved. The clinical pregnancy rate in women younger than 35 years, from whom we retrieved more than 10 immature GV oocytes, is 38% per cycle. As with IVF, clinical pregnancy and implantation rates decrease with increasing age[54]. In our practice, the clinical pregnancy rate for women younger than 35 years is 38% per oocyte retrieval and the implantation rate is 13%, while for women between 36 and 40 years old, the clinical pregnancy rate is 21% per retrieval and the implantation rate is 5%. Because of lower implantation rates, we transfer 1–2 more embryos compared with conventional IVF for women in comparable age groups without any increase in the multiple pregnancy rate.

In four centers performing IVM cycles, more than 1000 IVM cycles with hCG priming were done before oocyte collection, the pregnancy rates reached 30–35% and the implantation rates 10–15%[55].

In various published series, no increased rates of congenital malformations have been reported with IVM[56,57]. A recent analysis of the obstetric, neonatal, and infant outcome in our IVM conceptions showed a pregnancy outcome of 73% singleton, 24% twin, and 2.7% triplet. The median gestation age was 39 weeks for singletons and 37 weeks for multiple pregnancies. Similar reassuring results have been published by others[58].

IVM FOR OOCYTE DONATION

Oocyte donation is now a standard treatment for women who have diminished ovarian reserve and/or who are of advanced reproductive age; women affected by, or who are carriers of a significant genetic defect; and women with poor oocyte and/or embryo quality[59]. This method of treatment results in a high pregnancy rate for patients who would otherwise have a poor reproductive prognosis; the accumulated pregnancy rate may even increase up to 94.8% after four transfers[60]. Many potential oocyte donors may be deterred by the risk of OHSS, complications associated with oocyte collection, and concern about the inconvenience of a large number of hormone injections, as well as their possible long-term side-effects[61,62]. This perception has been supported by the results of a recent survey which indicate that three-quarters of potential donors declined after receiving information about the procedures involved[63]. Avoidance of ovarian stimulation would obviously eliminate the associated risks to oocyte donors and would drastically reduce the costs of donation cycles[64]. The first reported IVM pregnancy was, in fact, conceived from immature oocytes retrieved and donated to a woman with premature ovarian failure[65]. At our center, 12 oocyte donors (age 29 ± 4) with high antral follicle counts (29.6 ± 8.7) underwent immature oocyte collection without ovarian stimulation. Out of a mean of 12.8 ± 5.1 GV oocytes collected, 68% matured and were fertilized using ICSI. Of a total of 47 embryos transferred to 12 recipients, six (50%) were successfully conceived, four of which have resulted in live births[66]. Based on the foregoing evidence, it would therefore appear that collecting immature oocytes from the unstimulated ovaries of oocyte donors is both prudent and worthwhile.

IVM AND PGD

Preimplantation genetic diagnosis (PGD) is a procedure that allows the in-vitro testing of embryos produced by couples who are potential carriers of an inherited disease or genetic defect, or by patients who have had three or more unexplained miscarriages. Patients can now select only those embryos diagnosed as being unaffected for implantation in the woman's uterus, thus improving the chance of a successful pregnancy. PGD patients are generally required to undergo IVF treatment in order to generate multiple embryos for genetic analysis. However, we have recently used IVM as an alternative for selected PGD patients with PCO/PCOS in order to avoid the side-effects of fertility drugs and to eliminate the risk of OHSS. We recently treated a 35-year-old patient with recurrent miscarriage who had unsuccessfully undergone two intrauterine insemination cycles and two IVF cycles in Germany. We collected 14 GV and 1 MII oocytes and biopsied the eight embryos generated. After the transfer of two normal embryos following aneuploidy screening, she became

pregnant and we had the world's first live birth after combined IVM and PGD[67].

CONCLUSIONS

PCOS is the most common endocrinologic disorder among women of reproductive age as well as the most common cause of anovulatory infertility[15]. Patients with PCO or PCOS are particularly more prone to develop OHSS, with an incidence of up to 6%[9].

IVM is the maturation of oocytes in vitro from the GV stage to the MII stage of development. Because of the absence of OHSS and reduction in cost and complexity, IVM appears to be a promising treatment for infertility, especially for women with PCO or PCOS. The pregnancy rate in four centers performing IVM cycles in PCOS/PCO patients currently reaches 30–35%[54].

REFERENCES

1. Steptoe PC, Edwards RG. Birth after the preimplantation of a human embryo. Lancet 1978; 312: 366.

2. Tan SL, Royston P, Campbell S et al. Cumulative conception and livebirth rates after in-vitro fertilisation. Lancet 1992; 339: 1390–4.

3. Engmann L, Maconochie N, Bekir JS et al. Cumulative probability of clinical pregnancy and live birth after a multiple cycle IVF package: a more realistic assessment of overall and age-specific success rates? Br J Obstet Gynaecol 1999; 106: 165–70.

4. Brinsden PR, Wada I, Tan SL et al. Diagnosis, prevention and management of ovarian hyperstimulation syndrome. Br J Obstet Gynaecol 1995; 102: 767–72.

5. Child TJ, Phillips SJ, Abdul-Jalil AK et al. A comparison of in vitro maturation and in vitro fertilization for women with polycystic ovaries. Obstet Gynecol 2002; 100: 665–70.

6. Papanikolaou EG, Tournaye H, Verpoest W et al. Early and late ovarian hyperstimulation syn-

drome: early pregnancy outcome and profile. Hum Reprod 2005; 20: 636–41.

7. Semba S, Moriya T, Youssef EM et al. An autopsy case of ovarian hyperstimulation syndrome with massive pulmonary edema and pleural effusion. Pathol Int 2000; 50: 549–52.

8. Tan SL, Child TJ, Gulekli B. In-vitro maturation and fertilization of oocytes from unstimulated ovaries: predicting the number of immature oocytes retrieved by early follicular phase ultrasonography. Am J Obstet Gynecol 2002; 186: 684–9.

9. MacDougall MJ, Tan SL, Balen A et al. A controlled study comparing patients with and without polycystic ovaries undergoing in-vitro fertilization. Hum Reprod 1993; 8: 233–7.

10. Balen AH, Laven JSE, Tan SL et al. Ultrasound Assessment of the Polycystic Ovary: International Consensus Definitions. Hum Reprod Update 2003; 9: 505–14.

11. Baker TG. Oogenesis and ovulation. In Austin CR, Short RV, eds. Reproduction in Mammals, 2nd edn. Cambridge University Press, Cambridge, 1982: 17–45.

12. Hreinsson J, Rosenlund B, Friden B et al. Recombinant LH is equally effective as recombinant hCG in promoting oocyte maturation in a clinical in vitro maturation programme: a randomized study. Hum Reprod 2003; 18: 2131–6.

13. Chian RC, Ao A, Clarke HJ et al. Production of steroids from human cumulus cells treated with different concentrations of gonadotropins during culture in vitro. Fertil Steril 1999; 71: 61–6.

14. The Rotterdam ESHRE/ASRM-Sponsored PCOS consensus workshop group. Revised 2003 consensus on diagnostic criteria and long-term health risks related to polycystic ovary syndrome (PCOS). Hum Reprod 2004; 19: 41–7.

15. Carmina E, Lobo RA. Polycystic ovary syndrome (PCOS): arguably the most common endocrinopathy is associated with significant morbidity in women. J Clin Endocrinol Metab 1999; 84: 1897–9.

16. Polson DW, Adams J, Wadsworth J et al. Polycystic ovaries – a common finding in normal women. Lancet 1988; 331: 870–2.

17. Abdel Gadir A, Khatim MS, Mowafi RS, Alnaser HM et al. Implications of ultrasonically diagnosed polycystic ovaries. I. Correlations with basal hormonal profiles. Hum Reprod 1992; 7: 453–7.

18. Abdel Gadir A, Khatim MS, Mowafi RS, Alnaser HM et al. Implications of ultrasonically diagnosed polycystic ovaries. II. Studies of dynamic and pulsatile hormonal patterns. Hum Reprod 1992; 7: 458–61.

19. Engmann L, Maconochie N, Sladkevicius P et al. The outcome of in-vitro fertilization treatment in women with sonographic evidence of polycystic ovarian morphology. Hum Reprod 1999; 14: 167–71.

20. Tan SL, Child TJ. In-vitro maturation of oocytes from unstimulated polycystic ovaries. Reprod Biomed Online 2002; 4(Suppl 1): 18–23.

21. McClure N, Healy DL, Rogers PA et al. Vascular endothelial growth factor as capillary permeability agent in ovarian hyperstimulation syndrome. Lancet 1994; 344: 235–6.

22. Buckett WM, Bouzayen R, Watkin KL et al. Ovarian stromal echogenicity in women with normal and polycystic ovaries. Hum Reprod 1999; 14: 618–21.

23. Agrawal R, Conway G, Sladkevicius P et al. Serum vascular endothelial growth factor and Doppler blood flow velocities in in vitro fertilization: relevance to ovarian hyperstimulation syndrome and polycystic ovaries. Fertil Steril 1998; 70: 651–8.

24. Zaidi J, Jacobs H, Campbell S et al. Blood flow changes in the ovarian and uterine arteries in women with polycystic ovary syndrome who respond to clomiphene citrate: correlation with serum hormone concentrations. Ultrasound Obstet Gynecol 1998; 12: 188–96.

25. Tan SL, Balen A, el Hussein E et al. The administration of glucocorticoids for the prevention of ovarian hyperstimulation syndrome in in vitro fertilization: a prospective randomized study. Fertil Steril 1992; 58: 378–83.

26. Awonuga AO, Pitroff R, Zaidi J et al. Elective cryopreservation of all embryos in women at risk of developing ovarian hyperstimulation syndrome may not prevent the condition but reduces the livebirth rate. J Assist Reprod Genet 1996; 13: 401–6.

27. Buckett WM, Chian RC, Tan SL. Can we eliminate severe OHSS? Not completely. Hum Reprod 2005; 20: 2367.

28. Homburg R. Management of infertility and prevention of ovarian hyperstimulation in women with polycystic ovary syndrome. Best Pract Res Clin Obstet Gynaecol 2004; 18: 773–88.

29. Trounson A, Wood C, Kausche A. In vitro maturation and the fertilization and developmental competence of oocytes recovered from untreated polycystic ovarian patients. Fertil Steril 1994; 62: 353–62.

30. Barnes FL, Crombie A, Gardner DK et al. Blastocyst development and birth after in-vitro maturation of human primary oocytes, intracytoplasmic sperm injection and assisted hatching. Hum Reprod 1995; 10: 3243–7.

31. Suikkari AM, Tulppala M, Tuuri T et al. Luteal phase start of low-dose FSH priming of follicles results in an efficient recovery, maturation and fertilization of immature human oocytes. Hum Reprod 2000; 15: 747–51.

32. Cavilla JL, Kennedy CR, Baltsen M et al. The effects of meiosis activating sterol on in-vitro maturation and fertilization of human oocytes from stimulated and unstimulated ovaries. Hum Reprod 2001; 16: 547–55.

33. Barnes FL, Kausche A, Tiglias J et al. Production of embryos from in vitro-matured primary human oocytes. Fertil Steril 1996; 65: 1151–6.

34. Trounson A, Anderiesz C, Jones GM et al. Oocyte maturation. Hum Reprod 1998; 13(Suppl 3): 52–62.

35. Cha KY, Han SY, Chung HM et al. Pregnancies and deliveries after in vitro maturation culture followed by in vitro fertilization and embryo transfer without stimulation in women with polycystic ovary syndrome. Fertil Steril 2000; 73: 978–83.

36. Paulson RJ, Sauer MV, Francis MM et al. Factors affecting pregnancy success of human in vitro fertilization in unstimulated cycles. Hum Reprod 1994; 9: 1571–5.

37. Thornton MH, Francis MM, Paulson RJ. Immature oocyte retrieval: lessons from unstimulated IVF cycles. Fertil Steril 1998; 70: 647–50.

38. Chian RC, Buckett WM, Abdul Jalil AK et al. Natural-cycle in vitro fertilization combined with in vitro maturation of immature oocytes is a potential approach in infertility treatment. Fertil Steril 2004; 82: 1675–78.

39. Wynn P, Picton HM, Krapez JA et al. Pretreatment with follicle stimulating hormone promotes the numbers of human oocytes reaching metaphase II by in-vitro maturation. Hum Reprod 1998; 13: 3132–8.

40. Mikkelsen AL, Smith SD, Lindenberg S. In vitro maturation of human oocytes from regularly menstruating women may be successful without follicle stimulating hormone priming. Hum Reprod 1999; 14: 1847–51.

41. Trounson A, Anderiesz C, Jones G. Maturation of human oocytes in vitro and their developmental competence. Reproduction 2001; 121: 51–75.

42. Chian RC, Park SE, Park EL et al. Molecular and structural characteristics between immature human oocytes retrieved from unstimulated ovaries. In Gomel V, Leung PCK, eds. In vitro Fertilization and Assisted Reproduction. Bologna: Monduzzi, 1997: 315–19.

43. Chian RC, Buckett WM, Too LL et al. Pregnancies resulting from in vitro matured oocytes retrieved from patients with polycystic ovary syndrome after priming with human chorionic gonadotropin. Fertil Steril 1999; 72: 639–42.

44. Chian RC, Gulekli B, Buckett WM et al. Priming with human chorionic gonadotropin before retrieval of immature oocytes in women with infertility due to the polycystic ovary syndrome. N Engl J Med 1999; 341: 1624–6.

45. Chian RC, Buckett WM, Tulandi T et al. Prospective randomized study of human chorionic gonadotrophin priming before immature oocyte retrieval from unstimulated women with polycystic ovarian syndrome. Hum Reprod 2000; 15: 165–70.

46. Chian RC, Gulekli B, Buckett WM et al. Pregnancy and delivery after cryopreservation of zygotes produced by in-vitro matured oocytes retrieved from a woman with polycystic ovarian syndrome. Hum Reprod 2001; 16: 1700–2.

47. Hwang JL, Lin YH, Tsai YL et al. Oocyte donation using immature oocytes from a normal ovulatory

woman. Acta Obstet Gynecol Scand 2002; 81: 274–5.

48. Nagele F, Sator MO, Juza J et al. Successful pregnancy resulting from in-vitro matured oocytes retrieved at laparoscopic surgery in a patient with polycystic ovary syndrome: case report. Hum Reprod 2002; 17: 373–4.

49. Son WY, Yoon SH, Lee SW et al. Blastocyst development and pregnancies after IVF of mature oocytes retrieved from unstimulated patients with PCOS after in-vivo HCG priming. Hum Reprod 2002; 17: 134–6.

50. Buckett WM, Chian RC, Tan SL. Human chorionic gonadotropin for in vitro oocyte maturation: does it improve the endometrium or implantation? J Reprod Med 2004: 49: 93–8.

51. Soderstron AV, Makinen S, Tuuri T et al. Favourable pregnancy results with insemination of in vitro matured oocytes from unstimulated patients. Hum Reprod 2005; 20: 1534–40.

52. Philips SJ, Dean NL, Buckett WM et al. Consecutive transfer of day 3 embryos and of day 5–6 blastocyst increases overall pregnancy rates associated with blastocyst culture. J Assist Reprod Genet 2003; 20: 461–4.

53. Chian RC, Kuwayama M, Tan L et al. High survival rate of bovine oocytes matured in vitro following vitrification. J Reprod Dev 2004; 50: 685–96.

54. Chian RC. In-vitro maturation of immature oocytes for infertile women with PCOS. Reprod Biomed Online 2004; 8: 547–52.

55. Mikkelsen AL, Andersson AM, Skakkebaek NE et al. Basal concentrations of oestradiol may predict the outcome of in-vitro maturation in regularly menstruating women. Hum Reprod 2001; 16: 862–7.

56. Buckett WM, Chian RC, Holzer H et al. Congenital abnormalities and perinatal outcome in pregnancies following IVM, IVF, and ICSI delivered in a single center. 61st Annual Meeting of ASRM, Montreal, Canada. Fertil Steril 2005; 84(Suppl 1): S80–1.

57. Buckett WM, Chian RC, Barrington K et al. Obstetric, neonatal and infant outcome in babies conceived by in vitro maturation (IVM): initial five-year results 1998–2003. 60th Annual Meeting of ASRM, Philadelphia, USA, Fertil Steril 2004; 82(Suppl 2): S133.

58. Cha KY, Chung HM, Lee DR et al. Obstetric outcome of patients with polycystic ovary syndrome treated by in vitro maturation and in vitro fertilization–embryo transfer. Fertil Steril 2005; 83: 1461–5.

59. The American Society for Reproductive Medicine. Guidelines for oocyte donation. Fertil Steril 2004; 82: s13–15.

60. Remohi J, Gartner B, Gallardo E et al. Pregnancy and birth rates after oocyte donation. Fertil Steril 1997; 67: 717–23.

61. The American Society for Reproductive Medicine. Repetitive oocyte donation. Fertil Steril 2004; 82: s158–9.

62. Bennett SJ, Waterstone JJ, Cheng WC et al. Complications of transvaginal ultrasound-directed follicle aspiration: a review of 2670 consecutive procedures, J Assist Reprod Genet 1993; 10: 72–7.

63. Murray C, Golombok S. Oocyte and semen donation: a survey of UK licensed centres. Hum Reprod 2000; 15: 2133–9.

64. Scharf E, Chian RC, Abdul Jalil K et al. In vitro maturation of oocytes: a new option for donor oocyte treatment. Fertil Steril 2004; 82(Supp 2): 514.

65. Cha KY, Koo JJ, Ko JJ et al. Pregnancy after in vitro fertilization of human follicular oocytes collected from nonstimulated cycles, their culture in vitro and their transfer in a donor oocyte program. Fertil Steril 1991; 55: 109–13.

66. Holzer H, Chian RC, Scharf E et al. IVM oocyte donors: oocyte donation without ovarian stimulation. Fertil Steril (submitted).

67. Ao A, Jin S, Rao D et al. First successful pregnancy outcome after preimplantation genetic diagnosis for aneuploidy screening in embryos generated from natural-cycle in vitro fertilization combined with an in vitro maturation procedure. Fertil Steril 2006; 85: 1510 e9–e11.

CHAPTER 16

The first steps in the era of human in-vitro oocyte maturation

Frank L Barnes

...ova maturation and degeneration then proceed pari passu [at an equal pace], and the extent of the former is limited by the degree of advancement of the latter.

Gregory Pincus and Barbara Saunders, 1939

The purpose of this review is to point to the salient contributions to human immature oocyte collection (IOC) and in-vitro oocyte maturation (IVM) by the pioneers and investigators of our field as they are used in those procedures today. We are grateful to all investigators who have added to this body of knowledge. Any lack of reference to them here does not minimize their contribution.

Between 1935 and 1939, Gregory Pincus and coauthors EV Enzman and B Saunders conducted their studies on the maturation of mammalian oocytes[1,2]. In the rabbit pituitary hormones lead to ovulation of the ovarian follicle and the initiation of oocyte maturation in vivo. This was demonstrated by injecting bovine pituitary extracts into the doe. In vivo, mature ova are shed into the oviduct following copulation. When ova were removed from the follicle experimentally and cultured in vitro in the absence of hormones, they spontaneously resumed meiosis and progressed to metaphase II at a rate similar to that observed in vivo. When in-vitro fertilization was induced, the resulting zygotes underwent regular cleavage when allowed to develop in the living oviduct. Care was taken to maintain a proper temperature. High concentrations of sperm were required to bring about fertilization in vitro that in many instances led to polyspermy, which was visibly manifested by aborted early cleavage. That ova spontaneously resumed meiosis when removed from the follicle led to the hypothesis that the follicle may produce substances that inhibit maturation[1]. These findings were quickly extrapolated to the woman, studied, and described. Long and Mark (1911) and Long and Evans (1922) were credited by Pincus and Saunders as having observed that the first maturation division is achieved independent of copulation in spontaneously ovulating mammals[2]. Other investigators had isolated human ova previously; however, it was Pincus and Saunders who observed maturation of the human oocyte. Their studies confirmed that removal of human ova from the follicle initiated the resumption of meiosis and that external stimulation of explanted ova was not required. They concluded that the ability to resume meiosis is not necessarily linked to the ability to complete meiosis[2]. Resumption of meiosis occurs spontaneously upon removal from the follicle, and a 'positive [meiosis] inhibiting factor prevails in vivo.' Finally, oocyte removal from the follicle delays oocyte atresia[1,2]. They believed that the ability of ova to be rescued from advancing follicular atresia might be measured by their ability to mature and fertilize in vitro[2]. This misconception would be held by most investigators for the next 60 years as each would set new developmental thresholds as a measure of complete developmental potential short of live birth. Subsequent studies in years to come would show that the competence to succeed in development is acquired sequentially and, to a limited extent, is temporally associated with egg diameter and follicle size. Embryos derived from IVM ova that fertilize and undergo early cleavage are not all developmentally competent.

In 1965 Bob Edwards, predicted, 'with this technique [IVM] it should eventually be possible to study pre-ovulatory development, and perhaps fertilization and preimplantation development in various species including man'[3]. In his two publications on the topic that year he discussed the importance of selecting appropriate media and introduced TCM-199 to the IVM protocol. TCM-199 is still used widely for the IVM process today and arguably remains the medium of choice. The kinetics of IVM were described in detail for human primary oocytes as well as other species[3,4]. Resumption of meiosis with a synchronous progression, independent of both menstrual cycle day of recovery and gonadotropin support in the IVM medium, was found to occur in over 80% of oocytes. The progression of meiosis as reported is: germinal vesicle breakdown (GVBD) at approximately 25 hours postexplantation (hpe), diakinesis between 25 and 28 hpe, metaphase I between 28 and 35 hpe, and metaphase II between 36 and 43 hpe. Edwards reported that some ova were recovered from the follicle without cumulus and had progressed to metaphase II[4]. This observation suggests that

oocytes are triggered to resume, and in some cases complete, meiosis in the atretic follicle. This is in agreement with studies in cattle where it was subsequently found that oocytes within cohort follicles undergoing atresia spontaneously resume and complete meiosis within the follicle, a process termed pseudo-maturation[5]. Possibly the most important observation made was in his last sentence, 'human oocytes can be fertilized after maturation in vitro.'

Lucinda Veeck and coauthors, from the renowned Jones Clinic, reported an ongoing pregnancy and birth from in-vitro matured oocytes in 1983[6]. The resemblance of the stimulation protocol used in that investigation to FSH and hCG priming protocols used today is remarkable[7–9]. It would next be described in the literature in 1994 when used in cattle and again in 2001 in human IVM[10–13]. Starting on day 3, daily injections of human menopausal gonadotropin (HMG) were given to patients until follicle size reached 12–15 mm as determined by ultrasound. Ten thousand mIU of hCG were administered 50 h after the last hMG injection and followed by egg recovery via laparoscopy 36–38 h later. Immature oocytes were cultured for 22 to 35 hours and inseminated. Frequencies of IVM, fertilization, and the number of cleaving zygotes were at least 80%[6]. Their report suggests but does not specifically state, that many immature oocytes identified at the time of recovery matured within 24 h of in-vitro culture in gonadotropin free medium. This may be the first recorded observation indicating that maturation may progress from the germinal vesicle stage to metaphase II within 24 h of in-vitro culture if hCG is administered to the patient 36 h prior to IOC. The rate of maturation observed would agree with that reported by Chian et al. 16 years later using hCG priming[8]. This observation indicates that hCG administration does not lead to overt IVM in small to medium sized follicles. However, over the course of the ensuing 36 h before recovery it prepares the oocyte for what may appear to be accelerated maturation in-vitro. This suggests that gonadotropin supplementation of the IVM medium as used by subsequent investigators may not be required if the trigger to resume meiosis is initiated in vivo. Of note was that the recovery of immature oocytes occurred in the absence of a dominant follicle, a significant point that would recur and become a dominant theme in subsequent successful protocols. Assisted reproductive technology took a distinct turn away from IVM at this point to favor the more common strategy of recovering and fertilizing mature oocytes. In the late 1990s several groups would similarly report pregnancies from stimulated patients with and without administration of hCG[14–16]. Nonetheless, the threshold of producing a child from an IVM oocyte had been crossed.

Cha and coworkers (1991, also as a prize paper reported at American Society for Reproductive Medicine 1989) made the link between IVM protocols used in sheep and cattle to an experimental protocol used for the treatment of human infertility[17]. In their original work, oocytes were recovered from patients undergoing gynecologic surgery and subsequently donated to their IVF program. Performed in situ, aspiration of antral follicles occurred using a 21-gauge needle attached to a syringe containing medium supplemented with 10% fetal cord serum[17]. If oophorectomy was performed, oocytes were recovered by repeatedly slicing and subsequently rinsing the cortical tissue (personal communication). The maturation protocol used Ham's F10 medium supplemented with either 20% fetal cord serum or 50% mature follicular fluid (heat inactivated)[17]. Subsequent protocols from the same laboratory would use TCM-199 supplemented with pregnant mare serum gonadotropin with hCG or rFSH with hCG and estradiol[18]. A triplet pregnancy occurred after transfer of five embryos to a patient with premature ovarian failure. The paper was of particular importance as it renewed interest in using IVM as an infertility treatment modality[17].

Alan Trounson foresaw the significance of the IVM technology as it might apply to the treatment of infertile patients suffering from polycystic ovarian syndrome (PCOS)[19]. His enthusiasm for the technique and its possibilities was the inspiration for many lectures around the world during the 1990s. His historic understanding of IVM as it is applied to livestock gave him immediate insight into procedure development[20]. In cooperation with Cook Australia, Trounson, Carl Wood, and other colleagues at Monash IVF defined a protocol for ultrasound guided follicle aspiration of human immature oocytes. During their initial investigation, they developed a more rigid needle with a thicker wall and shorter bevel. The increased rigidity facilitated penetration of the ovarian cortical stroma of PCO patients; the shortened bevel allowed the entire lumen of the needle to be placed inside the antral cavity of small follicles. The aspiration pressure used at oocyte collection was reduced to half that used in standard IVF (7.5 kPa vs 15 kPa). This was believed to reduce the amount of granulosa cells that would be stripped from the oocyte during aspiration. Aspirates were recovered in Hepes buffered HTF medium supplemented with heparin[19]. Cumulus–oocyte complexes (COCs) were isolated by filtration through an embryo-concentrating filter, methodology originating from the bovine embryo transfer industry. Fresh medium was used to rinse away red blood cells and other debris then the filter retentant was poured into a 100 mm dish for COC isolation using a dissecting microscope. The collection and isolation protocol described by Trounson et al. has been used extensively in subsequent studies in other laboratories. The observation times used and rate of maturation observed were similar to that first reported by Edwards in 1965[4]. GVBD occurred in greater than 80% of oocytes at 21 to 22 h, with 81% mature by 48 to 54 h. Initially, insemination was performed at 44–54 h. It was noted that some oocytes were mature after only 23 to 25 h of culture. Postulating that early maturing oocytes would have the best developmental competence, subsequent insemination times were moved to ~35 h. Maturation and fertilization frequencies were similar across ovulatory and anovulatory polycystic ovary syndrome (PCO(S)) groups and ovulatory patients. The rate of embryo development in PCO patients was retarded, suggesting suboptimal culture conditions or intrinsic defects in developmental competence[19]. Their publications provided the essential methodology used in immature oocyte collection and IVM around the world today.

In a series of two publications, Barnes et al. from the Monash IVF laboratory would reintroduce the use of TCM 199, as first used by Edwards, to the maturation protocol[4,21,22]. They would also introduce intracytoplasmic sperm injection (ICSI), blastocyst culture, and assisted hatching and characterize embryo development of PCO(S) and ovulatory non-PCO(S) patients. Their publication indicated that IVM oocytes from ovulatory non-PCO(S) patients had equivocal early cleavage development when compared to stimulated patients where maturation occurred in vivo. A single pregnancy and live birth was reported from the study series; the outcome clearly indicated that good embryo morphology is not an adequate measure of oocyte developmental competence[21,22].

In 1999 Cobo et al.[23] and Mikkelsen et al.[7] simultaneously began focusing on the timing of immature oocyte collection, both having identified the trigger point for retrieval to be before the lead follicle achieves 10 mm. While Mikkelsen et al.[7] principally focused on the effect of FSH priming and would eventually demonstrate the merits of the protocol in subsequent publications, their consideration of follicle dominance in this initial work proved to be insightful. Cobo et al. principally focused on the time of aspiration, correlating it to the emergence of the dominant follicle. They postulated that the visible emergence of the dominant follicle may lead to changes in the follicular endocrine milieu of the cohort that would be detrimental to their subsequent developmental potential. The frequency of oocytes that were atretic, with cumulus cover, matured and fertilized in vitro, did not differ

between predominance and postdominance recovery groups. However, significantly more oocytes were recovered and development to blastocyst was improved in the predominance group with cumulus cover[23]. The point was made that early egg and embryo morphology is a poor predictor of developmental potential. The studies of Cobo and colleagues demonstrated that the trigger point for follicle aspiration is a critical component in the IOC/IVM procedure[23]. Mikkelsen and colleagues showed that by using dominant follicle selection to determine the time of IOC, developmentally competent oocytes and live births would result[7]. Both studies were successful for what appears to be the same reason.

Is it possible that oocytes lose developmental competence in the reverse order that they acquire it? Hypothetically, mRNA and proteins that have a specific purpose in early development have temporal limitations while other housekeeping mRNA and proteins are relatively stable. This may lead to the appearance of a reverse loss in the ability to develop. For example: early cleavage, up to the eight-cell stage, is driven by mRNA and proteins derived from the maternal genome. It is likely that embryonic development fails because advanced atresia induces a fundamental decay of these components. Studies using ultrasound (u/s) to evaluate follicle dynamics show that cohort follicles shrink in diameter dramatically within 1 to 2 days of the visible emergence of a dominant follicle[24], suggesting a rapidly advancing atretic process in that population. Therefore embryos derived from postdominance IVM oocytes maintain the ability to resume and complete meiosis, fertilize, and cleave into what we may perceive to be good embryos, but in fact have lost the ability to develop beyond those early cleavage stages. A difference in oocyte recovery of a mere 48 h may be all that separates developmentally competent from incompetent oocytes.

In further exploring the treatment of PCO(S) patients, Chian et al. introduced hCG priming[8]. PCO(S) patients were staged for IOC/IVM with progesterone induced withdrawal bleeding followed by u/s monitoring to exclude patients with a dominant follicle. Human chorionic gonadotropin was given 36 h prior to egg retrieval on cycle days 10 to 12. The principal finding was that hCG priming increased the number of immature oocytes that would progress from the germinal vesicle stage to the metaphase II stage within the first 24 h of IVM[8]. This suggests again that the signal initiating the resumption of meiosis is initiated in vivo.

There are essentially two methodologies that appear to lead to improved developmental competence of IVM oocytes. The first relies on the ability of an oocyte recovered at the time of dominant follicle selection to spontaneously resume and complete meiosis in vitro within approximately 24–30 h of culture. The second relies on hCG priming, which may recruit oocytes that also resume and complete meiosis in vitro within approximately 24–30 h. The paracrine signal resulting from dominant follicle selection or hCG priming likely prepares for and/or initiates the resumption of meiosis of the cohort in vivo. The resulting in-vitro accelerated maturation rate in both protocols provides a valuable selection method, optimizing oocyte developmental potential.

The first steps in the era of human IVM have, after nearly 70 years, achieved clinical significance. The methodology comes together in a recent work by Soderstrom-Anttiila and colleagues[25], which embraces the ideology of the investigators who preceded them. The ovary contains a large supply of developmentally competent oocytes that, upon explantation from ovarian follicles, can be matured and fertilized in vitro and develop into healthy children. The process of immature oocyte recovery and IVM should be simple and easy to apply and minimally invasive to the patient. Their clinical protocol starts with definitive parameters for when to recover immature oocytes: the day following the observation of a leading follicle (dominant follicle selection) in cycling patients or in PCO(S)

patients when endometrial thickness reaches 5 mm following progesterone-induced withdrawal bleeding but before dominant follicle selection. Maturation using TCM-199 supplemented with patient serum and gonadotropins is followed by in-vitro fertilization (by insemination or ICSI) of those oocytes that are mature within 30 h of culture. Finally the transfer of one or two morphologically superior embryos to the prepared endometrium (oral estrogen followed by vaginal progesterone) is performed[25]. As measured by implantation rates of greater than 20%, the success of this protocol would appear to equal that of current IVF protocols.

When selecting human oocytes with the potential for totipotent development, timing appears to be everything. While maturation in vitro can take 36–48 h, it is when oocytes mature within 24 h in vitro that reported pregnancy outcomes are best. The outlined studies suggest that it is when we collect primary oocytes and not how we mature them in vitro that ultimately leads to success. That oocytes acquire developmental competence briefly and lose it in the course of follicle atresia reflects the insight of Pincus and Saunders who stated[2] 'ova maturation and degeneration then proceed pari passu, and the extent of the former is limited by the degree of advancement of the latter.'

REFERENCES

1. Pincus G, Enzmann EV. The comparative behavior of mammalian eggs in vivo and in vitro. I The activation of ovarian eggs. J Exp Med 1935; 62: 665–75.

2. Pincus G, Saunders B. The comparative behavior of mammalian eggs in vivo and in vitro. VI The maturation of human ovarian ova. Anat Rec 1939; 75: 537–45.

3. Edwards RG. Maturation in vitro of mouse, sheep, cow, pig, rhesus monkey and human ovarian oocytes. Nature 1965; 208: 349–51.

4. Edwards RG. Maturation in vitro of human ovarian oocytes. Lancet 1965; 286: 926–9.

5. Assey RJ, Hyttel P, Greve T et al. Oocyte morphology in dominant and subordinate follicles. Mol Reprod Dev 1994; 37: 335–44.

6. Veeck LL, Wortham JWE, Witmyer J et al. Maturation and fertilization of morphologically immature human oocytes in a program of *in vitro* fertilization. Fertil Steril 1983; 39: 594–602.

7. Mikkelsen A, Smith S, Lindenberg S. In-vitro maturation of human oocytes from regularly menstruating women may be successful without follicle stimulating hormone priming. Hum Reprod 1999; 14: 1847–51.

8. Chian RC, Buckett WM, Too LL et al. Pregnancies resulting from *in vitro* matured oocytes retrieved from patients with polycystic ovary syndrome after priming with human chorionic gonadotropin. Fertil Steril 1999; 72: 639–42.

9. Suikkari AM, Tulppala M, Tuuri T et al. Luteal phase start of low-dose FSH priming of follicles results in an efficient recovery, maturation and fertilization of immature human oocytes. Hum Reprod 2000; 15: 747–51.

10. Looney CR, Lindsay BR, Gonseth CL et al. Commercial aspects of oocyte retrieval and *in vitro* fertilization (IVF) for embryo production in the problem cow. Theriogenology 1994; 41: 67–72.

11. Blondin P, Guilbault LA, Sirard MA. The time interval between FSH-P administration and slaughter can influence the developmental competence of beer heifer oocytes. Theriogenology 1997; 48: 803–13.

12. Sirard MA, Picard L, Dery M et al. The time interval between FSH aspiration and ovarian aspiration influences the development of cattle oocytes. Theriogenology 1999; 51: 699–709.

13. Mikkelsen AL, Lindenberg S. Benefit of FSH priming of women with PCOS to the *in vitro* maturation procedure and the outcome: a ramdomized prospective study. Reproduction 2001; 122: 587–92.

14. Nagy ZP, Janssenwillen C, Liu J et al. Pregnancy and birth after intracytoplasmic sperm injection of *in vitro* matured germinal-vesicle stage oocytes: case report. Fertil Steril 1996; 65: 47–50.

15. Jaroudi KA, Hollanders JM, Sieck UV et al. Pregnancy after transfer of embryos which were generated from in-vitro matured oocytes. Hum Reprod 1997; 12: 857–9.

16. Liu J, Katz E, Garcia JE et al. Successful *in vitro* maturation of human oocytes not exposed to human chorionic gonadotropin during ovulation induction, resulting in pregnancy. Fertil Steril 1997; 67: 556–8.

17. Cha KY, Koo JJ, Ko JJ et al. Pregnancy after *in vitro* fertilization of human follicular oocytes collected from non-stimulated cycles, their culture *in vitro* and their transfer in a donor oocyte program. Fertil Steril 1991; 55: 109–13.

18. Cha KY, Chung HM, Lee DR et al. Obstetric outcome of patients with polycystic ovary syndrome treated by *in vitro* maturation and *in vitro* fertilization–embryo transfer. Fertil Steril 2005; 83: 1461–5.

19. Trounson AO, Wood C, Kausche A. *In vitro* maturation and the fertilization and developmental competence of oocytes recovered from untreated polycystic ovarian patients. Fertil Steril 1994; 62: 353–62.

20. Moor RM, Trounson AO. Hormonal and follicular factors affecting maturation of sheep oocytes in vitro and their subsequent developmental capacity. J Reprod Fert 1977; 49: 101–9.

21. Barnes FL, Crombie A, Gardner DK et al. Blastocyst development and birth after in vitro maturation of human primary oocytes, intracytoplasmic sperm injection and assisted hatching. Hum Reprod 1995; 10: 3243–7.

22. Barnes FL, Kausche A, Tiglias J et al. Production of embryos from *in vitro* matured primary human oocytes. Fertil Steril 1996; 65: 151–6.

23. Cobo AC, Requena A, Neuspiller F et al. Maturation *in vitro* of human oocytes from unstimulated cycles: selection of the optimal day for ovum retrieval based on follicular size. Hum Reprod 1999; 14: 1864–8.

24. Baerwald AR, Adams GP, Pierson RA. A new model for ovarian follicular development during the human menstral cycle. Fertil Steril 2003; 80: 116–22.

25. Soderstrom-Anttiila V, Makinen S, Tuuri T et al. Favorable pregnancy results with insemination of *in vitro* matured oocytes from unstimulated patients. Hum Reprod 2005; 20: 1534–40.

CHAPTER 17

FSH priming in IVM cycles

Anne Lis Mikkelsen

BACKGROUND

The experience in handling immature oocytes has been obtained from two main groups. The first group is women suffering from polycystic ovarian syndrome (PCOS), as these women are extremely sensitive to stimulation with follicle stimulating hormone (FSH) in assisted reproduction, and they have a significant risk of developing ovarian hyperstimulation syndrome (OHSS). The second group is regularly cycling women with normal ovaries referred for in-vitro fertilization (IVF) or intracytoplasmic sperm injection (ICSI). In both groups aspiration of immature oocytes has been performed in unstimulated cycles and after priming with FSH, and/or after priming with human chorionic gonadotropin (hCG) before aspiration. In this chapter the experience obtained after handling immature oocytes after FSH priming is summarized.

Immature oocytes can be obtained from women who are undergoing routine superovulated IVF (rescue in-vitro maturation, IVM). During controlled ovarian hyperstimulation the oocyte population may be heterogeneous and this leads to retrieval of oocytes at different stages of maturation. About 15% of oocytes will remain in prophase I of meiosis. These oocytes can be matured in vitro and develop into viable embryos. In 1983, Veeck and co-workers[1] reported two pregnancies from transfer of embryos developed from immature oocytes obtained from stimulated cycles in their IVF program. Several groups have since made similar reports[2,3]. These oocytes failed to mature although the follicles were exposed to supraphysiologic concentrations of FSH and may represent an inferior population of oocytes. Therefore these clinical cases are not included in this review.

IMMATURE OOCYTES OBTAINED FROM WOMEN WITH PCOS

No priming

Trounson et al.[4] described the first pregnancy with immature oocyte retrieval and subsequent in-vitro maturation (IVM) in a woman with PCOS. The following year another pregnancy was reported in a patient with PCOS treated with IVM, combined with ICSI and assisted hatching[5,6]. Barnes et al.[6] compared rates of maturation, fertilization, and cleavage between untreated regularly ovulating and irregularly ovulating or anovulatory polycystic women. In almost all the parameters analyzed, oocytes from regularly cycling patients performed better. However, the reasons for this were not determined.

Later Cha et al.[7] reported a pregnancy rate of 27.1%. However this high pregnancy rate was obtained after transfer of an average 6.3 embryos per patient, and the implantation rate was still low (6.9%). To compensate for this, endogenous priming with FSH[8,9] or hCG[10,11] has been suggested before immature oocyte retrieval and subsequent IVM.

Priming with FSH

It has been postulated that FSH stimulation before oocyte retrieval might increase either the number of immature oocytes retrieved or the maturational potential and developmental competence of these oocytes. Suikkari et al.[8] proposed using low-dose (37.5 IU) recombinant FSH (rFSH) from the previous luteal phase until the leading follicle reached 10 mm. This resulted in maturation and fertilization rates in women with PCOS comparable with those in regularly cycling women, however no pregnancies were achieved in 12 patients.

A beneficial effect of higher dose FSH priming was, however, found in a later prospective randomized study[9]. Oocytes obtained after priming with rFSH (150 IU per day) for 3 days were compared with oocytes obtained in unstimulated cycles. FSH priming resulted in an improved pregnancy rate (29% vs. 0%) and implantation rate (21.6% vs. 0%) compared with the non-primed group. This was partly explained by the increased size of the folllicles in the primed group compared to the non-primed group. Previous studies have demonstrated that human oocytes appear to have a size dependent ability to resume meiosis and complete maturation[12].

Furthermore, it has been hypothesized that oocyte differentiation may be incomplete during follicular growth, and that oocytes from plateau phase follicles have increased competence[13]. Therefore, not only FSH priming but also the following FSH deprivation caused by withholding exogenous FSH should enhance the competence of the oocytes.

Priming with hCG

In 1999 Chian et al.[14] reported that giving 10 000 IU of hCG 36 hours before oocyte retrieval improved the maturation rate of immature oocytes from PCOS women. In a prospective randomized study they later demonstrated that hCG priming not only improved the maturation rate, but also hastened the maturation process[10]. Pregnancy rates of 30–35% and implantation rates of 10–15% have been reported using hCG priming[15,16]. Additional FSH priming (75 IU per day for 6 days initiated on day 3), however, did not further improve the pregnancy rate or the implantation rate[16].

IMMATURE OOCYTES FROM REGULARLY CYCLING WOMEN WITH NORMAL OVARIES

No priming

Control of the menstrual cycle is a complex process involving both the hypothalamic–pituitary axis as well as local (paracrine and endocrine) factors. The follicles destined to ovulate will be selected from a cohort of follicles, which enter the follicular phase of the menstrual cycles with a diameter of 2–6 mm. The selected follicle will grow to a diameter of 20–25 mm at the time of ovulation. Circulating levels of FSH and LH regulate the follicular growth and development. The rise in serum FSH levels during the early follicular phase causes a cohort of follicles responsive to FSH stimulation to grow and the dominant follicle can be distinguished from other cohort follicles by size (>10 mm diameter). Synthesis of estradiol is closely linked to development of the preovulatory follicle and the concentrations of estradiol in the follicle and serum correlate significantly with the size of the follicle. The increase in the concentration of estradiol is the principal factor for establishment of dominance. It has a negative feedback on the hypothalamus axis with a subsequent decrease in the level of FSH. The dominant follicle withstands this decline, while subordinate follicles are susceptible to a decline in gonadotropins and these follicles undergo atresia. The subordinate follicles, however, can be rescued and thereby avoid atresia by stimulatory treatments with FSH or by retrieval of these immature oocytes and their subsequent IVM.

The timing of oocyte aspiration in unstimulated cycles may be critical, allowing as many follicles as possible to reach sufficient size for cytoplasmic competence of the oocytes[17], while avoiding a prolonged negative effect of the developing dominant follicle. The first births from IVM of immature oocytes from unstimulated cycles used oocytes that had been retrieved at different times in the menstrual cycle[6,18–20].

Up to the point of dominant follicle selection all oocytes in the cohort undergo processes such as RNA transcription, protein synthesis, and organelle modifications and redistributions that prepare them for the potential of resumption of meiosis and eventual fertilization. Mikkelsen et al.[21–23] aimed to coincide oocyte collection with selection of the dominant follicle. Oocytes were aspirated after a leading follicle of 10 mm and an endometrial thickness of at least 5 mm were observed at ultrasound. A pregnancy rate of 18–24% per transfer was obtained in cycles with a detected increase in the level of estradiol on the day of aspiration. Oocytes originating from the ipsilateral ovary did not show an impaired competence to mature and cleave compared to oocytes originating from the contralateral ovary[23].

FSH priming

A few studies have examined the effect of priming with FSH before aspiration of immature oocytes in regularly menstruating women[8,16,23–25]. The series are small and a variety of stimulation regimens have been used, therefore only limited information can be drawn.

Wynn et al.[24] administered 600 IU rFSH to women over 5 days (300 IU on day 2, 150 IU on day 4, and 150 IU on day 6). A mean of 7.5 oocytes were retrieved from rFSH compared with 5.2 from unprimed women. Wynn et al.[24] did not perform fertilization of the oocytes and no conclusions concerning the developmental capacity of the oocytes can be drawn from that experiment.

Later studies of the treatment of women for 1 or 3 days with rFSH early in the follicular phase showed no difference in recovery rate of oocytes, or rates of maturation, fertilization, or cleavage in culture[17]. This was confirmed in a prospective randomized study[25]. In one group oocytes were aspirated after priming with rFSH (150 IU per day) for 3 days followed by deprivation for 2–3 days. In the other group oocytes were obtained in unstimulated cycles and the day of aspiration was fixed in the same way (after a follicle of 10 mm could be demonstrated). FSH priming did not increase the number of oocytes recovered and no benefit of FSH priming compared to the natural cycle on the maturation rate, fertilization rate, cleavage rate, or pregnancy rate could be demonstrated.

Studies in cattle indicate an advantage of using moderate follicle stimulation followed by a period of FSH deprivation to obtain optimal embryo production from bovine oocytes[13]. Similar studies in humans are lacking. Mikkelsen et al.[26] compared 2 vs. 3 days of priming and were unable to demonstrate any difference in the implantation rate between the two groups.

CONCLUSIONS

Recent data taken together suggest that in future immature oocyte retrieval combined with IVM could possibly replace standard stimulated IVF in selected patients. Priming with FSH for 3 days followed by deprivation for 2–3 days before harvesting of immature oocytes from patients with PCOS may improve the maturational potential of the oocytes and the implantation rate of the cleaved embryos. No beneficial effect of FSH priming has been observed in regularly cycling women[25]. In unstimulated cycles the recovery of oocytes has to coincide with selection of the dominant follicle. In stimulated cycles a time interval between FSH administration and aspiration has been found to improve the developmental capacity of oocytes.

REFERENCES

1. Veeck LL, Wortham JW, Witmeyer J et al. Maturation and fertilization of morphologically immature human oocytes in a program of in vitro fertilization. Fertil Steril 1983; 39: 594–602.

2. Nagy ZP, Cecile J, Liu J et al. Pregnancy and birth after intracytoplasmic sperm injection of *in vitro* matured germinal vesicle stage oocytes:case report. Fertil Steril 1996; 65: 1047–50.

3. Liu J, Katz E, Garcia JE et al. Successful in vitro maturation of human oocytes not exposed to human chorionic gonadotropin during ovulation induction, resulting in pregnancy. Fertil Steril 1997; 67: 566–8.

4. Trounson A, Wood C, Kausche A. In vitro maturation and the fertilization and developmental competence of oocytes recovered from untreated polycystic ovarian patients. Fertil Steril 1994; 62: 353–62.

5. Barnes FL, Crombie A, Gardner DK et al. Blastocyst development and birth after in vitro maturation of human primary oocytes, intracytoplasmic sperm injection and assisted hatching. Hum Reprod 1995; 10: 3243–7.

6. Barnes FL, Kausche A, Tiglias J et al. Production of embryos from in vitro matured primary human oocytes. Fertil Steril 1996; 65: 1151–6.

7. Cha KY, Han SY, Chung HM et al. Pregnancies and deliveries after in vitro maturation culture followed by in vitro fertilization and embryo transfer without stimulation in women with polycystic ovary syndrom. Fertil Steril 2000; 73: 978–83.

8. Suikkari A-M, Tulppala M, Tuuri T et al. Lutheal phase start of low-dose FSH priming of follicles results in an efficient recovery, maturation and fertilization of immature human oocytes. Hum Reprod 2000; 15: 747–51.

9. Mikkelsen AL, Lindenberg S. Benefit of FSH priming of women with PCOS to the in vitro maturation procedure and the outcome. A randomized prospective study. Reproduction 2001; 122: 587–92.

10. Chian RC, Buckett WM, Tulandi T et al. Prospective randomized study of human chorionic gonadotrophin priming before immature oocyte retrieval from unstimulated women with polycystic ovarian syndrome. Hum Reprod 2000; 15: 165–70.

11. Child TJ, Guleki B, Abdul-Jalil AK et al. In vitro maturation and fertilization of oocytes from unstimulated normal ovaries, polycystic ovaries, and women with polycystic ovarian syndrome. Fertil Steril 2001; 76: 936–42.

12. Durenzi KL, Wentz AC, Saniga EM et al. Follicle stimulating hormone effects on immature oocytes: in-vitro maturation and hormone production. J Assist Reprod Genet 1997; 14: 199–204.

13. Barnes FL, Sirard MA. Oocyte maturation. Semin Reprod Med 2000; 18: 123–31.

14. Chian RC, Gulekli B, Buckett WM et al. Priming with human chorionic gonadotropin before retrieval of immature oocytes in women with infertility due to polycystic ovary syndrome. N Engl J Med 1999; 341: 1624–6.

15. Chian RC. In-vitro maturation of immature oocytes for infertile women with PCOS. RBM Online 2004; 8: 547–52.

16. Lin YH, Hwang JL, Huang LW et al. Combination of FSH priming and hCG priming for in-vitro maturation of human oocytes. Hum Reprod 2003; 18: 1632–6.

17. Trounson A, Anderiesz C, Jones G. Maturation of human oocytes in vitro and their developmental competence. Reproduction 2001; 121: 51–75.

18. Russell JB, Knezevich KM, Fabian K et al. Unstimulated immature oocyte retrieval: early versus midfollicular endometrial priming. Fertil Steril 1997; 67: 616–20.

19. Thornton MH, Francis MM, Paulson RJ. Immature oocyte retrieval: lessons from unstimulated IVF cycles. Fertil Steril 1998; 70: 647–50.

20. Cobo AC, Requena A, Neuspiller F et al. Maturation in vitro of human oocytes from unstimulated cycles: selection of the optimal day for ovum retrieval based on follicular size. Hum Reprod 1999; 14: 1864–8.

21. Mikkelsen AL, Smith S, Lindenberg S. Impact of oestradiol and inhibin A concentrations on pregnancy rate in in-vitro oocyte maturation. Hum Reprod 2000; 15: 1685–90.

22. Mikkelsen AL, Andersson AM, Skakkebæk NE et al. Basal concentrations of oestradiol may predict the outcome of IVM in regular menstruating women. Hum Reprod 2001; 16: 862–7.

23. Mikkelsen AL, Lindenberg S. Influence of the dominant follicle on in vitro maturation of human oocytes. RBM Online 2001; 3: 199–204.

24. Wynn P, Picton HM, Krapez J et al. Pretreatment with follicle stimulating hormone promotes the number of human oocytes reaching metaphase II by in-vitro maturation. Hum Reprod 1998; 13: 3132–8.

25. Mikkelsen AL, Smith SD, Lindenberg S. In vitro maturation of human oocytes from regular menstruating women may be successful without FSH priming. Hum Reprod 1999; 14: 1847–51.

26. Mikkelsen AL, Høst E, Blaabjerg J et al. Time interval between FSH priming and aspiration of immature oocytes for in-vitro maturation: a prospective randomized study. RBM Online 2003; 16: 416–20.

CHAPTER 18

Combination of FSH priming and hCG priming in IVM cycles

Jiann-Loung Hwang and Yu-Hung Lin

INTRODUCTION

After birth, human oocytes remain at prophase I of meiosis until they are stimulated by gonadotropin to resume meiosis before ovulation. Throughout a woman's lifetime, only a few hundred oocytes will complete meiosis and maturation and be ovulated, while the majority of oocytes will undergo apoptosis. In conventional assisted reproductive technologies, ovarian stimulation is usually utilized to increase the number of available oocytes and embryos, and therefore the pregnancy rate. However, the use of stimulation drugs increases the patient's cost and suffering, and is associated with side-effects such as nausea, abdominal pain, mood swings, menopausal symptoms, ovarian hyperstimulation syndrome (OHSS), and a potential cancer risk. The recovery of immature oocytes followed by in-vitro maturation (IVM) and fertilization is an attractive alternative because it reduces the patient's cost and suffering and avoids the side-effects associated with ovarian stimulation.

Another application of IVM is preservation of women's fertility, especially for those who are going to undergo cancer treatment. Cryopreservation of immature oocytes or ovarian tissue, coupled with IVM, is a potential way to preserve fertility, although the successful cases are limited[1]. Immature oocytes can also be a new source of oocyte donation. Pregnancies resulting from immature oocyte donation have been reported from oophorectomy specimens[2], during cesarean section[3], and from woman with polycystic ovaries[4].

OOCYTE MATURATION

Oocyte maturation is a complex process that comprises nuclear maturation and cytoplasmic maturation. Nuclear maturation refers to the resumption of meiosis and progression from germinal vesicle breakdown (GVBD) to metaphase II (MII). Cytoplasmic maturation refers to the preparation of oocyte cytoplasm for fertilization and embryonic development[5]. GVBD is initiated by the preovulatory surge of LH. LH probably induces GVBD by an indirect action mediated by cumulus cells. The oocyte and the cumulus cells are coupled by gap junctions. Inhibitory factors are transported from the cumulus cells to the oocytes to maintain meiotic arrest of the oocytes. Some evidence suggests cyclic adenosine monophosphate (cAMP) as a potential inhibitor of meiotic resumption[6,7]. It was speculated that LH causes dissociation of the cumulus cells and the oocyte, and thus terminates the flow of the meiosis-inhibiting substances into the oocyte[5]. It is also possible that LH induces the production of a GVBD-inducing signal in the cumulus cells that is subsequently transferred to the oocyte through the gap junctions[8]. Cytoplasmic maturation involves complicated processes that prepare the oocyte for activation, fertilization, and development. During this process, RNA molecules, proteins, and imprinted genes are accumulated in the cytoplasm to regulate oocyte meiosis and development[9]. Insufficient cytoplasmic maturation will fail to promote male pronucleus formation and will increase chromosomal abnormalities after fertilization[10].

HISTORY OF HUMAN IVM

In 1935, Pincus and Enzmann found that rabbit oocytes, when liberated from Graafian follicles, would undergo spontaneous meiotic maturation in vitro[11]. Edwards demonstrated in 1965 that human oocytes removed from follicles could mature in medium supplemented with serum[12]. The first human birth resulting from IVM was reported by Cha et al. in 1991[2]. They obtained immature oocytes from oophorectomy specimens. After maturation in vitro, the oocytes were donated to a woman of premature menopause, and a set of triplets was born. In 1994, Trounson et al.[13] reported the first birth from IVM in PCOS women, and he developed a special aspiration needle for immature oocyte retrieval. However, the maturation rate of human IVM was about 30–50%[2,14,15], which was much lower than that of other species, and the pregnancies resulting from IVM were limited. In addition, Trounson et al.[16] demonstrated that the in-vitro matured human oocytes had reduced developmental competence. The poor outcome of human IVM was thought to be at least partly due to abnormalities of cytoplasmic maturation in in-vitro matured oocytes. Several treatment modalities have been proposed to improve the outcome of human IVM.

FSH PRIMING

The early studies on human IVM did not use gonadotropin before oocyte retrieval. Since FSH acts on cumulus cells and promotes steroid production, oocyte RNA, and protein synthesis[17], it has been postulated that pretreatment with FSH might increase either the number of immature oocytes recovered or the maturation potential and developmental competence of the oocytes.

In a study performed on rhesus monkeys, FSH priming for 6–7 days enhanced nuclear and cytoplasmic maturation of oocytes in vitro[18]. In comparison to the non-stimulated monkeys, greater percentages of oocytes completed meiotic maturation (74% vs. 41%), were fertilized (85% vs. 61%), and cleaved to the two–four-cell stage embryos (79% vs. 38%) in the FSH-primed monkeys.

The effects of FSH priming on human IVM were contradictory. Gómez et al.[19], in a small series, found that only 16.7% of immature oocytes obtained from non-stimulated ovaries reached MII after 48 h. The percentages of immature oocytes from stimulated cycles (with HMG) that reached MII were 50% at 24 hours and 87.5% at 48 hours, which were comparable with animal studies. They speculated that the intrafollicular environment induced by FSH may be able to generate the protein synthesis involved in oocyte maturation.

Wynn et al. gave a truncated course of 600 IU FSH (300 IU on day 2, 150 IU on days 4 and 6) to normal women; after which, a significantly greater percentage of oocytes completed meiotic maturation in vitro (71.1% vs. 43.5%) and higher serum estradiol (E_2) concentrations on the day of oocyte retrieval were found after FSH treatment (1049 ± 241 pg/ml vs. 154 ± 17 pg/ml). Immature oocyte numbers and endometrial thickness were not significantly different[20].

Cha and Chian[5] demonstrated that the time courses of germinal vesicle breakdown (GVBD) and oocyte maturation were faster in the oocytes retrieved from stimulated ovaries, although the final percentages of GVBD and MII oocytes were not different between stimulated and unstimulated ovaries. Mikkelsen and Lindenberg pretreated PCOS women with 150 IU FSH per day for 3 days from day 3, and they found that the maturation rate was significantly higher in the FSH-primed group (59%) compared with the non-primed group (44%). There were no significant differences in the rates of fertilization and embryo cleavage between the two groups[21]. However, in another similar study on normal cyclic women, FSH priming did not increase the number of oocytes obtained and did not improve the maturation and cleavage rates or embryo development[22]. Similarly, Trounson et al. found no significant differences in the number of oocytes recovered, maturation rate, fertilization rate, and embryo development in patients pretreated with 1 day or 3 days of 150 IU recombinant FSH compared to patients without treatment[16].

Jaroudi et al.[23] reported 21 IVM cycles in women who were at risk of OHSS (with too many follicles or high serum E_2 levels). The women were stimulated with gonadotropin-releasing hormone agonist (GnRHa) on long or short protocols. Oocyte retrieval was performed, without hCG injection, when leading follicles were <15 mm. No MII oocytes were obtained at oocyte retrieval. The maturation rate was 70.8%, and the fertilization rate was 58.7% with ICSI. However, only two pregnancies (9.5%) were obtained.

In a bovine study it was found that, although superovulation with FSH increased follicular size and decreased atresia, the oocytes were developmentally less competent[24]. It was speculated that superovulation forced the follicles into an accelerated growing phase, leaving the oocytes with insufficient time to acquire competence. In humans, it has also been found that HMG stimulation results in follicular asynchrony[25]. Therefore the role of FSH priming in IVM seems inconclusive and contradictory. Whether normal

women and PCOS women respond differently to FSH priming is also unknown.

hCG PRIMING

In the final stages of follicular maturation, the LH surge initiates the continuation of meiosis in the oocyte and luteinization of the granulosa cells. Because of their structural similarity, hCG has been used in assisted reproduction to mimic the endogenous LH surge. Since the LH surge or hCG injection induces final oocyte maturation, it is tempting to give hCG before oocyte retrieval in IVM cycles.

In 1999, Chian et al.[26] reported a series of 25 IVM cycles in PCOS women. By giving 10 000 IU of hCG 36 h before oocyte retrieval, they obtained an impressive pregnancy rate of 40%. In their other randomized study to compare the outcome of IVM with and without hCG priming, the maturation process was faster in the hCG-primed group[27]. At the time of oocyte retrieval, GVBD had occurred in 46.2% of oocytes in the hCG-primed group, but in none in the non-hCG-primed group. The percentage of MII oocytes after 48 h of culture was higher in the hCG-primed group (84.3%) than in the non-hCG-primed group (69.1%), although the rates of fertilization and cleavage and embryo quality were similar between the two groups.

The mechanism of hCG priming in improving the outcome of IVM is not clear. It was hypothesized that follicles might possess hCG receptors to respond to hCG priming[28]. During ovarian stimulation, hCG is used to substitute for LH to induce final oocyte maturation. Besides inducing GVBD, LH also causes cumulus expansion by secreting a hyaluronic acid-rich proteoglycan matrix[29]. Indeed, we found that many cumulus–oocyte complexes (COC) obtained after hCG priming were class 3 (slight expansion in outer layers of cumulus) in Hazeleger's classification of bovine COC[30], which was shown to have the highest developmental rate[31]. This is in contrast to our previous experience of IVM without hCG priming, in which most of the COC were cumulus compact. This implies that hCG can initiate the oocyte maturation process in small follicles.

Trounson et al.[32] questioned whether the oocytes obtained after hCG priming were really 'immature' since they have demonstrated that mature oocytes could be obtained even from 6-mm follicles. However, no oocytes obtained at oocyte retrieval were MII in Chian's studies and in our experience. Barnes et al. found that the maturation, fertilization, and cleavage rates were higher in women with regular cycles than in PCOS women. They thought the reason may be related to elevated androgen levels in follicular fluid in PCOS women[33]. It has also been shown with murine oocytes that testosterone significantly reduces their ability to mature and undergo normal embryonic development[34]. However, in the study of Child et al.[35] using hCG priming before oocyte retrieval, although the maturation rate at 24 h was higher in women with normal ovaries than in PCOS women, by 48 h the rates of maturation were similar. The fertilization and cleavage rates were also similar between the two groups. It seems therefore that hCG plays a more important role in oocyte maturation than FSH priming, and can overcome the deleterious effect of androgens.

COMBINATION OF FSH AND hCG PRIMING

Since Chian et al.[26,27] proposed hCG priming for IVM in PCOS patients, we followed their protocol and we obtained several pregnancies. However, if IVM is to be applied to regularly cycling women, a major limitation is the small number of antral follicles available. It has been shown that the pregnancy rate of IVM is correlated with the number of immature oocytes retrieved, with the highest in those with >10 immature oocytes[36]. Although Child et al.[35] obtained an average of 5.1 (± 3.7) immature

oocytes in normal, cyclic women, we rarely obtained more than 2 oocytes in these women. Futhermore, a thin endometrium (<7 mm) found in some PCOS women, which may be associated with a reduced pregnancy rate. In order to see if gonadotropin would stimulate follicular growth or enhance the growth of endometrium, we gave small doses of rFSH (Gonal-F, 75 IU per day, for 3 to 6 days) to 10 PCOS women whose endometrium was <7 mm on day 9. The endometrium thicknesses before and after rFSH stimulation were 5.2 mm and 7.9 mm, respectively. Two out 10 women became pregnant (20.0%). We then performed a randomized study on PCOS women in whom 35 cycles were pretreated with 75 IU of rFSH for 6 days and 33 cycles were not[37]; 10 000 IU of hCG was given 36 hours before oocyte retrieval. The overall maturation rate, fertilization rate, and pregnancy rate were 74.2%, 72.8%, and 33.8%, respectively. As shown in Table 18.1, serum E_2 level on the day of hCG injection was higher in the FSH-primed group, but the maturation rates, fertilization rates, and pregnancy rates were similar between the two groups. The numbers of oocytes obtained and endometrial thicknesses were also similar. It was concluded that, with hCG priming, FSH priming had no additional beneficial effect on IVM[37]. It should be noted, however, that this study was conducted on PCOS women. Whether the combination of FSH priming and hCG priming will improve the outcome of IVM in normal women is not known.

It has been shown in cows that withdrawing FSH stimulation before oocyte pick-up creates a 'coasting' period that provides a favorable follicular microenvironment for the oocyte to complete final maturation[38,39]. An interesting experiment was performed by Blondin et al.[40] in cows, in which FSH stimulation and different 'coasting' periods were compared. With four injections of FSH (200 IU in total) and 33 h of coasting, administration of LH 6 h before oocyte retrieval increased the percentage of blastocysts and the embryo production rate on days 7 and 8. However, if a 48-h coasting period was used,

Table 18.1 Clinical variables and outcome of FSH-priming and non-FSH-priming groups[37]

	FSH priming	Non-FSH priming	p
No of cycles	35	33	
Age (years)	30.1 ± 2.8	31.3 ± 4.1	NS
Day 3 FSH (mIU/ml)	5.10 ± 1.43	5.54 ± 1.55	NS
Day 3 LH (mIU/ml)	12.46 ± 7.37	11.63 ± 6.61	NS
E_2 on day of hCG (pg/ml)	102.78 ± 98.58	39.17 ± 14.52	0.001
Endometrial thickness on day of hCG (mm)	8.09 ± 1.49	7.77 ± 1.03	NS
No of immature oocytes per patient	21.9 ± 9.4	23.1 ± 11.0	NS
Mean MII oocytes	16.7 ± 7.6	16.6 ± 5.8	NS
Maturation rate at 24 h	43.2%	39.2%	NS
Maturation rate at 48 h	76.5%	71.9%	NS
2PN oocytes per patient	12.7 ± 6.2	11.6 ± 4.6	NS
Fertilization rate	75.8%	69.5%	NS
Cleavage rate	89.4%	88.1%	NS
No of transferred embryos	3.8 ± 1.0	3.8 ± 0.9	NS
Pregnancy rate	31.4%	36.4%	NS
Implantation rate	9.7%	11.3%	NS

LH injection did not affect the rates of blastocyst or embryo production on days 7 and 8. The best results were obtained when the cows received six doses of FSH (300 IU in total) with 48-h coasting, and the administration of LH did not affect the rates of blastocyst production. The results suggested that with four injections of FSH and 33-h coasting, follicles were still in the growing phase, so extending the coasting period to 48 h and LH administration allowed oocytes to acquire developmental competence in vivo. A standard FSH stimulation protocol and 48-h coasting, in association with LH administration, creates an optimal follicular environment for oocyte maturation. These results seem to contradict our study. In our study, rFSH was given from day 3 to day 8, and oocyte retrieval was performed after day 10, so there were at least 48 h of coasting. But we found that the combination of FSH priming and hCG priming is no better than hCG priming alone. It is not known if extended stimulation with FSH would be more helpful, but prolonged ovarian stimulation will offset the major benefit of IVM – namely avoiding the use of gonadotropins.

In our center, we use the traditional double-lumen aspiration needle (K-OPSD-1735-ET; Cook, Australia) for oocyte retrieval instead of the special aspiration needle for immature oocytes (K-OPS-1235-Wood; Cook, Australia) designed by Trounson et al.[13]. Because the COCs are tenacious and detachment from the follicle wall may be difficult, we always flush every follicle until a COC is found, or three times at most. Table 18.2 shows the mean numbers of COCs obtained in different studies. There is a trend to obtain more

COCs in PCOS women than in regularly cycling women. We obtained more COCs than other studies, probably because of follicular flushing. As shown in Tables 18.1 and 18.2, FSH priming does not increase the number of oocytes recovered. Mikkelsen et al. also found that extending FSH stimulation (150 IU/day) from 3 days to 6 days did not increase the number of oocytes obtained[22].

IVM IN STIMULATED CYCLES

IVM with FSH priming and hCG priming is similar to 'rescue' IVM in conventional IVF cycles, in which gonadotropin and hCG are used before oocyte recovery. After ovarian stimulation with gonadotropin and hCG, about 15% of oocytes are found in GV or MI stage at the time of oocyte retrieval. Veeck et al.[41] reported two pregnancies out of 15 cases resulting from transfer of in-vitro matured oocytes from stimulated cycles, but one of them ended up as a miscarriage. Nagy et al.[42]

reported a birth resulting from in-vitro matured GV oocytes from a woman in whom hCG was injected when the leading follicles were only 16 mm. Jaroudi et al.[43] reported a pregnancy resulting from IVM to prevent OHSS. In that case, 10 immature oocytes were obtained, without hCG injection, when the leading follicles were 13 mm. Unfortunately, the pregnancy was lost at 24 weeks. The outcome of rescue IVM in stimulated cycles, however, is very poor, and only limited cases have been reported[23,41–43].

The major difference of IVM and 'rescue IVM' is the timing of oocyte retrieval. In conventional IVF, hCG is given when the leading follicles reach 18 mm and the serum E_2 level is adequate. On the contrary, in the IVM program, we always retrieve oocytes before the leading follicles reach 12 mm. Cobo et al.[44] demonstrated that if follicles were aspirated when a dominant follicle was >10 mm, there was a significant decrease in the rate of oocyte retrieval (50.5%, compared to 70.8% when the follicle was <10 mm). Maturation rates and fertilization rates were similar between the

Table 18.2 Mean numbers of COCs obtained in various studies

Authors	Patients	Priming	Mean no of COCs
Trounson et al.[13] (1994)	PCOS	—	15.3
Wynn et al.[20] (1998)	Normal	FSH	8.9
Mikkelsen et al.[22] (1999)	Normal	—	3.7
Mikkelsen et al.[22] (1999)	Normal	FSH	4.0
Chian et al.[27] (2000)	PCOS	hCG	7.8
Cha et al.[57] (2000)	PCOS	—	13.6
Smith et al.[58] (2000)	Normal	—	5.6
Child et al.[35] (2001)	PCOS	hCG	11.3
Child et al.[35] (2001)	Normal	hCG	5.1
Mikkelsen and Lindenberg[21] (2001)	PCOS	FSH	7.5
Du et al.[54] (2004)	PCOS	hCG	11.4

COC, cumulus–oocyte complex

two groups. However, development to blastocyst stage was also lower in the group in which the follicle was >10 mm. Russell found a dramatic decrease in the rates of maturation, fertilization, and transfer of embryos among cycles in which immature oocytes were retrieved when a dominant follicle (>14 mm) was present at the time of oocyte retrieval[45].

It is generally thought that after dominant follicles have formed, the secondary follicles will become atretic. However, little is known about how dominant follicles affect the developmental potential of oocytes in the smaller follicles, and several recent studies refute this notion. Smith et al. showed that in cattle the developmental competence of oocytes from small antral follicles is not adversely affected by the presence of a dominant follicle[46]. Chian et al.[47] demonstrated with bovine ovaries that, although the number of oocytes obtained in the early follicular phase (before dominant follicles have formed) was higher than those from the late follicular and luteal phases, the rates of maturation and fertilization and embryo cleavage were not significantly different.

In humans, Thornton et al.[48] reported a series of IVM in natural-cycle IVF. Ovulation was triggered with 10 000 IU of hCG when follicle maturity was achieved. After 24 h, 32% GV oocytes matured in standard culture medium, and 30% GV oocytes matured in 50% follicular fluid. The fertilization rates were 62% and 77%, respectively, and two pregnancies resulted from the transfer of embryos derived from immature oocytes. Chian et al.[49] reported three pregnancies resulting from natural-cycle IVF combined with IVM. At the time of oocyte retrieval, the largest follicles were 14–19 mm, but the immature oocytes obtained could still be matured in vitro and produce embryos. These reports also suggest that the maturational and developmental competence of immature oocytes may not be affected by the presence of dominant follicles.

The GV oocytes obtained from superovulated ovaries are different from the GV oocytes in IVM cycles. Nogueira et al.[50] found that the in-vitro matured oocytes from stimulated cycles had a 21% incidence of non-cleavage after fertilization, and chromosomal anomalies were found in 78.5% of embryos analyzed. However, the incidence of aneuploidy or chromosome aberration in in-vitro matured oocytes from unstimulated cycles was about 20%[51,52], which was similar to that reported for in-vivo matured oocytes after gonadotropic stimulation in IVF cycles[51,53]. Besides, the approximate 200 babies after IVM did not show increased anomalies[28,37,54,55].

We think the GV oocytes from stimulated cycles behave differently from the GV oocytes in IVM cycles (either with or without FSH and hCG priming). The GV oocytes obtained from stimulated ovaries had a lower fertilization rate even with ICSI[56], and the resulting embryos had a high incidence of cleavage arrest and chromosome anomalies[50]. The problem does not lie in the dominant follicles, since there is no solid evidence to show that the formation of dominant follicles adversely affects the GV oocytes from smaller follicles. The oocytes remaining at the GV stage in spite of ovarian stimulation may be of inferior quality or there may be an intrinsic defect in the oocytes or follicles.

CONCLUSIONS

Human chorionic gonadotropin priming initiates oocyte maturation in vivo and produces a favorable outcome in IVM. The role of FSH priming is controversial. The combination of FSH priming and hCG priming does not produce additional benefit over hCG priming alone.

REFERENCES

1. Tucker MJ, Wright G, Morton PC et al. Birth after cryopreservation of immature oocytes with subsequent in vitro maturation. Fertil Steril 1998; 70: 578–9.

2. Cha KY, Koo JJ, Ko JJ et al. Pregnancy after *in vitro* fertilization of human follicular oocytes collected from nonstimulated cycles, their culture *in vitro* and their transfer in a donor oocyte program. Fertil Steril 1991; 55: 109–13.

3. Hwang JL, Lin YH, Tsai YL. Pregnancy after immature oocyte donation and intracytoplasmic sperm injection. Fertil Steril 1997; 68: 1139–40.

4. Hwang JL, Lin YH, Tsai YL et al. Oocyte donation using immature oocytes from a normal ovulatory woman. Acta Obstet Gynecol Scand 2002; 81: 274–5.

5. Cha KY, Chian RC. Maturation *in vitro* of immature human oocytes for clinical use. Hum Reprod Update 1998; 4: 103–20.

6. Downs SM. Factors affecting the resumption of meiotic maturation in mammalian oocytes. Theriogenology 1993; 39: 65–79.

7. Albertini DF, Carabatsos MJ. Comparative aspects of meiotic cell cycle control in mammals. J Mol Med 1998; 76: 796–9.

8. Downs SM, Daniel SAJ et al. Induction of maturation in cumulus cell-enclosed mouse oocytes by follicle-stimulating hormone and epidermal growth factor: evidence for a positive stimulus of somatic cell origin. J Exp Zool 1988; 234: 86–96.

9. De Sousa PA, Caveney A, Westhusin ME et al. Theriogenology 1998; 49: 115–28.

10. Thibault C, Gerard M, Menezo Y. Preovulatory and ovulatory mechanisms in oocyte maturation. J Reprod Fertil 1975; 45: 605–10.

11. Pincus G, Enzmann EV. The comparative behavior of mammalian eggs *in vivo* and *in vitro*. J Exp Med 1935; 62: 665–75.

12. Edwards RG. Maturation *in vitro* of mouse, sheep, cow, pig, rhesus monkey and human ovarian oocytes. Nature 1965; 208: 349–51.

13. Trounson A, Wood C, Kausche A. *In vitro* maturation and fertilization and developmental competence of oocytes recovered from untreated polycystic ovarian patients. Fertil Steril 1994; 72: 353–62.

14. Hwung JL, Lin YH, Tsai YL. In vitro maturation and fertilization of immature oocytes: a comparative study of fertilization techniques. J Assist Reprod Genet 2000; 17: 39–43.

15. Tsuji K, Sowa M, Nakano R. Relationship between human oocyte maturation and different follicular sizes. Biol Reprod 1985; 32: 413–17.

16. Trounson A, Anderiesz C, Jones GM et al. Oocyte maturation. Hum Reprod 1998; 13(Suppl 3): 52–62.

17. McGee E, Spears N, Minammi S et al. Preantral follicles in serum-free culture: suppression of apoptosis after activation of the cyclic guanosine 3′, 5′-monophosphate pathway and stimulation of growth and differentiation by follicle-stimulating hormone. Endocrinology 1997; 138: 2417–24.

18. Suikkari AM, Tulppala M, Tuuri T et al. Luteal phase start of low-dose FSH priming of follicles results in an efficient recovery, maturation and fertilization of immature human oocytes. Hum Reprod 2000; 16: 747–51.

19. Gómez E, Tarin J, Pellicer A. Oocyte maturation in humans: the role of gonadotropins and growth factors. Fertil Steril 1993; 60: 40–6.

20. Wynn P, Picton HM, Krapez JA et al. Pretreatment with follicle stimulating hormone promotes the numbers of human oocytes reaching metaphase II by in-vitro maturation. Hum Reprod 1998; 13: 3132–8.

21. Mikkelsen AL, Lindenberg S. Benefit of FSH priming of women with PCOS to the in vitro maturation procedure and the outcome: a randomized prospective study. Reproduction 2001; 122: 587–92.

22. Mikkelsen AL, Smith SD, Lindenberg S. In-vitro maturation of human oocytes from regularly menstruating women may be successful without follicle stimulating hormone priming. Hum Reprod 1999; 14: 1847–51.

23. Jaroudi KA, Hollanders JMG, Elnour AM et al. Embryo development and pregnancies from in-vitro matured and fertilized oocytes. Hum Reprod 1999; 14: 1749–51.

24. Blondin P, Coenen K, Guilbault LA et al. Superovulation can reduce the developmental competence of bovine embryos. Theriogenology 1996; 46: 1191–203.

25. Laufer N, Tarlatzis BC, De Cherney AH et al. Asynchrony between human cumulus–corona cell complex and oocyte maturation after human menopausal gonadotropin treatment for in vitro fertilization. Fertil Steril 1984; 42: 366–9.

26. Chian RC, Gulekli B, Buckett WM et al. Priming with human chorionic gonadotropin before retrieval of immature oocytes in women with infertility due to the polycystic ovary syndrome. N Engl J Med 1999; 341: 1624–6.

27. Chian RC, Buckett WM, Tulandi T et al. Prospective randomized study of human chorionic gonadotrophin priming before immature oocyte retrieval from unstimulated women with polycystic ovarian syndrome. Hum Reprod 2000; 15: 165–70.

28. Chian RC. In-vitro maturation of human oocytes. Reprod BioMed Online 2003; 8: 148–66.

29. Salustri A, Yanagishita M, Hascell VC. Synthesis and accumulation of hyaluronic acid and proteoglycans in the mouse cumulus cell–oocyte complex during follicle-stimulating hormone-induced mucification. J Biol Chem 1989; 64: 1380–7.

30. Hazeleger NL, Hill DJ, Walton JS et al. The interrelationship between the development of bovine oocytes in vitro and their follicular fluid environment. Theriogenology 1993; 39: 231.

31. Blondin P, Sirard MA. Oocyte and follicular morphology as determining characteristics for developmental competence in bovine oocytes. Mol Reprod Dev 1995; 41: 54–62.

32. Trounson A, Anderiesz C, Jones G. Maturation of human oocytes in vitro and their developmental competence. Reproduction 2001; 121: 51–75.

33. Barnes FL, Kausche A, Tiglias J et al. Production of embryos from in vitro-matured primary human oocytes. Fertil Steril 1996; 65: 1151–6.

34. Anderiesz C, Trounson AO. The effect of testosterone on the maturation and developmental capacity of murine oocytes in vitro. Hum Reprod 1995; 10: 2377–81.

35. Child TJ, Abdul-Jalil AK, Bulekli B et al. In vitro maturation and fertilization of oocytes from unstimulated normal ovaries, polycystic ovaries, and women with polycystic ovary syndrome. Fertil Steril 2001; 76: 936–42.

36. Tan SL, Child TJ, Gulekli B. In vitro maturation and fertilization of oocytes from unstimulated ovaries: predicting the number of immature oocytes retrieved by early follicular phase ultrasonography. Am J Obstet Gynecol 2002; 186: 684–9.

37. Lin YH, Hwang JL, Huang LW et al. Combination of FSH priming and hCG priming for in-vitro maturation of human oocytes. Hum Reprod 2003; 18: 1632–6.

38. Blondin P, Guibault LA, Sirard MA. The time interval between FSH-P administration and slaughter can influence the developmental competence of beef heifer oocytes. Theriogenology 1997; 48: 803–13.

39. Sirard MA, Picard L, Dery M et al. The time interval between FSH administration and ovarian aspiration influences the development of cattle oocytes. Theriogenology 1999; 51: 699–708.

40. Blondin P, Bousquet D, Twagiramungu H et al. Manipulation of follicular development to produce developmentally competent bovine oocytes. Biol Reprod 2002; 66: 38–43.

41. Veeck L, Edwards J, Witmyer J et al. Maturation and fertilization of morphologically immature oocytes in a program of in vitro fertilization. Fertil Steril 1983; 39: 594–602.

42. Nagy Z, Cecile J, Liu J et al. Pregnancy and birth after intracytoplasmic sperm injection of in vitro matured germinal vesicle stage oocytes: case report. Fertil Steril 1996; 65: 1047–50.

43. Jaroudi KA, Hollanders JMG, Sieck U et al. Pregnancy after transfer of embryos which were generated from in vitro matured oocytes. Hum Reprod 1997; 12: 857–9.

44. Cobo AC, Requena A, Neuspiller F et al. Maturation in vitro of human oocytes from unstimulated cycles: selection of the optimal day for ovum retrieval based on follicular size. Hum Reprod 1999; 14: 1864–8.

45. Russell JB. Immature oocyte retrieval with in-vitro oocyte maturation. Curr Opin Obstet Gynecol 1999; 11: 289–96.

46. Smith LC, Olivera-Angel M, Groome NP et al. Oocyte quality in small antral follicles in the

presence or absence of a large dominant follicle in cattle. J Reprod Fertil 1996; 106: 193–9.

47. Chian RC, Chung JT, Downey BR et al. Maturational and development competence of immature oocytes retrieved from bovine ovaries at different phases of folliculogenesis. Reprod Biomed Online 2002; 4: 127–32.

48. Thornton MH, Francis MM, Paulson RJ. Immature oocyte retrieval: lessons from unstimulated IVF cycles. Fertil Steril 1998; 70: 647–50.

49. Chian RC, Buckett WM, Jalil AKA et al. Natural-cycle *in vitro* fertilization combined with *in vitro* maturation of immature oocytes is a potential approach in infertility treatment. Fertil Steril 2004; 82: 1675–9.

50. Nogueira D, Staessen C, Van de Velde H et al. Nuclear status and cytogenetics of embryos derived from in-vitro matured oocytes. Fertil Steril 2000; 74: 295–8.

51. Gras L, McBain J, Trounson A et al. The incidence of chromosome aneuploidies in stimulated and unstimulated (natural) uninseminated human oocytes. Hum Reprod 1992; 7: 1396–401.

52. Racowsky C, Kaufman ML. Nuclear degeneration and meiotic aberrations observed in human oocytes matured in-vitro: analysis by light microscopy. Fertil Steril 1992; 58: 750–5.

53. Munné S, Lee A, Rozenwaks Z et al. Diagnosis of major chromosomal aneuploidies in human preimplantation embryos. Hum Reprod 1993; 8: 2185–91.

54. Du AL, Kadoch IJ, Bourcigaux N et al. *In vitro* oocyte maturation for the treatment of infertility associated with polycystic ovarian syndrome: the French experience. Hum Reprod 2005; 20: 420–4.

55. Cha KY, Chung HM, Lee DR et al. Obstetric outcome of patients with polycystic ovary syndrome treated by *in vitro* maturation and *in vitro* fertilization–embryo transfer. Fertil Steril 2005; 83: 1461–5.

56. Kim BK, Lee SC, Kim KJ et al. *In vitro* maturation, fertilization, and development of human germinal vesicle oocytes collected from stimulated cycles. Fertil Steril 2000; 74: 1153–8.

57. Cha KY, Han SY, Chung HM et al. Pregnancies and deliveries after in-vitro maturation culture followed by in-vitro fertilization and embryo transfer without stimulation in women with polycystic ovary syndrome. Fertil Steril 2000; 73: 978–83.

58. Smith SD, Mikkelsen AL, Lindenberg S. Development of human oocytes matured *in vitro* for 28 or 36 hours. Fertil Steril 2000; 73: 541–4.

CHAPTER 19

Immature oocyte collection

Bulent Gulekli, Ezgi Demirtas, and William M Buckett

INTRODUCTION

In-vitro maturation (IVM) of immature oocytes retrieved from women without any ovarian stimulation is a promising new treatment especially for women with polycystic ovary syndrome (PCOS) and/or polycystic ovaries (PCO), with many successful pregnancies reported worldwide. Although Cha et al.[1] reported the first birth using IVM of immature oocytes collected at cesarean section within an oocyte donation program in 1991, in 1994 it was Trounson and colleagues[2] who put IVM into clinical practice when they reported the first pregnancy using a woman's own immature oocytes collected by transvaginal ultrasound-guided follicle aspiration from a patient with polycystic ovaries.

Although the classic indication for IVM is PCOS/PCO, it is also for other indications today: poor responders, fertility preservation of cancer patients, normal responders with a history of poor oocyte/embryo quality, as well as for oocyte donation.

DEVELOPMENT OF OOCYTE RETRIEVAL FOR IVF

Before the first successful birth following in-vitro fertilization (IVF) and embryo transfer, the first culture and maturation of human oocytes in vitro were carried out on oocytes that were obtained by laparotomy. Similar experiments were done by Steptoe and Edwards and they introduced a laparoscopic method for aspirating oocytes from the ovarian follicles[3]. Laparoscopic oocyte retrieval may be performed either by the 2- or 3-puncture technique depending on the type of laparoscope and the experience of the surgeon. Each follicle is punctured and aspirated at an avascular site (Figure 19.1). The needle may be left in the follicle to permit flushing and re-aspiration in case an oocyte is not identified in the initial aspirate.

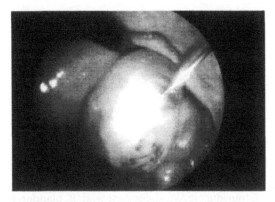

Figure 19.1 Laparoscopic oocyte retrieval (see color plate section)

Following those first few births via laparo-scopically aspirated oocytes, ultrasound-guided oocyte collection techniques were described. While laparoscopic oocyte retrieval is generally performed under general anesthesia with endo-tracheal intubation, the major advantages for the ultrasound-guided oocyte retrieval include decreased exposure to general anesthesia, lower risk for operative complications, and feasibility of performing on an outpatient basis. In addi-tion, laparoscopy identifies visible follicles on the ovarian surface whereas ultrasonography identifies intraovarian follicles, as well.

There are many different ultrasound-guided oocyte collection techniques. The first follicu-lar puncture under transabdominal ultrasound guidance was described in 1981 and the same group introduced transabdominal transvesi-cal ultrasound-directed oocyte recovery for the oocytes from the ovarian follicles a year later (Figure 19.2)[4,5]. Transabdominal oocyte retrieval under ultrasound guidance is still indicated in women with vaginal/müllerian agenesis[6]. Oocyte retrieval for IVF by ultrasonically guided

needle aspiration via the urethra was proposed by Parsons and coworkers in 1985 (Figure 19.3)[7]. The above techniques were in routine use dur-ing the days of conventional external ultrasound transducers. Gleicher et al.[8] described the first oocyte retrieval via the vaginal route; today's method using the transvaginal approach for both the scanning and the oocyte retrieval was intro-duced by Wickland et al.[9] and has become the worldwide method for oocyte recovery[10].

CURRENT TECHNIQUE FOR IVF OOCYTE RETRIEVAL

Anesthesia/analgesia

Today almost all oocyte retrievals are performed transvaginally. The transvaginal route is used both for the scanning and the retrieval. Generally, spinal or epidural anesthesia may be used for the procedure; however, in most cases intravenous sedation, opioid analgesia, and cervical blockage with local anaesthesia is sufficient for effective

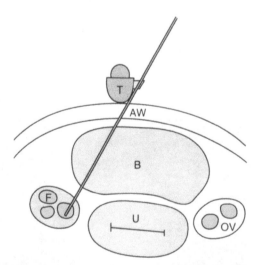

Figure 19.2 Transabdominal ultrasound-guided oocyte retrieval
T, transducer; AW, abdominal wall; B, bladder; F, follicle; U, uterus; OV, ovary

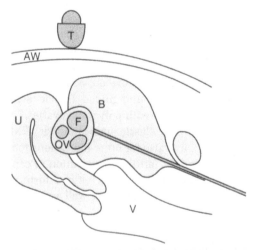

Figure 19.3 Transurethral oocyte retrieval under transabdominal ultrasound guidance
T, transducer; AW, abdominal wall; B, bladder; F, follicle; OV, ovary; U, uterus; V, vagina

pain relief. In the McGill Reproductive Center, 1–2 mg midazolam for intravenous sedation, 25 mg fentanyl every 10 minutes or according to the needs of the patient for analgesia, and 0.5% bupivacaine 10–20 ml for the cervical block are used and effective pain relief is maintained in most of the patients. Rarely, non-steroid anti-inflammatory drugs alone may provide sufficient analgesia in cases with a few follicles or in natural IVF cycles where there is only one follicle to be aspirated.

Cleaning and antisepsis

Normal saline is used for vaginal cleaning before the oocyte retrieval. When compared to vaginal cleaning with povidon iodine, no increase in infection risk is observed. However, povidon iodine may decrease the pregnancy rate[11], probably by an adverse effect on oocytes. Routine antibiotic prophylaxis is not recommended, however it may be administered in selected cases with endometriomas or hydrosalpinges.

Materials needed for the IVF oocyte retrieval

An ultrasound scanner with a 6 MHz or 7.5 MHz transvaginal probe, a sterile condom or plastic sheath to cover the probe, sterile ultrasound gel, a needle guide, a 15 or 16G single/double lumen aspiration needle, suction pump, test tubes, 1% heparinized saline, a heater block for the tubes, an inverted microscope plus heating plate, and petri dishes for oocyte identification in the laboratory are the materials necessary for an IVF oocyte retrieval. The test tubes, heparinized saline, and petri dishes are preheated to 37°C before the collection.

Needles

Single or double lumen needles of 15/16G are used for aspiration. Double lumen needles allow the follicle to be flushed through a separate route. Although routine flushing does not offer any advantage in terms of the number of retrieved oocytes, it may be needed in cases with one or a few follicles.

Ultrasound technique

Transvaginal scanning and oocyte retrieval is the routine oocyte retrieval method today. The procedure is easy to learn for physicians who have already been trained in transvaginal ultrasound examination. A 9.3 MHz transvaginal transducer is used for oocyte retrieval in our center. The high resolution is particularly helpful in IVM retrieval in which small follicles of less than 10 mm in diameter are aspirated. In IVF oocyte retrievals 6 MHz or 7.5 MHz ultrasound transducers and two-dimensional visualization are successfully used. Doppler or three-dimensional ultrasound may be helpful, but they are not essential.

Aspiration technique

The transvaginal ultrasound guided follicular aspiration technique has become the method of choice because of refinements in the instrumentation and the clinicians' growing experience. Over the past few years automatic aspiration and washing systems have been introduced and the follicles can be aspirated and, if necessary, washed with various systems.

The needle is first introduced in the follicle closest to the transducer through the vaginal vault with controlled stabbing, resembling popping a balloon. Vacuum pressure should be less then 150 mmHg to aspirate the follicular fluid and a suction pump is used to maintain the constant vacuum pressure. The tip of the needle is echogenic, so it can be watched on the ultrasound screen while the follicular fluid is aspirated. When follicular walls collapse onto the needle, the needle can be retracted and rotated to aspirate all the follicular fluid (Figure 19.4). Then the next follicle is stabbed and the needle is gently moved from one follicle to another

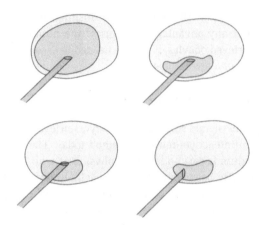

Figure 19.4 IVF oocyte retrieval: aspiration technique

after fully aspirating each follicle. Usually, only a single ovarian puncture is needed to aspirate all the follicles in one ovary. When all the follicles of one ovary have been aspirated the needle is withdrawn and flushed with the handling medium. If the needle is withdrawn before all the follicles in the ovary have been aspirated, it is flushed before puncturing the ovary a second time. The same procedure is repeated for the other ovary.

Flushing is not routinely recommended because no apparent improvement has been observed in the pregnancy rate[12]. However, as noted above, it may be needed in patients with few follicles.

Once a follicle has been aspirated the collection tube is handed over to the laboratory staff. If no oocyte is identified in the aspirate then the follicle may be flushed with the handling medium. Although the flushing can also be done with a single lumen needle, the oocyte may move back and forth in the dead space of the needle by repeated flushes and aspirations. Therefore it is recommended to use a double lumen needle in cases with a few follicles where flushing may be needed. The flushing volume should not exceed the aspiration volume in order not to rupture the follicle. Flushing can be done manually by using a syringe or by an automatic pump.

Heparinized saline or heparinized culture medium is used as the handling medium since there is no significant difference in fertilization rates between oocytes obtained after saline and culture medium flushing[13].

Risks

The complications of ultrasonically guided transvaginal oocyte collection are rare. Infection risk is around 0.25%. Serious pelvic infection – such as pelvic or ovarian abscess – is seen almost exclusively in women with either severe tubal disease or severe endometriosis and endometriomas which have been inadvertently punctured during oocyte retrieval. Serious intraperitoneal or vaginal bleeding is even rarer – with an estimated risk of 0.01%. Laparoscopy and very rarely laparotomy have been reported in cases of severe intra-abdominal bleeding[14].

DEVELOPMENT OF IVM

Today IVM has started to be routinely offered either to patients with PCOS or to normo-ovulatory patients with a high risk of developing OHSS (i.e. patients with PCO). As noted above, it has also been used for other indications: poor responders, fertility preservation in cancer patients, normal responders with a history of poor oocyte/embryo quality, and oocyte donation cycles. In these conditions immature oocyte retrieval may be performed in the presence of a few follicles. The only significant factor predicting the number of oocytes collected in unstimulated cycles is the antral follicle count[15]. Although the oocyte recovery rate in stimulated cycles is 70–80%, it is usually about 50% in IVM cycles and this oocyte recovery rate depends on the experience of the surgeon[16]. However, the reason could be that not all the follicles may be easily aspirated and/or oocytes may not be recovered from each follicle aspirated. Therefore good ultrasonographic visualization, accessibility of the ovaries, and the retrieval technique are even more important, particularly for those with a low antral follicle count.

IVM is improved by hCG priming[17]; hCG priming does not seem to increase the number of oocytes retrieved, but it reduces the time needed for IVM[18]. The dose of hCG was studied in a prospective, randomized, double blind study by our group and increasing the dose did not give any benefit in any of the outcomes, therefore current evidence suggests a benefit from 10 000 IU hCG administered 36 h before the collection[19].

In a typical IVM cycle all the follicles had to be <10 mm in diameter because data suggest that the presence of a dominant follicle at the time of immature oocyte retrieval is deleterious to the outcome in IVM[20,21]. The maximum diameter of the follicle on the day of oocyte recovery provides one of the main differences between IVF and IVM cycles. However, in natural cycle IVF/IVM treatments, in spite of the presence of a dominant follicle, where a mature oocyte is expected to be retrieved, immature oocytes have also been collected and matured in vitro and pregnancies and live births have been obtained[22]. The administration of short-term gonadotropins and hCG priming when the follicles reach 12–14 mm in diameter has also been suggested as another approach to IVM[23]. The combination of natural cycle IVF with IVM, or the short-term use of gonadotropin administration before immature oocyte retrieval, are modifications currently under investigation, and the criteria for their use are not yet well established[22,24].

Nevertheless, immature oocytes from follicles less than 10 mm in diameter should still be collected, even with these modifications. Thus in IVM collections, sometimes one or more follicles may be larger than 10 mm, and mature oocytes may be recovered from these follicles.

CURRENT TECHNIQUES FOR IVM OOCYTE RETRIEVAL

TVS-guided follicular aspiration has now become the preferred procedure of choice for oocyte retrieval in IVM cycles; it requires certain modifications compared to conventional IVF oocyte retrieval.

Anesthesia/analgesia

The mode of anesthesia is decided according to the accessibility of the ovaries. Although the initial cases were performed under general or spinal anesthesia, this is not needed for most cases.

Intravenous sedation with 2 mg midazolam and 50–200 mg fentanyl, and paracervical block with 20 ml of 1% bupivacaine, are used for immature egg retrieval in the McGill Reproductive Center. Intravenous propofol infusion may also be added in certain patients. However, because of the multiple ovarian punctures often needed in IVM, the immature oocyte retrieval is likely to be more painful than a conventional IVF oocyte collection. It has been shown that reducing the size of the needle used for oocyte collection from 15G (the standard IVF needle) to 19/20G reduces the pain without affecting the number of the oocytes collected.

Consequently, in patients who have had previous poor pain relief during oocyte retrieval or those where ovarian access is difficult, a general or spinal anesthesia may be more appropriate and, in our experience, is needed more frequently than for conventional IVF collections.

Cleaning and antisepsis

The same principles applied to IVF oocyte retrieval are also valid for IVM patients. Therefore the vagina is cleaned with sterile saline. In women at increased risk of pelvic sepsis – such as those with severe tubal disease or endometriosis – antibiotic prophylaxis is appropriate. It is unclear whether there is a role for routine antibiotic prophylaxis.

Collection needle

As discussed above, a smaller gauge needle (19G or 20G) is preferable. This causes less pain and less damage to the smaller follicles, thereby allowing greater numbers of immature oocytes to be collected. However, the finer gauge needles are more susceptible to blockage with stromal tissue or blood clots, and therefore require frequent removal and flushing through with fluid. Similarly, if ovarian access is difficult and the needle needs to pass through uterine tissue, care needs to be taken in order to avoid bending.

Aspiration pressure

Because the intrafollicular pressure is already higher in small follicles, the aspiration vacuum pressure is reduced to 75–80 mmHg, which is approximately half the conventional IVF aspiration pressure. A higher aspiration pressure provokes an increase in the number of denuded oocytes.

Tubes and blocks

The aspiration tubes are prepared with 2 ml heparinized saline before collection in the warm blocks. Heparinized saline is also used as the aspiration medium for flushing the needle. Some centers use IVM culture media rather than heparinized saline in the tubes and for flushing.

Aspiration technique

In unstimulated ovaries the follicles are small and often widespread throughout the ovarian stroma (Figure 19.5). Furthermore, polycystic ovaries are frequently mobile and external abdominal pressure and intravaginal pressure with the probe may be needed to fix the ovary in IVM oocyte retrieval.

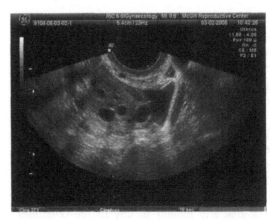

Figure 19.5 Ovary prior to commencing IVM collection. Note the widespread follicles throughout the stroma ranging from 4 mm to 11 mm mean diameter. A good quality ultrasound machine is needed at high magnification

The needle is introduced into the follicle with the bevel facing the larger part of the follicle, however it is probably less important than first thought. Because the needle slips easily into the surrounding stroma it should be stabbed into the follicle at 90° to the follicle wall. Also the needle is frequently removed to re-align it with the small follicles. The follicle should be completely emptied; rotating the needle could be of help. Although only a single puncture of the ovary is generally enough for IVF oocyte retrieval, multiple ovarian punctures are generally needed for IVM retrieval. The reason for this is that it is almost always impossible to reach all the follicles from the same puncture site (Figures 19.6, 19.7, and 19.8). In addition, the volume of the fluid aspirated from the follicles is very small and the single lumen aspiration needle tends to block frequently when passing through the dense ovarian stroma and follicular flushing is not performed. So, the needle is generally withdrawn after several follicles have been aspirated, and it is flushed with the heparinized saline. The collection takes, on average, longer than IVF oocyte retrieval because of the repeated flushing

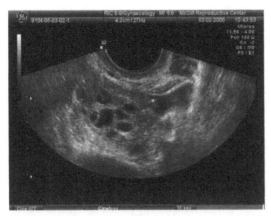

Figure 19.6 The commencement of an IVM oocyte retrieval. The needle tip is within the first follicle (6 mm) and a further three follicles can be aspirated on this puncture

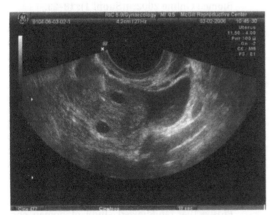

Figure 19.7 Towards the completion of one side. Two further antral follicles remain which will need to be aspirated with separate punc-

of the needle and the tubing in order to prevent the blockage[25,26].

Good ultrasonographic visualization is the key point for successful immature oocyte retrieval. Color-flow Doppler can help to differentiate intra-ovarian vessels from small antral follicles. The follicular sizes vary and certain follicles may be difficult to aspirate or, even if they are aspirated, no oocytes may be recovered, especially from the very small size follicles (<4 mm).

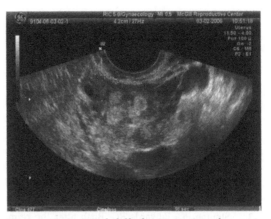

Figure 19.8 Final follicle (6 mm) to be aspirated. Note the hematomas in the previously emptied follicles

Follicles are isolated from follicular aspirates collected in tubes containing heparinized saline in the laboratory by using a stereomicroscope. The follicular aspirate is then filtered and rechecked for oocytes.

CONCLUSIONS

Although IVM oocyte collections may appear more challenging than conventional IVF oocyte collections, following the above guidelines and with appropriate experience they are relatively straightforward. The learning curve is relatively short and highly dependent on the clinician's already established skills in conventional IVF. The current techniques have been described here. However, one would expect further refinements over the next few years.

The basic principles for IVM oocyte retrieval can be summarized as the following:

- Adequate analgesia

- Multiple ovarian puncture

- Fine-bore aspiration needle

- Good quality ultrasound

- Frequent flushing of the needle and tubing.

REFERENCES

1. Cha KY, Koo JJ, Ko JJ et al. Pregnancy after *in vitro* fertilization of human follicular oocytes collected from nonstimulated cycles, their culture *in vitro* and their transfer in a donor oocyte program. Fertil Steril 1991; 55: 109–13.

2. Trounson AC, Wood C, Kausche A. In vitro maturation and the fertilization and developmental competence of oocytes recovered from untreated polycystic ovarian patients. Fertil Steril 1994; 64: 353–62.

3. Steptoe PC, Edwards RG. Birth after the reimplantation of a human embryo. Lancet 1978; 312: 366.

4. Lenz S, Lauritsen JG, Kjellow M. Collection of human oocytes for in vitro fertilisation by ultrasonically guided follicular puncture. Lancet 1981; 317: 1163–4.

5. Lenz S, Lauritsen JG. Ultrasonically guided percutaneous aspiration of human follicles under local anesthesia: a new method of collecting oocytes for in vitro fertilization. Fertil Steril 1982; 38: 673–7.

6. Damario MA. Transabdominal–transperitoneal ultrasound-guided oocyte retrieval in a patient with mullerian agenesis. Fertil Steril 2002; 78: 189–91.

7. Parsons J, Riddle A, Booker M et al. Oocyte retrieval for in-vitro fertilisation by ultrasonically guided needle aspiration via the urethra. Lancet 1985; 325: 1076–7.

8. Gleicher N, Friberg J, Fullan N et al. EGG retrieval for in vitro fertilisation by sonographically controlled vaginal culdocentesis. Lancet 1983; 322: 508–9.

9. Wikland M, Enk L, Hamberger L. Transvesical and transvaginal approaches for the aspiration of follicles by use of ultrasound. Ann NY Acad Sci 1985; 442: 182–94.

10. Sunde A, von During V, Kahn JA et al. IVF in the Nordic countries 1981–1987: a collaborative survey. Hum Reprod 1990; 5: 959–64.

11. van Os HC, Roozenburg BJ, Janssen-Caspers HA et al. Vaginal disinfection with povidon iodine and the outcome of in-vitro fertilization. Hum Reprod 1992; 7: 349–50.

12. Kingsland CR, Taylor CT, Aziz N et al. Is follicular flushing necessary for oocyte retrieval? A randomized trial. Hum Reprod 1991; 6: 382–3.

13. Biljan MM, Dean N, Hemmings R et al. Prospective randomized trial of the effect of two flushing media on oocyte collection and fertilization rates after in vitro fertilization. Fertil Steril 1997; 68: 1132–4.

14. Dicker D, Ashkenazi J, Feldberg D et al. Severe abdominal complications after transvaginal ultrasonographically guided retrieval of oocytes for in vitro fertilization and embryo transfer. Fertil Steril 1993; 59: 1313–15.

15. Tan SL, Child TJ. In-vitro maturation of oocytes from unstimulated polycystic ovaries. Reprod Biomed Online 2002; 4(Suppl 1): 18–23.

16. Tan SL, Child TJ, Gulekli B. In vitro maturation and fertilization of oocytes from unstimulated ovaries: predicting the number of immature oocytes retrieved by early follicular phase ultrasonography. Am J Obstet Gynecol 2002; 186: 684–9.

17. Chian RC, Gulekli B, Buckett WM et al. Priming with human chorionic gonadotropin before retrieval of immature oocytes in women with infertility due to the polycystic ovary syndrome. N Engl J Med 1999; 341: 1624–6.

18. Chian RC, Buckett WM, Tulandi T et al. Prospective randomized study of human chorionic gonadotrophin priming before immature oocyte retrieval from unstimulated women with polycystic ovarian syndrome. Hum Reprod 2000; 15: 165–70.

19. Gulekli B, Buckett WM, Chian RC et al. Randomized, controlled trial of priming with 10,000 IU versus 20,000 IU of human chorionic gonadotropin in women with polycystic ovary syndrome who are undergoing in vitro maturation. Fertil Steril 2004; 82: 1458–9.

20. Russell JB. Immature oocyte retrieval combined with in-vitro oocyte maturation. Hum Reprod 1998; 13(Suppl 3): 63–70, 71–5.

21. Cobo AC, Requena A, Neuspiller F et al. Maturation in vitro of human oocytes from

unstimulated cycles: selection of the optimal day for ovum retrieval based on follicular size. Hum Reprod 1999; 14: 1864–8.

22. Chian RC, Buckett WM, Abdul-Jalil AK et al. Natural-cycle in vitro fertilization combined with in vitro maturation of immature oocytes is a potential approach in infertility treatment. Fertil Steril 2004; 82: 1675–8.

23. Lim KS. IVM/F-ET in stimulated cycles for the prevention of OHSS. Fertil Steril 2002; 78(Suppl 1): S11.

24. Chian RC, Buckett WM, Tan SL. In-vitro maturation of human oocytes. Reprod Biomed Online 2004; 8: 148–66.

25. Child TJ, Abdul-Jalil AK, Sulekli B et al. In vitro maturation and fertilization of oocytes from unstimulated normal ovaries, polycystic ovaries, and women with polycystic ovary syndrome. Fertil Steril 2001; 76: 936–42.

26. Child TJ, Phillips SJ, Abdul-Jalil AK et al. A comparison of in vitro maturation and in vitro fertilization for women with polycystic ovaries. Obstet Gynecol 2002; 100: 665–70.

CHAPTER 20

Endometrial preparation for IVM

Anne-Maria Suikkari

INTRODUCTION

Implantation depends both on the quality of the embryo and the endometrium. Proliferation and secretory changes of the endometrium are directly and indirectly influenced by the steroid hormones estrogen and progesterone. An inadequate exposure of the endometrium to these hormones may lead to implantation failure[1]. In different assisted reproductive techniques (ART), such as in-vitro fertilization (IVF), oocyte donation, frozen-thawed embryo transfer, and in-vitro maturation (IVM), the aim is to achieve synchronization between the receptive endometrium and embryo development. In spontaneous cycles these events are related to ovulation and cyclic hormonal changes. This is not the case in IVM. Therefore artificial preparation of the endometrium is necessary to open the window of implantation.

Although Cha et al. were the first to achieve a live birth after IVM in a recipient of a donated oocyte[2], it was Trounson et al. who first successfully transferred embryos in the same cycle in which the immature oocytes were retrieved using ultrasound guided transvaginal aspiration of small follicles[3]. One of the challenges of this method is to prepare the uterus in only a few days between the oocyte retrieval and embryo transfer. Because immature oocytes are usually retrieved before the dominant follicle develops, the endometrium is exposed to relatively low levels of estradiol by the time of immature oocyte collection (IOC). As a result, there is a dyssynchrony between the phase of the endometrium and the cleaved embryo. This is thought to be one of the reasons for the low success of the early days of IVM development[4]. Since then the clinical outcome of IVM has greatly improved and protocols for endometrial preparation have been developed.

This chapter will discuss the quality of endometrium in different applications of ART, the rationale for endometrial preparation in IVM, and current protocols used for the preparation of endometrium.

WHAT IS A RECEPTIVE ENDOMETRIUM?

The development of a receptive endometrium is a complex process which involves the sex steroid hormones and various local factors and cell surface structures such as cell adhesion molecules, integrins, cytokines, extracellular matrix proteins, and pinopodes[5,6]. The only known undisputed marker for uterine receptivity in the human, however, is implantation[6]. Proliferation of the endometrium is regulated by estradiol produced by the granulosa cells of the growing follicle/s. The transformation into secretory and subsequently receptive endometrium requires adequate progesterone exposure from the corpus luteum. A mathematic calculation by Rogers et al. estimated that the uterine receptivity accounts for about 31–64% of implantation[7].

The morphologic changes of the endometrium during a spontaneous menstrual cycle were described by Noyes et al. in 1950 and are still considered as the gold standard today[8]. However, normal morphology does not always imply adequate functional capacity of the endometrium[9]. In estrogen/progesterone-supplemented cycles, there is a frequently observed glandular–stromal asynchrony in endometrial biopsies taken in the mid luteal phase[10]. Furthermore, endometrial morphology differs according to the hormone replacement preparation and route of administration[11].

Specific genes and molecular markers for implantation and endometrial receptivity have been investigated[5,12,13]. The roles of the various adhesion molecules, cytokines, and other factors are being debated[5,6]. The expression of, e.g., $\alpha_v\beta_3$ integrin and leukemia inhibitory factor (LIF) coincides with the implantation window, but their exact biological action remains unclear[6]. Pinopodes are ultrastructural formations of the receptive endometrium. The appearance of pinopodes lasts less than 48 h and they coincide with the implantation window on cycle days 20–22. Pinopodes tend to form earlier in stimulated cycles and later in hormone replacement cycles compared with natural cycles[14]. However, the appearance of pinopodes varies individually and evidence for direct involvement in embryo attachment is still lacking[6].

ENDOMETRIUM IN STIMULATED CYCLES FOR IVF

Ovarian stimulation for IVF is known to cause an advancement of 2–5 days in the histology of the late follicular phase endometrium and a dyssynchronous glandular and stromal differentiation in the midluteal phase in 45–90% of stimulated IVF cycles[1,6,15–18]. When this endometrial advancement exceeded 3 days, no pregnancies occurred[1,19]. In the mid luteal phase, on the other hand, a delay in endometrial development has been observed[20]. This asynchronous endometrial development during GnRH-agonist and gonadotropin stimulated IVF cycles is normalized with progesterone or human chorionic gonadotropin (hCG) supplementation in the late luteal phase[21]. A study on pinopodes further supports this shift in endometrial maturation in IVF cycles[14]. Albeit that the implantation rates are lower in IVF compared with natural cycles, the observed altered endometrial development in IVF and hormone replacement cycles is thought to have no major impact on actual endometrial receptivity, the endometrium playing only a generally permissive role[1,22].

Adequate proliferative and secretory changes are necessary for successful implantation to occur. Endometrial thickness can be regarded as a marker for proliferation and is easily measurable using an ultrasound scan. Conflicting reports exist concerning possible relationships between endometrial thickness and treatment outcome in IVF cycles[23]. The existing data suggest that endometrial thickness has no predictive value on the cycle outcome[23]. However, most studies have concluded that pregnancy rates drop when the endometrial thickness is less than 7 mm[6].

LESSONS FROM OOCYTE DONATION AND FROZEN-THAWED EMBRYO TRANSFER CYCLES

Endometrial proliferation is necessary to enable optimal progesterone receptor function and transition to receptive endometrium[24]. Neither endometrial thickness nor serum estradiol has been shown to predict optimal receptivity and outcome in an oocyte donation program[25]. In oocyte donation cycles the length of estrogen administration can be varied between the extremes of 6 and 100 days before progesterone addition. However, the miscarriage rate increases below 11 days and beyond 9 weeks[24]. Different durations of progesterone exposure between 1 and 9 days before day 2–3 embryo transfer have been reported[24]. Pregnancies have been achieved after 1–6 days of progesterone before day 2–3 embryo transfers in oocyte donation cycles[26]. Rosenwaks et al.[27] found that in recipients of donor oocytes, day 2 embryos are best transferred to the uterus on day 3 or 4 of progesterone exposure.

In estradiol/progesterone supplemented frozen-thawed embryo transfer cycles varying durations, preparations, and dosages of hormone administration have been reported[24]. It has been suggested that it is appropriate to start progesterone administration as soon as the endometrium is developed sufficiently, i.e. at least 8 mm in thickness with a trilaminar ultrasound appearance, and to perform the embryo transfer not before 3–4 days of progesterone treatment[24].

FORMS OF DRUGS USED FOR ENDOMETRIAL PREPARATION

The various forms of estrogen and progesterone delivery used in oocyte donation programs have been extensively discussed in a review by Devroey and Pados[10]. The oral route of estrogen administration results in less fluctuation in serum estrogen concentrations but a lower estradiol:estrone ratio than the transdermal route of delivery. Both are equally effective in terms of pregnancy rates[10]. Native progesterone, which is more effective in luteal support for implantation and pregnancy than other progesterone derivatives, can be administered orally, intravaginally, or intramuscularly[10]. The vaginal micronized progesterone suppositories and i.m. injections have been shown to be the most effective and best tolerated routes of progesterone delivery.

A meta-analysis of five prospective randomized trials suggests that there is no difference in pregnancy rates between luteal support with i.m. progesterone or i.m. hCG[28]. It is recommended that the luteal supplementation should be performed using progesterone rather than hCG, given the higher risk of ovarian hyperstimulation syndrome (OHSS) with hCG use[1]. The comparison between the delivery of native progesterone by the i.m. or vaginal route gives a relative ratio of 1.33 in favor of i.m. delivery[28]. The significance of this finding needs to be further evaluated. So far, there does not seem to be any major change in the clinical practice of luteal support in IVM programs. This may be due to the greater ease and simplicity of vaginal progesterone administration.

HOMORNE SUPPLEMENTATION IN IVM CYCLES

Optimal thickness of the endometrium

In a retrospective analysis of frozen-thawed embryo transfers in spontaneous cycles, Loh and Leong[29] showed better pregnancy rates if the endometrium thickness was at least 11 mm. In IVF cycles the consensus has been that the thicker the endometrium, the better the pregnancy rate. In natural cycles the opposite seems to be true. The mid proliferative and preovulatory endometrial thickness has been shown to be less in conception cycles compared with non-conception cycles[30,31]. An increased preovulatory endometrial thickness seems unfavorable for spontaneous conception, with a cut-off thickness of 12 mm and a mean thickness of 7.8 mm for pregnant and 9.1 mm for non-pregnant cycles with a leading follicle of 19 mm in diameter[31].

IVM is performed in a natural cycle either in the mid follicular phase of an ovulatory cycle or in the proliferative phase of an anovulatory cycle. By the time of IOC, the endometrium has started to proliferate, but has not yet reached the thickness of a mature preovulatory endometrium. Therefore the ultrasonographic data on optimal endometrial thickness from stimulated IVF, oocyte donation, and frozen-thawed embryo transfer cycles may not be relevant to IVM. Many women with PCOS have a thin endometrium on the day of IOC, yet comparable pregnancy rates to IVF have been reported[32,33]. Child et al.[33] found a small but significant difference in the mean endometrial thickness on the day of embryo transfer between conception and non-conception cycles in 155 IVM patients (10.2 versus 9.4 mm, respectively). However, there was no difference in the mean endometrial thickness on the day of IOC between pregnant (6.5 mm) and non-pregnant women (6.6 mm). Figure 20.1 shows the thickness of the endometrium on the day of IOC in 171 cycles with embryo transfer performed at the Infertility Clinic of the Family Federation of Finland in women with normal or polycystic ovaries[34]. No correlation between endometrial thickness and cycle outcome was found. An ongoing pregnancy and live birth was achieved when the endometrium was 3 mm on the day of oocyte retrieval.

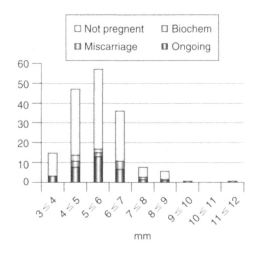

Figure 20.1 The number of ongoing pregnancies, miscarriages, biochemical pregnancies and non-pregnant cycles according to the endometrial thickness on the day of IOC

The effect of gonadotropin priming on the endometrium

The challenge with IVM is to retrieve immature oocytes before ovulation, usually in mid to late follicular phase, and then return a cleaving embryo a few days later into the uterus. The use of minimal FSH stimulation during the early follicular phase could potentially increase the endometrial thickness before IOC and thus improve the outcome. However, there does not seem to be any benefit of early follicular phase FSH priming in women with regular cycles and normal ovaries[35]. On the other hand, in PCOS patients with no spontaneous follicle development and subsequent endometrial proliferation, there were more pregnancies in the FSH primed group compared to the non-primed group, albeit no difference in the endometrial thickness at IOC between the groups was observed[36]. Others have not found any beneficial effect of FSH priming in PCOS patients[32,37].

In a case report, Barnes et al.[38] described a successful IVM cycle in the presence of an 18 mm dominant follicle; 1000 IU hCG was administered at the time of oocyte recovery followed by progesterone pessaries 300 mg/day 48 h later. Ultrasound assessment revealed a corpus luteum and a secretory endometrium of 9 mm at the time of embryo transfer. They speculated that the administration of hCG prior to IOC may enhance synchronization between the uterus and embryo. Administration of hCG has been shown to increase the endometrial thickness and implantation rate in recipients of donated oocytes[39]. The possible role of in-vivo administration of hCG on the uterus remains to be elucidated[40].

Start, dose, and duration of hormone supplementation

In IVM, the uterus has to be prepared and synchrony between the endometrium and embryo achieved in a greatly accelerated time schedule compared to other types of ART. At the time of IOC, the endometrium is still relatively thin owing to the low levels of estradiol secretion from the small antral follicles in the early to mid follicular phase. The start of progesterone administration at the time of insemination coincides with the rise of serum progesterone after ovulation in a natural cycle[35]. The first protocol used for endometrial preparation consisted of estradiol valerate 2–4 mg daily from the day of IOC and progesterone intravaginal suppositories 200–300 mg per day started 48 h later at the time of insemination[3,38].

Concerns for the short duration of estradiol priming and data from donor oocyte recipient studies suggesting that at least 6 days of estrogen priming before embryo transfer are needed to prepare the endometrium for implantation prompted Russell et al.[4] to compare two regimens of endometrial priming: an early follicular phase priming using 17β-estradiol 2 mg twice a day starting on cycle day 2 or 3 and a mid follicular priming of 2 mg of 17β-estradiol starting on cycle day 6 and increasing by 1–2 mg per day depending on the endometrial thickness on ultrasound scan. Both groups were continued on 8 mg per day from the day of IOC. Intramuscular progesterone 50 mg was started on the day following IOC and continued by 100 mg on the second day until the pregnancy test. Both estradiol and progesterone were continued, if the test was positive, until 70 days' gestation[4]. They concluded that a significant decrease in the maturation and cleavage rates was identified with immature oocytes exposed to early exogenous estrogens[41].

The hypothesis of potentially inadequate endometrial preparation in the IVM cycle by the Trounson method[3] was addressed in a study by Suikkari et al.[37] in which IVM embryos at both pronucleus and cleaved stage were cryopreserved to be replaced in either a natural or hormone supplemented frozen-thawed embryo transfer cycle. Unfortunately, the cryosurvival of the IVM embryos was found to be significantly decreased compared to conventional IVF

and ICSI embryos and no conclusions on the efficacy of endometrial preparation could be drawn[37].

Prospective studies comparing different protocols for optimal endometrial preparation in IVM cycles are lacking. Based on the insights into the physiology of endometrial preparation from oocyte donation and frozen-thawed embryo transfer programs, the groups performing IVM with embryo transfers have conjured slightly different estrogen/progesterone supplementation protocols, shown in Table 20.1. The differences in the pregnancy results are likely to be due to factors other than the endometrial priming protocols used. Figure 20.2 shows a schematic presentation of the timing of hormone supplementation in IVM cycles used by several groups[33–35]. In general, the administration of oral estrogen is started on the day of IOC and the dose is adjusted to the thickness of the endometrium on the day. Vaginal progesterone pessaries are commenced at the time of insemination or intracytoplasmic sperm injection (ICSI). The time of embryo transfer may vary between day 2 and day 5 after insemination or ICSI. Both estrogen and progesterone are continued after a positive pregnancy test until 7–12 weeks of gestation.

Mikkelsen et al.[42] have used a standard protocol for endometrial preparation in all their studies including women with regular cycles and normal ovaries and women with polycystic ovaries with or without follicular phase FSH

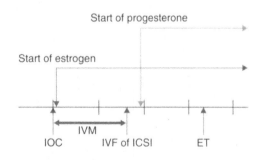

Figure 20.2 Protocol for endometrial preparation in IVM cycle (see color plate section)

Table 20.1 Endometrial preparation protocols for IVM in the patient's own transfer cycle

Reference	Estrogen preparation	Dose, route	Start	Progesterone preparation	Dose, route	Start	Continued until	PR/ET (%)
Trounson et al.[3], 1994	Estradiol valerate	2 mg/d, oral	Day of IOC	Progesterone pessaries			Not identified	Not identified
Barnes et al.[38], 1996	Estradiol valerate	4 mg/d, oral	Day of IOC	Progesterone pessaries	300 mg/d, vaginal	48 hours after IOC at the time of insemination	Not identified	Not identified
Russell et al.[4], 1997	Estradiol valerate	4 mg/d or incremental increase from 2 mg/d, oral	Cycle day 2–3 or 6	Progesterone	50 mg increasing to 100 mg on the second day, intramuscular	Day after IOC	10 gw	1/14 (7)*
Mikkelsen et al.[35], 1999	Estradiol valerate	6 mg/d, oral	Day of IOC	Micronized progesterone	300 mg/d, vaginal	2 days after IOC	7 gw	5/20 (25)*
Child et al.[43], 2001	Estradiol valerate	6–10 mg/d, oral	Day of IOC	Progesterone	400 mg/d, vaginal	Day of ICSI	12 gw	34/169 (20)*
Lin et al.[32], 2003	Estradiol valerate	6–10 mg/d, oral	Day of IOC	Micronized progesterone	800 mg/d, vaginal	Day of ICSI	12 gw	23/68 (34)*
Le Du et al.[46], 2005	Estradiol hemihydrate	6–10 mg/d, oral	Day of IOC	Progesterone	Not identified	Day of IOC	12 gw	9/40 (23)*
Son et al.[47], 2005	Estradiol valerate	6 mg/d, oral	Day of IOC	Progesterone cream	100 mg/d, vaginal	Day of IOC	9–10 gw	24/47 (51)*
Söderström-Anttila et al.[34], 2005	Estradiol valerate	6 mg/d, oral	Immediately after IOC	Micronized progesterone capsules	600 mg/d, vaginal	Evening of the day of insemination or ICSI	9–10 gw	49/184 (27)*

* percentage of pregnancies/embryo transfer
PR/ET, pregnancies/embro transfer; gw, gestation week.

priming. The administration of 17β-estradiol 2 mg orally three times daily was started on the day of oocyte retrieval. If endometrial thickness was <6 mm at ultrasound on the day of aspiration, the cycle was cancelled. Two days later the luteal phase was supported by vaginal micronized progesterone suppositories 100 mg three times daily. Both estrogen and progesterone were continued until the pregnancy test, and if it was positive hormone supplementation was continued until 50 days, i.e. 7 weeks of gestation.

The McGill group in Montreal has used individualized protocols adjusted to the endometrial thickness at IOC. The patients have been given estradiol valerate in divided doses, starting on the day of oocyte retrieval. If the endometrial thickness on the day of oocyte retrieval was less than 6 mm, a 10 mg dose of estradiol was given; if it was more than 6 mm, a 6 mg dose was given[43,44]. Luteal support was provided by 200 mg intravaginal progesterone twice daily, starting on the day of ICSI and continued along with estradiol until 12 weeks of gestation[43]. On the day of embryo transfer, the endometrial thickness was measured again and if it was less than 7 mm, the couples were offered embryo cryopreservation and transfer in a subsequent cycle[45]. Other groups around the world working closely with the McGill group have adopted slightly different estrogen/progesterone treatment regimens[46,47]. The French group reported their results in infertile women with PCOS. They used an endometrial thickness of 5 mm as a cut-off to give 10 mg of estradiol, otherwise they gave 6 mg estradiol per day. Unlike in other programs, progesterone was started on the day of IOC. Their results showed an endometrial thickness of 8–13 mm at embryo transfer in all patients and a clinical pregnancy rate of 23% (9/40) per embryo transfer[46]. A group in South Korea has published high pregnancy and implantation rates (51% and 24%, respectively) after blastocyst transfers in patients with a risk of OHSS in previous IVF cycles. For endometrial preparation they gave estradiol valerate 6 mg and progesterone 100 mg daily from the day after IOC. The medication was continued until 9–10 weeks of pregnancy[47].

After our preliminary study[37], we have adopted the estrogen/progesterone supplementation protocol described by Mikkelsen et al.[35] Endometrial proliferation is enhanced by commencing oral estradiol valerate 6 mg per day (Progynova, Schering, Finland) immediately after IOC to ensure as long an estrogen exposure as possible before the start of progesterone. Vaginal micronized progesterone 300 mg twice daily (Lugesteron, Leiras, Finland) is commenced in the evening of the following day, which is the day of insemination or ICSI. Both estrogen and progesterone are continued until the first pregnancy ultrasound at 7 weeks of gestation. If a healthy pregnancy is found, the estrogen and progesterone doses are tapered over the following 2 weeks and discontinued at 9–10 weeks of gestation[34].

IVM combined with natural cycle IVF

The combination of a natural cycle IVF and IVM offers an interesting alternative to improve the pregnancy rates of conventional IVM. Thornton et al.[48] found that at the oocyte pick-up in unstimulated IVF cycles, immature oocytes were observed in 48% of the cases. These metaphase I and GV oocytes could be matured and fertilized in vitro, resulting in 'extra' embryos available for transfer. In a natural cycle there is a cohort of follicles developing alongside the dominant follicle. These follicles have been thought to undergo atresia under the increasing steroid hormone secretion from the dominant follicle[49]. This hypothesis is being questioned by Chian et al.[50], who found that developing follicles of about 12 mm in diameter seemed to be able to respond to exogenous hCG administration and mature oocytes could be retrieved from these follicles. As the endometrial thickness increases with increasing estradiol levels from the growing follicles, exogenous hormonal supplementation may not be necessary in these cases[50].

SUMMARY AND CONCLUSIONS

In an IVM cycle, the physiologic periovulatory hormonal and endometrial changes of a natural cycle are missing at the time of oocyte retrieval. Adequate endometrial proliferation has to be achieved in just 2 days before the start of progesterone administration in order to open the window of implantation for the embryo. Basically, identical protocols for endometrial preparation have been used both in women with regular cycles and normal appearing ovaries and in women with polycystic ovaries with or without follicular phase priming with FSH or hCG[34–36,42].

There are only minor differences in the estrogen/progesterone supplementation protocols between the groups performing clinical IVM today. In general, estrogen is commenced on the day of IOC because of the evidence that excessive estrogen exposure in the early follicular phase may be deleterious to the oocytes[41]. In order to allow as long an estrogen exposure as possible before the progesterone is administered, it is advisable to start estrogen tablets immediately after the oocyte pick-up. Progesterone is usually started 36–48 h later. Both estrogen and progesterone are continued until 7–12 weeks of gestation (Table 20.1). The pregnancy rates vary between 20 and 51% in different reports[32,34–36,43–47]. It is likely that other factors such as patient selection, hormonal priming, oocyte aspiration technique, and culture method have more impact on the results than the current endometrial preparation protocols. However, to further increase the efficacy of IVM, it is important to focus on ways of improving the endometrial preparation.

ACKNOWLEDGMENTS

I am grateful to Dr Viveca Söderström-Anttila for her critical comments while preparing the manuscript.

REFERENCES

1. Devroey P, Bourgain C, Macklon NS et al. Reproductive biology and IVF: ovarian stimulation and endometrial receptivity. Trends Endocrinol Metab 2004; 15: 84–90.

2. Cha KY, Koo JJ, Ko JJ et al. Pregnancy after *in vitro* fertilization of human follicular oocytes collected from nonstimulated cycles, their culture *in vitro* and their transfer in a donor oocyte program. Fertil Steril 1991; 55: 109–13.

3. Trounson A, Wood C, Kausche A. *In vitro* maturation and the fertilization and developmental competence of oocytes recovered from untreated polycystic ovarian patients. Fertil Steril 1994; 62: 353–62.

4. Russell JB, Knezevich KM, Fabian KF et al. Unstimulated immature oocyte retrieval: early versus midfollicular endometrial priming. Fertil Steril 1997; 67: 616–20.

5. Lessey BA. The role of the endometrium during embryo implantation. Hum Reprod 2000; 15(Suppl 6): 39–50.

6. Bourgain C, Devroye P. The endometrium in stimulated cycles for IVF. Hum Reprod Update 2003; 9: 515–22.

7. Rogers P, Milne B, Trounson A. A model to show uterine receptivity and embryo viability following ovarian stimulation for *in vitro* fertilizaion. J In Vitro Fertil Embryo Transf 1986; 3: 93–8.

8. Noyes RW, Hertig AJ, Rock J. Dating the endometrial biopsy. Fertil Steril 1950; 1: 3–25.

9. Younis JS, Simon A, Laufer N. Endometrial preparation: lessons from oocyte donation. Fertil Steril 1996; 66: 873–84.

10. Devroey P, Pados G. Preparation of endometrium for egg donation. Hum Reprod Update 1998; 4: 856–61.

11. Sauer MV, Stein AL, Paulson RJ et al. Endometrial responses to various hormone replacement regimens in ovarian failure patients preparing for embryo donation. Int J Gynaecol Obstet 1991; 35: 61–8.

12. Kao LC, Tulac S, Lobo S et al. Global gene profiling in human endometrium during the win-

dow of implantation. Endocrinology 2002; 143: 2119–38.

13. Horcajadas JA, Riesewijk A, Martin J et al. Global gene expression profiling of human endometrial receptivity. J Reprod Immunol 2004; 63: 41–9.

14. Nikas G, Develioglu OH, Toner JP et al. Endometrial pinopodes indicate a shift in the window of receptivity in IVF cycles. Hum Reprod 1999; 14: 787–92.

15. Basir GS, O WS, Ng EH et al. Morphometric analysis of peri-implantation endometrium in patients having excessively high oestradiol concentrations after ovarian stimulation. Hum Reprod 2001; 16: 435–40.

16. Garcia JE, Acosta AA, Hsiu JG et al. Advanced endometrial maturation after ovulation induction with human menopausal gonadotropin/human chorionic gonadotropin for in vitro fertilization. Fertil Steril 1984; 41: 31–5.

17. Lass A, Peat D, Avery S et al. Histological evaluation of endometrium on the day of oocyte retrieval after gonadotropin-releasing hormone agonist–follicle stimulating hormone ovulation induction for in-vitro fertilization. Hum Reprod 1998; 13: 3203–5.

18. Marchini M, Fedele L, Bianchi S et al. Secretory changes in preovulatory endometrium during controlled ovarian hyperstimulation with buserelin acetate and human gonadotropins. Fertil Steril 1991; 55: 717–21.

19. Ubaldi F, Bourgain C, Tournaye H et al. Endometrial evaluation by aspiration biopsy on the day of oocyte retrieval in the embryo transfer cycles in patients with serum progesterone rise during the follicular phase. Fertil Steril 1997; 67: 521–6.

20. Smitz J, Devroye P, Camus M et al. The luteal phase and early pregnancy after combined GnRH-agonist/HMG treatment for superovulation in IVF or GIFT. Hum Reprod 1988; 3: 585–90.

21. Balasch J, Jove I, Marquez M et al. Hormonal and histological evaluation of the luteal phase after combined GnRH-agonist/gonadotropin treatment for superovulation and luteal phase support in in vitro fertilization. Hum Reprod 6: 914–17.

22. Damario MA, Lesnick TG, Lessey TG et al. Endometrial markers of uterine receptivity utilizing the donor oocyte model. Hum Reprod; 16: 1893–9.

23. Friedler S, Schenker JG, Herman A et al. The role of ultrasonography in the evaluation of endometrial receptivity following assisted reproductive treatments: a critical review. Hum Reprod Update 1996; 2: 323–35.

24. Nawroth F, Ludwig M. What is the 'ideal' duration of progesterone supplementation before the transfer of cryopreserved-thawed embryos in estrogen/progesterone replacement protocols? Hum Reprod 2005; 5: 1127–34.

25. Remohi J, Ardiles G, Garcia-Velasco JA et al. Endometrial thickness and serum oestradiol concentrations as predictors of outcome in oocyte donation. Hum Reprod 1997; 12: 2271–6.

26. Navot D, Bergh PA, Williams M et al. An insight into early reproductive processes through the in vivo model of ovum donation. J Clin Endocrinol Metab 1991; 72: 408–14.

27. Rosenwaks Z. Donor eggs: their application in modern reproductive technologies. Fertil Steril 1987; 47: 895–909.

28. Pritts E, Atwood A. Luteal phase support in infertility treatment: a meta-analysis of the randomised trials. Hum Reprod 2002; 17: 2287–99.

29. Loh SK, Leong NK. Factors affecting success in an embryo cryopreservation programme. Ann Acad Med Singapore 1999; 2: 260–5.

30. Gonen Y, Calderon I, Dirnfeld M et al. The impact of sonographic assessment of the endometrium and meticulous hormonal monitoring during natural cycles in patients with failed donor artificial insemination. Ultrasound Obstet Gynecol 1991; 1: 122–6.

31. Keulers MJ, Hamilton CJCM. Preovulatory endometrial thickness as predictor of spontaneous pregnancy in natural cycles. Hum Reprod 2005; 20(Suppl 1): i69.

32. Lin YH, Hwang JH, Huang LW et al. Combination of FSH priming and hCG priming for in-vitro maturation of human oocytes. Hum Reprod 2003; 18: 1632–6.

33. Child T, Gulekli B, Sylvestre C et al. Ultrasonographic assessment of endometrial receptivity at embryo transfer in an *in vitro* maturation of oocyte program. Fertil Steril 2003; 79: 656–7.

34. Söderström-Anttila V, Mäkinen S, Tuuri T et al. Favourable pregnancy results with insemination of *in vitro* matured oocytes from unstimulated patients. Hum Reprod 2005; 20: 1534–40.

35. Mikkelsen AL, Smith SD, Lindenberg S. In-vitro maturation of human oocytes from regularly menstruating women may be successful without follicle stimulating hormone priming. Hum Reprod 1999; 14: 1847–51.

36. Mikkelsen AL, Lindenberg S. Benefit of FSH priming of women with PCOS to the *in vitro* maturation procedure and the outcome: a randomized prospective study. Reproduction 2001; 122: 587–92.

37. Suikkari A-M, Tulppala M, Tuuri T et al. Luteal phase start of low-dose FSH priming of follicles results in an efficient recovery, maturation and fertilization of immature human oocytes. Hum Reprod 2000; 15: 747–51.

38. Barnes FL, Crombie A, Gardner DK et al. Blastocyst development and birth after in-vitro maturation of human primary oocytes, intracytoplasmic sperm injection and assisted hatching. Hum Reprod 1995; 10: 3243–7.

39. Tesarik J, Hazout A, Mendoza C. Luteinizing hormone affects uterine receptivity independently of ovarian function. Reprod Biomed Online 2003; 7: 59–64.

40. Filicori M, Fazleabas A, Huhtaniemi I et al. Novel concepts of human chorionic gonadotropin: reproductive system interactions and potential in the management of infertility. Fertil Steril 2005; 84: 275–84.

41. Russell JB. Immature oocyte retrieval with in-vitro oocyte maturation. Curr Opin Obstet Gynecol 1999; 11: 289–96.

42. Mikkelsen AL. Strategies in in-vitro maturation and their clinical outcome. Reprod Biomed Online 2005; 10: 593–9.

43. Child TJ, Abdul-Jalil AK, Gulekli B et al. *In vitro* maturation and fertilization of oocytes from unstimulated normal ovaries, polycystic ovaries, and women with polycystic ovary syndrome. Fertil Steril 2001; 76: 936–42.

44. Chian RC, Buckett WM, Tan S-L. In-vitro maturation of human oocytes. Reprod Biomed Online 2004; 8: 148–66.

45. Chian RC, Buckett WM, Tulandi T et al. Prospective randomized study of human chorionic gonadotrophin priming before immature oocyte retrieval from unstimulated women with polycystic ovarian syndrome. Hum Reprod 2000; 15: 165–70.

46. Le Du A, Kadoch IJ, Bourcigaux N et al. *In vitro* oocyte maturation for the treatment of infertility associated with polycystic ovarian syndrome: the French experience. Hum Reprod 2005; 20: 420–4.

47. Son WY, Lee SY, Lim JH. Fertilization, cleavage and blastocyst development according to the maturation timing of oocytes in *in vitro* maturation cycles. Hum Reprod 2005; 20: 3204–7.

48. Thornton MH, Francis MM, Paulson RJ. Immature oocyte retrieval: lessons from unstimulated IVF cycles. Fertil Steril 1998; 70: 647–50.

49. Gougeon A. Regulation of ovarian follicular development in primates: facts and hypothesis. Endocrine Rev 1996; 17: 121–55.

50. Chian R-C, Buckett WM, Abdul-Jalil AK et al. Natural-cycle *in vitro* fertilization combined with *in vitro* maturation of immature oocytes is a potential approach in infertility treatment. Fertil Steril 2004; 82: 1675–8.

CHAPTER 21

Laboratory aspects of IVM treatment

Ri-Cheng Chian

INTRODUCTION

To date, assisted reproductive technology (ART) has helped thousands and thousands of women to overcome infertility problems. Although initial attempts at human oocytes with in-vitro maturation (IVM) and in-vitro fertilization (IVF) were undertaken as far back as the 1940s[1,2], it was not until the 1960s that landmark work was done on IVM of immature human oocytes[3-5]. Laparoscopy was introduced in the late 1960s to collect human oocytes from the Graafian follicle, resulting in the first live birth from human IVF produced from an in-vivo matured oocyte[6]. This natural cycle IVF treatment was gradually replaced by ovarian stimulation IVF because it was believed that the number of oocytes retrieved relate to the embryos available for transfer which, in turn, directly affected the achievement of a successful pregnancy. At the beginning, relatively inexpensive medications, such as clomiphene citrate, were used to stimulate ovaries to produce multiple follicles. However, current ovarian stimulation protocols use the much more expensive gonadotropin-releasing hormone (GnRH) agonists or antagonists in combination with gonadotropins to generate multiple follicles in the ovaries. Some women are extremely sensitive to stimulation

with exogenous gonadotropins and are at an increased risk of developing ovarian hyperstimulation syndrome (OHSS), which is a life-threatening condition[7]. In addition, there is concern that the long-term side-effects of repeated ovarian stimulation may increase the risk of ovarian, endometrial, and breast cancers[8,9].

Since Cha et al.[10] reported the first pregnancy from in-vitro matured oocytes derived from a cesarean section donor, fertilization, embryo development, and pregnancy by immature human oocytes matured in vitro have been successfully achieved in women with polycystic ovary syndrome (PCOS)[11,12]. Recent improvements in culture condition and transfer techniques have demonstrated that immature oocyte retrieval followed by IVM is an effective treatment for women with polycystic ovaries (PCO) or polycystic ovary syndrome (PCOS) related infertility because there are numerous antral follicles within the ovaries in this group of patients. In general, clinical pregnancy and implantation rates for infertile women with PCO or PCOS have reached approximately 35% and 15%, respectively[13,14].

Recovery of immature oocytes followed by IVM of these oocytes is a potentially useful treatment for women with infertility. Compared to women with normal ovaries, women with

PCO or PCOS have a significantly higher risk of developing OHSS when stimulated with exogenous gonadotropins. Although immature oocyte retrieval followed by IVM might be useful for approximately 35% of women undergoing IVF treatment who have polycystic-like ovaries seen on ultrasound scan, it is important to mention here that IVM technology is an attractive alternative for women with all types of infertility. In comparison with conventional IVF, the major advantages of IVM treatment include: (i) avoidance of the side-effects resulting from gonadotropin stimulation including the risk of OHSS, (ii) reduced cost, and (iii) simplified treatment.

Theoretically, all infertile women are candidates for IVM treatment. However, pregnancy rates are directly related to the number of oocytes retrieved and embryos available for transfer. Therefore, the best candidates for IVM treatment are women under 35 years of age who have polycystic-like ovaries seen on ultrasound scan because younger women have a greater number of follicles that continue to grow through to the preovulatory stage of development during each menstrual cycle.

There is an increasing interest in natural cycle IVF among patients because it produces fewer side-effects and less discomfort. Although natural cycle IVF may result in low success rates per oocyte collection due to a lack of oocytes and embryos available for transfer, by using life table analysis to calculate cumulative success rates of stimulated cycle IVF over the same time span, it becomes evident that the cumulative probability of achieving pregnancy is 46% after four natural cycle IVF treatments[15]. It is therefore possible to offer a treatment that combines natural cycle IVF with immature oocyte retrieval followed by IVM to women with all types of infertility, thereby eliminating the need to resort to ovarian stimulation and providing reasonable pregnancy and implantation rates. However, it is important to individualize natural cycle IVF treatment combined with IVM treatment for each patient in order to optimize the success rates.

For IVM treatment or IVF combined with IVM treatment, the patients normally are given an injection of 10 000 IU human chorionic gonadotropin (hCG) 36 hours before oocyte retrieval, because it has been demonstrated that hCG priming before immature oocyte retrieval benefits the treatment cycle[16]. Oocyte retrieval is usually performed between days 10 and 14 of the menstrual cycle, depending upon the thickness of the endometrial lining and the size of the follicles. It is extremely important to prevent ovulation from the dominant follicle due to a natural LH surge. Our experience indicates that hCG can be administered up to and before the maximum size of the dominant follicle reaches 14 mm in diameter. Most oocytes collected from the dominant follicle are at metaphase II (MII) stage.

IN-VITRO MATURATION OF IMMATURE HUMAN OOCYTES

Human oocytes acquire a series of competences during follicular development (oocyte growth and maturation) that play critical roles at fertilization and subsequent early embryonic development. Early studies have shown that nuclear maturation can occur spontaneously following culture in vitro of animal and human immature oocytes. However, the developmental competence after fertilization of these oocytes is questionable. Oocyte maturation in vitro is profoundly affected by culture conditions. The percentage of oocytes that can develop to the blastocyst stage is practically considered a suitable indication of developmental competence. However, recent data from animal studies suggested that 'blastocyst formation' is a limited predictor of development[17]. The successful production of morphologically normal blastocyst stage embryos has not proved reliable in indicating whether a successful pregnancy will be established. Therefore, expression of these genes could provide potentially important markers for assessing embryo viability and implantation. However, it is difficult for clinical practice to use these important markers at the present time. Further research is required to develop reliable markers for assessing oocyte and embryo viability.

Follicular size

During folliculogenesis, the human oocyte grows from 35 μm to 120 μm in diameter[18]. At the end of oocyte growth, the antrum is formed and the oocyte has acquired the capacity to resume meiosis. Most of the mRNA and protein is synthesized during the period of oocyte growth. Normally, it is believed that the ability to complete maturation to MII and developmental competence is acquired progressively with increasing follicular size. In mice, it has been reported that developmental competence is dependent on both the size of the follicle and the size of the oocytes[19]. Although it has been reported that the human oocyte has a size-dependent ability to resume meiosis from 90 to 120 μm in diameter[20], non-full-size oocytes should not be considered when assessing developmental competence, because the non-full-size oocytes have fewer products (mRNA and protein) stored in the cytoplasm during oocyte growth. Sometimes, small-size oocytes can be collected from antral follicles and matured to MII following proper in-vitro culture. Therefore, it seems that these oocytes are still growing in size during antrum formation in humans and some animal species[21].

Early studies indicated that the size-dependent ability for meiotic competence depends not only on the sizes of the follicle and oocyte but also on the stage of the menstrual cycle[22]. In the follicular phase of the menstrual cycle, the percentage of oocyte maturation in the large follicle group (9–15 mm in diameter; 34.5%) was significantly ($p < 0.05$) higher than that of the small follicle group (3–4 mm; 8.8%). During the follicular phase, normally the largest healthy follicle (5.5–8.2 mm in diameter) appears to be selected[23]. The selected follicle becomes the dominant follicle

and will be destined to ovulate. The remaining cohort of follicles will be terminated by atresia. The mechanism of the selection of the follicle for ovulation is still unclear, but it has been suggested that it may be related to FSH-induced aromatase activity of the granulosa cells[24]. Prolonged exposure to androgens in the remaining cohort of follicles may have an adverse effect on mouse oocyte viability and developmental competence[25]. However, it has been reported that the developmental competence of bovine oocytes from the small antral follicles is not adversely affected by the presence of a dominant follicle[26]. Furthermore, the results from our laboratory indicate that rates of oocyte maturation, fertilization, and early embryonic development are not affected by the phases of folliculogenesis when the immature bovine oocytes are aspirated from the size of follicles between 2 and 8 mm in diameter[27]. Therefore, further investigation is needed to understand when the remaining cohort of follicles undergoes atresia. Our experience indicates that the immature human oocytes from the small follicles (between 3 and 8 mm in diameter) were healthy when hCG was primed as the leading follicular size reached 14 mm in diameter in infertile women with regular menstrual cycles and non-PCO ovaries.

In current gonadotropin-stimulated IVF protocols, gonadotropins are used to induce multiple follicular development and oocyte maturation in vivo. FSH is necessary for the growth of preovulatory follicles. LH supports follicular growth by providing androgen substrate for the granulosa cell aromatase and also triggers the resumption of oocyte maturation. The use of exogenous gonadotropins has resulted in follicle asynchrony[28]. Mature oocytes are retrieved by transvaginal aspiration 36 h post-hCG administration. The size of the leading follicle does not affect the fertilization and cleavage rates of cohort oocytes from gonadotropin-stimulated cycles[29]. However, it has been reported that fertilization rates are lower in oocytes obtained from follicles less than 10 mm in diameter than in those retrieved from larger follicles[30,31]. It has been shown that the development of embryos in cohort follicles from stimulated cycles appears to be independent of the diameter of the leading follicle at the time of hCG injection[32,33]. It must be noted, however, that immature oocytes are retrieved frequently after hCG administration even from follicles of diameter >10 mm, and these immature oocytes can be matured and developed in vitro[12,34].

Basis of IVM medium

Although numerous data have been accumulated from animal studies, the current rationale for choosing a specific medium for IVM of immature human oocytes appears to stem largely from adapting methods developed from culturing other cell types. Complex culture media, such as tissue culture medium 199 (TCM-199), Ham's-F10, and Chang's medium buffered with bicarbonate or HEPES (N-2-hydroxyethylperazine N-2-ethane sulfonic acid), supplemented with various sera, gonadotropins (FSH and LH), and estradiol, have been most widely used in research or the clinical application of oocyte IVM[35]. Although major beneficial components seem to be already present in these media[36], more research is necessary to determine specific metabolic needs and optimal culture conditions required by maturing oocytes for appropriate gene expression and regulation.

Different energy substrates and nutrients can greatly influence oocyte meiotic and cytoplasmic maturation[37,38]. Glucose, pyruvate, and lactate are the main substrates for energy metabolism in somatic cells and oocytes. Glutamine can also serve as an energy substrate to improve in-vitro nuclear maturation of hamster[39] and rabbit[40] oocytes. Oocyte utilization of pyruvate is closely dependent upon cumulus cells that can convert glucose or lactate into pyruvate to be used by oocytes[41]. Pyruvate or oxaloacetate, but not glucose, lactate, or phosphoenolpyruvate, supports the maturation of denuded mouse oocytes

through meiosis to MII[42]. It has been confirmed that mitochondrial oxidative metabolism is much more important than anaerobic glucose metabolism for energy production in the mammalian oocytes[43]. Synthesis of pyruvate from glucose in the cumulus cells provides additional evidence that these cells are able to influence the nutritional environment of the maturing oocytes[44]. It has been shown that sodium pyruvate in non-serum maturation medium supports and promotes nuclear maturation of bovine cumulus-denuded oocytes[45]. However, it has been reported that pyruvate alone is insufficient for oocyte cytoplasmic maturation[46]. Nevertheless, it has been indicated that the expression pathway of glycolytic metabolism reflects the presence of different mechanisms involved in gene expression/regulation at the transcriptional and translational level and their accumulation during human oocyte maturation[47]. In addition, it has been indicated that metabolism of glucose through the Embden–Meyerhof pathway is important during bovine oocyte maturation in vitro[48]. There is no direct information about human oocytes.

Spontaneous mouse oocyte maturation in-vitro, in either the presence or the absence of meiotic inhibitor, is associated with a decrease in oocyte cAMP levels[49]. In mice, glucose treatment of cumulus–oocyte complexes (COCs) produced elevated cAMP levels, which is associated with a decreased incidence of germinal vesicle breakdown (GVBD) in hypoxanthine-supplemented medium[50]. Pyruvate directly affects nuclear maturation in mouse oocytes[51]. Although it has been indicated that glucose may have an inhibitory effect on cumulus-free human oocyte maturation during culture in vitro[52], the results from our laboratory indicate that oocyte maturation medium with glucose is beneficial to bovine and human oocyte nuclear and cytoplasmic maturation in vitro with proper concentrations[34,38].

Essential and/or non-essential amino acids are commonly added to serum-supplemented or serum-free culture media for mammalian embryo development in vitro. In many species, it has been known that addition of amino acids to the culture medium is beneficial for embryonic development[53]. Apart from amino acid use for protein synthesis, they play important roles as osmolytes[54], intracellular buffers[55], heavy metal chelators, and energy sources[56], as well as precursors for versatile physiologic regulators, such as nitric oxide and polyamines[57]. It has also been shown that culture medium enriched with amino acids affects glucose metabolism in mouse blastocysts in vitro[53]. Although it has been shown that amino acids support rabbit[40], hamster[39], porcine[58], and bovine[37] oocyte maturation, amino acid requirements for human oocyte maturation in culture are not fully understood. The data from our laboratory indicate that essential amino acids supplemented to a simple chemically defined medium are absolutely required for bovine oocyte cytoplasmic maturation to support subsequent embryonic development, and non-essential amino acids with essential amino acids have a synergic effect on oocyte cytoplasmic maturation[59,60].

It has been reported that the addition of water-soluble vitamins, particularly inositol, to the embryo culture medium enhances the hatching of rabbit and hamster blastocysts[61,62]. Vitamins affect glucose metabolism in mouse[53] and sheep embryos[63]. However, there is a paucity of information about the effects of vitamins in culture medium on the maturational and developmental competence of immature oocytes. The results from this laboratory demonstrate that the presence of vitamins in the oocyte maturation medium is important for subsequent bovine embryonic development[64]. Based on the animal model study, we have designed a new IVM medium and shown that this is beneficial for nuclear and cytoplasmic maturation of immature human oocytes derived from both stimulated IVF and unstimulated cycles[34].

Supplements

Serum

Earlier studies cultured immature human oocytes with TCM-199 or Ham's F-10 supplemented with 10% fetal calf serum (FCS) or fetal bovine serum (FBS). Normally, successful oocyte maturation media for animals contain a large quantity of FBS[65]. FBS is considered crucial for animal oocyte maturation and may also contain factors essential for human oocyte maturation. The important factors in serum for oocyte maturation could be many growth factors. Although a few pregnancies and live births were achieved when using 50% human follicular fluid (HFF) or 50% human peritoneal fluid (HPF) as supplements in the oocyte maturation medium[10,66], rates of oocyte maturation were relatively low. In the pregnancy and first birth of a normal baby occurring in an anovulatory PCOS patient following immature oocyte maturation in vitro, TCM-199 plus 10% FBS supplemented with gonadotropins was used[11]. It has been confirmed that FBS can be replaced by the patient's own serum for immature human oocyte maturation in vitro[67]. Therefore, the concerns about potential transmission of infectious agents could be resolved in the clinical application of oocyte maturation in vitro. Recent results indicate that the patient's serum could be replaced by human serum albumin (HSA) (Coopersurgical/SAGE IVM-Kit, USA). Therefore, it has been confirmed that serum is not an essential supplement for IVM of immature human oocytes.

Gonadotropins

As mentioned, gonadotropins (FSH and LH) play an important role in the development and function of preantral, antral, and preovulatory follicles in vivo. However, it is important to determine whether these gonadotropins could play the same role in promoting oocyte maturation in vitro. Currently most IVM protocols do supplement FSH, or LH, or a combination, in the culture medium. However, the effect of gonadotropins and their relative importance to oocyte maturation and subsequent fertilization and early development are still controversial. While the rationale behind using FSH and LH is based on the physiologic role of FSH and LH in oocyte maturation in vivo, it is most likely that the mechanisms of oocyte maturation are different between the in-vitro and in-vivo cases, because most IVM experiments are performed with oocytes derived from small and medium size follicles. Those follicles differ in many aspects from preovulatory follicles. In in-vitro conditions, LH probably acts to induce GVBD by an indirect action mediated by cumulus cells. It has been reported that mRNAs for FSH and LH receptors are present in mouse oocytes, zygotes, and pre-implantation embryos, indicating a potential role for gonadotropins in the modulation of meiotic resumption and the completion of oocyte maturation[68]. Recently the same authors reported that mRNAs for FSH and LH receptors are observed in human oocytes and preimplantation embryos at different stages[69].

It has been indicated that only FSH, not LH, influences the IVM of bovine oocytes[36], suggesting that the contradictory reports supporting LH as a major hormone involved in IVM are most likely caused by FSH contamination of the applied LH preparations[70,71]. However, it has been shown that FSH does not have a beneficial effect on mouse oocyte development in vitro[72]. Therefore, FSH and LH, apart from regulating oocyte growth and ovulation, must also directly or indirectly act on oocyte or cumulus cells to promote cytoplasmic maturation. The addition of FSH to oocyte culture medium does not significantly increase the ability of the human oocyte to reach MII[73]. However, maturation medium with FSH significantly increases oocyte fertilization of rhesus monkeys[74]. The ability of FSH to increase the developmental capacity of mouse oocytes maturing in vitro varies depending on the age and prior gonadotropin priming

in vivo[19]. Addition of FSH into culture medium does not increase the nuclear maturation of rat[75], monkey[74], or human[73] oocytes and FSH initially has an inhibitory action on mouse oocyte maturation[76]. It has been reported that mouse oocyte GVBD is inhibited by FSH due to its effect on the rise in the levels of cAMP in the cumulus cells[77]. FSH levels in the follicular fluid of MI and MII oocytes were found to be significantly higher than in follicles containing GV oocytes in women undergoing oocyte retrieval for stimulated IVF cycles[78]. The results from our laboratory using recombinant FSH (rFSH) indicate that supplementation of FSH into IVM medium is beneficial to both oocyte maturation and subsequent embryonic development in bovine and human oocytes (unpublished data).

IVM of bovine oocytes in the presence of LH resulted in increased embryonic development after IVF[79]. Denuded cumulus cells from oocytes do not respond to LH, thereby implicating the cumulus cells as the mediator of the LH effect[79]. One mechanism by which LH enhances IVM of bovine oocytes is through changing glucose metabolism in cumulus-enclosed oocytes and through modifying the nutritional environment of the oocyte[80]. It has been reported that increased pyruvate and lactate production from rat cumulus and granulosa cells occurs in response to LH[81,82]. It has been reported that LH-enhanced IVM of bovine oocytes needs the presence of either 20% FBS or 3 mg/ml bovine serum albumin (BSA)[79]. To achieve efficient FSH- and LH-dependent steroid production, cumulus cells require the presence of FBS[83]. Therefore, these data suggest that the beneficial effect of LH on the oocytes during IVM involves many possible pathways to effect oocyte and cytoplasmic maturation. The results from our laboratory using rFSH and LH indicate that both FSH and LH added to oocyte maturation medium are beneficial to oocyte maturation and subsequent early embryonic development (unpublished data).

The concentrations of FSH and LH in the oocyte maturation medium should be the same as in the follicular fluid containing fully mature oocytes. Nevertheless, an extremely high concentration of FSH and LH in the oocyte maturation medium has been used by some investigators[84,85]. Our understanding is that there is no specific reason for using such high concentrations (10 IU/ml) of pregnant mare's serum gonadotropin (PMSG) and hCG in the maturation medium. PMSG has approximately 50:50 FSH and LH bioactivity. The optimal condition for IVM of immature human oocytes should be similar to the physiologic concentration of gonadotropins in follicular fluid that contains fully mature oocytes. In addition, exposure of immature oocytes to different ratios of FSH:LH during maturation in vitro may result in different developmental competence. It has been reported that exposure of cattle and human oocytes to a 1:10 ratio of FSH:LH resulted in significantly higher developmental competence, evident by increased development to the blastocyst stage in vitro compared with FSH alone or no gonadotropins[86]. However, a report from an animal study indicated that the ratio of FSH:LH is not important for oocyte maturation and subsequent embryonic development[87]. Furthermore, our previous results indicated that culture medium supplemented with a physiologic concentration of FSH stimulated estradiol secretion from the cumulus cells derived from mature and immature human oocytes, suggesting that it may not be necessary to add estradiol to the oocyte maturation medium when the oocytes are cultured with the cumulus cells[83].

Steroids

Estradiol and progesterone are mediators of normal mammalian ovarian function. Estradiol may be important not only in regulating oocyte maturation, but also by its involvement in subsequent embryonic development[88]. Progesterone is required for fertilization and maintenance of luteal function[89]. There is evidence to support the hypothesis that levels of progesterone in follicular fluid are closely associated with oocyte matu-

rity[90]. The actions of estradiol and progesterone on oocyte maturation might be mediated rapidly through the non-genomic mechanism via cell membrane proteins as described in *Xenopus*[91]. Morrison et al.[92] indicated that in *Xenopus*, progesterone operates through a membrane associated tyrosine kinase to activate phospholipase.

Inhibition of steroid synthesis in whole cultured follicles from sheep impairs subsequent fertilization and developmental capacity following oocyte maturation[93]. The presence of estradiol in the culture medium of in-vitro matured human oocytes had no effect on the progression of meiosis, but improved the fertilization and cleavage rate[88]. To consider the effect of estradiol in bovine culture medium, the consensus appears to be a concentration of 1.0 µg/ml, which is the concentration in the follicular fluid of preovulatory follicles shortly after the LH peak[94]. As mentioned, estradiol is produced during culture of COCs[83], therefore it does not seem necessary to supplement exogenous estradiol during oocyte maturation if the oocytes were cultured with the cumulus and granulosa cells. There is little information about the effect of progesterone contained in the culture medium on human oocyte maturation. The results from our laboratory indicated a negative effect of progesterone on bovine oocyte cytoplasmic maturation when it was added to culture medium with gonadotropins (FSH and LH) and estradiol (unpublished data).

Growth factors

There are several growth factors and their receptors in follicular fluid. The intraovarian regulators include epidermal growth factor (EGF)/transforming growth factor beta (TGF-β) and members of the TGF-β superfamily (TGF-βs, inhibin, and activin). In-vitro studies using growth factors have shown that meiotic resumption in COCs can be induced by EGF[95], TGF-α and TGF-βs[96,97], and activin-A[98]. EGF alone and in association with gonadotropins induces cumulus expansion and promotes nuclear and cytoplasmic maturation of immature oocytes during culture in vitro[99]. Nuclear maturation was not affected when denuded oocytes were cultured with EGF, indicating that EGF action is mediated by the cumulus cells[95,100]. It seems that stimulating the activity of EGF is independent of the cAMP pathway[97]. Recent results from our laboratory indicated that there were no beneficial effects on oocyte maturation when bovine and human COCs were cultured in the presence of EGF and insulin (unpublished data).

Insulin is an anabolic hormone involved with energy storage. Primarily, this action is manifested as an increase in glucose and amino acid transport into cells and the stimulation of conversion of these precursors into storage forms, such as glycogen, protein, and triglycerides. Insulin and its receptor (IR), are both expressed on many different cell types, where they are likely to regulate glucose homeostasis and gene expression[101]. The IR is tyrosine kinase linked, but many of its actions require accessory molecules known as insulin receptor substrates (IRS-1, IRS-2, and IRS-3). Mural granulosa cells contain IR, and insulin can bind to the IGF-I receptor (IGF-IR). The IGF-IR is a heterotetramer with two α- and two β-subunits in a structure similar to that of the insulin receptor. Insulin can bind to the α-subunit ligand-binding domain and activate the β-subunit[102]. Thus, insulin can modulate ovarian cellular functions either through its own receptor or through the IGF-IR[103]. Although insulin and IGF-I seem to stimulate oocyte maturation and morphologic development of mouse[104] and bovine blastocysts[105], its action on human oocyte maturation is largely unknown.

MEDIA FOR IVM TREATMENT

IVM media are now commercially available. In our IVF Center, we are using the products from Cooper Surgical/SAGE Inc. The product described by Cooper Surgical/SAGE as the IVM-Kit contains three major culture media. The first is oocyte-washing medium, the second, oocyte-maturation medium, and the third, embryo-maintenance medium.

Oocyte-washing medium

This medium is used for washing immature oocytes, COCs, collected from the follicles before maturation in culture. This medium is buffered with HEPES, therefore the medium pH is not markedly changed at room temperature and atmosphere. This medium is ready for use following preincubation for at least 60 minutes at 37°C.

Oocyte-maturation medium

This medium is used for maturation in culture of immature oocytes in an incubator at 37°C under an atmosphere of 5% CO_2 in air and high humidity. An incubator with a triple gas mixture (90% N_2, 5% CO_2, and 5% O_2) and 100% humidity is also suitable for maturation in culture of immature oocytes, COCs.

Embryo-maintenance medium

This medium is used for fertilization and embryonic culture following insemination by intracytoplasmic sperm injection (ICSI). Although it is known that the fertilization rate of in-vitro matured oocytes is not affected by IVF, it is preferable to perform ICSI for in-vitro matured oocytes because it can be guaranteed that more than 65–70% of oocytes will be fertilized if the sperm used have a normal morphology.

IMMATURE OOCYTE RETRIEVAL

Flushing medium

COCs are collected in 10 ml culture tubes (Falcon) containing approximately 2–3 ml of heparinized warm flushing medium (usually containing

2 IU/ml of heparin). Any commercially available flushing medium, such as modified human tubal fluid (mHTF) or Ham's F-10 medium, can be used. However, it is important to make sure that the medium used contains heparin to prevent clouding (solidification) of the aspirates. It is also possible to use 0.9% saline containing 2 IU/ml heparin (Baxter, Toronto, Ontario, Canada) as flushing medium (Figure 21.1).

Identification of immature oocytes

There are two ways to look for and collect COCs from follicular aspirates: (1) Dish research: the follicular aspirates are poured directly into a petri dish (or tissue culture dish) and examined for COCs under a stereomicroscope. (2) Cell strainer: the follicular aspirates are filtered through a cell strainer (Falcon, Cell Strainer 352350, 70 μm nylon; Figure 21.2). After filtering, the collected aspirates can be rinsed with prewarmed IVM washing medium and transferred to a petri dish (Falcon, 60 × 15 mm) to search for COCs under a stereomicroscope. All handling procedures should be conducted on warm stages or plates at 37°C (Figure 21.3).

In order to determine whether the oocyte is mature or not, a special observation technique called 'sliding' can be employed. Briefly, the COC is allowed to slide slowly from one side to

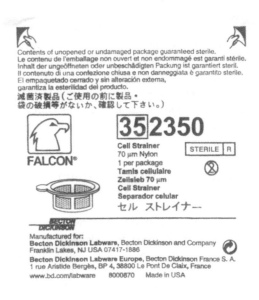

Figure 21.2 Labeling on cell strainer (Falcon, Becton Dickinson and Company, USA)

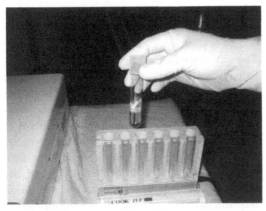

Figure 21.1 Follicular aspirates collected into tubes (10 ml, Falcon) containing approximately 2–3 ml of heparinized warm (37°C) flushing medium (0.9% saline containing 2 IU/ml heparin; Baxter, Toronto, Ontario, Canada)

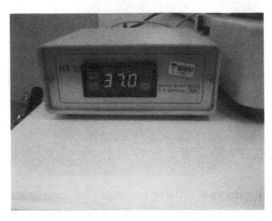

Figure 21.3 All handling procedures for culture dishes should be performed on warm stages or plates at 37°C

the other on the bottom of the petri dish, while being observed under the stereomicroscope (Figure 21.4). During COC sliding, it is possible to observe clearly whether or not the oocyte cytoplasm contains a germinal vesicle (GV) or if the oocyte has extruded a first polar body (1PB) into the perivitelline space (PVS). If neither a GV is seen in the oocyte cytoplasm nor a 1PB is found in the PVS, the oocyte is defined as GVBD or metaphase I stage (MI) (Figure 21.5). If any mature oocytes are found, they should be inseminated by either IVF or ICSI within 3 hours after collection.

Preparation of oocyte-washing medium

Oocyte-washing medium must be prepared at least 1 hour before oocyte collection and kept at 37°C. Briefly, three petri dishes (Falcon, 35 × 10 mm), each containing approximately 2.0–2.5 ml of oocyte-washing medium under mineral oil, are prepared for every patient. If a cell strainer is to be used to collect COCs, a flask (Falcon, 50 ml) containing approximately

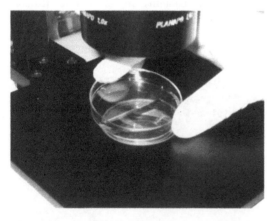

Figure 21.4 Sliding technique for observation of oocyte maturity. COCs are allowed to slide slowly from one side to the other on the bottom of the petri dish, while being observed under the stereomicroscope

25–30 ml of oocyte-washing medium must also be prepared for each patient and kept in an incubator.

To use a cell strainer, each tube of follicular aspirate is poured through the cell strainer immediately after collection. The cell strainer can be placed in a petri dish (Falcon, 60 × 15 mm) containing 3–5 ml of oocyte-washing medium on a warm stage or plate in order to prevent the COCs from drying in the strainer between the time of follicular aspiration and tube collection. Once follicular aspiration has been completed, the COCs contained in the cell strainer are collected with a pipette, then immediately transferred into petri dishes for scanning of the COCs under a stereomicroscope. To identify the status of oocyte maturity, the sliding technique of observation is then used as described previously. COCs are transferred to oocyte-washing medium to be washed three times and then are transferred to oocyte-maturation medium for maturation in culture (Figure 21.6).

IVM OF IMMATURE OOCYTES

Preparation of oocyte-maturation medium

The immature COCs (maximum of 10) are incubated in an organ tissue culture dish (Falcon, 60 × 15 mm) containing 1 ml oocyte-maturation medium supplemented with a final concentration of 75 mIU/ml FSH and 75 mIU/ml LH at 37°C in an incubator with an atmosphere of 5% CO_2 and 95% air with high humidity (or with triple gas mixture, 90% N_2, 5% CO_2, and 5% O_2, and 100% humidity). Oocyte-maturation medium should be prepared for equilibration at least 2 hours before immature oocyte retrieval (practically, it can be made one day before). A brief description of the procedures involved in the preparation of oocyte-maturation medium follows (Figure 21.7):

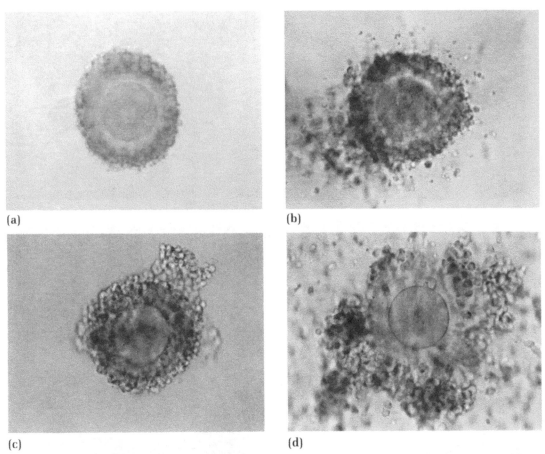

(a)

(b)

(c)

(d)

Figure 21.5   During COC sliding, it is possible to observe clearly whether or not the oocyte cytoplasm contains a germinal vesicle (GV) (a and b) or whether the oocyte has extruded a first polar body (1PB) intc the perivitelline space (PVS) (c). If neither a GV is seen in the oocyte cytoplasm nor a 1PB is found in the PVS, then the oocyte is defined as germinal vesicle breakdown (GVBD) or metaphase I stage (MI) (d) (see color plate section)

(1)   Place 10.0 ml of oocyte-maturation medium into a test tube (**a** in Figure 21.7).

(2)   Completely dissolve 1 ampoule of 75 IU FSH and 75 IU LH into tube **a**.

(3)   Place 9.9 ml of fresh oocyte-maturation medium into a test tube (**b** in Figure 21.7).

(4)   Take 100 µl of the FSH and LH solution from tube **a** and transfer to tube **b**.

(5)   Prepare three organ tissue culture dishes for each patient. In each dish, the inner well contains 1 ml and the outer well 2 ml of medium from tube b.

(6)   Cover the organ culture dish with the dish cover and place it in the incubator.

Sperm preparation

Semen can be collected and prepared for insemination on the day of oocyte retrieval if a mature oocyte has been retrieved from the dominant follicle. Otherwise, semen collection and prepara-

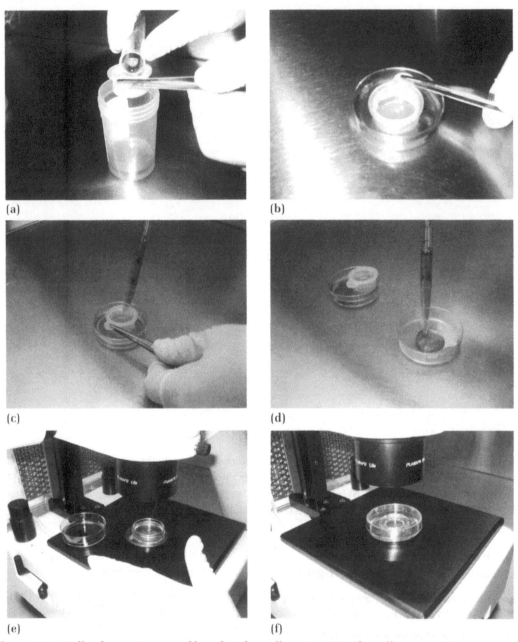

Figure 21.6 Follicular aspirates are filtered with a cell strainer (a). The cell strainer is kept in a petri dish (Falcon, 60 × 15 mm) containing the oocyte-washing medium between tube collection and filtering (b). After filtering, the collected aspirates can be rinsed and transferred into another petri dish in order to search for COCs under a stereomicroscope (c and d). After washing two or three times with prewarmed oocyte-washing medium in a washing dish (Falcon, 30 × 10 mm) (e), COCs are transferred to the oocyte-maturation medium for maturation in culture (f)

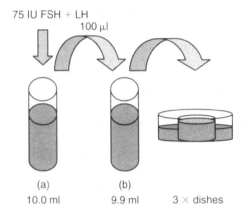

75 IU FSH + LH
100 μl

(a)
10.0 ml

(b)
9.9 ml

3 × dishes

Figure 21.7 Preparation of the oocyte-maturation medium. Take two tubes, the first tube (a) contains 10.0 ml of the oocyte-maturation medium, and the second tube (b) contains 9.9 ml of the oocyte-maturation medium, respectively. Using the medium from tube (a) dissolve 75 IU of FSH and 75 IU of LH (gonadotropin stock). Place 100 μl of the gonadotropin stock into the second tube (b). Prepare three organ tissue culture dishes (Falcon, 60 × 15 mm) with tube (b) for each patient, the inner well containing 1 ml of the oocyte-maturation medium and the outer well 2 ml of the oocyte-maturation medium

tion should be performed the day after oocyte retrieval. If possible, a fresh sperm sample should be obtained which can then be prepared for the insemination. Since the procedure is identical to that used for sperm preparation for IVF or ICSI, it will not be repeated here.

Stripping oocytes 24 h after culture

The immature COCs are cultured in the oocyte-maturation medium in the incubator and allowed to begin the maturation process for 24 to 48 hours. Twenty-four hours after maturation in culture, all of the COCs are stripped for identification of oocyte maturity (Figure 21.8). COCs are denuded using a finely drawn glass pipette following one minute of exposure to a commer-

cially available hyaluronidase solution. The mature oocytes are then subjected to insemination by either IVF or ICSI after stripping. The remaining immature oocytes (GV and MI) will continue to mature in culture for another 24 h. At this point, it is not necessary to change the oocyte-maturation medium.

Identification of mature oocytes 48 h after culture

Forty-eight hours after oocyte retrieval (or oocyte maturation in culture), the remaining stripped oocytes are re-examined and, if any have matured (MII) at this point, they will be inseminated immediately by either IVF or ICSI.

INSEMINATION OF MATURE OOCYTES

Preparation of embryo-maintenance medium

Embryo-maintenance medium must be prepared at least 1 hour before ICSI and kept at 37°C in an incubator with an atmosphere of 5% CO_2 and 95% air with high humidity or with a triple gas mixture (90% N_2, 5% CO_2, and 5% O_2) and

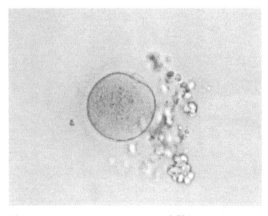

Figure 21.8 Mature oocyte following in-vitro culture 24 h in the oocyte-maturation medium after partially stripping the cumulus cells from the oocyte

100% humidity. Briefly, it is appropriate to prepare each droplet with 20 µl of embryo-maintenance medium under mineral oil in a petri dish (Falcon, 35 × 10 mm). The number of dishes used for each patient will depend upon the number of mature oocytes obtained after maturation in culture.

Insemination by ICSI

ICSI is recommended for the insemination of in-vitro matured oocytes because we believe that this method offers a greater chance of successful fertilization than does IVF. ICSI is a common procedure for this reason (Figure 21.9). Although it is preferable to prepare sperm freshly before ICSI, it does not appear problematic to use sperm prepared on the day of egg collection or the day after for oocytes matured 48 h after egg retrieval. Commercially available ICSI medium and polyvinylpyrrolidone (PVP) solution can be used to prepare the ICSI dish. It is also appropriate to use the oocyte-washing medium for preparation of the ICSI droplets because the pH of the oocyte-washing medium is quite stable at room temperature and atmosphere. However, it is important to note that the ICSI dish should

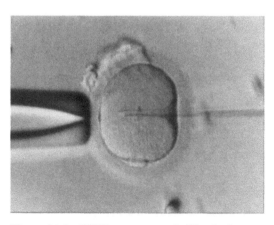

Figure 21.9 ICSI is recommended for the insemination of in-vitro matured oocytes because we believe that this method offers a greater chance of successful fertilization than does IVF

be prepared at least 1 hour before ICSI and kept at 37°C in the incubator or on a warm stage or plate for equilibration. After ICSI, the individual oocyte is transferred into a droplet (20 µl) of the embryo-maintenance medium in a petri dish for culture in the incubator.

Identification of fertilization

Between 16 and 18 hours after ICSI, fertilization of the oocytes is checked under a microscope for the appearance of two distinct pronuclei (2PN) and two polar bodies (sometimes the polar bodies are fragmented). Pronuclear scoring can be carried out by rating embryos as 'good' if they have aligned nucleoli, a cytoplasmic halo, and abutting pronuclei or other systems. However, at this point it is not necessary to transfer the fertilized oocytes (2PN embryos) into another medium (dish) for continued culture.

Embryo culture

The fertilized oocytes are cultured in the droplets (20 µl) under mineral oil for 1 or 2 additional days, depending upon the number and quality of embryos achieved. If blastocyst culture is requested, the cleaved embryos should be transferred to new droplets (20 µl) in a petri dish containing the same embryo-maintenance medium under mineral oil 2 days after ICSI. The cleaved embryos can be cultured until the blastocyst stage in this embryo-maintenance medium.

EMBRYVO TRANSFER

Embryo developing stage

It seems that most embryo transfers (ET) in IVM treatment can be done on day 2 or day 3 after ICSI because no extra benefit is derived by culturing the embryos to blastocyst stage if the available number of embryos is small. In general, ET should be performed on day 2 after ICSI if the number of embryos obtained is ≤3; ET should be performed on day 3 after ICSI if the number of embryos obtained is ≥4. ET with blastocysts should only be considered if a total of more than four good quality four-cell stage embryos are achieved on day 2 of embryo assessment after ICSI.

Scoring embryos

The scoring of cleavage-stage embryos for transfer is crucial for pregnancy potential. Since the oocytes may not be matured and inseminated at the same time following maturation in culture, the developmental stages of embryos may be variable in the same patient. Therefore, before ET, all embryos for each patient should be pooled and selected for transfer (Figure 21.10). The final outcome of pregnancy may depend to a great extent on the experience of the embryologist. The cleavage speed of embryos and the morphologic marker of each cleaved blastomere are usually used for scoring the quality of embryo generated from in-vitro matured oocytes. It is recommended that a maximum of three embryos be transferred into the uterus, based on the quality of embryos, or, if blastocysts are obtained, the number of embryos for transfer should be only one or two. It is not true that transferring a greater number of poor-quality embryos increases pregnancy and implantation rates.

Thickness of endometrium

On the day of ET, endometrial thickness should be measured by transvaginal ultrasound scan. At this point, the endometrial thickness should be at least ≥7.0 mm. If the endometrial thickness is <7.0 mm, the embryo should be cryopreserved and transferred in a subsequent cycle.

Embryo loading and transfer

It seems that selecting a good ET catheter is important for establishing successful pregnancy. The ideal ET catheter should be very soft and its tip should be rounded to prevent any trauma to the endometrial lining. In addition, it should be easy to aspirate embryos through the tip under the microscope without air bubbles. Furthermore, the ET catheter should be smooth enough to prevent the embryos from getting stuck to the inner wall of the catheter. Rinsing the inner wall of the catheter with a syringe is very important prior to ET. At this point, the oocyte-washing medium (2–3 ml) contained in a test tube can be used for rinsing the inner wall of the catheter with a syringe. The volume of the embryo (average 3.0 ± 1.0) plus transfer medium loaded into the ET catheter should not exceed 10 µl (Figure 21.11).

One of the final key contributory factors to a successful pregnancy is embryo transfer. Careful

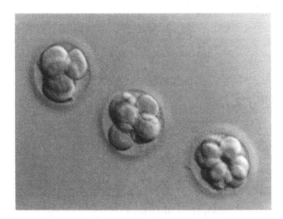

Figure 21.10 Embryos are pooled together 2 or 3 days after ICSI. Note that the embryos are at different stages of development

Approximately 10 µl medium with embryos

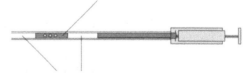

Approximately 1.0 cm length of air

Figure 21.11 A diagram of embryo loading in an ET catheter. The volume of the embryo plus transfer medium loaded into the ET catheter should be approximately 10 µl

attention must be paid to both the scientific and clinical aspects of this event. A trial or mock transfer prior to the actual transfer provides very useful information to ensure a curved cervical canal, ascertain the position of the uterus, and avert any foreseeable problems during the actual transfer. It is important that as much mucus as possible is removed from the cervix with a sterile cotton bud before ET. An abdominal ultrasound-guided ET may be recommended in selected cases in order to confirm that the embryos with the fluid contents of the catheter are in the uterus.

CONCLUSIONS

The size of the follicles may be an important feature for subsequent embryonic development, but the developmental competence of oocytes derived from small antral follicles seems not to be adversely affected by the presence of a dominant follicle. It is important to identify the maturity of oocytes at egg collection in order to maximize the success rate of infertility treatment. Although it seems that the laboratory is the 'key' for IVM treatment, other clinical aspects have to be taken into account for a successful pregnancy.

ACKNOWLEDGMENTS

The work described in this chapter was part of the Program on Oocyte Health funded under the Healthy Gametes and Great Embryos Strategic Initiative of the Canadian Institutes of Health Research (CIHR), Institute of Human Development, Child and Youth Health (IHDCYH), grant number HGG62293 and was supported by the Natural Sciences and Engineering Research Council (NSERC) of Canada, grant number RGPIN 227107.

REFERENCES

1. Rock J, Menkin MF. *In vitro* fertilization and cleavage of human ovarian eggs. Science 1946; 100: 105–7.

2. Menkin MF, Rock J. *In vitro* fertilization and cleavage of human ovarian eggs. Am J Obst Gynecol 1948; 55: 440–2.

3. Edwards RG. Maturation *in vitro* of mouse, sheep, cow, pig, rhesus monkey and human ovarian oocytes. Nature 1965; 208: 349–51.

4. Edwards RG. Maturation *in vitro* of human ovarian oocytes. Lancet 1965; II: 926–9.

5. Edwards RG, Bavister BD, Steptoe PC. Early stages of fertilization in vitro of human oocytes matured in vivo. Nature 1969; 221: 632–5.

6. Steptoe PC, Edwards RG. Birth after the reimplantation of a human embryo. Lancet 1978; 312: 366.

7. Beerendonk CCM, van Dop PA, Braat DDM et al. Ovarian hyperstimulation syndrome: facts and fallacies. Obstet Gynecol Surv 1998; 53: 439–49.

8. Tarlatzis BC, Grimbizis G, Bontis J et al. Ovarian stimulation and ovarian tumours: a critical reappraisal. Hum Reprod Update 1995; 1: 284–301.

9. Duckitt K, Templeton AA. Cancer in women with infertility. Curr Opin Obstet Gynecol 1998; 10: 199–203.

10. Cha KY, Koo JJ, Ko JJ et al. Pregnancy after in vitro fertilization of human follicular oocytes collected from nonstimulated cycles, their culture *in vitro* and their transfer in a donor oocyte program. Fertil Steril 1991; 55: 109–13.

11. Trounson A, Wood C, Kausche A. *In vitro* maturation and the fertilization and developmental competence of oocytes recovered from unstreated polycystic ovarian patients. Fertil Steril 1994; 62: 353–62.

12. Cha KY, Chian RC. Maturation *in vitro* of immature human oocytes for clinical use. Hum Reprod Update 1998; 4: 103–20.

13. Chian RC, Buckett WM, Tan SL. *In vitro* maturation of human oocytes. RBM Online 2004; 8: 148–66.

14. Chian, RC, Lim JH, Tan SL. State of the art in in-vitro oocyte maturation. Curr Opin Obstet Gynecol 2004; 16: 211–19.

15. Nargund G, Waterstone J, Bland JM et al. Cumulative conception and live birth rates in natural (unstimulated) IVF cycles. Hum Reprod 2001; 16: 259–62.

16. Chian RC, Buckett WM, Tulandi T et al. Prospective randomized study of human chorionic gonadotrophin priming before immature oocyte retrieval from unstimulated women with polycystic ovarian syndrome. Hum Reprod 2000; 15: 165–70.

17. Duranthon V, Renard JP. The developmental competence of mammalian oocytes: a convenient but biologically fuzzy concept. Theriogenology 2001; 55: 1277–89.

18. Gougeon A. Regulation of ovarian follicular development in primates: facts and hypotheses. Endocrinol Rev 1996; 17: 121–55.

19. Eppig JJ, Schroeder AC, O'Brien MJ. Developmental capacity of mouse oocytes matured in vitro: effect of gonadotrophic stimulation, follicular origin and oocyte size. J Reprod Fertil 1992; 95: 119–27.

20. Durinzi KL, Saniga EM, Lanzendorf SE. The relationship between size and maturation in vitro in the unstimulated human oocyte. Fertil Steril 1995; 63: 404–6.

21. Fair T, Hyttel P, Greve T. Bovine oocyte diameter in relation to maturational competence and transcriptional activity. Mol Reprod Dev 1995; 42: 437–42.

22. Tsuji K, Sowa M, Nakano R. Relationship between human oocyte maturation and different follicular sizes. Biol Reprod 1985; 32: 413–17.

23. Gougeon A, Lefevre B. Evolution of the diameters of the largest healthy and atretic follicles during the human menstrual cycle. J Reprod Fertil 1983; 69: 497–502.

24. Hillier SG. Sex steroid metabolism and follicular development in the ovary. Oxford Rev Reprod Biol 1985; 7: 168–222.

25. Anderiesz C, Trounson AO. The effect of testosterone on the maturation and developmental capacity of murine oocytes in vitro. Hum Reprod 1995; 10: 2377–81.

26. Smith LC, Olivera-Angel M, Groome NP et al. Oocyte quality in small antral follicles in the presence or absence of a large dominant follicle in cattle. J Reprod Fertil 1996; 106: 193–9.

27. Chian RC, Chung JT, Downey BF et al. Maturational and developmental competence of immature oocytes retrieved from ovaries at different phases of folliculogenesis: bovine model study. RBM Online 2002; 4: 127–32.

28. Bomsel-Helmreich O, Huyen LVN, Durand-Gasselin I et al. Mature and immature oocytes in large and medium follicles after clomiphene citrate and human menopausal gonadotropin stimulation without human chorionic gonadotropin. Fertil Steril 1987; 48: 596–604.

29. Wittmaack FM, Kreger DO, Blasco L et al. Effect of follicular size on oocyte retrieval, fertilization, cleavage and embryo quality in in vitro fertilization cycles: a 6-year data collection. Fertil Steril 1994; 62: 1205–10.

30. Dubey AK, Wang HA, Duffy P et al. The correlation between follicular measurements, oocyte morphology and fertilization rates in an in vitro fertilization program. Fertil Steril 1995; 64: 787–90.

31. Salha O, Abusheika N, Sharma V. Dynamics of human follicular growth and in vitro oocyte maturation. Hum Reprod Update 1998; 4: 816–32.

32. Jones GM, Trounson AO, Gardner DK et al. Evolution of a culture protocol for successful blastocyst development and pregnancy. Hum Reprod 1998; 13: 169–77.

33. Trounson A, Anderiesz C, Jones G. Maturation of human oocytes in vitro and their developmental competence. Reproduction 2001; 121: 51–75.

34. Chian RC, Tan SL. Maturational and developmental competence of cumulus-free immature human oocytes derived from stimulated and intracytoplasmic sperm injection cycles. RBM Online 2002; 5: 125–32.

35. Trounson AO, Anderiesz C, Jones GM et al. Oocyte maturation. Hum Reprod 1998; 13: 52–62.

36. Bevers MM, Dieleman SJ, van den Hurk R et al. Regulation and modulation of oocyte maturation in the bovine. Theriogenology 1997; 47: 13–22.

37. Rose-Hellekant TA, Libersky-Williamson EA, Bavister BD. Energy substrates and amino acids provided during *in vitro* maturation of bovine oocytes alter acquisition of developmental competence. Zygote 1998; 6: 285–94.

38. Chung JT, Tan SL, Chian RC. Effect of glucose on bovine oocyte maturation and subsequent fertilization and early embryonic development in vitro. Biol Reprod 2002; 66(Suppl): 177.

39. Gwatkin RBL, Haidri AA. Requirements for the maturation of hamster oocytes in vitro. Exp Cell Res 1973; 76: 1–7.

40. Bae IH, Foote RH. Utilization of glutamine for energy and protein synthesis by cultured rabbit follicular oocytes. Exp Cell Res 1975; 90: 432–6.

41. Leese HJ, Barton AM. Production of pyruvate by isolated mouse cumulus cells. J Exp Zool 1985; 234: 231–6.

42. Biggers JD, Whittingham DG, Donahue RP. The pattern of energy metabolism in the mouse oocyte and zygote. Proc Natl Acad Sci USA 1967; 58: 560–7.

43. Gandolfi F, Milanesi E, Pocar P et al. Comparative analysis of calf and cow oocytes during in vitro maturation. Mol Reprod Dev 1998; 49: 168–75.

44. Leese HJ, Barton AM. Pyruvate and glucose uptake by mouse ova and preimplantational embryos. J Reprod Fertil 1984; 72: 9–13.

45. Geshi M, Takenouchi N, Yamauchi N et al. Effects of sodium pyruvate in nonserum maturation medium on maturation, fertilization, and subsequent development of bovine oocytes with or without cumulus cells. Biol Reprod 2000; 63: 1730–4.

46. Zheng P, Wang H, Bavister BD et al. Maturation of rhesus monkey oocytes in chemically defined culture media and their functional assessment by IVF and embryo development. Hum Reprod 2001; 16: 300–5.

47. Mouatassim SEL, Hazout A, Bellec V et al. Glucose metabolism during the final stage of human oocyte maturation: genetic expression of hexokinase, glucose phosphate isomerase and phosphofructokinase. Zygote 1999; 7: 45–50.

48. Krisher RL, Bavister BD. Enhanced glycolysis after maturation of bovine oocytes in vitro is associated with increased developmental competence. Mol Reprod Dev 1999; 53: 19–26.

49. Downs SM, Daniel SAJ, Bornslaeger EA et al. Maintenance of meiotic arrest in mouse oocytes by purines: modulation of cAMP levels and cAMP phosphodiesterase activity. Gamete Res 1989; 23: 323–34.

50. Downs SM. The influence of glucose, cumulus cells, and metabolic coupling on ATP levels and meiotic control in the isolated mouse oocyte. Devel Biol 1995; 167: 502–12.

51. Haekwon K, Schuetz AW. Regulation of nuclear membrane assembly and maintenance during in vitro maturation of mouse oocytes: role of pyruvate and protein synthesis. Cell Tissue Res 1991; 265: 105–12.

52. Cekleniak NA, Combelles CMH, Ganz DA et al. A novel system for in vitro maturation of human oocytes. Fertil Steril 2001; 75: 1185–93.

53. Lane M, Gardner DK. Amino acids and vitamins prevent culture-induced metabolic perturbations and associated loss of viability of mouse blastocysts. Hum Reprod 1998; 13: 991–7.

54. Biggers JD, Lawwitts JA, Lechene CP. The protective action of betaine on the deleterious effects of NaCl on preimplantation mouse embryos in vitro. Mol Reprod Dev 1993; 34: 380–90.

55. Edwards LJ, Williams DA, Gardner DK. Intracellular pH of the mouse preimplantation embryo: amino acids act as buffers of intracellular pH. Hum Reprod 1998; 13: 344–8.

56. Bavister BD. Culture of preimplantation embryos: facts and artifacts. Hum Reprod Update 1995; 1: 91–148.

57. Wu G, Morris SM Jr. Arginine metabolism: nitric oxide and beyond. Biochem J 1998; 336: 1–17.

58. Ka HH, Sawai K, Wang WH et al. Amino acids in maturation medium and presence of cumulus cells at fertilization promote male pronuclear formation in porcine oocytes matured and penetrated in vitro. Biol Reprod 1997; 57: 1478–83.

59. Rezaei N, Abdul-Jalil AK, Chung JT et al. Role of essential and non-essential amino acids contained in maturation medium on bovine oocyte maturation and subsequent fertilization and early embryonic development in vitro. Theriogenology 2003; 59: 497.

60. Rezaei N, Chian RC. Effects of essential and non-essential amino acids on in-vitro maturation, fertilization and development of immature bovine oocytes. Iran J Reprod Med 2005; 3: 36–41.

61. Kane MT, Bavister BD. Vitamins requirements for development of eight-cell hamster embryos to hatching blastocysts in vitro. Biol Reprod 1988; 39: 1137–43.

62. Fahy MM, Kane MT. Inositol stimulates DNA and protein synthesis, and expansion by rabbit blastocysts in vitro. Hum Reprod 1992; 7: 550–2.

63. Gardner DK, Lane M, Spitzer A et al. Enhanced rates of cleavage and development for sheep zygotes cultured to the blastocyst stage in vitro in the absence of serum and somatic cells: amino acids, vitamins, and culturing embryos in groups stimulate development. Biol Reprod 1994; 50: 390–400.

64. Abdul Jalil AK, Rezaei N, Chung JT et al. Effect of vitamins during oocyte maturation on subsequent embryonic development in vitro. 48th Ann Meeting CFAS 2002; TP-24.

65. Younis AI, Brackett BG, Fayrer-Hosken RA. Influence of serum and hormones on bovine oocyte maturation and fertilization in vitro. Gamete Res 1989; 23: 189–201.

66. Cha KY, Do BR, Chi HJ et al. Viability of human follicular oocytes collected from unstimulated ovaries and matured and fertilized in vitro. Reprod Fertil Dev 1992; 4: 695–701.

67. Chian RC, Buckett WM, Too LL et al. Pregnancies resulting from in vitro matured oocytes retrieved from patients with polycystic ovary syndrome after priming with human chorionic gonadotropin. Fertil Steril 1999; 72: 639–42.

68. Patsoula E, Loutradis D, Drakakis P et al. Expression of mRNA for the LH and FSH receptors in mouse oocytes and preimplantation embryos. Reproduction 2001; 121: 455–61.

69. Patsoula E, Loutradis D, Drakakis P et al. Messenger RNA expression for the follicle-stimulating hormone receptor and luteinizing hormone receptor in human oocytes and preimplantation-stage embryos. Fertil Steril 2003; 79: 1187–93.

70. Harper KM, Brackett BG. Bovine blastocyst development after in vitro maturation in a defined medium with epidermal growth factor and low concentrations of gonadotropins. Biol Reprod 1993; 48: 409–16.

71. Harper KM, Brackett BG. Bovine blastocyst development after in vitro maturation in a defined medium with epidermal growth factor and low concentrations of gonadotropins. Biol Reprod 1993; 48: 409–16.

72. Eppig JJ, Hose M, O'Brien MJ et al. Conditions that affect acquisition of developmental competence by mouse oocytes in vitro: FSH, insulin, glucose and ascorbic acid. Mol Cell Endocrinol 2000; 163: 109–16.

73. Durinzi KL, Wentz AC, Saniga EM et al. Follicle stimulating hormone effects on immature human oocytes: in vitro maturation and hormone production. J Assist Reprod Genet 1997; 14: 199–204.

74. Morgan PM, Warikoo PK, Bavister BD. In vitro maturation of oocytes from unstimulated rhesus monkeys: assessment of cytoplasmic maturity by embryonic development after in vitro fertilization. Biol Reprod 1991; 45: 89–93.

75. Vanderhyden BC, Armstrong DT. Role of cumulus cells and serum on the in vitro maturation, fertilization, and subsequent development of rat oocytes. Biol Reprod 1989; 40: 720–8.

76. Downs SM, Daniel SAJ, Eppig JJ. Induction of maturation in cumulus cell-enclosed mouse oocytes by follicle-stimulating hormone and epidermal growth factor: evidence for a positive stimulus of somatic cell origin. J Exp Zool 1988; 245: 86–96.

77. Schultz RM, Montgomery R, Ward-Bailey PF et al. Regulation of oocyte maturation in the mouse: possible roles of intercellular communication, cAMP and testosterone. Devel Biol 1983; 95: 294–304.

78. Laufer N, Tarlatzis BC, De Cherney AH. Asynchrony between human cumulus–corona cell complex and oocyte maturation after human

menopausal gonadotropin treatment for in vitro fertilization. Fertil Steril 1984; 42: 366–9.

79. Zuelke KA, Brackett BG. Luteinizing hormone-enhanced in vitro maturation of bovine oocytes with and without protein supplementation. Biol Reprod 1990; 43: 784–7.

80. Zuelke KA, Brackett BG. Effects of luteinizing hormone on glucose metabolism in cumulus enclosed bovine oocytes matured in vitro. Endocrinology 1992; 131: 2690–6.

81. Hillensjo T. Oocyte maturation and glycolysis in isolated pre-ovulatory follicles of PMS-injected immature rats. Acta Endocrinol 1976; 82: 809–30.

82. Billig H, Hedin L, Magnusson C. Gonadotrophins stimulate lactate production by rat cumulus and granulose cells. Acta Endocrinol 1983; 103: 562–6.

83. Chian RC, Ao A, Clarke HJ et al. Production of steroids from human cumulus cells treated with different concentrations of gonadotropins during culture in vitro. Fertil Steril 1999: 71: 61–6.

84. Nagy ZP, Cecile J, Liu J et al. Pregnancy and birth after intracytoplasmic sperm injection of in vitro matured germinal vesicle stage oocytes: case report. Fertil Steril 1996; 65: 1047–50.

85. Liu J, Katz E, Garcia JE et al. Successful in vitro maturation of human oocytes not exposed to human chorionic gonadotropin during ovulation induction, resulting in pregnancy. Fertil Steril 1997; 67: 566–8.

86. Anderiesz C, Ferraretti AP, Magli C et al. Effect of recombinant human gonadotrophins on human, bovine and murine oocyte meiosis, fertilization and embryonic development in vitro. Hum Reprod 2000; 15: 1140–8.

87. Choi YH, Carnevale EM, Seidel Jr GE et al. Effects of gonadotropins on bovine oocytes matured in TCM–199. Theriogenology 2001; 56: 661–70.

88. Tesarik J, Mendoza C. Nongenomic effects of 17β-estradiol on maturing human oocytes: relationship to oocyte developmental potential. J Clin Endocrinol Metab 1995; 80: 1438–43.

89. Hibbert M, Stouffer RL, Wolf DP et al. Midcycle administration of a progesterone synthesis inhibitor prevents ovulation in primates. Proc Natl Acad Sci USA 1996; 93: 1897–901.

90. Seibel MM, Smith D, Dlugi AM et al. Periovulatory follicular fluid hormone levels in spontaneous human cycles. J Clin Endocrinol Metab 1989; 68: 1073–7.

91. Bayaa M, Booth RA, Sheng Y et al. The classical progesterone receptor mediates Xenopus oocyte maturation through a nongenomic mechanism. Proc Natl Acad Sci USA 2000; 7: 12607–12.

92. Morrison T, Waggoner L, Whitworth-Langley L et al. Nongenomic action of progesterone: activation of Xenopus oocyte phospholipase C through a plasma membrane-associated tyrosine kinase. Endocrinology 2000; 141: 214–52.

93. Moor RM, Polge C, Willadsen SM. Effects of follicular steroids on the maturation and fertilization of mammalian oocytes. J Embryol Exp Morph 1980; 56: 319–35.

94. Dieleman SJ, Kruip ThAM, Fontijne P et al. Changes in oestradiol, progesterone and testosterone concentrations in follicular fluid and in the micromorphology of preovulatory bovine follicles relative to the peak of luteinizing hormone. J Endocrinol 1993; 97: 31–42.

95. Lorenzo PL, Illera MJ, Illera JC et al. Enhancement of cumulus expansion and nuclear maturation during bovine oocyte maturation in vitro by the addition of epidermal growth factor and insulin-like growth factor I. J Reprod Fertil 1994; 101: 697–701.

96. Brucker C, Alexander NJ, Hodgen GD et al. Transforming growth factor-alpha augments meiotic maturation of cumulus cell-enclosed mouse oocytes. Mol Reprod Dev 1991; 28: 94–8.

97. Coskun S, Lin YC. Mechanism of action of epidermal growth factor-induced porcine oocyte maturation. Mol Reprod Dev 1995; 42: 311–17.

98. Coskun S, Lin YC. Effects of transforming growth factors and activin-A on in vitro porcine oocyte maturation. Mol Reprod Dev 1994; 38: 153–9.

99. De La Fuente R, O'Brien MJ, Eppig JJ. Epidermal growth factor enhances preimplantation developmental competence of maturing mouse oocytes. Hum Reprod 1999; 14: 3060–8.

100. Wang WH, Niwa K. Synergetic effects of epidermal growth factor and gonadotropins on the cytoplasmic maturation of pig oocytes in a serum-free medium. Zygote 1995; 3: 345–50.

101. Wozniak M, Rydzewski B, Baker SP et al. The cellular and physiological actions of insulin in the central nervous system. Neurochem Int 1993; 22: 1–10.

102. Voutilainen R, Franls S, Mason HD et al. IGF-binding protein, and IGF receptor messenger ribonucleic acid in normal and polycystic ovaries. J Clin Endocrinol Metab 1996; 81: 1003–8.

103. Giudice L. The insulin-like growth factor system in normal and abnormal human ovarian follicle development. Am J Med 1995; 16: 48–54S.

104. Reed ML, Estrada JL, Illera MJ et al. Effects of epidermal growth factor, insulin-like growth factor-1, and dialyzed porcine follicular fluid on porcine oocyte maturation in vitro. J Exp Zool 1993; 266: 74–8.

105. Ocana-Quero JM, Pinedo-Merlin M, Ortega-Mariscal E et al. Infuence of human and bovine insulin on in vitro maturation, fertilization and cleavage rates of bovine oocytes. Arch Zootec 1998; 47: 85–93.

CHAPTER 22

Human embryonic development in vitro

David K Gardner

INTRODUCTION

Human embryo culture systems have improved significantly over the past two decades. The overall increase in pregnancy rates within the USA as reported by the Centers for Disease Control (CDC) (Figure 22.1) is a direct reflection of our improved ability to culture (and select) viable human embryos. Furthermore, as well as increasing the outcome of an IVF cycle following embryo transfer at the pronuclear and cleavage stages, with the advent of more physiologic culture media, it is now also possible to culture the human embryo to the blastocyst stage as a matter of routine. This in turn has been responsible for further increases in implantation rates (and decreases in pregnancy losses). The aim of this chapter is therefore to review the current systems available to culture the human embryo and also to guide the reader to factors outside of a media bottle that can affect the outcome of an IVF cycle.

THE EMBRYO CULTURE SYSTEM

In Figure 22.2 some of the factors that can affect the outcome of an IVF cycle are highlighted. It can be seen that the embryo culture system

is composed of more than the type of culture medium chosen to sustain the embryo in vitro, and that several of these factors can impact the outcome of an IVF cycle. In order to optimize outcome one must therefore consider

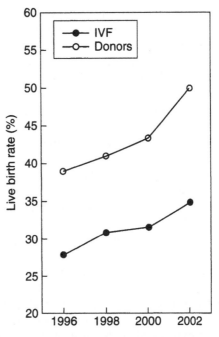

Figure 22.1 Live birth rates following IVF and oocyte donation in the USA from 1996 to 2002 (source: the Centers for Disease Control (CDC))

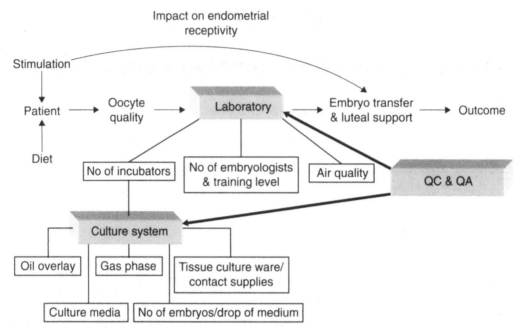

Figure 22.2 A holistic analysis of human IVF. This figure serves to illustrate the complex and interdependent nature of human IVF treatment. For example, the stimulation regimen used not only impacts oocyte quality (hence embryo physiology and viability), but can also affect subsequent endometrial receptivity. Furthermore, the health and dietary status of the patient can have a profound effect on the subsequent developmental capacity of the oocyte and embryo. The dietary status of patients attending IVF is typically not considered as a compounding variable, but growing data would indicate otherwise.

In this schematic, the laboratory has been broken down into its core components, only one of which is the culture system. The culture system has in turn been broken down into its components, only one of which is the culture medium. Therefore, it would appear rather simplistic to assume that by changing only one part of the culture system (i.e. culture medium), that one is going to mimic the results of a given laboratory or clinic.

A major determinant of the success of a laboratory and culture system is the level of quality control and quality assurance in place. For example, one should never assume that anything coming into the laboratory that has not been pretested with a relevant bioassay (e.g. mouse embryo assay) is safe merely because a previous lot has performed satisfactorily. Only a small percentage of the contact supplies and tissue culture ware used in IVF comes suitably tested. Therefore it is essential to assume that everything entering the IVF laboratory without a suitable pretest is embryo toxic until proven otherwise.

In our program, the one-cell mouse embryo assay (MEA) is employed to prescreen every lot of tissue culture ware that enters the program, i.e. plastics that are approved for tissue culture. Around 25% of all such material fails the one-cell MEA (in a simple medium lacking protein after the first 24 h). Therefore, if one does not perform quality control (QC) to this level, one in four of all contact supplies used clinically could compromise embryo development. In reality many programs cannot allocate the resources required for this level of QC, and when embryo quality is compromised in the laboratory, it is the media that are held responsible, when in fact the tissue culture ware is more often the culprit. (Modified from reference 28 with permission from Reproductive Healthcare Ltd)

each component of the culture system in turn. Subsequently, sufficient resources must also be made available for adequate quality control (QC) and quality assurance (QA), to ensure the establishment of optimum conditions within the laboratory, and the appropriate monitoring of laboratory performance.

MEDIA

It is evident that the composition of the medium used has a significant effect on embryo development and viability[1–4]. Today, unlike a decade ago, one can purchase ready to use embryo culture media from several companies. All but gone are days of in-house media preparation. One reason for this is the impact of regulatory bodies that are looking to restrict such practice. Another reason is that modern embryo culture media have increased in complexity and are therefore considerably more difficult to prepare and to ensure the highest quality. Consequently, it is important that embryologists know what media are composed of in order to make an informed decision regarding their use.

Initially, human IVF media were either those used for tissue culture (i.e. Ham's F10) or were derived from the original culture media developed for F1 mice embryos back in the 1970s[1]. Neither of the approaches can be considered optimal and, in the mid 1980s, media designed specifically for the human embryo started to appear[5,6]. Subsequently there was a resurgence of interest in mammalian embryo culture and, in the following years, several changes to media were made. One of the most significant developments in embryo culture media was the recognition that amino acids fulfill several important niches during the pre-implantation developmental period. The laboratories of Gwatkin[7,8], Pedersen[9], Bavister[10], and Gardner[11,12] all determined that specific amino acids had a positive impact on embryo development, while interestingly some amino acids actually exhibited a negative effect. What also became clear was that during the preimplantation period the embryo changes its utilization of amino acids. A developing theme was that the cleavage stage embryo is stimulated by those amino acids present at high levels in oviduct fluid, while at later stages the postcompacted embryo requires a wider array of amino acids.

Amongst those amino acids found to stimulate the cleavage stage embryo were alanine, glutamate, glycine, proline, serine, and taurine. Interestingly, such amino acids are used by simple and unicellular organisms to assist in the regulation of intracellular homeostasis, such as the regulation of pH and osmolytes[13–15]. In-vitro studies on the cleavage stage mammalian embryo have revealed that such amino acids are in fact used by the embryo to regulate such intracellular functions[16,17]. Furthermore, postcompaction, when the embryo has created a transporting epithelium, such amino acids are not required to regulate intracellular function. This indicates that the embryo postcompaction is, far more robust an entity than during the cleavage stages[18].

Of general interest, those amino acids that appear at high levels within the mammalian oviduct have a striking homology to those found in Eagle's non-essential amino acids[19], defined as those amino acids not required by somatic cells in culture. Subsequently there have been numerous publications covering the non-essential group and their effects on mammalian preimplantation embryos. However, it must be pointed out that this term has nothing to do with embryology, and with hindsight perhaps a more suitable name should have been adopted. In contrast to non-essential amino acids, those termed essential (i.e. required by somatic cells in culture) cannot substitute for the non-essential amino acids prior to compaction in fulfilling these important intracellular niches[17].

Lessons learned from such work include that the oocyte, pronucleate oocyte, and cleavage stages are dependent on specific amino acids to regulate intracellular function. It is therefore paramount that such amino acids are included in all media that the oocyte and early embryos are exposed to. Subsequently, should one wish to culture embryos to the blastocyst stage then a more comprehensive array of amino acids is required.

As with amino acids, the preimplantation mammalian embryo also changes with regard to its uptake and metabolism of carbohydrates[20,21]. Specifically, prior to compaction the embryo utilizes the carboxylic acids pyruvate and lactate as its preferred energy substrates. Glucose at this time is only consumed at low levels, and is used primarily for biosynthetic purposes and not as an energy source. By the blastocyst stage, the embryo utilizes glucose preferentially by the processes of oxidation and aerobic glycolysis. Control of nutrient uptake and utilization by the embryo is complex and changes as development proceeds[3,13,22,23]. Interestingly, in vivo the embryo is exposed to gradients of nutrients within the human female reproductive tract[24,25]. These gradients of relatively high levels of the carboxylic acids pyruvate and lactate, and low levels of glucose in the oviduct compared to the uterus, reflect the changes in carbohydrate uptakes and subsequent metabolism during preimplantation development as determined through in-vitro analysis of embryos.

Consequently, two schools of thought exist. One is that embryos should be cultured in successive media to accommodate the changes in nutrient preferences in metabolism[26]. The second is that one simply needs to provide the embryo with all the nutrients at one concentration throughout the entire preimplantation period and then let the embryo use what it requires[4]. In our experience, although the latter approach does support blastocyst development in a number of species[27], by applying a more dynamic approach to embryo culture, i.e. using media in sequence (or sequential media), one gets faster

growing embryos that result in blastocysts with more cells and higher viability[28,29].

For the past decade, sequential media have been used clinically by numerous Assisted Reproductive Techniques (ART) programs. Although it can be difficult to compare data from different clinics, due to potential differences in patient populations, etc., one can derive a good indication of the efficacy of a clinic by examining their oocyte donor data. In such cases the oocytes are typically from women under 30 years old, and therefore represent a source of gametes with high viability. Oocyte donors are not only an excellent means to quantify the ability of a laboratory to culture human embryos, but they also serve as an invaluable group of patients for use in quality management. Using sequential culture media, combined with blastocyst transfer, implantation rates (fetal heart beat) of 65% can be attained, with a clinical pregnancy rate of greater than 85% when two embryos are transferred[30]. Clearly such physiologic sequential media are highly effective in a clinical setting[31].

PROBLEMS WITH STATIC CULTURE IN VITRO

Although embryo culture media have become more physiologic, for example with the inclusion of amino acids, and as a result have become more effective, one still faces the problems of working outside the female reproductive tract in a polystyrene culture dish. This can hardly be considered physiologic. This means that culture in vitro can lead to the development of artifacts that could harm the embryo. The best documented example of this is the production of ammonium from amino acids[11,32].

Although amino acids are metabolized by embryos and subsequently release ammonium in vivo, one anticipates that this ammonium is subsequently removed by the epithelial cells of the female reproductive tract, then passes through the circulation and is subsequently detoxified by the urea cycle in the liver. However, in a static culture system any ammonium produced by embryonic metabolism simply builds up in the medium[11]. To add insult to injury, the amino acids themselves (especially glutamine) are labile at 37°C and spontaneously deaminate to release ammonium[11] (Figure 22.3). The reason that this is a cause for concern is that ammonium has been documented to affect several cellular processes in mouse and human embryos, including decreased blastocyst development, impaired inner cell mass formation, perturbed metabolism, increased apoptosis, and altered gene expression[18,32–34]. More alarmingly, if

mouse embryos are transferred after exposure to ammonium in culture the resultant fetuses may be retarded, and in some cases exhibit neural tube defects[12,35].

Several possible remedies to this problem have been attempted, including in-situ transamination of free amino acids to glutamate using the addition of enzymes and substrates to the medium[36]. Although effective, this approach is far from practical. An alternative approach is to remove the most labile amino acid, glutamine, and replace it with a stable dipeptide form such as alanyl or glycyl glutamine[37,38]. This approach greatly decreases the release of ammonium into the medium (Figure 22.3). However, even if this is done it is still important to change the medium every 48 h as there appears to be sufficient deamination of other amino acids to produce dangerous levels of ammonium[12,38].

SUPPLEMENTS

Although embryo culture media containing amino acids do not necessarily require the addition of a macromolecule to support embryo development, embryo culture is easier and the outcome improved by supplementation with the appropriate macromolecule. The most common supplement is human serum albumin (HSA), typically in the form of albumin derived from blood. Although effective, such a source of albumin carries with it the finite possibility of disease transmission, especially in the form of prions. An alternative to blood-derived albumin is recombinant albumin. This has been shown not only to be equally as effective[39], but has the added advantage of increasing the ability of embryos to survive cryopreservation[40].

Other components of human serum documented to be effective supplement to albumin are the α and β globulins[41]. However, their efficiency has yet to be determined in prospective randomized trials. The most abundant macromolecules within the oviduct are mucins[42]. However, their

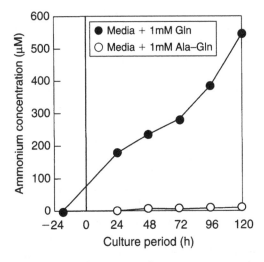

Figure 22.3 The release of ammonium into the culture medium by the deamination of amino acids. A base culture medium was supplemented with either 1 mM glutamine or 1 mM of the heat stable dipeptide alanyl-glutamine. Media were placed in the incubator at 37°C at 4:00 pm to simulate the pre-equilibration of media for use the next morning. Time zero (0 h) represents the time when an embryo would be placed in such media. However, in this example, no embryos were present. After just 48 h of culture in the presence of 1 mM GLn, embryos would be exposed to an ammonium concentration of >200 μM

role in embryo development remains to be elucidated. Another macromolecule present within the female reproductive tract, and present at increasing levels in the uterus at the time of implantation in the mouse, is the glycosaminoglycan hyaluronan. Unlike other glycosaminoglycans, hyaluronan contains no protein moieties and can therefore be synthesized in vitro under FDA approved conditions using recombinant technology. The supplementation of hyaluronan to embryo-culture media results not only in increased cryotolerance of the embryos[40], but enhances implantation post-transfer[43]. One supplement that was popular in the early days of IVF, serum, is no longer considered favorable. The exposure of gametes and embryos to serum induces trauma, resulting in altered organelle ultrastructure, perturbed metabolism (specifically loss of oxidative capacity), altered gene expression, aberration of genomic imprinting, and ultimately altered fetal development[44–46]. It is therefore the humble opinion of this author that no gamete or embryo should be exposed to whole serum.

Another supplement to culture media for the early embryo is ethylenediaminetetraacetic acid (EDTA), which was first shown to alleviate the so called 'two-cell block' in mouse embryos cultured in a simple medium[47]. Subsequently, there has been an extensive analysis on the effects of EDTA on mouse embryo metabolism and viability[48]. The effects of 1, 10, and 100 μM EDTA at two different glucose concentrations, 0.5 and 3.15 mM (i.e. the concentrations present in the human oviduct and uterus, and in the sequential media G1 and G2), were investigated. It was determined that at 0.5 mM glucose both 10 and 100 μM EDTA significantly reduced glycolytic activity in the eight-cell embryo, but at 3.15 mM glucose the inhibition of glycolysis by EDTA was diminished. However, subsequent analysis of the glycolytic enzyme 3-phosphoglycerate kinase in two-cell, eight-cell, and blastocyst stage embryos revealed that enzyme activity was significantly reduced by 10 μM EDTA as well as by 100 μM

EDTA. Given that Hewitson and Leese[49] have determined that the inner cell mass uses glycolysis exclusively, it would appear fitting to remove EDTA from the second phase media to prevent interfering with ICM physiology, which in turn could affect fetal development.

GAS PHASE, pH AND INCUBATION CHAMBERS

Embryo culture media typically utilize a bicarbonate/CO_2 buffering system to regulate the pH. This is achieved by the inclusion of 20–25 mM $NaHCO_3$ in the culture medium and the use of a 5–7% CO_2 atmosphere using a tissue culture chamber. Historically, embryo culture media are used at pH 7.4. However, analysis of the intracellular pH (pHi) of the mammalian embryo has revealed that it is actually around 7.2 to 7.3[50–52]. Therefore there has been a trend to decrease the pH of human embryo culture medium to 7.2 to 7.35.

Interestingly, the actual pH of the culture medium does not necessarily reflect that of the oocyte and the embryo[50]. Rather, by including specific amino acids in the culture medium, the embryo is able to buffer itself from changes in medium pH[17]. Furthermore, the ratios of the carboxylic acids lactate and pyruvate also impact intracellular pH[50]. However, it would appear prudent to have a medium pH of 7.2–7.35, as one does not wish to exceed a pH of 7.4. If one sets the medium pH to 7.4, then it quickly increases when the embryo's culture dish is taken out of the incubator, culminating in a rapid increase in medium pH in a bicarbonate buffer system that will affect embryonic development.

It is therefore important to monitor the pH of the medium and CO_2 environment within the incubator. The pH of a CO_2/bicarbonate buffered medium is not easy to quantitate. A pH electrode can be used, but one must be quick and the same technician must take all readings to ensure consistency. Solid-state probes are now available with a higher degree of accuracy. An alternative approach is to take samples of medium and measure the pH with a blood-gas analyzer. A final method necessitates the presence of phenol red in the culture medium and the use of Sorensons's phosphate buffer standards. This method allows visual inspection of a medium's pH with a tube in the incubator, but is accurate to only 0.2 pH units[37]. Typically, Fyrite has been employed to quantitate CO_2 within the chamber used. However, the accuracy of such a procedure is rather low. Fortunately, there are now available new hand held infra red (IR) CO_2 analysis meters with very high accuracy (to 0.1%) (e.g. Vaisala, Helsinki, Finland).

Historically, embryo culture has been performed at ambient O_2, which is around 20%. This is in spite of the fact that the levels of O_2 in the female reproductive tract are significantly less, at only around 5–7%[53–56]. Furthermore, in several mammalian species it has been demonstrated that embryo development and subsequent viability are increased when embryos are cultured in an O_2 concentration of just 5%[57–61]. The pathologies associated with the use of high O_2 include retarded embryo development, altered metabolism, perturbed gene expression, and a changed proteome, culminating in loss of viability[18,61,62].

Some clinics have been deterred from employing a low O_2 environment because of the concerns of the cost associated with having to purchase new incubators capable of regulating both CO_2 and O_2 concentrations. However, compared to a conventional CO_2 incubator, multi-gas incubators are not that much more expensive (only around 10–20%). Furthermore, the modern multi-gas incubator uses considerably less N_2, one or two cylinders a week. Their capacity to maintain their internal environment is further enhanced by the inclusion of inner glass doors, which prevents the gas phase from being totally disrupted throughout the chamber when the main door is opened. Alternatives to multi-gas are modular chambers or even desiccators. Such

chambers are purged with the gas from a mixed cylinder (e.g. 5% O_2, 6% CO_2, 89% N_2). Inside such chambers embryos are effectively isolated from the laboratory and environment within the incubator[61]. Although effective, this approach is not very practical for a busy IVF clinic. For practicality, multi-gas chambers are the preferred method. Realistically one should have two chambers per 40 to 50 patients[63], one chamber for medium equilibration in dishes or test tubes, the other chamber for gamete and embryo culture only. However, there is a role for modular chambers and desiccators in the IVF lab (see the section on quality control below). Should one go with a tissue culture incubator, ensure that the CO_2 sensor is IR and not a thermocouple type, as the latter can be responsible for too much pH drift due to fluctuations in humidity. The O_2 concentration in multi-gas chambers is regulated by the injection of N_2 to purge the ambient O_2 down to that required, typically 5–7%. Such N_2 can be supplied from N_2 cylinders, a liquid N_2 tank with an appropriate regulator, or an N_2 generator. Your choice will be influenced by the number of chambers required, which in turn is determined by patient volume.

INCUBATION VOLUME AND NUMBER OF EMBRYOS PER DROP

The optimum volume of culture medium and the number of embryos per drop has not been effectively established for the human embryo. In animal models, such as the mouse and cow, growing embryos in decreased volumes (i.e. 10–50 µl as apposed to 800 µl) and in groups (typically 4–10 embryos per drop) has been shown to stimulate embryonic development[64–67]. Hence it would appear prudent to culture human embryos in groups within decreased volumes; a typical situation is five embryos in a 40 µl drop. However, it is acknowledged that culturing groups means that a lot of information regarding embryo morphology is lost as one cannot readily track individual embryos. Therefore, should one move to single embryo culture in order to track individual embryos, it is imperative that smaller volumes be employed, i.e. around 5 µl. However, decreasing volumes of medium results in an increase in the surface area to volume ratio of the drop, which can have significant negative impacts if there is a problem with the oil overlay. Therefore, there is an absolute requirement for oils of the highest quality.

OIL

There are numerous suppliers of oil an embryologist can choose from. The benefits of working with an oil overlay include better control of pH and osmolality by preventing evaporation of the water in the medium. Both aspects are very important. As indicated above, embryo development is enhanced in smaller volumes of culture medium. To ensure the oils used for microdrop cultures are suitable, especially at volumes between 2 and 20 µl, it is essential that such oils be tested rigorously using a suitable bioassay (see section below on quality control)[68]. Oils must be tested with a one-cell mouse embryo assay (MEA), as opposed to a two-cell test, and such oils should maintain embryos when media are used in small microliter volumes.

QUALITY CONTROL

To ensure all aspects of the culture system are optimized, it is important to use an appropriate model to screen all components individually. The MEA can be used to great effectiveness providing it is performed under conditions that maximize sensitivity. Therefore, it is important to perform such assays from the early one-cell stage, in media lacking amino acids, EDTA, and albumin (at least after the first cleavage division) and in 20% O_2. It is evident that such culture conditions are contrary to those described ear-

lier; however, it is important to stress the embryo in order to maximize the sensitivity of the assay. Rather than a single endpoint of blastocyst development, it is important to assess development at set time points, and evaluate the blastocyst for signs of necrosis (this can be visualized easily on an inverted but not a stereomicroscope[68]). Furthermore, it is most important that the cell number of the resulting blastocysts are determined. One can readily obtain 80% blastocyst development on day 5, but it is also important to note how embryos form blastocysts in the afternoon of day 4 (i.e. on time development), and to determine the cell numbers of the resultant blastocysts is. There is a significant difference in the viability of blastocysts with 40 vs. 80 cells.

Using such an approach to testing, one can pick up subtle problems that can exist with a medium, or more typically with contact supplies. It is important to note that just because a lot number of culture dishes has been approved safe for use in somatic cell tissue culture, it does not automatically mean that it can support gametes or embryos (Figure 22.2).

With regard to determining the suitability of laboratory air, there is a quick and effective means to determine whether a problem exists in the general laboratory environment. As discussed above, the use of modular chambers or dessicators facilitates the isolation of the embryo from the rest of the laboratory. Therefore, by using a premixed cylinder, which tend to be of excellent gas quality, one can culture embryos in the IVF laboratory, but at the same time isolate the embryos from the impact of the air handling system.

HUMAN EMBRYO CULTURE PROTOCOL

The protocol described below is based on the assumption that the media in question will be renewed after 48 h. As discussed above, this is paramount whether one is using a biphasic or non-sequential system. The protocol has been validated using the media and consumables listed. Any change to the protocol, whether it be a different source of oil or media, needs to be validated carefully. When using the sequential media G1 and G2[28], embryos should be cultured in a gas phase of 5% O_2 and 6% CO_2. Remember, human embryos will grow at 20% O_2, but development is superior at lower oxygen tensions.

Pronucleate stage embryos to day 3 culture

All manipulations of oocytes and embryos should be performed using a pulled Pasteur pipette, glass capillary, or a displacement pipette. It is important to use a pipette with the appropriate size tip. For example, once the cumulus is removed (day 1 to 3) a bore of around 275–300 μm is required. Using the appropriate size tip minimizes the volumes of culture medium moved with each embryo, which typically should be less than a microliter. Such volume manipulation is a prerequisite for successful culture.

Around 4:00 pm on the day of oocyte retrieval, label 60 mm Falcon Primaria dishes with the patient's name. Using a single-wrapped tip, first rinse the tip then place 6×25 μl drops of G1 into the plate. Four drops should be at the 3, 6, 9, and 12 o'clock positions (for embryo culture), the fifth and sixth drops should be in the middle of the dish (wash drops). Immediately cover the drops with 9 ml of tested oil (such as Ovoil, Vitrolife). Prepare no more than two plates at one time. Using a new tip for each drop, first rinse the tip and then add a further 25 μl of medium to each original drop. Place the dish in the incubator at 5% O_2 and 6% CO_2. Gently remove the lid of the dish and set at an angle on the side of the plate. Dishes must gas in the incubator for a minimum of 4 h (this is the minimum measured time for the medium to reach the correct pH under oil). For each patient, set up a wash dish at the same time as the culture dishes. Place 1 ml of medium G1 into the center of an organ well dish, place 2

ml of medium into the outer well and then place the dish in the incubator. If working outside an isolette use a MOPS or HEPES buffered medium with amino acids. This should not be placed in a CO_2 incubator, but rather warmed on a heated stage.

Following removal of the cumulus cells, embryos are transferred to the organ well dish and washed in the center well drop of medium in the dish. Washing involves picking up the embryo 2–3 times and moving it around within the well. Embryos should then be washed in the two center drops in the culture dish and up to five embryos placed in each drop of G1. This will result in no more than 20 embryos per dish. Return the dish to the incubator immediately. It is advisable to culture embryos in groups of at least two. Therefore, for example, for a patient with six embryos it is best to culture in two groups of three, and not four and two or five and one. On day 3, embryos can be transferred to the uterus in a hyaluronan enriched medium[43].

Day 3 embryos to the blastocyst stage

On day 3, before 8:30 am, label a 60 mm dish with the patient's name. Using a single-wrapped tip rinse the tip then place 6×25 μl drops of G2 onto the plate. Immediately cover with 9 ml of oil. Never prepare more than two plates at one time. Using a new tip for each drop, rinse the tip and then add a further 25 μl of medium to each original drop. Place the dish in the incubator and gently remove the lid and set on the side of the plate.

For each patient, set up one wash dish per 10 embryos. Place 1 ml of medium G2 into the center of an organ well dish. Place 2 ml of medium into the outer well. Place into the incubator. Dishes must gas in the incubator for a minimum of 4 h. If working outside an isolette use MOPS or HEPES buffered medium with amino acids. This should not be placed in a CO_2 incubator, but rather warmed on a heated stage. Set up one sorting dish before 8:30 am. Place 1 ml of medium G2 into the center of an organ well dish. Place 2 ml of medium into the outer well. Place immediately into the incubator.

Moving embryos from G1 to G2 should occur between 10:00 am and 2:00 pm. Wash embryos in the organ well. Washing entails picking up the embryo 2–3 times and moving it around within the well. Transfer the embryos to the sorting dish and group like stage and quality embryos together. Rinse through the wash drops of medium and again place up to five embryos in each drop of G2. Return the dish to the incubator immediately. If working outside an isolette use HEPES/MOPS buffered medium with amino acids in the sorting dish. This should not be placed in a CO_2 incubator, but rather warmed on a heated stage.

On the morning of day 5, embryos should be scored (see below) and the top one or two scoring embryos selected for transfer. Manipulation of blastocysts requires the use of a capillary bore of 275–300 μm. Transfers should be performed in a hyaluronan-enriched medium[43]. Any blastocysts not transferred can be cryopreserved. Should an embryo not have formed a blastocyst by day 5 it should be cultured in a fresh drop of G2 for 24 h and assessed on day 6.

EMBRYO GRADING

Assessment of pronucleate embryos

Tesarik and Greco[69] proposed that the morphology of the pronuclei was related to the viability of human embryos. Analysis of the number and distribution of nucleolar precursor bodies (NPBs) in each pronucleus of fertilized zygotes was subsequently related to implantation potential. Features of pronucleate oocytes that had 100% implantation success were that the number of NPBs in both pronuclei never differed by more than three, and that the NPBs were always polarized or not-polarized in both pronuclei, but never polarized in one pronucleus and not in the other.

Other features examined in the zygote were pronuclear orientation and size and the presence of a cytoplasmic halo. All the above features have been linked to increased pregnancy rates to certain degrees[70–72].

Assessment of cleavage stage embryos

Hardy et al.[73] showed a correlation between multi-nucleation and poor embryo development in humans. This parameter has been used in both single and double embryo transfers. Van Royen et al.[74] reported that multi-nucleated embryos had a decreased implantation rate: 5.7% in double embryo transfers. In the double embryo transfer group, two multinucleated embryos resulted in a 4.3-fold lower implantation rate than transfers of non-multi-nucleated embryos.

Another key parameter is the speed of embryo development, which can be quantitated initially at the first cleavage division. Cleavage to the two-cell stage at 24–27 h after insemination or microinjection has been shown to be a critical time point for selecting embryos for transfer[75,76]. Sakkas and colleagues have shown that early cleavage is effective in improving pregnancy rates[77]. Scott and Smith[78] devised an embryo scoring method on day 1 on the basis of alignment of pronuclei and nucleoli, the appearance of the cytoplasm, nuclear membrane breakdown, and cleavage to the two-cell stage. Patients who had an overall high embryo score (≥15) had a pregnancy and implantation rate of 34 out of 48 (71%) and 49 out of 175 (28%), respectively, compared with only 4 out of 49 (8%) and four out of 178 (2%) in the low embryo score group. Interestingly, in their study, in order to obtain a high score the embryos had to be fast cleaving; this therefore further supports the use of early cleavage as an indicator of embryonic viability.

Subsequently, Salumets et al.[79] analyzed 178 elective single embryo transfer procedures. They found that a significantly higher clinical pregnancy rate was observed after transfer of early cleaving two-cell embryos (50%) than non-early cleaving embryos (26.4%). Van Montfoort et al.[80] have also reported a significantly higher pregnancy rate after 165 single embryo transfers of single early cleaving embryos compared with single non-early cleaving embryos (46 versus 18%). In the same study the benefit of transferring early cleaving two-cell embryos was confirmed after double embryo transfer with two early cleaving two-cell embryos as compared with two non-early cleaving embryos (45 versus 25%). In addition, the blastocyst formation of early cleaving two-cell embryos compared with non-early cleaving embryos (66 versus 40%) was significantly higher. Logistic regression showed that early cleaving two-cell embryos were an independent predictor for both pregnancy and blastocyst development in addition to cell morphology and number.

With the aim of transferring one or two embryos on day 3, Gerris and colleagues[81,82] used strict embryo criteria to select single embryos for transfer. The necessary characteristics of their 'top' quality embryos were established by retrospectively examining embryos that had very high implantation potential[82]. These top quality embryos had the following characteristics: four or five blastomeres on day 2 and at least seven blastomeres on day 3 after fertilization, absence of multinucleated blastomeres, and less than 20% fragmentation on days 2 and 3 after fertilization. Recently, the same group has reported impressive pregnancy rates after transfer of a single embryo in a selected patient population. A total of 370 single top quality embryo transfers in patients younger than 38 years of age resulted in 192 pregnancies (51.9%). Of these, 57 failed to progress and 135 (36.5%) cycles resulted in ongoing pregnancies[83].

Assessment of the blastocyst

As with the scoring of embryos during the cleavage stages, time and morphology play an impor-

tant part in selecting the best blastocyst. The scoring assessment for blastocysts devised by Gardner and Schoolcraft[84] is based on the expansion state of the blastocyst and on the consistency of the inner cell mass and trophectoderm cells (Figure 22.4). Using their grading system, when two high scoring blastocysts (>3AA), i.e. expanded blastocoel with compacted inner cell mass and cohesive trophectoderm epithelium, were transferred, clinical pregnancy and implantation rates of 59/68 (86.7%) and 95/136 (69.9%) were achieved[85]. When two blastocysts not achieving these scores (<3AA) were transferred, the clinical pregnancy and implantation rates were significantly lower, 7/16 (43.8%) and 9/32 (28.1%).

The time of blastocyst formation is also crucial. When we compared cases where only day 5 and 6 frozen blastocysts were transferred compared to those frozen on or after day 7 and transferred, the pregnancy rates were 7/18 (38.9%) and 1/16 (6.2%), respectively[86]. In these cases, expanded blastocysts with a definable inner cell mass and trophectoderm were frozen. These results showed that even though blastocysts could be obtained, the crucial factor was when they became blastocysts. When taking this into account, the best blastocysts would be those that have developed by day 5.

SEQUENTIAL SCORING TECHNIQUES

By including several of the scoring criteria above, continuous scoring systems, whereby multiple parameters are used to select the best embryo, have been developed[87]. A number of these have been proposed, including one looking at day 2 and 3 assessment, using strict embryo criteria to select single embryos for transfer[81,88]. An extension of this technique was proposed by Fisch et al.[89], who used the graduated embryo score to evaluate parameters from the first 3 days of development. Finally, Neuber et al.[90] examined parameters on all 5 days of

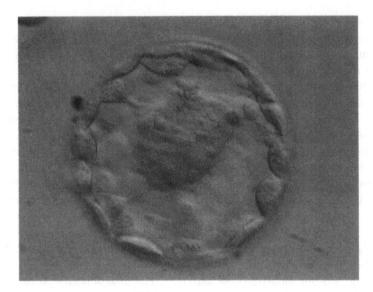

Figure 22.4 Scoring system for human blastocysts. Initially blastocysts are given a numerical score from 1 to 6 based upon their degree of expansion and hatching status:

(1)   Early blastocyst; the blastocoel being less than or equal to half the volume of the embryo.
(2)   Blastocyst; the blastocoel being greater than half of the volume of the embryo.
(3)   Full blastocyst; the blastocoel completely fills the embryo.
(4)   Expanded blastocyst; the blastocoel volume is now larger than that of the early embryo and the zona is thinning.
(5)   Hatching blastocyst; the trophectoderm has started to herniate through the zona.
(6)   Hatched blastocyst; the blastocyst has completely escaped from the zona.

The initial phase of the assessment can be performed using a dissection microscope. The second step in scoring the blastocysts should be performed under an inverted microscope. For blastocysts graded as 3 to 6 (i.e. full blastocysts onwards) the development of the inner cell mass (ICM) and trophectoderm can then be assessed.

ICM grading

A.   Tightly packed, many cells
B.   Loosely grouped, several cells
C.   Very few cells.

Trophectoderm grading

A.   Many cells forming a cohesive epithelium
B.   Few cells forming a loose epithelium
C.   Very few large cells.

The photomicrograph is of a human blastocyst (score 4AA on the morning of day 5). The blastocoel cavity is expanding and the zona is thinning (score of 4). The ICM is clearly made up of many cells (score of A). The trophectoderm can be seen to be composed of numerous cells (score of A)

development as a means of performing sequential embryo assessment using morphologically based parameters. All the above studies reported improved pregnancy rates when these techniques were utilized.

ON WHICH DAY SHOULD EMBRYO TRANSFER BE PERFORMED?

The possible benefits of blastocyst transfer are listed in Table 22.1. From such a list, it would appear that blastocyst transfer on day 5 offers several advantages over the convention of transferring early embryos on days 1 to 3 of development. However, many clinics around the world have yet to adopt extended culture and blastocyst transfer. In a review on blasto-

Table 22.1 Potential benefits of blastocyst transfer

- Embryo selection; ability to identify those embryos with limited, as well as those with the highest developmental potential
- Synchronization of embryonic stage with the female tract; reduces cellular stress on the embryo
- Minimize exposure of embryo to the hyperstimulated uterine environment
- Reduction in uterine contractions; reduces chance of embryo being expelled
- Ability to undertake cleavage stage embryo biopsy without the need for cryopreservation when analysis of the biopsied blastomere requires more than 24 hours
- Assessment of true embryo viability; assessing the embryo post-genome activation
- High implantation rates; reduces the need to transfer multiple embryos
- Increased ability to survive cryopreservation
- Increase in overall efficiency of IVF

---

cyst vs. cleavage stage transfer[91], it was noted that in most papers published on blastocyst transfer, very little information regarding the culture system, save the medium type, was ever reported. This in turn makes comparing various studies rather problematic. An analysis of 16 prospective randomized trials published to date revealed that eight studies found a positive outcome from blastocyst transfer compared to transfers on day 2 or day 3, with only one study reporting a negative outcome. The remaining seven demonstrated equivalency between days of transfer. However, more and more reports are now erring on the side of blastocyst transfer, especially with regard to single embryo transfer[92,93]. Furthermore, it appears that cryopreservation of human embryos is most effective at the blastocyst stage[94,95]. Consequently, extended culture, facilitated by the methodological advances outlined in this chapter, may represent a way to increase the overall efficiency of human IVF.

CONCLUSIONS

In this chapter the significance of the media and other components of an embryo culture system have been presented. Understanding why media contain the components they do will assist the embryologist in making an informed decision as to which media to use in their own laboratory. Furthermore, by taking a more holistic look at an embryology laboratory (and clinic), one can further improve the efficacy of the culture system, leading to increased implantation and pregnancy rates.

With regards to blastocyst transfer, more information regarding the embryo can be obtained prior to transfer. This is perhaps best exemplified following in-vitro maturation (IVM), when extended culture can assist in identifying those embryos which may arrest at the eight-cell stage, due to suboptimal oocyte maturation[96].

REFERENCES

1. Gardner DK, Lane M. Embryo Culture systems. In Trounson A, Gardner DK, eds. Handbook of In Vitro Fertilization. Boca Raton, Florida: CRC Press, 1993: 85–114.

2. Bavister BD. Culture of preimplantation embryos: facts and artifacts. Hum Reprod Update 1995; 1: 91–148.

3. Gardner DK, Pool TB, Lane M. Embryo nutrition and energy metabolism and its relationship to embryo growth, differentiation, and viability. Semin Reprod Med 2000; 18: 205–18.

4. Summers MC, Biggers JD. Chemically defined media and the culture of mammalian preimplantation embryos: historical perspective and current issues. Hum Reprod Update 2003; 9: 557–82.

5. Quinn P, Kerin JF, Warnes GM. Improved pregnancy rate in human in vitro fertilization with the use of a medium based on the composition of human tubal fluid. Fertil Steril 1985; 44: 493–8.

6. Menezo Y, Testart J, Perrone D. Serum is not necessary in human in vitro fertilization, early embryo culture, and transfer. Fertil Steril 1984; 42: 750–5.

7. Gwatkin RB. Amino acid requirements for attachment and outgrowth of the mouse blastocyst in vitro. J Cell Comp Physiol 1966; 68: 335–44.

8. Gwatkin RB, Haidri AA. Requirements for the maturation of hamster oocytes in vitro. Exp Cell Res 1973; 76: 1–7.

9. Spindle AI, Pedersen RA. Hatching attachment, and outgrowth of mouse blastocysts in vitro: fixed nitrogen requirements. J Exp Zool 1973; 186: 305–18.

10. Bavister BD, McKiernan SH. Regulation of hamster embryo development in vitro by amino acids. In: Bavister BD, ed. Preimplantation Embryo Development. Springer-Verlag, New York, 1992, p. 57–72.

11. Gardner DK, Lane M. Amino acids and ammonium regulate mouse embryo development in culture. Biol Reprod 1993; 48: 377–85.

12. Lane M, Gardner DK. Increase in postimplantation development of cultured mouse embryos by amino acids and induction of fetal retardation and exencephaly by ammonium ions. J Reprod Fertil 1994; 102: 305–12.

13. Gardner DK. Changes in requirements and utilization of nutrients during mammalian preimplantation embryo development and their significance in embryo culture. Theriogenology 1998; 49: 83–102.

14. Lane M. Mechanisms for managing cellular and homeostatic stress in vitro. Theriogenology 2001; 55: 225–36.

15. Lane M, Gardner DK. Understanding cellular disruptions during early embryo development that perturb viability and fetal development. Reprod Fertil Dev 2005; 17: 371–8.

16. Dawson KM, Collins JL, Baltz JM. Osmolarity-dependent glycine accumulation indicates a role for glycine as an organic osmolyte in early preimplantation mouse embryos. Biol Reprod 1998; 59: 225–32.

17. Edwards LJ, Williams DA, Gardner DK. Intracellular pH of the mouse preimplantation embryo: amino acids act as buffers of intracellular pH. Hum Reprod 1998; 13: 3441–8.

18. Gardner DK, Lane M. Ex vivo early embryo development and effects on gene expression and imprinting. Reprod Fertil Dev 2005; 17: 361–70.

19. Eagle H. Amino acid metabolism in mammalian cell cultures. Science 1959; 130: 432–7.

20. Biggers JD, Whittingham DG, Donahue RP. The pattern of energy metabolism in the mouse oocyte and zygote. Proc Natl Acad Sci USA 1967; 58: 560–7.

21. Leese HJ, Barton AM. Pyruvate and glucose uptake by mouse ova and preimplantation embryos. J Reprod Fertil 1984; 72: 9–13.

22. Lane M, Gardner DK. Lactate regulates pyruvate uptake and metabolism in the preimplantation mouse embryo. Biol Reprod 2000; 62: 16–22.

23. Lane M, Gardner DK. Mitochondrial malate–aspartate shuttle regulates mouse embryo nutrient consumption. J Biol Chem 2005; 280: 18361–7.

24. Gardner DK, Lane M, Calderon I et al. Environment of the preimplantation human

embryo *in vivo*: metabolite analysis of oviduct and uterine fluids and metabolism of cumulus cells. Fertil Steril 1996; 65: 349–53.

25. Harris SE, Gopichandran N, Picton HM et al. Nutrient concentrations in murine follicular fluid and the female reproductive tract. Theriogenology 2005; 64: 992–1006.

26. Gardner DK, Leese HJ. Concentrations of nutrients in mouse oviduct fluid and their effects on embryo development and metabolism *in vitro*. J Reprod Fertil 1990; 88: 361–8.

27. Gardner DK, Lane M. Development of viable mammalian embryos *in vitro*: evolution of sequential media. In: Cibelli R, Lanza K, Campbell AK, West MD, eds. Principles of Cloning: Academic Press: San Diego, 2002, p. 187–213.

28. Gardner DK, Lane M. Towards a single embryo transfer. Reprod Biomed Online 2003; 6: 470–81.

29. Reed LC, Lane M, Gardner DK. *In vivo* rates of mouse embryo development can be attained *in vitro*. Theriogenology 2003; 59: 349.

30. Schoolcraft WB, Gardner DK. Blastocyst culture and transfer increases the efficiency of oocyte donation. Fertil Steril 2000; 74: 482–6.

31. Wilson M, Hartke K, Kiehl M et al. Transfer of blastocysts and morulae on day 5. Fertil Steril 2004; 82: 327–33.

32. Virant-Klun I, Tomazevic T, Vrtacnik-Bokal E et al. Increased ammonium in culture medium reduces the development of human embryos to the blastocyst stage. Fertil Steril 2006; 85: 526–8.

33. Lane M, Gardner DK. Ammonium induces aberrant blastocyst differentiation, metabolism, pH regulation, gene expression and subsequently alters fetal development in the mouse. Biol Reprod 2003; 69: 1109–17.

34. Zander DL, Thompson JG, Lane M. Perturbations in mouse embryo development and viability caused by ammonium are more severe after exposure at the cleavage stages. Biol Reprod 2006; 74: 288–94.

35. Sinawat S, Hsaio WC, Flockhart JH et al. Fetal abnormalities produced after preimplantation exposure of mouse embryos to ammonium chloride. Hum Reprod 2003; 18: 2157–65.

36. Lane M, Gardner DK. Removal of embryo-toxic ammonium from the culture medium by in situ enzymatic conversion to glutamate. J Exp Zool 1995; 271: 356–63.

37. Gardner DK, Lane M. Embryo Culture systems. In: Trounson A, Gardner DK, eds. Handbook of In-Vitro Fertilization, 2nd edn. CRC Press, Boca Raton, FL, 1999, p. 205–64.

38. Biggers JD, McGinnis LK, Lawitts JA. Enhanced effect of glycyl-L-glutamine on mouse preimplantation embryos *in vitro*. Reprod Biomed Online 2004; 9: 59–69.

39. Bungum M, Humaidan P, Bungum L. Recombinant human albumin as protein source in culture media used for IVF: a prospective randomized study. Reprod Biomed Online 2002; 4: 233–6.

40. Lane M, Maybach JM, Hooper K et al. Cryo-survival and development of bovine blastocysts are enhanced by culture with recombinant albumin and hyaluronan. Mol Reprod Dev 2003; 64: 70–8.

41. Weathersbee PS, Pool TB, Ord T. Synthetic serum substitute (SSS): a globulin-enriched protein supplement for human embryo culture. J Assist Reprod Genet 1995; 12: 354–60.

42. Pool TB. Recent advances in the production of viable human embryos in vitro. Reprod Biomed Online 2002; 4: 294–302.

43. Gardner DK, Rodriegez-Martinez H, Lane M et al. Fetal development after transfer is increased by replacing protein with the glycosaminoglycan hyaluronan for mouse embryo culture and transfer. Hum Reprod 1999; 14: 2575–80.

44. Gardner DK. Mammalian embryo culture in the absence of serum or somatic cell support. Cell Biol Int 1994; 18: 1163–79.

45. Thompson JG, Gardner DK, Pugh PA et al. Lamb birth weight is affected by culture system utilized during *in vitro* pre-elongation development of ovine embryos. Biol Reprod 1995; 53: 1385–91.

46. Khosla S, Dean W, Brown D et al. Culture of pre-implantation mouse embryos affects fetal devel-

opment and the expression of imprinted genes. Biol Reprod 2001; 64: 918–26.

47. Abramczuk J, Solter D, Koprowski H. The beneficial effect EDTA on development of mouse one-cell embryos in chemically defined medium. Dev Biol 1977; 61: 378–83.

48. Lane M, Gardner DK. Inhibiting 3-phosphoglycerate kinase by EDTA stimulates the development of the cleavage stage mouse embryo. Mol Reprod Dev 2001; 60: 233–40.

49. Hewitson LC, Leese HJ. Energy metabolism of the trophectoderm and inner cell mass of the mouse blastocyst. J Exp Zool 1993; 26: 337–43.

50. Edwards LJ, Williams DA, Gardner DK. Intracellular pH of the preimplantation mouse embryo: effects of extracellular pH and weak acids. Mol Reprod Dev 1998; 50: 434–42.

51. Lane M, Baltz JM, Bavister BD. Regulation of intracellular pH in hamster preimplantation embryos by the sodium hydrogen (Na+/H+) antiporter. Biol Reprod 1998; 59: 1483–90.

52. Phillips KP, Leveille MC, Claman P et al. Intracellular pH regulation in human preimplantation embryos. Hum Reprod 2000; 15: 896–904.

53. Mastroianni L, Jr., Jones R. Oxygen tension within the rabbit fallopian tube. J Reprod Fertil 1965; 147: 99–102.

54. Ross RN, Graves CN. O$_2$ levels in female rabbit reproductive tract. J Anim Sci 1974; 39: 994.

55. Maas DH, Stein B, Metzger H. PO$_2$ and pH measurements within the rabbit oviduct following tubal microsurgery: reanastomosis of previously dissected tubes. Adv Exp Med Biol 1984; 169: 561–70.

56. Fischer B, Bavister BD. Oxygen tension in the oviduct and uterus of rhesus monkeys, hamsters and rabbits. J Reprod Fertil 1993; 99: 673–9.

57. Quinn P, Harlow GM. The effect of oxygen on the development of preimplantation mouse embryos in vitro. J Exp Zool 1978; 206: 73–80.

58. Harlow K, Quinn P. Foetal and placenta growth in the mouse after pre-implantation development in vitro under oxygen concentrations of 5 and 20%. Aust J Biol Sci 1979; 32: 363–9.

59. Thompson JG, Simpson AC, Pugh PA et al. Effect of oxygen concentration on in-vitro development of preimplantation sheep and cattle embryos. J Reprod Fertil 1990; 89: 573–8.

60. Batt PA, Gardner DK, Cameron AW. Oxygen concentration and protein source affect the development of preimplantation goat embryos in vitro. Reprod Fertil Dev 1991; 3: 601–7.

61. Gardner DK, Lane M. Alleviation of the '2-cell block' and development to the blastocyst of CF1 mouse embryos: role of amino acids, EDTA and physical parameters. Hum Reprod 1996; 11: 2703–12.

62. Katz-Jaffe MG, Linck DW, Schoolcraft WB et al. A proteomic analysis of mammalian preimplantation embryonic development. Reproduction 2005; 130: 899–905.

63. Gardner DK, Lane M. Culture systems for human embryo. In Gardner DK, Weissman A, Howles C, Shoham Z, eds. Textbook of Assisted Reproductive Techniques. Laboratory and Clinical Perspectives, 2nd edn. Taylor and Francis, London and New York, 2004, pp. 211–34.

64. Wiley LM, Yamami S, Van Muyden D. Effect of potassium concentration, type of protein supplement, and embryo density on mouse preimplantation development in vitro. Fertil Steril 1986; 45: 111–19.

65. Paria BC, Dey SK. Preimplantation embryo development in vitro: cooperative interactions among embryos and role of growth factors. Proc Natl Acad Sci USA 1990; 87: 4756–60.

66. Lane M, Gardner DK. Effect of incubation volume and embryo density on the development and viability of mouse embryos in vitro. Hum Reprod 1992; 7: 558–62.

67. Gardner DK, Lane M, Spitzer A et al. Enhanced rates of cleavage and development for sheep zygotes cultured to the blastocyst stage in vitro in the absence of serum and somatic cells: amino acids, vitamins, and culturing embryos in groups stimulate development. Biol Reprod 1994; 50: 390–400.

68. Gardner DK, Reed L, Linck D et al. Quality control in human in vitro fertilization. Semin Reprod Med 2005; 23: 319–24.

69. Tesarik J, Greco E. The probability of abnormal preimplantation development can be predicted

by a single static observation on pronuclear stage morphology. Hum Reprod 1999; 14: 1318–23.

70. Ebner T, Moser M, Tews G. Developmental potential of human pronuclear zygotes in relation to their pronuclear orientation. Hum Reprod 2004; 19: 1925–6.

71. Nagy ZP, Dozortsev D, Diamond M et al. Pronuclear morphology evaluation with subsequent evaluation of embryo morphology significantly increases implantation rates. Fertil Steril 2003; 80: 67–74.

72. Kattera S, Chen C. Developmental potential of human pronuclear zygotes in relation to their pronuclear orientation. Hum Reprod 2004; 19: 294–9.

73. Hardy K, Winston RM, Handyside AH. Binucleate blastomeres in preimplantation human embryos in vitro: failure of cytokinesis during early cleavage. J Reprod Fertil 1993; 98: 549–58.

74. Van Royen E, Mangelschots K, Vercruyssen M et al. Multinucleation in cleavage stage embryos. Hum Reprod 2003; 18: 1062–9.

75. Sakkas D, Shoukir Y, Chardonnens D et al. Early cleavage of human embryos to the two-cell stage after intracytoplasmic sperm injection as an indicator of embryo viability. Hum Reprod 1998; 13: 182–7.

76. Shoukir Y, Campana A, Farley T et al. Early cleavage of in-vitro fertilized human embryos to the 2-cell stage: a novel indicator of embryo quality and viability. Hum Reprod 1997; 12: 1531–6.

77. Sakkas D, Percival G, D'Arcy Y et al. Assessment of early cleaving in vitro fertilized human embryos at the 2-cell stage before transfer improves embryo selection. Fertil Steril 2001; 76: 1150–6.

78. Scott LA, Smith S. The successful use of pronuclear embryo transfers the day following oocyte retrieval. Hum Reprod 1998; 13: 1003–13.

79. Salumets A, Hyden-Granskog C, Makinen S et al. Early cleavage predicts the viability of human embryos in elective single embryo transfer procedures. Hum Reprod 2003; 18: 821–5.

80. Van Montfoort AP, Dumoulin JC, Kester AD et al. Early cleavage is a valuable addition to existing embryo selection parameters: a study using single embryo transfers. Hum Reprod 2004; 19: 2103–8.

81. Gerris J, De Neubourg D, Mangelschots K et al. Prevention of twin pregnancy after in-vitro fertilization or intracytoplasmic sperm injection based on strict embryo criteria: a prospective randomized clinical trial. Hum Reprod 1999; 14: 2581–7.

82. Van Royen E, Mangelschots K, De Neubourg D et al. Characterization of a top quality embryo, a step towards single-embryo transfer. Hum Reprod 1999; 14: 2345–9.

83. De Neubourg D, Gerris J, Mangelschots K et al. Single top quality embryo transfer as a model for prediction of early pregnancy outcome. Hum Reprod 2004; 19: 1476–9.

84. Gardner DK, Schoolcraft WB. In vitro culture of human blastocyst. In Jansen R, Mortimer D, eds. Towards Reproductive Certainty: Fertility and Genetics Beyond 1999. Parthenon Publishing, Carnforth, UK, 1999, pp. 378–88.

85. Gardner DK, Lane M, Stevens J et al. Blastocyst score affects implantation and pregnancy outcome: towards a single blastocyst transfer. Fertil Steril 2000; 73: 1155–8.

86. Shoukir Y, Chardonnens D, Campana A et al. The rate of development and time of transfer play different roles in influencing the viability of human blastocysts. Hum Reprod 1998; 13: 676–81.

87. Sakkas D, Gardner DK. Evaluation of embryo quality: sequential analysis of embryo development with the aim of single embryo transfer. In: Gardner DK, Weissman A, Howles CM, Shoham Z, eds. Textbook of Assisted Reproductive Techniques. Laboratory and Clinical Perspectives. Second edition ed. Taylor and Francis Group, London and New York, 2004, pp. 235–45.

88. Gerris J, De Neubourg D, Mangelschots K et al. Elective single day 3 embryo transfer halves the twinning rate without decrease in the ongoing pregnancy rate of an IVF/ICSI programme. Hum Reprod 2002; 17: 2626–31.

89. Fisch JD, Rodriguez H, Ross R et al. The Graduated Embryo Score (GES) predicts blastocyst formation and pregnancy rate from cleavage-stage embryos. Hum Reprod 2001; 16: 1970–5.

90. Neuber E, Rinaudo P, Trimarchi JR et al. Sequential assessment of individually cultured human embryos as an indicator of subsequent good quality blastocyst development. Hum Reprod 2003; 18: 1307–12.

91. Gardner DK, Balaban B. Choosing between day 3 and day 5 embryo transfers. Clin Obstet Gynecol 2006; 49: 85–92.

92. Papanikolaou EG, D'Haeseleer E, Verheyen G et al. Live birth rate is significantly higher after blastocyst transfer than after cleavage-stage embryo transfer when at least four embryos are available on day 3 of embryo culture. A randomized prospective study. Hum Reprod 2005; 20: 3198–203.

93. Papanikolaou V. Early pregnancy loss is significantly higher after day 3 single embryo transfer than after day 5 single blastocyst transfer in GnRH antagonist stimulated IVF cycles. Reprod Biomed Online 2006; 12: 60–5.

94. Veeck LL. Does the developmental stage at freeze impact on clinical results post-thaw? Reprod Biomed Online 2003; 6: 367–74.

95. Anderson AR, Weikert ML, Crain JL. Determining the most optimal stage for embryo cryopreservation. Reprod Biomed Online 2004; 8: 207–11.

96. Barnes FL, Crombie A, Gardner DK et al. Blastocyst development and birth after in-vitro maturation of human primary oocytes, intracytoplasmic sperm injection and assisted hatching. Hum Reprod 1995; 10: 3243–7.

CHAPTER 23

Pregnancy and neonatal outcome following IVM

William M Buckett

INTRODUCTION

Immature oocyte retrieval and subsequent oocyte maturation in vitro (IVM) without the need for any ovarian stimulation is a promising new development in assisted reproductive technology (ART). Many successful pregnancies have been reported and IVM is successfully performed in many parts of the world[1-5].

IVM gives the benefits of ovarian stimulation – namely more oocytes – without the risks of ovarian stimulation. Ovarian hyperstimulation syndrome (OHSS) is a potentially life-threatening condition associated with ovarian stimulation. Severe OHSS affects 1–2% of all women undergoing ART and up to 6% of women with polycystic ovaries (PCO) or polycystic ovary syndrome (PCOS)[6]. The only way to avoid OHSS totally is to avoid ovarian stimulation[7].

Any new development in assisted reproduction must also be accompanied by data concerning congenital abnormality, perinatal outcome, and later developmental sequelae.

Early data concerning pregnancies resulting from IVM have been generally reassuring so far[8-10]. This chapter will outline the currently available data, as well as data from the McGill series, concerning congenital abnormality, neonatal outcome, and obstetric outcome following IVM. The importance, as with all ART, of continuing surveillance and ideally centralized data collection will also be highlighted.

CONGENITAL ABNORMALITY

Although the collection of immature oocytes without any ovarian stimulation at all avoids the costs, side-effects, increased monitoring, and short- and possible long-term risks associated with ovarian stimulation, IVM also involves an additional 1 or 2 days' culture of the oocyte in vitro from the immature germinal vesicle, or metaphase I stage, to the metaphase II stage when fertilization can take place. Recent concerns regarding the possible effects of in-vitro gamete and embryo culture on congenital abnormalities in general and of imprinting disorders in particular[11,12] highlight the importance of continued reporting of any congenital abnormalities following IVM. To date, however, data are limited to four published series[8-10,13].

From a total of over 150 babies born following IVM, six major congenital abnormalities have been reported (Table 23.1). This rate – just under 4% – is similar to that reported following other ARTs[14] and slightly higher than that in spontaneously conceived controls. A comparative study[13]

Table 23.1 Major congenital abnormalities following IVM ($n = 155$)

Omphalocele ($n = 1$)
Cleft palate ($n = 2$)
Ventriculo-septal defect ($n = 2$)
45XO/46XY mosaic ($n = 1$)

n, number of babies

shows a similar odds ratio when IVM is compared with IVF and with ICSI (Figure 23.1).

Minor congenital abnormalities – those which are not life-threatening, do not impair function, and do not require corrective treatment – are often not reported. However, in the most recent McGill series, these affected 3/55 babies (5.4%) – two cases were unilateral congenital dislocation of the hip and one was a patent ductus arteriosus which closed spontaneously without requiring any corrective treatment.

MULTIPLE PREGNANCY

All ART treatments are associated with a significantly increased risk of multiple pregnancy[15,16]. The major determinant of multiple pregnancy is the number of embryos transferred. National differences in legislation account for the major differences in practice in differing parts of the world. Therefore one would expect lower incidences of multiple pregnancy in many European and Scandinavian countries following IVM compared with countries where many embryos are transferred.

All series report a high incidence of multiple pregnancy following IVM when compared with spontaneously conceived controls. Multiple pregnancy is the single most important factor leading to an increased perinatal risk with all ART. Rates of preterm delivery, stillbirth, neonatal loss, and later developmental sequelae are all more frequent following multiple pregnancy compared with singleton pregnancies.

At McGill, when IVM was compared with IVF and with ICSI, then multiple pregnancy rates were similar. The triplet pregnancy rate was 5% for IVM, 3% for IVF, and 3% for ICSI. The twin pregnancy rate was 21% for IVM, 20% for IVF, and 17% for ICSI – our rate of twin pregnancy is 1.3% in the general population.

There are no significant differences in the multiple pregnancy rates between IVM and other ART pregnancies. Nevertheless, couples undergoing IVM need to be aware of the risks

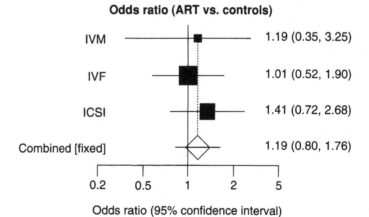

Figure 23.1 Odds ratio (fixed effects model) of any congenital abnormality following conception with IVM, IVF, and ICSI

and consequences of multiple pregnancy when more than one embryo is transferred and to balance these risks against the increased likelihood of live birth associated with two and three embryo transfer compared with single embryo transfer in IVM.

MODE OF DELIVERY

More ART pregnancies are delivered by cesarean section. Although much of this increased intervention is the result of the higher rate of multiple pregnancy, the cesarean section rate is still increased in singleton ART pregnancies. The reasons for this are unclear – although some studies have reported higher incidences of malpresentation and also of placenta praevia in pregnancies conceived as a result of IVF or ICSI[15,17]. Other authors have suggested that the threshold for recourse to cesarean section is lower in women who have conceived following ART[18,19].

The McGill data shows no demonstrable difference in the rates of cesarean section following IVM, IVF, or ICSI conceptions. Overall cesarean section rates are higher following ART (Figure 23.2).

Overall rates of instrumental delivery following IVM are similar to those in the general population at around 10% of deliveries.

BIRTHWEIGHT

Mean birthweight of all babies – singletons and multiples – following ART is lower than spontaneously conceived babies. The major reason for this is the high rate of multiple pregnancy. However, even in singleton pregnancies following ART, there is an increased incidence of lower birthweight babies[16].

Data from IVM are too early to determine whether or not the incidence of low birthweight babies is increased compared with spontaneously conceived babies. Some data suggest it is similar to other ART, whereas other data suggest that birthweight is similar to the general population[13]. That IVM singleton pregnancies are not associated with lower birthweight could either be as a result of the patients undergoing IVM – usually those with PCOS or those with ultrasound-only PCO – or because the number of pregnancies is still too small to demonstrate a difference.

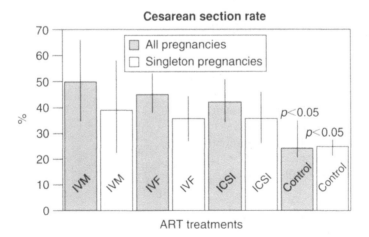

Figure 23.2 Cesarean section rates (95% CI) in all pregnancies (shaded) and singleton pregnancies (clear) following IVM, IVF, and ICSI treatments and spontaneously conceived controls

Similarly, when the proportion of macrosomic babies from singleton pregnancies is compared, there is no significant difference between any of the ART groups. This is important as some animal studies have suggested there may be an increased incidence of large-offspring syndrome following IVM[20].

GESTATIONAL AGE AT DELIVERY

Similarly the mean gestational age at delivery of all babies – singletons and multiples – following ART is lower than in spontaneously conceived pregnancies. As discussed above, the major reason for this is the high rate of multiple pregnancy. However, even in singleton pregnancies following ART, there is an increased incidence of preterm and extreme preterm birth[16].

Data from IVM are too early to determine whether or not the incidence of preterm delivery is increased compared with spontaneously conceived babies. Early data amongst the different ART treatments suggest that there is no significant difference between the proportion of premature deliveries before 37 weeks or before 34 weeks[13].

APGAR SCORES AND CORD pH LEVELS

For babies conceived following IVM compared with gestational age-matched controls, no studies so far have shown any difference in the median Apgar scores at 1 and 5 minutes, the proportion of babies with an Apgar score of 6 or less at 1 and 5 minutes, the mean cord pH, and the proportion of babies with mild acidosis (cord pH <7.2) or severe acidosis (cord pH <7.05).

WEIGHT FOR GESTATIONAL AGE

Weight for gestational age is determined by calculating the ratio between the birthweight at delivery and the standard norm for that gestation. This is an indirect measure of intrauterine growth retardation[21].

Babies conceived following IVF or ICSI have a slightly lower mean birthweight ratio than spontaneously conceived controls[16]. Also the proportion of all babies with a weight for their gestational age below the 5th centile (birthweight ratio <0.8) is higher in babies conceived following IVF or ICSI compared with the general population. Early data suggest that this is the same for babies conceived following IVM[13].

PREGNANCY COMPLICATIONS

The rate of gestational diabetes is higher in pregnancies which resulted from IVM compared with other ART and with spontaneously conceived controls (Figure 23.3).

This is more likely to be a result of the inherent predisposing risk of women undergoing IVM – namely those with PCO/PCOS who already have a higher risk of gestational diabetes[22,23] rather than as a direct result of the IVM treatment modality.

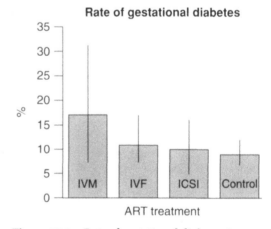

Figure 23.3 Rate of gestational diabetes in pregnancies conceived as a result of IVM, IVF, ICSI, and spontaneously

The rates of other pregnancy complications, including pre-eclampsia, do not appear increased following IVM when compared with other ART or when compared with spontaneously conceived controls.

CONCLUSIONS

The data presented here are generally reassuring for women undergoing IVM. Previously published evidence demonstrates higher rates of multiple pregnancy, earlier delivery, and lower birthweight – even in singleton pregnancies following established ART treatments (IVF or ICSI). The obstetric and perinatal outcomes following IVM are comparable to these established treatments, and may be associated with fewer low birthweight babies, although the data are still early. Continued ongoing surveillance – as with any ART modality – is important so that the risks and benefits of all infertility treatments can be appropriately compared.

Furthermore, all ART treatments show a trend towards a slight increase in the occurrence of any congenital abnormality, and this is most marked for babies conceived following ICSI. This is consistent with increasing evidence from large ART-based studies which show an increased prevalence of major malformations[14,24], chromosomal anomalies[25], and, more recently, imprinting disorders[26]. Whether ART has a direct causative effect, however, is still equivocal owing to the many confounding variables – particularly the effect of infertility per se on the risk of developing congenital abnormalities[27,28]. Similarly, multiple pregnancy – whether spontaneous or following ART – is itself associated with an increase in the incidence of congenital abnormalities, particularly congenital cardiac malformations[29].

In conclusion, when ART is indicated, IVM offers a reduction in the risks of ovarian stimulation and, based on current data, no increased risk of congenital abnormality or perinatal outcome over that already accepted for IVF or ICSI. For an 80% power and a 5% alpha, with a probability of congenital abnormality in the population of 3% and a factor of 1.5, over 1000 IVM babies and over 3000 controls would be needed. The establishment of national and international registries for babies born following IVM, continued data collection and matched studies, and the results from ongoing child development longitudinal studies are essential as the use of IVM as a clinical treatment continues to expand.

REFERENCES

1. Trounson A, Wood C, Kausche A. *In vitro* maturation and the fertilization and developmental competence of oocytes recovered from untreated polycystic ovarian patients. Fertil Steril 1994; 62: 353–62.

2. Chian RC, Gulekli B, Buckett WM et al. Priming with human chorionic gonadotrophin before retrieval of immature oocytes in women with infertility due to the polycystic ovary syndrome. N Engl J Med 1999; 341: 1624–6.

3. Mikkelsen AL, Smith SD, Lindenberg S. *In vitro* maturation of human oocytes from regularly menstruating women may be successful without follicle stimulation hormone priming. Hum Reprod 1999; 14: 1847–51.

4. Cha KY, Han SY, Chung HM et al. Pregnancies and deliveries after *in vitro* maturation culture followed by *in vitro* fertilization and embryo transfer without stimulation in women with polycystic ovary syndrome. Fertil Steril 2000; 73: 978–83.

5. Soderstrom-Anttila V, Makinen S, Tuuri T et al. Favourable pregnancy results with insemination of *in vitro* matured oocytes from unstimulated patients. Hum Reprod 2005; 20: 1534–40.

6. MacDougall MJ, Tan SL, Balen A et al. A controlled study comparing patients with and without polycystic ovaries undergoing *in vitro* fertilization. Hum Reprod 1993; 8: 233–7.

7. Buckett WM, Chian RC, Tan SL. Can we eliminate severe ovarian hyperstimulation syndrome? Not completely. Hum Reprod 2005; 20: 2367.

8. Mikkelsen AL, Ravn SH, Lindenberg S. Evaluation of newborns delivered after in vitro maturation. Hum Reprod 2003; 8(Suppl 1): xviii.

9. Buckett WM, Chian RC, Barrington K et al. Obstetric, neonatal and infant outcome in babies conceived by in-vitro maturation (IVM): initial five-year results 1998–2003. Fertil Steril 2004; 82(Suppl 2): S133.

10. Cha KY, Chung HM, Lee DR et al. Obstetric outcome of patients with polycystic ovary syndrome treated by in vitro maturation and in vitro fertilization–embryo transfer. Fertil Steril 2004; 83: 1462–5.

11. DeBaun MR, Niemitz EL, Feinberg AP. Association of in vitro fertilization with Beckwith–Wiedemann syndrome and epigenetic alterations of *LIT1* and *H19*. Am J Hum Genet 2003; 72: 156–60.

12. Ørstavik KH, Eiklid K, van der Hagen CB et al. Another case of imprinting defect in a girl with Angelman syndrome who was conceived by intracytoplasmic sperm injection. Am J Hum Genet 2003; 72: 218–9.

13. Buckett WM, Chian RC, Holzer H et al. Congenital abnormalities and perinatal outcome in pregnancies following IVM, IVF, and ICSI delivered in a single center. Fertil Steril 2005; 84 (Suppl 2): S180.

14. Hansen M, Kurinczuk JJ, Bower C et al. The risk of major birth defects after intracytoplasmatic sperm injection and in vitro fertilization. N Engl J Med 2002; 346: 725–30.

15. Tan SL, Doyle P, Campbell S et al. Obstetric outcome of in vitro fertilization pregnancies compared with normally conceived pregnancies. Am J Obstet Gynecol 1992; 167: 778–84.

16. Helmerhorst FM, Perquin DAM, Donker D et al. Perinatal outcome of singletons and twins after assisted conception: a systematic review of controlled studies. Br Med J 2004; 328: 261.

17. Jackson RA, Gibson KA, Wu YW et al. Perinatal outcomes in singletons following in vitro fertilization: a meta-analysis. Obstet Gynecol 2004; 103: 551–63.

18. Saunders DH, Mathew M, Lancaster PAL. The Australian Register: current research and future role. A preliminary report. Ann NY Acad Sci 1988; 541: 7–21.

19. Goeverts I, Devreker F, Koenig I et al. Comparison of pregnancy outcome after intracytoplasmic sperm injection and in vitro fertilization. Hum Reprod 1998; 13: 1514–8.

20. Lazzari G, Wrenzycki C, Hermann D et al. Cellular and molecular deviations in bovine in-vitro produced embryos are related to the large offspring syndrome. Biol Reprod 2002; 67: 767–75.

21. Kramer MS, Olivier M, McLean FH et al. Impact of intra-uterine growth retardation and body proportionality on fetal and neonatal outcome. Pediatrics 1990; 86: 707–13.

22. Antilla L, Karjala K, Penttila RA et al. Polycystic ovaries in women with gestational diabetes. Obstet Gynecol 1998; 92: 13–16.

23. Glueck CJ, Wang P, Goldenberg N et al. Pregnancy outcomes among women with polycystic ovary syndrome treated with metformin. Hum Reprod 2002; 17: 2858–64.

24. Koivurova S, Kartikainen AL, Gissler M et al. Neonatal outcome and congenital malformations in children born after in in-vitro fertilization. Hum Reprod 2002; 17: 1391–8.

25. Bonduelle M, Van Assche E, Joris H et al. Prenatal testing in ICSI pregnancies: incidence of chromosomal anomalies in 1586 karyotypes and relation to sperm parameters. Hum Reprod 2002; 17: 2600–14.

26. Gosden R, Trasler J, Lucifero D et al. Rare congenital disorders, imprinting genes, and assisted reproductive technology. Lancet 2003; 361: 1975–7.

27. Ludwig M, Katalinic A, Gross S et al. Increased prevalence of imprinting defects in patients with Angelman syndrome born to subfertile couples. J Med Genet 2005; 42: 289–91.

28. McDonald SD, Murphy K, Beyene J et al. Perinatal outcome of singleton pregnancies achieved by in vitro fertilization: a systematic review and meta-analysis. J Obstet Gynaecol Can 2005; 27: 449–59.

29. Berg KA, Astemborski JA, Boughman JA et al. Congenital cardiovascular malformations in twins and triplets from a population-based study. Am J Dis Child 1989; 143: 1461–3.

CHAPTER 24

How do we improve implantation rate following in-vitro maturation of oocytes?

Antoine Torre, Nelly Achour-Frydman, Estelle Feyereisen, Renato Fanchin, and Réné Frydman

INTRODUCTION

Many years have passed since the in-vitro maturation (IVM) of animal oocytes was first performed by Edwards[1] in the 1960s. In-vitro maturation of human oocytes has now been technically mastered for a decade[2]. Substantial improvements in efficacy have been achieved so that the technique has really quit the research sphere and entered routine clinical use about 5 years ago.

In 2004, Chian et al.[3] estimated that more than 300 healthy infants have been born following immature oocyte retrieval and IVM. About 30–35% of infertile women with polycystic ovary syndrome (PCOS) who undergo IVM treatment achieve clinical pregnancies.

However, in spite of these encouraging results, implantation rates (typically 10–15%) tend to be lower than in conventional in-vitro fertilization (IVF) with ovarian stimulation. In our experience we also have a high miscarriage rate following establishment of clinical pregnancies. These raise concerns regarding the implantation of embryos generated from in-vitro matured oocytes. This appears to be the principal drawback of IVM.

Two main hypothesis can be put forward as an explanation:

- Embryo quality (which can be patient-determined or as a result of the process of in-vitro oocyte maturation and culture).

- Endometrial quality (which can also be patient-determined or a result of asynchronous steroid hormone preparation).

The continued spread of IVM as a real alternative to classical IVF will only be possible if it proves to have comparable outcomes. Hence, we must determine how to improve implantation rate following IVM.

POLYCYSTIC OVARY SYNDROME

As with any new technique, IVM has been tried in numerous reproductive diseases. After 10 years of experience, IVM has been successfully applied in:

- Women with PCOS[4].

- Rescue of oocytes which have failed to mature in conventional IVF stimulated cycles[5].

- Unexplained poor-quality embryos following conventional IVF[6].

- Oocyte donation[7].

- Fertility preservation prior to potentially sterilizing treatments (e.g. chemotherapy[8]).

Even though encouraging successes have been described for the last four indications, the small number of pregnancies make these arguably anecdotal. On the other hand, PCOS patients represent the large majority of women who undergo IVM and also therefore the majority of clinical pregnancies and live births follow IVM to women with PCOS.

Definition of PCOS

This reproductive syndrome is:

- One of the oldest reproductive diseases known (first described by Stein and Leventhal in 1935)[9].

- The commonest cause of anovulatory infertility (75%)[10].

- The commonest endocrinopathy among reproductive age women[11].

Its definition has been heterogeneous until relatively recently. Since 2003 and the Consensus of Rotterdam, this syndrome needs two out of three of the following criteria:

- Polycystic ovaries (PCO): ≥12 follicles/ovary measuring 2 to 9 mm and/or ovarian volume >10 ml

- Troubles of the menstrual cycle (oligo-amenorrhea)

- Hyperandrogenism (hirsutism, acne, alopecia, raised serum testosterone or androstenedione)

without other evident causes (deficiency of 21-hydroxylase, Cushing's syndrome, hyperprolactinemia, acromegaly, virilizing adrenal or ovarian neoplasms)[12].

The epidemiologic importance has often been overestimated by numerous selection biases in published studies[13]. Based on an unselected sample of American women between 18 and 35 years old, Knochenhauer et al. found this syndrome in only 4.7% of Caucasian women and 3.4% of African-American women[14].

Reproductive abnormalities

Oligo-amenorrhea and infertility

These common symptoms push many women with PCOS to consult their gynecologist. Indeed, among PCOS patients, oligomenorrhea (defined as <8 periods/year) is found in 29% to 47% of women with PCOS and total amenorrhea in 19% to 51%. Between 20% and 74% of PCOS patients also suffer from infertility[13].

Miscarriage

One author recently did cast doubt on the increased risk of miscarriage related to PCOS, suggesting a detection/selection bias[15,16]. Indeed, several reports found no association between recurrent pregnancy loss and PCOS as an independent factor[17].

Nevertheless, PCOS is accepted by many authorities as a significant risk factor for early pregnancy loss (for example, according to the Royal College of Obstetricians and Gynaecologists, amongst women with recurrent early miscarriage, PCO is found in 56%, while PCO represents only 22% in the general population). Moreover, women with PCOS seem to suffer a higher rate of early pregnancy loss (30 to 50%) compared to regularly cycling women (10 to 15%)[18]. A confounding factor (such as obesity) could explain these findings. However, most would agree that women with PCOS suffer from a high early pregnancy loss rate no matter whether it is directly or indirectly linked to the PCOS physiology.

Several mechanisms have been suggested to explain this predisposition to miscarriage: obesity (as noted above)[19], low luteal phase progesterone concentration[20], high tonic LH levels (thought to be associated with early pregnancy loss, independently of PCOS)[18], elevated plasminogen activator inhibitor 1 (PAI 1) – related to insulin resistance which could be responsible for a thrombophilic state, and decreased serum IGFbp1 and glycodelin (which could impair placentation)[21,22].

ASSISTED REPRODUCTIVE TECHNOLOGY (ART) STRATEGY

Many treatments have proved either their safety or their efficiency in overcoming PCOS-related infertility and a balance between benefits and risks must be taken into account before determining appropriate treatment. In an editorial, Norman gave his thoughts about which treatment should be proposed for PCOS and in which order[15]. Hence, as an invasive heavy technique, IVM should not be used as a first line treatment (Figure 24.1).

Lifestyle modification (diet and exercise)

Obesity is known to impair the success of classical assisted reproduction, increasing the risk

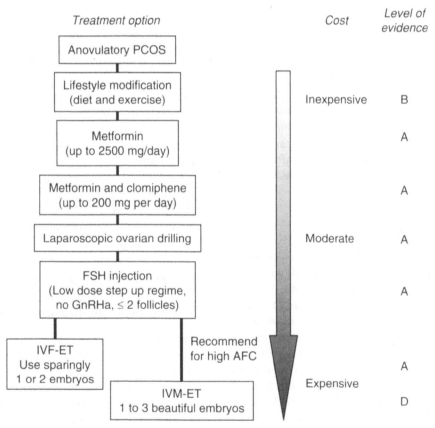

Figure 24.1 A cost-effective and evidence-based approach to the anovulatory woman with polycystic ovary syndrome (PCOS) who is seeking to become pregnant. In-vitro maturation and embryo transfer (IVM-ET) as in-vitro fertilization and embryo transfer (IVF-ET) are last lines of treatment and might depend on antral follicular count (AFC). Ovulation induction by clomiphene citrate or follicle-stimulating hormone (FSH) should be carried out with careful monitoring. Adapted from Norman[15]

of miscarriage and the gonadotropin consumption[23]. A 5–10% decrease of the body mass index (BMI) restores spontaneous reproductive function in 55–100% of women[24].

Clomiphene citrate

This is the uncontested first line of treatment for PCOS with oligo-amenorrhea and permits restoration of ovulation in 80% and a pregnancy rate of 40%[24].

Metformin

This insulin-sensitizing drug has been shown to improve clomiphene citrate efficacy on ovulation induction and pregnancy rates in infertile women with PCOS by two meta-analyses[25,26] and should be largely used as a pretreatment with clomiphene citrate. This same use could also decrease excessive follicular development during ovulation monitoring[27] and increase the biochemical pregnancy rate (pregnancy diagnosed only by hCG measurements) during conventional IVF/ICSI treatment in lean women with PCOS[28].

Gonadotropins

This efficient technique is also associated with a much increased risk of excessive follicular development – and therefore an increased risk of cycle cancellation or high-order multiple pregnancy. GnRH agonists which exacerbate this risk should be avoided in PCOS and a low-dose step-up protocol should be used[29]. For patients with very high numbers of antral follicles (AFC) in the early follicular phase, we counsel regarding the risks and benefits of ovulation induction with gonadotropins compared to the more invasive IVM.

Ovarian drilling

This old treatment is still useful and may be an alternative to IVM, although it carries the risks associated with general anesthesia and the surgical risks associated with laparoscopy. Between 43% and 84% of patients with clomiphene-resistant PCOS could achieve a pregnancy[12], especially non-obese (lean) patients and those with low testosterone and high LH levels[30]. Followed by conventional IVF, it could also increase pregnancy rate, decrease gonadotropin dose, and avoid complications, such as OHSS[31].

In-vitro fertilization

A meta-analysis of comparative studies between PCOS and non-PCOS infertile women concluded that there was an increased cancellation rate but more oocytes were retrieved at each oocyte collection. The authors concluded that the benefits (namely good response and generation of multiple good quality embryos) were balanced by the risks (namely cycle cancellation as a result of OHSS risk). The pregnancy rates were similar in both groups (around 30%)[32].

Furthermore the incidence of OHSS is higher in women with PCOS undergoing conventional IVF (10–19% versus almost 0%)[33,34]. Therefore, IVM must be discussed each time IVF is planned on a woman with PCOS.

Advantages of in-vitro maturation

Ovarian hyperstimulation syndrome

The major advantage of IVM is to avoid OHSS in women with PCOS. This complication of ovarian stimulation is known to lead to a hospitalization rate of 2%[35]. In exceptional cases, OHSS can even be fatal[36]. Because IVM does not use any ovarian stimulation, this technique cannot be complicated by OHSS. A recent review of 10 publications concluded a significant and consistent relationship between women with PCO undergoing ovarian stimulation and the development of OHSS. Indeed, when PCO was present, the combined odds ratio of developing OHSS was 6.8 (95% CI 4.9–9.6)[37]. Although no formal relationship between AFC and the risk of OHSS has been determined, one may logically assume that the higher the AFC's, the higher the risk for OHSS exists. This may therefore be the best determinant for IVM.

Economical benefits

Because IVM does not use any ovarian stimulation, it has been suggested that there may be an economic benefit to IVM. Although this may be the case for the couple undergoing treatment, by charging set prices, most of the centers offering IVM do not take into account a likely longer oocyte retrieval and the additional laboratory work. What is acceptable for a small number of cases or proportion of the workload may not be realistic as IVM becomes more widespread. We suggest that any economic benefit is less important than initially thought.

Other advantages

The absence of ovarian stimulation makes IVM comfortable and rules out the hypothetical risk of ovarian cancer attributed to ovarian stimulation. On the other hand, oocyte retrieval is technically more demanding and may need a deeper anesthesia.

PROBLEMS ASSOCIATED WITH IN-VITRO MATURATION

Results from several centers performing IVM have been published and reviewed[38]. Cha et al.[39] recently reported their experience and the obstetric outcome in women with PCOS who conceived following IVM and further data are available in an earlier report[40]. The Family Federation of Finland recently reported a comparison of insemination with or without ICSI in their IVM program[41]. These results and ours

brought up to date are presented in Table 24.1. Numerous similarities attest to the representativeness of these data. Unfortunately, we are missing data on cycle cancellation, embryo quality, and often miscarriage rate. Hence, as we feel these features are of crucial importance in the improvement of IVM outcome, we will describe our experience without being able to corroborate it.

Cycle cancellation

Since July 2002, 138 new attempts of IVM took place in 75 couples in our center. According to the consensus of Rotterdam, 60% of our women had PCOS, 21% had PCO, and 19% had no ovulatory/ovarian abnormality. Among these attempts, 11.6% were cancelled or commuted into an IVF in a natural cycle because of bleeding (2.9%) or development of a dominant follicle (8.7%). When adding logistic and male factor cancellations, in our experience, more than one patient out of five will not have her IVM as initially planned. Before considering IVM use on a large scale, solutions must be found to improve this high cancellation/delay rate.

Poor embryo quality

Among our 526 embryos obtained by IVM, 19% of them were of A or B quality, while 47% were C quality, and 34% were D quality. Because we always perform ICSI for the fertilization of IVM oocytes, we compared these results with conventional IVF/ICSI. Embryos from IVM oocytes seem different from our usual ICSI embryos in which 42% are A or B quality embryos, 35% are C quality embryos, and 23% are D quality embryos. This spread of low quality embryos obtained from IVM has repercussions on the quality of embryos transferred after IVM: 35% of embryos transferred were of A or B quality, while 54% were C quality, and 9% were D quality. With our conventional ICSI program, at embryo transfer

Table 24.1 Summary of the published outcomes of IVM. Our results are brought up to date (without frozen embryos). Those of the Montreal, Taipei, and Maria Infertility Hospital of Seoul groups are from a review by Chian et al.[38]. Those of The Family Federation of Finland can be roughly deduced from a recent article[41]. Finally, clinical data from Cha et al.[39] have been published recently, while his biological data (*) from a smaller number of patients in an older paper[40] given in brackets

ART Service		A Beclere, Paris	McGill, Montreal[38]	Shin Kong Wu Ho-Su Memorial Hospital, Taipei[38]	The Family Federation of Finland, Helsinki[41]	Infertility Medical center of Cha, Seoul[39,40]	Maria Infertility Hospital Seoul[38], Embryo transfer	Maria Infertility Hospital Seoul[38], Blastocyst transfer
Cycles (n)		138	254	68	239	203	419	80
Oocytes retrieved	Total (n)	1406	3079	1528	971	3148	6860	2108
	Mean ± sd	12.1 ± 7.7	11.9 ± 6.2	22.5 ± 10.1	8.0 ± 5.2	15.5 ± 8.2	16.4 ± 7.1	26.4 ± 9.9
Maturation rate (%)		61.7	78.8	74.2	58.6	(55.3)*	73.2	77
Fertilization rate (%)		62	69.2	72.8	51.3	(75.1)*	79.0	79.3
Cleavage rate (%)		95.2	89.9	88.8		(88)*		36.3
Embryo transfer	Total (n)	230	865	258	287	926	1816	246
	Mean ± sd	2.4 ± 0.7	3.4 ± 0.9	3.8 ± 0.9		5.0 ± 2.1	4.3 ± 0.9	3.1 ± 0.4
Implantation rate (%)		10.9	11.1	10.5	18.5	5.5	11.6	27.2
Clinical pregnancy rate per oocyte retrieval (%)		24.5	24.0	33.8	26.6	21.9	32.7	53.8
Miscarriage rate (%)		42.3			26.5	36.8		

61% of embryos transferred are of A or B quality, 31% are C quality, and 3% are D quality. Consequently, the number of frozen embryos following IVM is very low (7.2%).

This fact could explain the low implantation rate observed in IVM. However, we must say that the quality of embryos involved in several of our clinical pregnancies was surprisingly low.

Low implantation rate

The implantation rate has always been low since the initial clinical experience with IVM. Improvements have occurred as the early practitioners reported implantation rates of around 5%[40] and most studies now report implantation rates of around 10% (Table 24.1). However, no study has been able to link this improvement to any precise practice adopted. Information about different centers' results changing is not available.

This low implantation rate (10.9% in our center when our usual implantation rate during ICSI is 27%) might either be part of the IVM technique or related to a detection bias explained by the PCOS. We will see that many convincing arguments support this low implantation rate as an intrinsic drawback of IVM rather than a PCOS characteristic.

Related to PCOS

The only argument supporting PCOS itself as a possible cause for the low implantation rate in IVM is the results from the oocyte donation program of McGill University – this center reported a 50% pregnancy rate per cycle in recipients of IVM egg donation[7]. Nevertheless, as recipients of IVM egg donation do not have PCOS (rather premature ovarian failure) and the oocyte donors do have PCO/PCOS, it is possible that implantation might be improved when the recipient does not have PCOS.

On the other hand, when comparing outcomes of 251 matched patients with and without PCOS, undergoing conventional IVF, MacDougall et al.[34] could find no difference between the implantation rates[34]. In another prospective study, Child et al[51]. compared the outcomes of 144 women with normal ovaries, PCO, and PCOS. This time, the pregnancy rate and the implantation rate were significantly lower in women with normal ovaries compared to those with PCO and PCOS[42]. These last findings do not support the implication of PCOS itself in the low implantation rate associated with IVM.

Related to the IVM technique

In another case-controlled study, Child et al.[43] compared 107 IVM cycles with 107 matched conventional IVF cycles in women with PCO. The implantation rate of IVF-derived embryos was significantly higher (17.7% vs. 9.5%) than that of IVM (p <0.01). Even if more data are needed, most of the arguments support the low implantation rate as an intrinsic drawback of IVM rather than a characteristic of PCOS.

High miscarriage rate

The high frequency of early pregnancy loss in IVM is not of common knowledge. Even so, the few published figures speak for themselves, with miscarriage rates from 26.5% to 42.3%. These figures are similar to what could be the 'background' miscarriage rate of women with PCOS. However, this higher miscarriage rate is not noticed when women with PCOS undergo conventional IVF treatment[32]. On the other hand, in an oocyte donation program, Copperman et al. noted a miscarriage rate of 33% for PCOS patients compared to 6% for non-PCOS patients[44]. In this case, the high early pregnancy loss rate may be linked to PCOS.

IMPROVEMENTS IN IN-VITRO MATURATION

Patient selection

Oocytes from normo-ovulatory young women are known to show a higher developmental capability than oocytes from women with PCOS.[45] Nevertheless, Child et al.[42] compared the outcomes of 144 women with normal ovaries, PCO, and PCOS in a prospective study and found a tendency to a better maturation and fertilization rate, but a pregnancy rate and an implantation rate significantly lower in women with normal ovaries than with PCO and PCOS. Obviously, IVM seems best suited to women with PCOS.

As in every ART procedure, age is important and younger age (particularly below 35 years) is associated with a higher pregnancy and live birth rate (Smitz et al., unpublished data).

The antral follicle count (AFC) is known to be the best predictor of the number of immature oocytes retrieved and of the likelihood of clinical pregnancy following IVM[46].

Finally, over-responders during conventional ovarian stimulation for IVF can be commuted to IVM rather than cancelled. In this way, Lim[49] administered human chorionic gonadotropin (hCG) to patients undergoing IVF with a high response when the leading follicle reached 12–14 mm in diameter. IVM-ICSI was performed with a 47.1% pregnancy rate and no OHSS.

FSH and hCG priming

FSH priming may improve oocyte yield and maturational competence, although there are conflicting results[38,45]. Although the use of FSH was not thought to affect implantation, one study suggested it may do[47]. So the effect of FSH priming is still unclear and further research is needed.

On the other hand, hCG priming shows fewer conflicting results. It has been shown to hasten oocyte maturation and to increase matu-

ration rate[38,45]. In a randomized controlled trial, comparing IVM with and without hCG priming in 20 women with PCOS, Buckett et al. noticed an increased number of oocytes retrieved with hCG priming, but no effect on the endometrium[48]. Hence, hCG priming is unlikely to affect implantation.

A combination of FSH and hCG priming does not any add benefit[49]. Most centers practice hCG priming before IVM oocyte retrieval; over 200 healthy infants have been born following hCG priming[38].

Technical improvements

In the animal model, increasing the aspiration pressure tended to reduce the proportion of oocytes with intact cumulus so that almost every center now practices immature oocyte retrieval with a reduced vacuum pressure (7.5 kPa). Further animal studies noted the deleterious effect of cooling ovaries or oocytes and suggested that a temperature higher than 30°C should always be used for oocyte culture[50].

FUTURE POSSIBLE IMPROVEMENTS

Estradiol priming

While comparing a pregnant cohort to a nonpregnant cohort following IVM, Child et al. observed a statistical significance difference between endometrial thicknesses: greater than 10 mm on the day of embryo transfer was a good predictor of pregnancy[51]. Hence, endometrial preparation is necessary and must take place in a very short period of time unless it begins before oocyte retrieval (Figure 24.2). Starting 17β-estradiol early in the cycle could permit a better endometrial preparation and may improve the cancellation rate. However, the prospective work of Russell[52] suggested that early exposure of ovaries to 17β-estradiol could impair oocyte maturation, fertilization, and cleavage. The

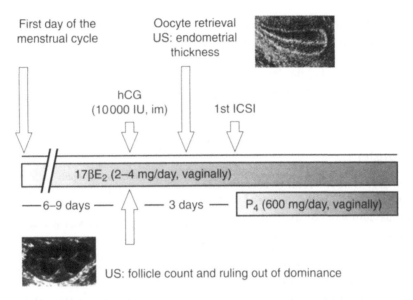

Figure 24.2 A protocol of immature oocyte retrieval and IVM designed to improve endometrial thickness. 17β-Estradiol (17βE₂) might be given from the first day of the patient's menstrual cycle. This picture represents a protocol of immature oocyte retrieval and IVM which might improve the endometrium. Ultrasound (US) is performed to rule out dominance and to measure endometrial thickness. Progesterone (P₄) is begun on the day of ICSI

global effect will depend on the improvement of the implantation rate induced by 17β-estradiol.

Metformin

This fashionable insulin-sensitizing drug has been recently tried for many aspects of ART, sometimes without any conclusive benefit[15,16]. Two observational retrospective studies with metformin alone and one with the addition of enoxaparin suggest that metformin could decrease the miscarriage rate of PCOS when continued at the beginning of the pregnancy[53,54]. On the other hand, one other observational retrospective study was unable to demonstrate this benefit[55].

Mechanisms put forward to explain this are a decrease in serum androgens, an improvement in uterine vasculature (decreasing PAI 1 and increasing IGFbp1 and glycodeline)[21],

weight loss, or an improved luteal phase progesterone[20].

Metformin could be carefully assessed in PCOS patients undergoing IVM, as we have seen that the miscarriage rate is high and it could be related to endocrinologic disturbance of PCOS that may be improved by metformin.

On the other hand, we have seen that the low implantation rate observed in IVM must be an intrinsic drawback of IVM rather than a PCOS characteristic. Even if a recent study found a beneficial effect of metformin over porcine oocytes in vitro[56], it may not improve overall implantation rates.

GnRH pumps or GnRH agonists

A meta-analysis was unable to determine any significant effect of the GnRH pump when used in PCOS patients (the patient numbers were too small)[57]. However, the pump has been shown to normalize LH levels in an observational study of 13 anovulatory PCOS women[58]. As the high miscarriage rate observed in PCOS has been linked to high LH levels, it may be possible to improve implantation rates and decrease miscarriage rates.

Blastocyst transfer

The experience of IVM in The Family Federation of Finland is novel. In this center, the use of ICSI is reserved for masculine infertility. This restrictive use of ICSI decreases the fertilization rate and the number of embryo transfers, but the clinical pregnancy rate per embryo transfer is much higher so that the clinical pregnancy rate per immature oocyte retrieval is not significantly different[41].

Blastocyst transfer shows a high implantation rate when used in conventional IVF, presumably by better selection of embryos with the greatest developmental potential. Prolonged culture may be a good selection tool for the developmental potential of embryos generated from IVM oocytes.

CONCLUSIONS

Because it avoids OHSS and because it is less expensive, IVM might become an alternative to conventional IVF. Outcomes have already improved. However, the main drawbacks remain a high cancellation rate, a low implantation rate, and a high miscarriage rate. 17β-Estradiol and metformin may be of help, but the future must go to embryo selection by prolonged (blastocyst) culture.

REFERENCES

1. Edwards RG. Maturation in vitro of mouse, sheep, cow, pig, rhesus monkey and human ovarian oocytes. Nature 1965; 208: 349–51.

2. Trounson A, Wood C, Kausche A. In vitro maturation and the fertilization and developmental competence of oocytes recovered from untreated polycystic ovarian patients. Fertil Steril 1994; 62: 353–62.

3. Chian RC, Lim JH, Tan SL. State of the art in in-vitro oocyte maturation. Curr Opin Obstet Gynecol 2004; 16: 211–19.

4. Le Du A, Kadoch IJ, Bourcigaux N et al. In vitro oocyte maturation for the treatment of infertility associated with polycystic ovarian syndrome: the French experience. Hum Reprod 2005; 20: 420–4.

5. Liu J, Lu G, Qian Y et al. Pregnancies and births achieved from in vitro matured oocytes retrieved from poor responders undergoing stimulation in in vitro fertilization cycles. Fertil Steril 2003; 80: 447–9.

6. Chian RC, Bucket WM, Abdul Jalil AK et al. Natural-cycle in vitro fertilization combined with in vitro maturation of immature oocytes is a potential approach in infertility treatment. Fertil Steril 2004; 82: 1675–8.

7. Rao DG, Tan SL. In vitro maturation of oocytes. Semin Reprod Med 2005; 23: 242–7.

8. Oktay K, Buyuk E. Fertility preservation in women undergoing cancer treatment. Lancet 2004; 363: 1830.

9. Adams J, Polson DW, Franks S. Prevalence of polycystic ovaries in women with anovulation and idiopathic hirsutism. Br Med J (Clin Res Ed) 1986; 293: 355–9.

10. Carmina E, Lobo RA. Polycystic ovary syndrome (PCOS): arguably the most common endocrinopathy is associated with significant morbidity in women. J Clin Endocrinol Metab 1999; 84: 1897–9.

11. Rotterdam ESHRE/ASRM-Sponsored PCOS Consensus Workshop Group. Revised 2003 consensus on diagnostic criteria and long-term health risks related to polycystic ovary syndrome. Fertil Steril 2004; 81: 19–25.

12. Gomel V, Yarali H. Surgical treatment of polycystic ovary syndrome associated with infertility. Reprod Biomed Online 2004; 9: 35–42.

13. Hart R, Hickey M, Franks S. Definitions, prevalence and symptoms of polycystic ovaries and

polycystic ovary syndrome. Best Pract Res Clin Obstet Gynaecol 2004; 18: 671–83.

14. Knochenhauer ES, Key TJ, Kahsar-Miller M et al. Prevalence of the polycystic ovary syndrome in unselected black and white women of the southeastern United States: a prospective study. J Clin Endocrinol Metab 1998; 83: 3078–82.

15. Norman RJ. Editorial: Metformin – comparison with other therapies in ovulation induction in polycystic ovary syndrome. J Clin Endocrinol Metab 2004; 89: 4797–800.

16. Norman RJ, Wang JX, Hague W. Should we continue or stop insulin sensitizing drugs during pregnancy? Curr Opin Obstet Gynecol 2004; 16: 245–50.

17. Porter TF, Scott JR. Evidence-based care of recurrent miscarriage. Best Pract Res Clin Obstet Gynaecol 2005; 15: 85–101.

18. Regan L, Owen EJ, Jacobs HS. Hypersecretion of luteinising hormone, infertility, and miscarriage. Lancet 1990; 336: 1141–4.

19. Al-Azemi M, Omu FE, Omu AE. The effect of obesity on the outcome of infertility management in women with polycystic ovary syndrome. Arch Gynecol Obstet 2004; 270: 205–10.

20. Meenakumari KJ, Agarwal S, Krishna A et al. Effects of metformin treatment on luteal phase progesterone concentration in polycystic ovary syndrome. Braz J Med Biol Res 2004; 37: 1637–44.

21. McCarthy EA, Walker SP, McLachlan K et al. Metformin in obstetric and gynecologic practice: a review. Obstet Gynecol Surv 2004; 59: 118–27.

22. Cheang KI, Nestler JE. Should insulin-sensitizing drugs be used in the treatment of polycystic ovary syndrome? Reprod Biomed Online 2004; 8: 440–7.

23. Urman B, Tiras B, Yakin T. Assisted reproduction in the treatment of polycystic ovarian syndrome. Reprod Biomed Online 2004; 8: 419–30.

24. Homburg R. The management of infertility associated with polycystic ovary syndrome. Reprod Biol Endocrinol 2003; 1: 109.

25. Kashyap S, Wells GA, Rosenwaks Z. Insulin-sensitizing agents as primary therapy for patients with polycystic ovarian syndrome. Hum Reprod 2004; 19: 2474–83.

26. Lord JM, Flight IH, Norman RJ. Metformin in polycystic ovary syndrome: systematic review and meta-analysis. Br Med J 2003; 327: 951–3.

27. Palomba S, Falbo A, Orro F Jr. et al. A randomized controlled trial evaluating metformin pretreatment and co-administration in non-obese insulin-resistant women with polycystic ovary syndrome treated with controlled ovarian stimulation plus timed intercourse or intrauterine insemination. Hum Reprod 2005; 10: 2879–86.

28. Kjotrod SB, von During V, Carlsen SM. Metformin treatment before IVF/ICSI in women with polycystic ovary syndrome; a prospective, randomized, double blind study. Hum Reprod 2004; 19: 1315–22.

29. Christin-Maitre S, Hugues JN. A comparative randomized multicentric study comparing the step-up versus step-down protocol in polycystic ovary syndrome. Hum Reprod 2003; 18: 1626–31.

30. Amer SA, Li TC, Ledger WL. Ovulation induction using laparoscopic ovarian drilling in women with polycystic ovarian syndrome: predictors of success. Hum Reprod 2004; 19: 1719–24.

31. Tozer AJ, Al-Shawaf T, Zosmer A et al. Does laparoscopic ovarian diathermy affect the outcome of IVF-embryo transfer in women with polycystic ovarian syndrome? A retrospective comparative study. Hum Reprod 2001; 16: 91–5.

32. Heijnen EM, Eijkemans MJ, Huges EG et al. A meta-analysis of outcomes of conventional IVF in women with polycystic ovary syndrome. Hum Reprod Update 2005; 12: 13–21.

33. Dor J, Shulman A, Levron D et al. The treatment of patients with polycystic ovarian syndrome by in-vitro fertilization and embryo transfer: a comparison of results with those of patients with tubal infertility. Hum Reprod 1990; 5: 816–18.

34. MacDougall MJ, Tan SL, Balen A et al. A controlled study comparing patients with and without polycystic ovaries undergoing in-vitro fertilization. Hum Reprod 1993; 8: 233–7.

35. Papanikolaou EG, Tournaye H, Verpoest W et al. Early and late ovarian hyperstimulation syn-

drome: early pregnancy outcome and profile. Hum Reprod 2005; 20: 636–41.

36. Semba S, Moriya T, Youssef EM et al. An autopsy case of ovarian hyperstimulation syndrome with massive pulmonary edema and pleural effusion. Pathol Int 2000; 50: 549–52.

37. Tummon I, Gavrilova-Jordan L, Allemand MC et al. Polycystic ovaries and ovarian hyperstimulation syndrome: a systematic review. Acta Obstet Gynecol Scand 2005; 84: 611–16.

38. Chian RC, Buckett WM, Tan SL. In-vitro maturation of human oocytes. Reprod Biomed Online 2004; 8: 148–66.

39. Cha KY, Chung HM, Lee DR et al. Obstetric outcome of patients with polycystic ovary syndrome treated by in vitro maturation and in vitro fertilization-embryo transfer. Fertil Steril 2005; 83: 1461–5.

40. Cha KY, Han SY, Chung HM et al. Pregnancies and deliveries after in vitro maturation culture followed by in vitro fertilization and embryo transfer without stimulation in women with polycystic ovary syndrome. Fertil Steril 2000; 73: 978–83.

41. Soderstrom-Anttila V, Makinen S, Tuuri T et al. Favourable pregnancy results with insemination of in vitro matured oocytes from unstimulated patients. Hum Reprod 2005; 20: 1534–40.

42. Child TJ, Abdul-Jalil AK, Gulekli B et al. In vitro maturation and fertilization of oocytes from unstimulated normal ovaries, polycystic ovaries, and women with polycystic ovary syndrome. Fertil Steril 2001; 76: 936–42.

43. Child TJ, Phillips SJ, Abdul-Jalil AK et al. A comparison of in vitro maturation and in vitro fertilization for women with polycystic ovaries. Obstet Gynecol 2002; 100: 665–70.

44. Copperman A. The egg or the endometrium: why do PCO patients have higher rates of miscarriage? Fertil Steril 2000; 73(Suppl 1): S101.

45. Papanikolaou EG, Platteau P, Albano C et al. Immature oocyte in-vitro maturation: clinical aspects. Reprod Biomed Online 2005; 10: 587–92.

46. Tan SL, Child TJ, Gulekli B. In vitro maturation and fertilization of oocytes from unstimulated

ovaries: predicting the number of immature oocytes retrieved by early follicular phase ultrasonography. Am J Obstet Gynecol 2002; 186: 684–9.

47. Mikkelsen AL, Lindenberg S. Benefit of FSH priming of women with PCOS to the in vitro maturation procedure and the outcome: a randomized prospective study. Reproduction 2001; 122: 587–92.

48. Buckett WM, Chian RC, Tan SL. Human chorionic gonadotropin for in vitro oocyte maturation: does it improve the endometrium or implantation? J Reprod Med 2004; 49: 93–8.

49. Lim YH, Hwang JL, Huang LW et al. Combination of FSH priming and hCG priming for in-vitro maturation of human oocytes. Hum Reprod 2003; 18(8): 1632–6.

50. Yuge M, Otoi T, Nii M et al. Effects of cooling ovaries before oocyte aspiration on meiotic competence of porcine oocytes and of exposing invitro matured oocytes to ambient temperature on in vitro fertilization and development of the oocytes. Cryobiology 2003; 47: 102–8.

51. Child TJ, Gulekli B, Sylvestre C et al. Ultrasonographic assessment of endometrial receptivity at embryo transfer in an in vitro maturation of oocyte program. Fertil Steril 2003; 79: 656–8.

52. Russell JB, Knezevich KM, Fabian KF, Dickson JA. Unstimulated immature oocyte retrieval: early versus midfollicular endometrial priming. Fertil Sterile 1997; 67: 616–20.

53. Glueck CJ, Wang P, Goldenberg N et al. Pregnancy outcomes among women with polycystic ovary syndrome treated with metformin. Hum Reprod 2002; 17: 2858–64.

54. Jakubowicz DJ, Iuorno MJ, Jakubowicz S et al. Effects of metformin on early pregnancy loss in the polycystic ovary syndrome. J Clin Endocrinol Metab 2002; 87: 524–9.

55. Glueck CJ, Wang P, Goldenberg N et al. Pregnancy loss, polycystic ovary syndrome, thrombophilia, hypofibrinolysis, enoxaparin, metformin. Clin Appl Thromb Hemost 2004; 10: 323–34.

56. Lee MS, Kang SK, Lee BC et al. The beneficial effects of insulin and metformin on in vitro

developmental potential of porcine oocytes and embryos. Biol Reprod 2005; 73: 1264–8.

57. Bayram N, van Wely M, van der Veen F. Pulsatile gonadotrophin releasing hormone for ovulation induction in subfertility associated with polycystic ovary syndrome. Cochrane Database Syst Rev 2004: CD000412.

58. Grana-Barcia M, Liz-Leston J, Lado-Abeal J. Subcutaneous administration of pulsatile gonadotropin-releasing hormone decreases serum follicle-stimulating hormone and luteinizing hormone levels in women with polycystic ovary syndrome: a preliminary study. Fertil Steril 2005; 83: 1466–72.

CHAPTER 25

IVM as an alternative for poor responders

Jiayin Liu, Jin-Ho Lim, and Ri-Cheng Chian

INTRODUCTION

In conventional in-vitro fertilization (IVF) treatment, infertile women are treated with gonadotropin-releasing hormone (GnRH)-agonist or -antagonist in combination with gonadotropins for approximately 2 or 3 weeks to induce the development of ovarian follicles, because the number of oocytes retrieved determines the number of embryos available for transfer, which in turn directly affects the pregnancy rate.

However, many patients respond poorly to ovarian stimulation. It has been estimated that up to 15% of all patients treated for IVF are poor responders to stimulation with exogenous gonadotropins[1]. Reports have indicated that, amongst patients undergoing IVF treatment, the prevalence of poor response to gonadotropin stimulation is between 9 and 24%[2]. Therefore, this has become a frequently encountered problem in all IVF treatment centers.

Poor response to gonadotropin stimulation occurs more often in older women, but may also present in young women with both an abnormal and a normal endocrinologic profile[3]. These patients are characterized typically by low estradiol concentrations combined with markedly reduced numbers of follicles in spite of stimulation with massive doses of gonadotropins[4]. Other patients appear to respond to gonadotropin stimulation but have a low estrogen level or few or slow-growing follicles. Finally, in some patients, the number of follicles in the ovaries seems normal following ovarian stimulation, but their size remains less than 12 mm in diameter on day 15 of the treatment cycle[5,6]. Oocyte quality is often compromised in these groups of patients and results in diminished clinical pregnancy rates, increased spontaneous abortion rates, and lower implantation rates when compared with age-matched controls.

A modified stimulation regimen may help to overcome poor ovarian response and oocyte growth retardation, but most patients still require longer stimulation time and higher gonadotropin doses. These patients seem resistant to gonadotropin stimulation. However, a higher dose of gonadotropin may negatively affect fertilization and pregnancy outcome[7]. Furthermore, many women also experience a higher cycle cancellation rate because of the smaller number and size of follicles.

Since the first successful live birth from in-vitro maturation (IVM) of immature oocytes was reported from a woman with polycystic ovary syndrome (PCOS)[8], immature oocyte retrieval followed by IVM has been applied as a clinical treatment, especially for infertile women with

PCOS[9]. Liu et al.[10] reported a 37.5% pregnancy rate following immature oocyte retrieval and IVM, suggesting that IVM may be a viable alternative to cancellation in this group of patients[11].

DEFINITION OF POOR RESPONDERS

There is no universal standard definition for 'poor responder' in the field of assisted reproductive technology (ART). However, it is common sense that such patients are characterized by lower-than-expected numbers of follicles and oocytes recruited in the face of exogenous gonadotropin stimulation. Several criteria have been used frequently to characterize poor responders: (1) the number of developed follicles in the ovaries; (2) the concentration of estradiol during the gonadotropin stimulation; (3) the increased basal FSH level; (4) other factors.

Number of follicles

The proposed number of follicles varies among the different reports. However, most reports indicate that less than three to five dominant follicles on the day of human chorionic gonadotropin (hCG) administration should be considered 'poor responders' in gonadotropin-stimulated IVF treatment cycles[12-16].

Estradiol level

Estradiol level is correlated with the number and size of follicles. A peak estradiol level of 300–660 pg/ml has been proposed as an important criterion for defining poor response to ovarian stimulation[15,17-19]. It also has been suggested that an estradiol level of less than 100 pg/ml on day 5 of stimulation should be defined as 'poor response'[16]. Poor response to ovarian stimulation for IVF treatment has been defined as a plasma estradiol level of less than 1000 pg/ml on the day of hCG administration and no more than four oocytes retrieved[20].

Basal FSH level

An age-related decline in fecundity is observed as women progress through reproductive life and ovarian reserves decline. It has been suggested that the age-related decline in oocyte quantity and quality is the result of defects in the follicle originating from development in the fetal ovary. There is a premature reduction in follicle numbers in 'poor responders'[21] and it is identifiable by a rise in FSH level in the early follicular phase[22], that reflects an effort by the pituitary gland to maintain the normal follicle response[23]. Therefore, it has been suggested that the basal FSH level is increased from 6.5 mIU/ml to 15.0 mIU/ml (average 10.0 mIU/ml) in 'poor responders'[24-26].

Other factors

Some other indicators have been also implicated in poor responders. These are a failed response to the 'clomiphene challenge test'[27] and the 'lupron screening test'[28], an advanced patient age of more than 40 years[25], at least one previous cancelled IVF treatment cycle[29], increased numbers of gonadotropin ampoules used (more than 300 IU/day)[26], and a prolonged duration of gonadotropin stimulation[30]. Recent studies have shown convincingly that poor ovarian response is a first sign of ovarian aging (early ovarian failure or early menopause)[31-33].

In a variety of studies, these criteria have been used either alone or in combination, thereby highlighting the complexity, the lack of uniformity in definitions, and also the major difficulties encountered when comparing the different strategies proposed to overcome this problem.

PREDICTION OF POOR RESPONDERS

There is no accurate prediction of low ovarian response. Despite the multitude of predictive tests for low ovarian response, the 'poor responder' is revealed definitively only during ovarian stimulation. However, multivariate analyses involving basal FSH and inhibin levels combined with antral follicle count may significantly improve the prediction of poor ovarian response in IVF treatment[34].

An increased serum FSH level on day 3 of the menstrual cycle is a biomarker for ovarian reserve decline and is believed to indicate a reduced reproductive potential[35]. Women with elevated FSH levels may require consistently more gonadotropin stimulation than women with a low range of FSH levels[36]. It has been known that women with higher basal FSH levels have a poor outcome compared with those with a normal range of FSH levels[37,38]. As FSH levels rise, there is a progressive decline in the pregnancy rate, suggesting that basal FSH is a better predictor than age with regard to pregnancy and cancellation rates[39]. Therefore, basal serum FSH level is the most widely used test of ovarian reserve and is strongly associated with poor ovarian response to gonadotropin stimulation[40]. However, there remains a group of young women with an apparently normal basal FSH level and ovarian reserve who do not respond well. In this case, the small antral follicle counting may be a better prognostic indicator of poor response before controlled ovarian stimulation for IVF treatment[41]. Another ultrasound marker of ovarian response may be ovarian volume[42].

An additional biomarker of ovarian reserve and response is inhibin. Inhibin-A and inhibin-B are secreted by granulosa cells of the developing follicles and exert a suppressive effect on FSH. It has been reported that lower inhibin-B levels are associated with fewer oocytes, higher cancellation rates, and lower pregnancy rates compared with patients with normal inhibin-B levels[34,43]. Although other biochemical markers of ovarian reserve and response have been proposed[44,45], it seems that no biomarker is absolute for the prediction of poor response to ovarian stimulation. Therefore, an accurate prediction of poor response should be based on multivariate analyses.

ETIOLOGIES OF POOR RESPONDERS

The mechanism of a poor response to gonadotropin stimulation is still unclear. Although several possible etiologies have been suggested, a diminished ovarian reserve is still thought to be the principal reason for poor ovarian response[6]. Alternatively some other factors, such as a decreased number of FSH receptors available in the granulosa cells[46], defective signal transduction after FSH receptor binding[47], an inappropriate local vascular network for the distribution of gonadotropins[5], premature luteinization due to an abnormal negative ovarian feedback at the level of the anterior pituitary, and the presence of autoantibodies against granulosa cells, as well as lowered circulating gonadotropin surge-attenuating factor (GnSAF) bioactivity[48], have all been suspected. In addition, vascularization around ovaries appears to play a very important role in the recruitment, growth, and maturation of follicles in both natural and stimulated IVF cycles[49], suggesting that the severe adhesions caused by previous pelvic infection or inflammation may result in an encumbrance for this process.

In general, it is accepted that the elevated FSH levels represent quantitative and qualitative limitations in follicle development, but do not always occur simultaneously[50]. It has been reported that the ovarian response to FSH stimulation is dependent upon the FSH receptor genotype, in which is expressed a less active FSH receptor requiring higher levels of FSH for stimulation[51]. Different isoforms of FSH have been described with differing receptor binding immunoactivity[52]. FSH binding inhibitors or FSH antibodies may affect the binding and result in a low ovarian response to FSH.

A frequently occurring variant of the FSH receptor has been reported in which the enzyme asparagine of the receptor protein is replaced by serine at position 680[51]. This change leads to a slightly less active FSH receptor that requires higher FSH levels for normal function and is probably not related to reproductive aging[53].

Therefore, it has been proposed that in cases of elevated FSH further investigations should be made, such as FSH receptor genotyping, dynamic ovarian testing, measurement of antral follicle count, and another potential biochemical marker – anti-Müllerian hormone[54,55].

MANAGEMENT OF POOR RESPONDERS

High dose of gonadotropins

Most authorities recommend a high dose of gonadotropins for poor responders. However, the results remain controversial. Some reports indicate that the increased dose of gonadotropins would improve oocyte yield[56–58]. Although some reports indicate that there is no benefit from the increase in FSH dose[12,16,24–26], large prospective randomized trials are needed to elucidate this issue further.

The type of gonadotropin used has been suggested to have the different potencies of ovarian response as a result of its increased purity and isoform properties[15,59]. The combination of FSH and LH may also benefit poor responders as compared with FSH alone[60]. Clomiphene citrate, when administered in conjunction with exogenous gonadotropins, may be a more potent stimulator of FSH than mid luteal GnRH-agonist among poor responders who failed responding to other ovarian stimulation protocols[61,62], indicating that the number of oocytes is not increased but the follicular growth and oocyte quality seem to be improved.

Downregulation with GnRH-agonist

Initially a GnRH-agonist was used to avoid a premature LH surge during ovarian stimulation. It was initially thought that using GnRH for downregulation might improve the response of poor responders[63]. However, using a GnRH-agonist for downregulation depletes endogenous FSH and LH, making it more difficult to achieve an adequate follicular response[64]. Therefore, modified GnRH-agonist downregulation protocols have been proposed.

The GnRH-agonist flare, or the short protocol, has been applied to poor responders to avoid the suppressive effects of GnRH-agonist downregulation on endogenous gonadotropins. This may benefit the initial pituitary release of FSH and LH in response to GnRH-agonist initiation. Although there is an improvement in oocyte quality seen by this modification of GnRH-agonist downregulation, there is little or no improvement in clinical outcome[65–67].

A microdose of GnRH-agonist flare protocol has the advantages of the standard flare. At least in theory, the regimens of microdose of GnRH-agonist flare would be suited to patients with a low ovarian response. Because approximately 1% of the normal GnRH-agonist dose could initiate pituitary release of gonadotropins, it results in delayed desensitization of the pituitary and allows for significant follicular recruitment and response[68]. Several microdoses of GnRH-agonist flare protocols have been tested, and most studies conducted to assess the standard dose flare protocols demonstrate a degree of improvement[16,69]. A significant improvement was demonstrated with the use of the microdose of GnRH-agonist regimens[70]. However, further clinical investigations are needed to confirm its outcome.

GnRH-antagonist protocols

The relatively new GnRH-antagonist regimens were brought into clinical use for eliminating the premature LH surge. A GnRH-antagonist offers potential advantages for the treatment of poor responders. Use of a GnRH-antagonist avoids the suppression of the early follicular phase endogenous gonadotropins by a GnRH-agonist. The synergic effect of endogenous FSH with high-dose exogenous gonadotropins may maximize the delivery of gonadotropin to the cohort of recruitable follicles in the early follicular phase.

Therefore, the use of a GnRH-antagonist regimen probably reduces the duration of ovarian stimulation in comparison with the conventional GnRH-agonist regimens[20]. However, asynchrony of the follicular cohort can result in the development of a single dominant follicle and is a potential problem of the GnRH-antagonist protocol. This risk may be avoided by taking the oral contraceptive pill[71,72]. Although a randomized control trial comparing microdoses of GnRH-agonist and GnRH-antagonist protocols demonstrated equivalent rates of treatment cancellation, pregnancy, and implantation[73], another report indicated that the GnRH-agonist flare protocol appears to be more effective than the GnRH-antagonist protocol in terms of mature oocytes retrieved, fertilization rate, and high-quality embryos transferred in poor responders[74].

Growth hormone

It was hypothesized that growth hormone (GH) can stimulate ovarian steroidogenesis and follicular development, and enhances the ovarian response to FSH[75]. The action of GH is believed to be mediated via insulin-like growth factor-1 (IGF-1) that acts in synergy with FSH, amplifying its effects on the granulosa cells[76]. It has been reported that GH-releasing hormone (GH-RH) causes an increase in endogenous GH secretion[77]. However, use of GH-RH seems not to improve the final cancellation and pregnancy rates compared to the controls. Pyridostigmine is an acetylcholinesterase inhibitor that can increase GH secretion by enhancing the action of acetylcholine[78]. Nevertheless, the published data so far do not support any benefit from using GH, GH-RH, or pyridostigmine as adjuvant therapy in poor responders.

Oral contraceptive pill

Oral contraceptive pill pretreatment (OCP) might benefit the ovarian response of poor responders. OCP administration is now widely used to suppress endogenous gonadotropins before controlled ovarian stimulation. OCP pretreatment seems to generate and to sensitize more estrogen receptors, and OCP administration prior to the GnRH-agonist protocol was associated with a higher pregnancy rate and lower cancellation rate[79]. However, a recent study indicated that pretreatment with OCP appears to be associated with no significant difference in ongoing pregnancy rate compared to controls and a significantly higher rate of early pregnancy loss[80]. Therefore, conclusive results are still awaited.

Low-dose aspirin treatment

Antiphospholipid antibodies (APAs) have clinical significance because of their association with thromboembolic events and adverse pregnancy outcome[81]. Among patients who have recurrent spontaneous abortions, prednisolone and low-dose aspirin therapy have been proven to be effective in maintaining and prolonging pregnancy in women with autoimmune conditions, including those with positive APA[82]. Many studies have indicated that the number of follicles, oocyte yield, and implantation and pregnancy rates are improved with a low dose of aspirin combined with either prednisolone or immunoglobulin G[83–85]. However, more recent studies indicate that low-dose aspirin does not improve ovarian stimulation, endometrial response, or pregnancy rates for IVF treatment[86–88]. Therefore, a well-designed clinical trial is needed to confirm the benefit of low-dose aspirin treatment for poor responders.

IVM FOR POOR RESPONDERS

No hCG priming prior to oocyte retrieval

Regardless of the modification of stimulation protocol, poor responders still experience a higher cancellation rate because of the small number or size of follicles. It has been reported that an acceptable pregnancy rate was obtained following immature oocyte retrieval and IVM without hCG administration before oocyte collection, suggesting that IVM may be a viable alternative to cancellation in poor responders to conventional stimulated IVF cycles[10,11]. As mentioned above, poor response to gonadotropin stimulation occurs more often in older women, but may also be present in young women with an abnormal or normal endocrinologic profile. Some poor responders appear to respond to stimulation but have a low estrogen level or few or slow growing follicles. These groups of patients require a prolonged stimulation time and higher doses of gonadotropins. Following gonadotropin stimulation, the number of follicles may be normal, but their size may be smaller than in the usual treatment cycles[89]. In these cases, IVM treatment may be a novel

Table 25.1 Results of in-vitro maturation and fertilization of oocytes retrieved from poor responders during stimulation cycles without hCG priming*

No of cycle (couples)	19 (18)
Age	30.6 ± 3.7
No of oocytes retrieved	
Total	170
Mean	9.0 ± 8.1
No of oocytes matured (%)	135 (79.4)
No of oocytes fertilized (%)	96 (71.1)
No of embryos cleaved (%)	89 (92.7)
No of embryos transferred	
Total	45
Mean	2.4 ± 0.9
No of clinical pregnancy (%)	6 (31.6)
No of implantation (%)	7 (15.6)

* Data from IVF Center, Nanjing Medical University, China

option for the patients instead of longer gonadotropin stimulation or treatment cancellation. Our experience demonstrates that acceptable pregnancy rates are obtained when IVM treatment is applied to these poor responders before treatment cancellation (Table 25.1). Prior to immature oocyte retrieval, the patients can have priming either with or without hCG. Indeed, there were also two pregnancies following IVM when immature oocytes were retrieved after hCG administration from such poor responders before treatment cancellation[90].

hCG priming prior to oocyte retrieval

It has been reported that the IVM pregnancy rate is potentially improved by priming with hCG prior to immature oocyte retrieval[91–93]. It is possible that priming with 10 000 IU hCG 36 hours before oocyte retrieval followed by IVM would optimize the successful pregnancy rate in such poor responders because at least some in-vivo matured oocytes can be collected after hCG administration. Indeed, these mature oocytes pooled together with IVM of immature oocytes will maximize successful IVF treatment without cycle cancellation. Recently, Maria Infertility Hospital, Seoul, Korea, has tried this alternative IVM treatment for poor responders after hCG priming, and the results are promising (Table 25.2). As a criterion for this alternative, the size of follicles was still less than 10 mm in diameter after stimulation for more than 7 days. The patients were given 10 000 IU of hCG and oocyte collection was performed 36 h later. Interestingly, approximately 15% (1.7 ± 0.5) mature oocytes were retrieved at collection. These in-vivo matured oocytes pooled with in-vitro matured oocytes will give a higher chance for embryo transfer and potential pregnancy. Reasonable clinical pregnancy and implantation rates (40.4% and 15.8%) have been achieved by application of hCG priming in poor responders who are undergoing ovarian stimulation.

Table 25.2 Results of mature and immature oocytes retrieved followed by IVM from poor responders during stimulation cycles with hCG priming*

No of patients (cycles)	50 (55)
Age (mean ± SD)	32.3 ± 3.4
No of oocytes retrieved (mean ± SD)	641 (11.7 ± 8.3)
No of oocytes matured on collection day (%)	94 (14.7)
No of immature oocytes retrieved (%)	547 (85.3)
No of oocytes matured following culture (%)	406 (74.2)
Total no of oocytes matured (%)	500 (78.0)
No of oocytes fertilized (%)	359 (71.8)
No of cycles completed (%)	52 (94.6)
No of embryos transferred (mean ± SD)	203 (3.9 ± 1.1)
No of clinical pregnancies (%)	21 (40.4)
No of embryos implanted (%)	32 (15.8)

* Data from Maria Infertility Hospital, Seoul, Korea

SUMMARY

Although poor responders have been identified in conventional stimulation IVF cycles, the mechanism to this poor response to gonadotropin stimulation is still unclear. The chance of achieving pregnancy in this group of patients seems significantly reduced. Patients with a poor or retarded response to stimulation seem not to benefit from a stimulation protocol of higher dose gonadotropin, and a higher dose of gonadotropin may negatively influence oocyte quality, fertilization, and pregnancy outcome. Therefore, an increased cancellation rate and decreased pregnancy rates are also noted among these poor responders. The results from the data presented suggest that IVM treatment may be a viable alternative to cancellation of IVF treatment cycles in these poor responders from the conventional stimulation IVF cycles. In conclusion, mature and immature oocyte retrieval following hCG priming from poor responders during stimulation cycles following by IVM is a novel method for this group of patients.

REFERENCES

1. Pellicer A, Lightman A, Diamond MP et al. Outcome of *in vitro* fertilization in woman with low response to ovarian stimulation. Fertil Steril 1987; 47: 812–15.

2. Keay SD, Liversedge NH, Mathur RS et al. Assisted conception following poor ovarian response to gonadotrophin stimulation. Br J Obstet Gynaecol 1997; 104: 521–7.

3. Lashen H, Ledgey W, Lopez-Bernal A et al. Poor responders to ovulation induction: is proceeding to in-vitro fertilization worthwhile? Gynecol Reprod Biol 2001; 97: 202–7.

4. Muasher SJ. Controversies in assisted reproduction – treatment of low responders. J Assist Reprod Genet 1993; 10: 112–14.

5. Pellicer A, Ballester MJ, Serrano MD et al. Aetiological factors involved in the low response to gonadotrophins in infertile women with normal basal serum follicle stimulating hormone levels. Hum Reprod 1994; 9: 806–11.

6. Pellicer A, Ardiles G, Neuspiller F et al. Evaluation of the ovarian reserve in young low

responders with normal basal FSH levels using three-dimensional ultrasound. Fertil Steril 1998; 47: 812–15.

7. Van Hooff F, Alberda AT, Huisman GJ et al. Doubling the human menopausal gonadotropin dose in the course of an *in vitro* fertilization treatment cycles in low responders: a randomized study. Hum Reprod 1993; 8: 364–9.

8. Trounson A, Wood C, Kausche A. *In vitro* maturation and the fertilization and developmental competence of oocytes recovered from unstimulated polycystic ovarian patients. Fertil Steril 1994; 62: 353–62.

9. Chian RC. *In vitro* maturation of immature oocytes for infertile women with PCOS. Reprod Biomed Online 2004; 8: 547–52.

10. Liu J, Lu G, Qian Y et al. Pregnancies and births achieved from *in vitro* matured oocytes retrieved from poor responders undergoing stimulation in *in vitro* fertilization cycles. Fertil Steril 2003; 80: 447–9.

11. Chian RC, Lim JH, Tan SL. State of the art in in-vitro oocyte maturation. Curr Opin Obstet Gynecol 2004; 16: 211–19.

12. Land JA, Yarmolinskaya MI, Dumoulin JCM et al. High-dose human menopausal gonadotropin stimulation in poor responders does not improve *in vitro* fertilization outcome. Fertil Steril 1996; 65: 961–5.

13. Rombauts L, Suikkari AM, MacLachlan V et al. Recruitment of follicles by recombinant human follicle-stimulating hormone commencing in the luteal phase of the ovarian cycle. Fertil Steril 1998; 69: 665–9.

14. Surrey ES, Bower J, Hill DM et al. Clinical and endocrine effects of a microdose GnRH agonist flare regimen administered to poor responders who are undergoing *in vitro* fertilization. Fertil Steril 1998; 69: 419–24.

15. Raga F, Bonilla-Musoles F, Casan EM et al. Recombinant follicle stimulating hormone stimulation in poor responders with normal basal concentrations of follicle stimulating hormone and oestradiol: improved reproductive outcome. Hum Reprod 1999; 14: 1431–4.

16. Schoolcraft W, Schlenker T, Gee M et al. Improved controlled ovarian hyperstimulation

in poor responder in vitro fertilization patients with a microdose follicle-stimulating hormone flare, growth hormone protocol. Fertil Steril 1997; 67: 93–7.

17. Hughes JN, Torresani T, Herve F et al. Interest of growth hormone-releasing hormone administration for improvement of ovarian responsiveness to gonadotropins in poor responder women. Fertil Steril 1991; 55: 945–51.

18. Scott RT, Navot D. Enhancement of ovarian responsiveness with microdoses of gonadotropin-releasing hormone agonist during ovulation induction for in vitro fertilization. Fertil Steril 1994; 61: 880–5.

19. Ibrahim ZH, Matson PL, Buck et al. The use of biosynthetic human growth hormone to augment ovulation induction with buserelin acetate/human menopausal gonadotropin in women with a poor ovarian response. Fertil Steril 1991; 55: 202–4.

20. Nikolettos N, Al-Hasani S, Felberbaum R et al. Gonadotropin-releasing hormone antagonist protocol: a novel method of ovarian stimulation in poor responders. Eur J Obstet Gynecol Reprod Biol 2001; 97: 202–7.

21. Faddy MJ, Gosden RG, Gougeon A et al. Accelerated disappearance of ovarian follicles in mid-life: implications for forecasting menopause. Hum Reprod 1992; 7: 1342–6.

22. Lee SJ, Lenton EA, Sexton L et al. The effect of age on the cyclical patterns of plasma LH, FSH, oestradiol and progesterone in women with regular menstrual cycles. Hum Reprod 1988; 3: 851–5.

23. Anasti JN. Premature ovarian failure: an update. Fertil Steril 1998; 70: 1–15.

24. Karande VC, Jones GS, Veek LL et al. High-dose follicle-stimulating hormone stimulation at the onset of the menstrual cycle does not improve the *in vitro* fertilization outcome in low-responder patients. Fertil Steril 1990; 53: 486–9.

25. Karande V, Morris R, Rinehart J et al. Limited success using the 'flare' protocol in poor responders in cycles with low basal follicle-stimulating hormone levels during *in vitro* fertilization. Fertil Steril 1997; 67: 900–3.

26. Faber BM, Mayer J, Cox B et al. Cessation of gonadotropin-releasing hormone agonist therapy combined with high-dose gonadotropin stimulation yields favorable pregnancy results in low responders. Fertil Steril 1998; 69: 826–30.

27. Navot D, Rosenwaks Z, Margalioth EJ et al. Prognostic assessment of female fecundity. Lancet 1987; 330: 645–7.

28. Katayama KP, Roesler M, Gunnarson C et al. Short-term use of gonadotropin-releasing hormone agonist (leuprolide) for *in vitro* fertilization. J In Vitro Fert Embryo Transf 1988; 5: 332–4.

29. Schachter M, Friedler S, Raziel A et al. Improvement of IVF outcome in poor responders by discontinuation of GnRH analogue during the gonadotropin stimulation phase – a function of improved embryo quality. J Assist Reprod Genet 2001; 18: 197–204.

30. Toth TL, Awwad JT, Veeck LL et al. Suppression and flare regimens of gonadotropin-releasing hormone agonist. Use in women with different basal gonadotropin values in an *in vitro* fertilization program. J Reprod Med 1996; 41: 321–6.

31. Nikolettos N, Al-Hasani S, Felberbaum R et al. Gonadotropin-releasing hormone antagonist protocol: a novel method of ovarian stimulation in poor responders. Eur J Obstet Gynecol Reprod Biol 2001; 97: 202–7.

32. Beckers NG, Macklon NS, Eijkemans MJ et al. Women with regular menstrual cycles and a poor response to ovarian hyperstimulation for *in vitro* fertilization exhibit follicular phase characteristics suggestive of ovarian aging. Fertil Steril 2002; 78: 291–7.

33. de Boer EJ, den Tonkelaar I, te Velde ER et al. A low number of retrieved oocytes at *in vitro* fertilization treatment is predictive of early menopause. Fertil Steril 2002; 77: 978–85.

34. Bancsi LF, Broekmans FJ, Eijkemans MJ et al. Predictors of poor ovarian response in *in vitro* fertilization: a prospective study comparing basal markers of ovarian reserve. Fertil Steril 2002; 77: 328–36.

35. Scott RT, Toner JP, Muasher SJ et al. Follicle-stimulating hormone levels on cycle day 3 are predictive of *in vitro* fertilization outcome. Fertil Steril 1989; 51: 651–4.

36. Cahill DJ, Prosser CJ, Wardle PG et al. Relative influence of serum follicle stimulating hormone, age and other factors on ovarian response to gonadotrophin stimulation. Br J Obstet Gynaecol 1994; 101: 999–1002.

37. Cameron IT, O'Shea FC, Rolland JM et al. Occult ovarian failure: a syndrome of infertility, regular menses, and elevated follicle-stimulating hormone concentrations. J Clin Endocrinol Metab 1988; 67: 1190–4.

38. Tinkanen H, Blauer M, Laippala P et al. Prognostic factors in controlled ovarian hyperstimulation. Fertil Steril 1999; 72: 932–6.

39. Toner JP, Philput CB, Jones GS et al. Basal follicle-stimulating hormone level is a better predictor of *in vitro* fertilization performance than age. Fertil Steril 1991; 55: 784–91.

40. Akende VA, Fleming CF, Hunt LP et al. Biological versus chronological ageing of oocytes, distinguishable by raised FSH levels in relation to the success of IVF treatment. Hum Reprod 2002; 17: 2003–8.

41. Chang MY, Chiang CH, Hsieh TT et al. Use of the antral follicle count to predict the outcome of assisted reproductive technologies. Fertil Steril 1998; 69: 505–10.

42. Syrop CH, Willhoite A, Van Voorhis BJ. Ovarian volume: a novel outcome predictor for assisted reproduction. Fertil Steril 1995; 64: 1167–71.

43. Seifer DB, Lambert-Messerlian G, Hogan JW et al. Day 3 serum inhibin-B is predictive of assisted reproductive technologies outcome. Fertil Steril 1997; 67: 110–14.

44. Winslow KL, Toner JP, Brzyski RG et al. The gonadotropin-releasing hormone agonist stimulation test – a sensitive predictor of performance in flare-up *in vitro* fertilization cycle. Fertil Steril 1991; 56: 711–17.

45. Fanchin R, de Ziegler D, Olivennes F et al. Exogenous follicle stimulating hormone ovarian reserve test (EFORT): a simple and reliable screening test for detecting 'poor responders' in in-vitro fertilization. Hum Reprod 1994; 9: 1607–11.

46. Zeleznik AJ. Premature elevation of systemic estradiol reduces serum levels of follicle-stimulating hormone and lengthens the follicular phase of the menstrual cycle in rhesus monkeys. Endocrinology 1981; 109: 352–5.

47. Hernandez ER, Hurwitz A, Botero L et al. Insulin-like growth factor receptor gene expression in the rat ovary: divergent regulation of distinct receptor species. Mol Endocrinol 1991; 5: 1799–805.

48. Martinez F, Barri PN, Coroleu B et al. Women with poor response to IVF have lowered circulating gonadotrophin surge-attenuating factor (GnSAF) bioactivity during spontaneous and stimulated cycles. Hum Reprod 2002; 17: 634–40.

49. Weiner Z, Thaler I, Levron J et al. Assessment of ovarian and uterine blood flow by transvaginal color Doppler in ovarian-stimulated women: correlation with the number of follicles and steroid hormone levels. Fertil Steril 1993; 59: 743–9.

50. van Rooij IA, Bancsi LF, Broekmans FJ et al. Women older than 40 years of age and those with elevated follicle-stimulating hormone levels differ in poor response rate and embryo quality in in vitro fertilization. Fertil Steril 2003; 79: 482–8.

51. Perez Mayorga M, Gromoll J, Behre HM et al. Ovarian response to follicle-stimulating hormone (FSH) stimulation depends on the FSH receptor genotype. J Clin Endocrinol Metab 2000; 85: 3365–9.

52. Zambrano E, Zarinan T, Olivares A et al. Receptor binding activity and in vitro biological activity of the human FSH charge isoforms as disclosed by heterologous and homologous assay systems: implications for the structure–function relationship of the FSH variants. Endocrine 1999; 10: 113–21.

53. Sudo S, Kudo M, Wada S et al. Genetic and functional analyses of polymorphisms in the human FSH receptor gene. Mol Hum Reprod 2002; 8: 893–9.

54. De Vet F, Laven JS, de Jong JF et al. Antimullerian hormone serum levels: a putative marker for ovarian aging. Fertil Steril 2002; 77: 357–62.

55. Lambalk CB. Value of elevated basal follicle-stimulating hormone levels and the differential diagnosis during the diagnostic subfertility work-up. Fertil Steril 2003; 79: 489–90.

56. Chong AP, Rafael RW, Forte CC. Influence of weight in the induction of ovulation with human menopausal gonadotropin and human chorionic gonadotropin. Fertil Steril 1986; 46: 599–603.

57. Crosignani PG, Ragni G, Lombroso GC et al. IVF: induction of ovulation in poor responders. J Steroid Biochem 1989; 32: 171–3.

58. Hofmann GE, Toner JP, Muasher SJ et al. High-dose follicle-stimulating hormone (FSH) ovarian stimulation in low-responder patients for in vitro fertilization. J In Vitro Fert Embryo Transf 1989; 6: 285–9.

59. Out HJ, Mannaerts BM, Driessen SG et al. Recombinant follicle stimulating hormone (rFSH; Puregon) in assisted reproduction: more oocytes, more pregnancies. Results from five comparative studies. Hum Reprod Update 1996; 2: 162–71.

60. De Placido G, Mollo A, Alviggi C et al. Rescue of IVF cycles by HMG in pituitary down-regulated normogonadotrophic young women characterized by a poor initial response to recombinant FSH. Hum Reprod 2001; 16: 1875–9.

61. Grochowski D, Wolczynski S, Kuczynski W et al. The results of an in vitro fertilization program: two regimens of superovulation. Gynecol Endocrinol 1995; 9: 59–62.

62. D'Amato G, Caroppo E, Pasquadibisceglie A et al. A novel protocol of ovulation induction with delayed gonadotropin-releasing hormone antagonist administration combined with high-dose recombinant follicle-stimulating hormone and clomiphene citrate for poor responders and women over 35 years. Fertil Steril 2004; 81: 1572–7.

63. Serafini P, Stone B, Kerin J et al. An alternate approach to controlled ovarian hyperstimulation in 'poor responders': pretreatment with a gonadotropin-releasing hormone analog. Fertil Steril 1988; 49: 90–5.

64. Horvath PM, Styler M, Hammond JM et al. Exogenous gonadotropin requirements are increased in leuprolide suppressed women undergoing ovarian stimulation. Fertil Steril 1988; 49: 159–62.

65. Loumaye E, Vankrieken L, Depreester S et al. Hormonal changes induced by short-term

administration of gonadotropin-releasing hormone agonist during ovarian hyperstimulation for *in vitro* fertilization and their consequences for embryo development. Fertil Steril 1989; 51: 105–11.

66. San Roman GA, Surrey ES, Judd HL et al. A prospective randomized comparison of luteal phase versus concurrent follicular phase initiation of gonadotropin-releasing hormone agonist for *in vitro* fertilization. Fertil Steril 1992; 58: 744–9.

67. Dirnfeld M, Fruchter O, Yshai D et al. Cessation of gonadotropin-releasing hormone analogue (GnRH-a) upon down-regulation versus conventional long GnRH-a protocol in poor responders undergoing *in vitro* fertilization. Fertil Steril 1999; 72: 406–11.

68. Novot D, Rosenwaks Z, Anderson F et al. Gonadotropin-releasing hormone agonist-induced ovarian hyperstimulation: low-dose side effects in women and monkeys. Fertil Steril 1991; 55: 1069–75.

69. Scott RT, Navot D. Enhancement of ovarian responsiveness with micro-doses of GnRH-agonist during ovulation induction for *in vitro* fertilization. Fertil Steril 1991; 55: 1069–75.

70. Schoolcraft WB. Evaluation and treatment of the poor responder. Clin Obstet Gynecol 2006; 49: 23–33.

71. Fanchin R, Salomon L, Castelo-Branco A et al. Luteal estradiol pretreatment coordinates follicular growth during controlled ovarian hyperstimulation with GnRH antagonists. Hum Reprod 2003; 18: 2698–703.

72. Fanchin R, Cunha-Filho JS, Schonauer LM et al. Coordination of early antral follicles by luteal estradiol administration provides a basis for alternative controlled ovarian hyperstimulation regimens. Fertil Steril 2003; 79: 316–21.

73. Akman MA, Erden HF, Tosun SB et al. Comparison of agonistic flare-up protocol and antagonist multiple dose protocol in ovarian stimulation of poor responders: results of a prospective randomized trial. Hum Reprod 2001; 16: 868–70.

74. Malmusi S, La Marca A, Giulini S et al. Comparison of a gonadotropin-releasing hormone (GnRH) antagonist and GnRH agonist flare-up regimen in poor responders undergo-

ing ovarian stimulation. Fertil Steril 2005; 84: 402–6.

75. Jia XC, Kalmijn J, Hsueh AJ. Growth hormone enhances follicle-stimulating hormone-induced differentiation of cultured rat granulosa cells. Endocrinology 1986; 118: 1401–9.

76. Adashi EY, Resnick CE, Rosenfeld RG et al. Insulin-like growth factor (IGF) binding protein-1 is an antigonadotropin: evidence that optimal follicle-stimulating hormone action in ovarian granulosa cells is contingent upon amplification by endogenously-derived IGFs. Adv Exp Med Biol 1993; 343: 377–85.

77. Howles CM, Loumave E, Germond M et al. Does growth hormone-releasing factor assist follicular development in poor responder patients undergoing ovarian stimulation for in-vitro fertilization? Hum Reprod 1999; 14: 1939–43.

78. Hoeck HC, Vestergaard P, Jakobsen PE et al. Diagnosis of growth hormone (GH) deficiency in adults with hypothalamic–pituitary disorders: comparison of test results using pyridostigmine plus GH-releasing hormone (GHRH), clonidine plus GHRH, and insulin-induced hypoglycemia as GH secretagogues. J Clin Endocrinol Metab 2000; 85: 1467–72.

79. al-Mizyen E, Sabatini L, Lower AM et al. Does pretreatment with progestogen or oral contraceptive pills in low responders followed by the GnRH-a flare protocol improve the outcome of IVF-ET? J Assist Reprod Genet 2000; 17: 140–6.

80. Kolibianakis EM, Papanikolaou EG, Camus M et al. Effect of oral contraceptive pill pretreatment on ongoing pregnancy rates in patients stimulated with GnRH antagonists and recombinant FSH for IVF. A randomized controlled trial. Hum Reprod 2006; 21: 352–7.

81. Cowchock FS, Reece EA, Balaban D et al. High fetal losses associated with antiphospholipid antibodies: a collaborative randomized trial comparing prednisone with low-dose heparin treatment. Am J Obstet Gynecol 1992; 166: 1318–23.

82. Hasegawa I, Takakuwa K, Goto S et al. Effectiveness of prednisolone/aspirin therapy for recurrent aborters with antiphospholipid antibody. Hum Reprod 1992; 7: 203–7.

83. Sher G, Maassarani G, Zouves C et al. The use of combined heparin/aspirin and immunoglobulin G therapy in the treatment of *in vitro* fertilization patients with antithyroid antibodies. Am J Reprod Immunol 1998; 39: 223–5.

84. Hasegawa I, Yamanoto Y, Suzuki M et al. Prednisolone plus low-dose aspirin improves the implantation rate in women with autoimmune conditions who are undergoing *in vitro* fertilization. Fertil Steril 1998; 70: 1044–8.

85. Geva E, Amit A, Lerner-Geva L et al. Prednisone and aspirin improve pregnancy rate in patients with reproductive failure and autoimmune antibodies: a prospective study. Am J Reprod Immunol 2000; 43: 36–40.

86. Stern C, Chamley L, Norris H et al. A randomized, double-blind, placebo-controlled trial of heparin and aspirin for women with *in vitro* fertilization implantation failure and antiphospholipid or antinuclear antibodies. Fertil Steril 2003; 80: 376–83.

87. Lok IH, Yip SK, Cheung LP et al. Adjuvant low-dose aspirin therapy in poor responders undergoing *in vitro* fertilization: a prospective, randomized, double-blind, placebo-controlled trial. Fertil Steril 2004; 81: 556–61.

88. Pakkila M, Rasanen J, Heinonene S et al. Low-dose aspirin does not improve ovarian responsiveness or pregnancy rate in IVF and ICSI patients: a randomized, placebo-controlled double-blind study. Hum Reprod 2005; 20: 2211–14.

89. Lashen H, Ledger W, Lopez-Baernal A et al. Poor responders to ovulation induction: is proceeding to in-vitro fertilization worthwhile? Hum Reprod 1999; 14: 964–9.

90. Check ML, Brittingham D, Check JH et al. Pregnancy following transfer of cryopreserved-thawed embryos that had been a result of fertilization of all *in vitro* matured metaphase or germinal stage oocytes. Case report. Clin Exp Obstet Gynecol 2001; 28: 69–70.

91. Chian RC, Buckett WM, Too LL et al. Pregnancies resulting from *in vitro* matured oocytes retrieved from patients with polycystic ovary syndrome after priming with human chorionic gonadotropin. Fertil Steril 1999; 72: 639–42.

92. Chian RC, Buckett WM, Tulandi T et al. Prospective randomized study of human chorionic gonadotropin priming before immature oocyte retrieval from unstimulated women with polycystic ovarian syndrome. Hum Reprod 2000; 15: 165–70.

93. Son WY, Yoon SH, Lee SW et al. Blastocyst development and pregnancies after IVF of mature oocytes retrieved from unstimulated patients with PCOS after in-vivo HCG priming. Hum Reprod 2002; 17: 134–6.

CHAPTER 26

IVM as an alternative for over-responders

Kyung-Sil Lim, San-Hyun Yoon, and Jin-Ho Lim

INTRODUCTION

Polycystic ovary syndrome (PCOS) is one of the most common reproductive disorders in women of childbearing age. It has a heterogeneous presentation, which is clinically characterized by anovulation and hyperandrogenism, and pelvic ultrasound examination shows numerous antral follicles within the ovaries[1]. Women with PCOS often present with anovulatory infertility with a significant proportion being resistant to induction of ovulation by clomiphene citrate. Although ovulation can be induced successfully in 75% of clomiphene-citrate non-responders with human menopausal gonadotropin (HMG), gonadotropin use requires intensive monitoring. In addition, many patients ovulate but do not achieve pregnancy even after their anovulation has been corrected. For these women, in-vitro fertilization (IVF) is the standard treatment but there is a significantly higher risk of ovarian hyperstimulation syndrome (OHSS) compared with IVF treatment in women with normal ovaries[2].

Some women are extremely sensitive to stimulation with exogenous gonadotropins and are at increased risk of developing OHSS that, sometimes, is a potentially life-threatening complication[3]. In general, the incidence of OHSS ranges from 0.6% to 14% in women undergoing ovarian stimulation for IVF[4]. Several preventive strategies have been proposed to reduce the incidence and severity of OHSS, including cancellation of treatment cycle, cryopreservation of all embryos, or intravenous administration of albumin or other plasma-expanding agents[5–7]. However, these methods are not efficient in preventing OHSS. Another popular strategy is withholding gonadotropin stimulation, the 'coasting' method. The advantage of coasting is that the treatment cycle is not necessarily cancelled and that no additional procedure is needed[8–10]. But coasting cannot be applied when the signs and symptoms predictive of OHSS are observed early in the stimulation phase of the cycle, because premature withholding of gonadotropin may result in arrest of follicular growth and atresia of oocytes. In addition, with coasting, frequent estimations of serum estradiol level and ultrasound scans are needed in order to determine the time of hCG administration[11]. Furthermore, the crucial timing of hCG administration has not been well defined.

Following the first successful live birth from in-vitro maturation (IVM) of immature oocytes in women with PCOS-related infertility[12], immature oocyte retrieval followed by IVM has been applied as a clinical treatment, often in women with PCOS[13,14]. In comparison with conventional IVF treatment, the major advantages of IVM treatment include reduced cost, simplified treatment, and eliminated side-effects from gonadotropins, particularly avoidance of the risk of OHSS. Furthermore, recently it has been reported that mature oocytes were collected from infertile women with PCOS when the leading follicle reached a mean diameter of 12 to 14 mm following administration of hCG[15,16]. This finding suggests that limited ovarian stimulation can result in retrieval of mature oocytes and may prevent the recurrence of severe forms of OHSS without reducing the clinical pregnancy rate from that of conventional IVF treatment. We report a new strategy for OHSS prevention during conventional IVF treatment that results in efficient elimination of OHSS among infertile women with PCOS.

OVARIAN STIMULATION

Women with PCOS receive the oral contraceptive pill, Mercilon (Organon, Netherlands), 1 tablet a day for 21 days, in order to induce menstrual bleeding. After withdrawal menstrual bleeding, the patients underwent either the 'long protocol' of downregulation with a GnRH-agonist for IVF or the GnRH-antagonist protocol.

For women undergoing the 'long protocol', pituitary downregulation was confirmed by demonstrating an endometrial thickness of <5.0 mm with a transvaginal ultrasound scan after at least 2 weeks of GnRH-agonist and the absence of any ovarian cysts. The initial dose of gonadotropin for ovarian stimulation is individualized according to the age of patients, day 3 serum FSH level, body mass index, and previous response to ovarian stimulation. The GnRH-antagonist protocol involved starting gonadotropins on day 3 of the menstrual cycle. Transvaginal ultrasound monitoring was commenced on day 5 of ovarian stimulation and repeated every 2–3 days. Serum estradiol con-

centrations were not measured routinely in our IVF program.

IDENTIFYING THE OVER-RESPONDER PATIENTS

A woman is considered an 'over-responder' when there are more than 20 follicles with a mean diameter >10 mm in both ovaries following gonadotropin stimulation for at least 5 days. In our study, a total of 123 patients, who were undergoing conventional IVF treatment and who over-responded with this sign, were included in this alternative treatment. The mean age of the patients was 28.1 ± 3.4 years.

MATURE AND IMMATURE OOCYTE RETRIEVAL

When the leading follicle reached 12–14 mm in diameter, 10 000 IU of human chorionic gonadotropin (hCG) was administered, and oocyte collection was performed 36 hours later. Transvaginal ultrasound-guided aspiration was conducted with a 19G aspiration needle (Cook, Eight Mile Plains, Queensland, Australia). A portable aspiration pump was connected to the aspiration needle with a pressure between 80 and 100 mmHg. The aspirates were collected in tubes (10 ml) containing prewarmed heparinized Ham's F-10 medium buffered with Hepes. Cumulus–oocyte complexes (COCs) were isolated by filtering the follicular aspirates through a mesh filter (diameter 70 μm, Falcon 1060, USA). In order to remove erythrocytes and small cellular debris, the filtrates were washed with Hepes-buffered Ham's F-10 medium. The retained COCs were then re-suspended in the medium. The maturity of oocytes at the time of oocyte retrieval was evaluated under a stereomicroscope. Oocyte maturation was assessed by the presence of the first polar body (1PB) in the pelliviteline space (PVS).

OOCYTE IN-VITRO FERTILIZATION AND IN-VITRO MATURATION

The collected mature oocytes (metaphase II) were subjected to insemination 2 or 3 h later using intracytoplasmic sperm injection (ICSI). The remaining immature oocytes (at germinal vesicle or metaphase I stages) were further cultured in oocyte IVM medium. We used YS-medium as oocyte IVM medium, containing 30% human follicular fluid (HFF) supplemented with 1 IU/ml FSH, 10 IU/ml hCG, and 10 ng/ml rhEGF (Daewoong Pharmaceutical Co, Korea)[17,18]. The HFF was prepared using the method reported by Chi et al.[19]. The immature oocytes were cultured in maturation medium at 37°C in 5% CO_2, 5% O_2, and 90% N_2. After 1 day of culture, COCs were denuded of the cumulus cells using 0.03% hyaluronidase (Sigma, St Louis, MO, USA) in Hepes buffered Ham's F-10 medium and mechanical pipetting. At 24 and 48 h of culture, the mature oocytes were inseminated by ICSI, respectively. Fertilization was assessed 17–19 h after ICSI to detect the appearance of two distinct pronuclei and two polar bodies. The zygotes were co-cultured with the cumulus cells prepared on the day of oocyte retrieval in 10 μl of YS medium supplemented with 10% HFF[20].

EMBRYO TRANSFER AND ENDOMETRIAL PREPARATION

Embryo transfer (ET) was performed on day 4 or 6 after oocyte retrieval. Blastocyst transfer was performed in some patients if they had more than three good-quality embryos examined on day 2 after insemination. Before transfer, all embryos for each patient were pooled together and selected for transfer. For endometrial preparation, 6 mg estradiol valerate (Progynova®, Schering, Korea) was administered daily, starting on the day of oocyte retrieval, and luteal support in the form of 100 mg progesterone in oil (Progest®, Samil Pharm Co, Ansan, Korea)

was injected daily, starting on the day after oocyte collection. A pregnancy test by measuring the level of serum β-hCG was performed on day 16 after oocyte retrieval, and clinical pregnancy was determined by visualization of the fetal heartbeat using an ultrasound scan. Differences between fertilization and cleavage in each group were compared using the χ^2-test (statistical analysis system, SAS Institute, Cary, NC, USA).

PREGNANCY OUTCOME

For each patient, the average dose of gonadotropins used for controlled ovarian hyperstimulation (COH) was 1228.6 ± 655.6 IU, and the mean duration of COH was 7 ± 2.8 days (Table 26.1). The average thickness of endometrium on the day of hCG administration was 10.5 ± 1.8 mm. As shown in Table 26.2, a total of 1554 oocytes were retrieved from 123 patients (12.6 ± 6.9); 293 (18.9%) oocytes were mature at the time of oocyte retrieval and the remaining 1261 oocytes were at either metaphase I (MI) or germinal vesicle (GV)-stages. Following culture, 764 (60.6%) oocytes matured at 24 h and another 188 (14.9%) oocytes were matured at 48 h. A total of 952 (75.5%) oocytes were matured following IVM. Together with 293 in-vivo mature oocytes, a total of 1245 (80.1%) mature oocytes were obtained from those 123 patients (10.7 ± 6.9).

A total of 967 (77.7%) oocytes were fertilized following ICSI (Table 26.2), and the cleavage rate was 93.5% (904/967). Following transfer, a mean of 4.2 ± 1.5 embryos per patient, the clinical pregnancy and implantation rates were 36.6% (45/123) and 11.3% (58/514); respectively. As shown in Table 26.2, 17 patients underwent blastocyst transfer and 8 (47.1%) of them became pregnant. The implantation rate was 23.6% (13/55). Among this group of patients, no patients suffered from severe symptoms of OHSS during the treatment cycle and pregnancy.

Table 26.1 Detailed information of the patients who underwent ovarian stimulation

	Value (range)
No of patients	123
Age (mean ± SD)	28.1 ± 3.4 (27–36)
Ampoules of gonadotropins used (mean ± SD)	16.4 ± 8.8 (8–52)
Dose (IU) of gonadotropins used (mean ± SD)	1228.6 ± 655.6 (600–3900)
Duration (days) of ovaries stimulated (mean ± SD)	7.0 ± 2.8 (4–14)
Endometrial thickness (mm) on day of hCG priming (mean ± SD)	10.5 ± 1.8 (8–15)

Table 26.2 Pregnancy outcome of the patients who underwent oocyte retrieval followed by in-vitro maturation

	Embryo transfer at		
	Day 3	Day 5	Total
No of patients (cycles)	106 (106)	17 (17)	123 (123)
Age (mean ± SD)	27.9 ± 3.4	29.2 ± 3.0	28.1 ± 3.4
No of oocytes retrieved (mean ± SD)	1236 (11.7 ± 6.5)	318 (18.7 ± 6.9)	1554 (12.6 ± 6.9)
No of mature oocytes retrieved at collection (%)	201 (14.2)	92 (28.9)	293 (18.9)
No of immature oocytes retrieved (mean ± SD)	1035 (9.8 ± 5.9)	226 (13.3 ± 7.3)	1261 (10.3 ± 6.2)
No of oocytes matured in-vitro 24 h postculture (%)	617 (59.6)	147 (65.0)	764 (60.6)
No of oocytes matured in-vitro 48 h postculture (%)	159 (15.4)	29 (12.8)	188 (14.9)
Total number of oocytes matured (%)	977 (79.0)	268 (84.3)	1245 (80.1)
No of oocytes fertilized (%)	760 (77.8)	207 (77.2)	967 (77.7)
No of embryos cleaved (%)	718 (94.5)	186 (89.9)	904 (93.5)
No of embryos transferred (mean ± SD)	459 (4.3 ± 1.6)	55 (3.2 ± 0.8)	514 (4.2 ± 1.5)
No of clinical pregnancies (%)	37 (34.9)	8 (47.1)	45 (36.6)
No of embryos implanted (%)	45 (9.8)	13 (23.6)	58 (11.3)

As shown in Figure 26.1, fertilization rates were not different between in-vivo (81.6% = 239/293) and in-vitro (24 h: 77.1% = 589/764; 48 h: 73.9% = 139/188) matured oocytes. However, the embryo cleavage rate was significantly lower ($p < 0.05$) in 48 h in-vitro matured oocytes (78.4% = 109/139) compared with in-vivo matured (96.2% = 230/239) and 24 h in-vitro matured (95.9% = 565/589) oocytes (Figure 26.2).

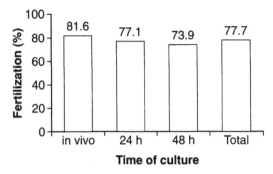

Figure 26.1 Comparison of fertilization rates in the oocytes matured in vivo (0 h), 24 h and 48 h following in-vitro maturation. There are no differences among groups

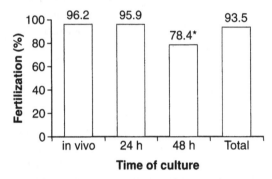

Figure 26.2 Comparison of cleavage rates in the oocytes matured in vivo (0 h), 24 h and 48 h following in-vitro maturation. Cleavage rate is significantly lower (*$p < 0.05$) in the oocytes matured 48 h following in-vitro maturation compared with other groups

CAN OHSS BE PREVENTED BY IVM TREATMENT?

OHSS is a serious and potentially life-threatening complication in patients who undergo ovarian stimulation for IVF treatment. Even in the mild cases of OHSS, ovarian enlargement, abdominal distension, and weight gain may occur. In severe cases of OHSS, ascites, pleural effusion, hypovolemia with oliguria, pericardial effusion, the adult respiratory distress syndrome (ARDS), hypercoagulability with thromboembolic sequelae, and multi-organ failure may occur[4]. There are several risk factors associated with the development of OHSS during ovarian stimulation for women undergoing IVF treatment. These include young age, low body weight, a high level of estradiol, and large numbers of follicles during gonadotropin stimulation. Anovulatory women with PCOS are especially at an increased risk for OHSS.

The mechanism of OHSS induced by gonadotropin stimulation is not fully understood. However, it is known that OHSS is triggered by hCG administration and is associated with very high levels of estradiol, subsequently increased capillary permeability, and extravasations of fluid in the abdominal cavity. Interestingly, hCG administration did not lead to OHSS in these patients when the size of the leading follicles reached 12–14 mm in diameter. The range of gonadotropins used in these patients was from 600 IU to 3900 IU (average: 1228.6 ± 655.6 IU). The mean stimulation period with gonadotropin for the group of patients was 7.0 ± 2.8 days (ranging from 4 days to 14 days) (Table 26.1).

Various strategies for preventing or diminishing OHSS and its severity have been suggested. The first approach is to abandon the treatment cycle[21]. The second, in view of the increased risk of OHSS associated with pregnancy, is to cryopreserve all resulting embryos[22]. In order to reduce the incidence of severe OHSS without compromising pregnancy rates in the treatment cycles, some other approaches, such as minimizing the dose of gonadotropin[23,24], reducing the dose of hCG for triggering ovulation[25], giving intravenous administration of albumin[26] or other plasma-expanding agents before or during oocyte retrieval[5,6], and withholding gonadotropin (coasting) during COH, have been proposed. Among these, it is suggested that coasting is an effective measure in the prevention of OHSS without jeopardizing the pregnancy outcome[27]. Recently, it has been reported that the use of GnRH antagonists/agonists instead of hCG to trigger ovulation may prevent OHSS[28]. However, OHSS will never be completely eliminated by these proposed methodologies, suggesting that the only way to avoid iatrogenic OHSS is to avoid ovarian stimulation using gonadotropins[29].

El-Sheikh et al.[15] reported that OHSS might be efficiently prevented by limited ovarian stimulation (LOS) in women with PCOS. Interestingly, they retrieved mature oocytes when the leading follicles reached a mean diameter of 12 mm following hCG administration, resulting in eight clinical pregnancies out of 20 patients. At the same time, the incidence and severity of OHSS were efficiently reduced[16]. In contrast, the results of the present study indicate that hCG administration triggers maturation of oocytes in some small follicles. Our results show that 18.9% of oocytes were mature at the time of oocyte retrieval when hCG was given once the follicles had reached a diameter of 12–14 mm (Table 26.2). This implies that these medium size follicles possess luteinizing hormone (LH) receptors that respond to the LH surge for oocyte maturation in vivo in women with PCOS. Yang et al.[30] reported that the pattern of cumulus cells at the time of oocyte collection plays a predictive role in the maturation of oocytes recovered from patients with PCOS in hCG-primed IVM cycles. They indicated that there were LH receptors in cumulus cells as detected by semiquantitative reverse transcription polymerase chain reaction (RT-PCR)[30].

It was reported that the cleavage and blastocyst development rates are different among oocytes matured in vivo, 24 h and 48 h following IVM[31], suggesting that the oocytes reaching MII faster following IVM have better embryonic developmental competence. In this study, we confirm that although fertilization rates were not different between groups (Figure 26.1), the cleavage rates were significantly different between in-vivo matured and in-vitro matured oocytes and between 24 h and 48 h in-vitro matured oocytes (Figure 26.2). Also, we found that the quality of embryos differed among oocytes matured in vivo and in vitro and among the oocytes matured at different times following IVM. More interestingly, among these 123 patients, 17 of them underwent blastocyst transfer. Eight of them became pregnant following blastocyst transfer.

Although it is hard to tell whether the implanted embryos were produced from in-vivo or in-vitro matured oocytes, the results from the present study indicate an improvement of clinical pregnancy rate (36.6%) when using embryos generated from both in-vivo and in-vitro matured oocytes. Our previous experiences with IVF alone (using mature oocytes only) in women who were over-responders and who had a high risk of OHSS during ovarian stimulation cycles resulted in only a 10–15% chance of clinical pregnancy per embryo transfer.

SUMMARY

Mature and immature oocyte retrieval followed by IVM is an efficient method for the prevention of OHSS during ovarian stimulation without compromising the pregnancy outcome for IVF treatment cycles in women with PCOS. The important criteria for this alternative is to stop gonadotropin stimulation when there are ultrasonographic signs of OHSS risk, where there are more than 20 growing follicles with a mean diameter >10 mm, and to administer hCG when the leading follicle reaches 12–14 mm in diameter.

REFERENCES

1. Adams J, Polson D, Franks S. Prevalence of polycystic ovaries in women with anovulation or idiopathic hirsutism. Br Med J 1986; 293: 355–9.

2. MacDougall MJ, Tan SL, Balen A et al. A controlled study comparing patients with and without polycystic ovaries undergoing *in vitro* fertilization. Hum Reprod 1993; 8: 233–7.

3. Beerendonk CCM, van Dop PA, Braat DDM et al. Ovarian hyperstimulation syndrome: facts and fallacies. Obstet Gynecol Surv 1998; 53: 439–49.

4. Whelan JG 3rd, Vlahos NF. The ovarian hyperstimulation syndrome. Fertil Steril 2002; 73: 883–96.

5. Delvigne A, Rozenberg S. Preventive attitude of physicians to avoid OHSS in IVF patients. Hum Reprod 2001; 16: 2491–5.

6. Isik AZ, Vicdan K. Combined approach as an effective method in the prevention of severe ovarian hyperstimulation syndrome. Eur J Obstet Gynecol Reprod Biol 2001; 97: 208–12.

7. Wiener M. Impact of cryopreservation and subsequent embryo transfer on the outcome of *in vitro* fertilization in patients at high risk for ovarian hyperstimulation syndrome. Fertil Steril 2002; 78: 201–3.

8. Al-Shawaf T, Zosmer A, Hussain S et al. Prevention of severe ovarian hyperstimulation syndrome in IVF with or without ICSI and embryo transfer: a modified 'coasting' strategy based on ultrasound for identification of high-risk patients. Hum Reprod 2001; 16: 24–30.

9. Delvigne A, Carlier C, Rozenberg S. Is coasting effective for preventing ovarian hyperstimulation syndrome in patients receiving a gonadotropin-releasing hormone antagonist during an *in vitro* fertilization cycle? Fertil Steril 2001; 76: 844–6.

10. Isaza V, Garcia-Velasco JA, Aragones M et al. Oocyte and embryo quality after coasting: the experience from oocyte donation. Hum Reprod 2002; 17: 1777–82.

11. Al-Shawaf T, Zosmer A, Tozer A et al. Value of measuring serum FSH in addition to serum estradiol in a coasting programme to prevent severe OHSS. Hum Reprod 2002; 17: 1217–21.

12. Trounson AO, Wood C, Kausche A. *In vitro* maturation and the fertilization and developmental competence of oocytes recovered from untreated polycystic ovarian patients. Fertil Steril 1994; 62: 353–62.

13. Chian RC. In-vitro maturation of immature oocytes for infertile women with PCOS. RBM Online 2004; 8: 547–52.

14. Chian RC, Lim JH, Tan SL. State of the art in in-vitro oocyte maturation. Curr Opin Obstet Gynecol 2004; 16: 211–19.

15. El-Sheikh MM, Hussein M, Sheikh AA et al. Limited ovarian stimulation results in the recovery of mature oocytes in polycystic ovarian disease patients: a preliminary report. Eur J Obstet Gynecol Reprod Biol 1999; 83: 81–3.

16. El-Sheikh MM, Hussein M, Fouad S et al. Limited ovarian stimulation (LOS), prevents the recurrence of severe forms of ovarian hyperstimulation syndrome in polycystic ovarian disease. Eur J Obstet Gynecol Reprod Biol 2001; 94: 245–9.

17. Son WY, Park SJ, Hyun CS et al. Successful birth after transfer of blastocysts derived from oocytes of unstimulated woman with regular menstrual cycle after IVM approach. J Assist Reprod Genet 2002; 19: 541–3.

18. Son WY, Lee SY, Lim JH. Fertilization, cleavage and blastocyst development according to the maturation timing of oocytes in *in vitro* maturation cycle. Hum Reprod 2005; 20: 3204–7.

19. Chi HJ, Kim DH, Koo JJ et al. The suitability and efficiency of human follicular fluid as a protein supplement in human *in vitro* fertilization programs. Fertil Steril 1998; 70: 871–7.

20. Yoon HG, Yoon SH, Son WY et al. Pregnancies resulting from *in vitro* matured oocytes collected from women with regular menstrual cycle. J Assist Reprod Genet 2001; 18: 249–53.

21. Serous GI, Aboulghar M, Mansour R et al. Complication of medically assisted conception in 3,500 cycles. Fertil Steril 1998; 70: 638–42.

22. Navot D, Bergh PA, Laufer N. Ovarian hyperstimulation syndrome in novel reproductive technologies: prevention and treatment. Fertil Steril 1992; 58: 249–61.

23. Golan A, Ron-EI R, Herman A et al. Ovarian hyperstimulation syndrome following D-Trp-6 luteinising hormone releasing hormone microcapsules and menotrophin for *in vitro* fertilization. Fertil Steril 1988; 50: 912–16.

24. Macklon NS, Fauser BC. Gonadotropin therapy for the treatment of anovulation and for ovarian hyperstimulation for IVF. Mol Cell Endocrinol 2000; 55: 159–61.

25. Abdalla HI, Ah-Moye M, Brinsden P et al. The effect of the dose of hCG and the typed gonadotropin stimulation on oocyte recovery rates in an IVF program. Fertil Steril 1987; 48: 958–63.

26. Asch RH, Ivery G, Goldsman M et al. The use of intravenous albumin in patients at high risk for severe ovarian hyperstimulation syndrome. Hum Reprod 1993; 8: 1015–20.

27. Mansour R, Aboulghar M, Serour G et al. Criteria of a successful coasting protocol for the prevention of severe ovarian hyperstimulation syndrome. Hum Reprod 2005; 20: 3167–72.

28. Orvietto R. Can we eliminate severe ovarian hyperstimulation syndrome? Hum Reprod 2005; 20: 320–2.

29. Buckett W, Chian RC, Tan SL. Can we eliminate severe ovarian hyperstimulation syndrome? Not completely. Hum Reprod 2005; 20: 2367.

30. Yang SH, Son WY, Yoon SH et al. Correlation between *in vitro* maturation and expression of LH receptor in cumulus cells of the oocytes collected from PCOS patients in HCG-primed IVM cycles. Hum Reprod 2005; 20: 2097–103.

31. Son WY, Yoon SH, Lee SW et al. Blastocyst development and pregnancies after IVF of mature oocytes retrieved from unstimulated patients with PCOS after in-vivo HCG priming. Hum Reprod 2002; 17: 134–6.

CHAPTER 27

Combination of natural cycle IVF with IVM as infertility treatment

Jin-Ho Lim, Seo-Yeong Park, San-Hyun Yoon, Seong-Ho Yang, and Ri-Cheng Chian

INTRODUCTION

The first live birth following in-vitro fertilization (IVF) resulted from natural cycle IVF[1]. However, this has been gradually replaced by ovarian stimulation combined with IVF, because it is believed that the number of oocytes retrieved relates to the embryos available for transfer, and that this directly affects the probability of successful pregnancy[2–4]. At the beginning, the relatively inexpensive clomiphene citrate was used to stimulate ovaries to produce multiple follicles, but currently ovarian stimulation protocols use the much more expensive gonadotropin-releasing hormone (GnRH) agonist or antagonist in combination with gonadotropins to generate multi-follicles in the ovaries. Some women are extremely sensitive to stimulation with exogenous gonadotropins and are at increased risk of developing ovarian hyperstimulation syndrome (OHSS), which, on rare occasions, can be a life-threatening condition[5]. In addition, there is anxiety that the long-term side-effects of repeated ovarian stimulation may increase the risk of ovarian, endometrial, and breast cancers[6–8]. Although these problems are not encountered in natural cycle IVF treatment, a number of other problems arise, including an increased risk that no oocytes will be retrieved during oocyte col-

lection and that no embryos will be available for transfer.

Literature reports for pregnancy rates per embryo transfer in natural cycle IVF vary between 0 and 30%[9–11]. However, there is an increasing interest in natural cycle IVF among patients, primarily because it is more comfortable and there are fewer side-effects, particularly the unknown long-term effects of repeated ovarian stimulation with GnRH and gonadotropins. Furthermore, in recent years, the efficiency of IVF technology has improved markedly[12]. It has been reported that, although the pregnancy rate was lower in natural cycle IVF treatment compared to ovarian stimulated IVF cycles, the implantation and birth rates achieved per started cycle were very similar[13]. Interestingly, Nargund et al.[12] indicated that when life-table analysis was performed to calculate the cumulative success rates after successive cycles of treatment, the cumulative probability of pregnancy was 46% with an associated live birth rate of 32% after four natural cycles of IVF treatment. Therefore, it is important to ask which infertility treatment we should offer primarily to our patients at the beginning.

In women, although only a single follicle usually grows to the preovulatory stage and releases its oocyte for potential fertilization, many small follicles also develop during the same follicular phase of the menstrual cycle. It is believed that more than 20 antral follicles are selected and continue to the preovulatory stages of development during each cycle[14]. It has been documented that there are two or three waves of ovarian follicular development in women during each menstrual cycle based on daily transvaginal ultrasonography, challenging the traditional theory of a single cohort of antral follicles that grow only during the follicular phase of the menstrual cycle[15,16]. In addition, it seems that atresia does not occur in the non-dominant follicles even after the dominant follicle is selected in the ovary during folliculogenesis, because immature oocytes retrieved from non-dominant follicles have been successfully matured in vitro, fertilized, and have resulted in several pregnancies and healthy live births[10,17,18]. Therefore, one very attractive possibility for enhancement of the success of natural cycle IVF treatment is its combination with immature oocyte retrieval and in-vitro maturation (IVM)[19]. When we are successful in maturing the immature oocytes from small follicles that are collected along with the mature oocyte from the dominant follicle and producing several viable embryos, the chances of pregnancy are greatly increased.

PREGNANCY OUTCOME FROM IVM TREATMENT

Immature oocyte retrieval followed by IVM was shown to be a successful treatment for infertile women with polycystic ovaries (PCO) because there are numerous antral follicles within the ovaries in this group of patients. Immature oocyte retrieval followed by IVM might be useful in 20–37% of women undergoing IVF treatment who have polycystic ovaries as seen on ultrasound scan[20,21]. However, it is important to apply IVM technology for women with various causes of infertility. In general, clinical pregnancy and implantation rates for women who have polycystic ovaries and for hyper- and poor

responders have reached 35–40% and 15–20%, respectively. These results demonstrate that IVM is an efficient clinical treatment for some infertile women. Thus, it is important to introduce this new approach, namely, the combination of natural cycle IVF and IVM, for all types of infertile women without any ovarian stimulation, if possible.

PATIENT SELECTION FOR IVF/IVM TREATMENT

All patients should be under 40 years of age and should have intact ovaries and regular menstrual cycles. The basal serum FSH level should be under 10 IU/l on day 2 or 3 of the menstrual cycle.

Baseline ultrasound scans

The treatment cycle is initiated by a baseline ultrasound scan on day 2 to 3 of the menstrual cycle to ensure that there are more than seven antral follicles present in the ovaries. Transvaginal ultrasound scans are repeated on day 6 or 8 of the menstrual cycle. At this point, the development of follicles and endometrial thickness are assessed.

hCG priming

When a leading follicle has reached 12–14 mm in diameter and endometrial thickness is ≥6.0 mm, then 10 000 IU of human chorionic gonadotropin (hCG) will be administered intramuscularly and oocyte retrieval will be performed 36 h later. In cases where the leading follicle size is <12 mm in diameter, the patient can wait for 1 or 2 days for another ultrasound scan, and can then be given an hCG injection. Our experience indicates that the day of oocyte collection ranges between days 9 and 19 of the menstrual cycle, depending upon the individual patient.

MATURE AND IMMATURE OOCYTE RETRIEVAL

Transvaginal ultrasound-guided aspiration is performed using a 19G aspiration needle (Cook, Eight Mile Plains, Queensland, Australia). A portable aspiration pump is connected to the aspiration needle with a pressure between 80 and 100 mmHg. The aspirates are collected in tubes (10 ml) containing prewarmed heparinized flushing medium (Ham's F-10 medium) buffered with Hepes. Cumulus–oocyte complexes (COCs) are isolated by filtering the follicular aspirates through a mesh filter (diameter 70 μm, Falcon 1060, USA). In order to remove erythrocytes and small cellular debris, the filtrate is washed with Hepes-buffered Ham's F-10 medium. The retained COCs are then re-suspended in Ham's F-10 medium. The atretic and denuded COCs are discarded. The maturity of oocytes at the time of oocyte retrieval is evaluated under a stereomicroscope. Oocyte maturation is assessed by the presence of the first polar body (1PB) in the pelliviteline space (PVS). Mature and immature oocytes can be retrieved at the same time. As shown in Figure 27.1a, the mature oocyte was identified by extrusion of 1PB into PVS,

and Figure 27.1b shows the immature oocyte assessed by containing germinal vesicle (GV) in the cytoplasm. Our experience indicates that the mature oocytes can be retrieved from follicles as small as 10 mm in diameter.

IVF AND IVM OF IMMATURE OOCYTES

The mature oocytes are subjected to insemination 2 or 3 h later by intracytoplasmic sperm injection (ICSI), and the remaining immature oocytes (at germinal vesicle or metaphase I stages) are further cultured in maturation medium[22]. The immature oocytes are cultured in maturation medium at 37°C in 5% CO_2, 5% O_2, and 90% N_2. After one day of culture, all COCs are denuded of the cumulus cells using 0.03% hyaluronidase (Sigma, St Louis, MO, USA) in Hepes-buffered Ham's F-10 medium and mechanical pipetting. At 24 and 48 h of culture, the mature oocytes are inseminated by ICSI. Fertilization is assessed 17–19 hours after ICSI in order to detect the appearance of two distinct pronuclei and two polar bodies. The zygotes are cultured in 10 μl of embryo development medium[23].

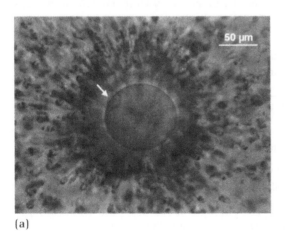

(a)

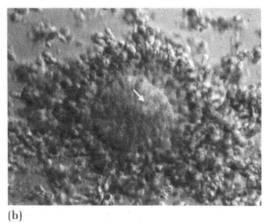

(b)

Figure 27.1 Mature (a) and immature (b) oocytes were retrieved at the time of oocyte collection for combination of natural cycle IVF with IVM treatment. Arrows indicate first polar body and germinal vesicle respectively

ENDOMETRIUM PREPARATION AND EMBRYO TRANSFER

For endometrial preparation, 6 mg estradiol valerate (Progynova®, Schering, Korea) is administered daily, starting on the day of oocyte retrieval, and luteal support of 100 mg of progesterone in oil (Progest®; Samil Pharm Co, Ansan, Korea) is injected daily, starting on the day of ICSI. Embryo transfer (ET) is performed on day 3 or 4 after oocyte retrieval, depending on whether or not mature oocytes are retrieved. Before transfer, each patient's embryos are pooled together and selected for transfer. Pregnancy is determined by the level of serum β-hCG on day 15 or 16 after oocyte retrieval, and clinical pregnancy is established by the appearance of a gestational sac on ultrasound scan 6 weeks after ET.

OUTCOME FROM IVF/IVM TREATMENT

We recruited 129 patients who underwent natural cycle IVF combined with IVM treatment. The completion of natural cycle IVF combined with IVM treatment is outlined in Table 27.1; 95.4% (123/129) of patients completed the treatment cycles. The mean number of embryos available for transfer was 4.0 ± 1.6. The clinical pregnancy rate was 29.3% per embryo transfer, and the implantation rate 10.4%. Both mature and immature oocytes were retrieved from 74.0% (91/123) of the patients, and immature oocytes only from 26.0% (32/123).

A total of 123 patients completed 123 treatment cycles of natural cycle IVF combined with IVM (Table 27.2). Further analysis of these completed cycles for IVF/IVM treatment indicated that both mature and immature oocytes were retrieved from 91 patients, while immature oocytes only were collected from 32 patients. Out of the 32 patients in the latter group, 8 had already experienced premature ovulation at the time of egg collection. Regardless of whether or not mature oocytes were collected, the average number of oocytes retrieved from both groups was similar (8.1 ± 0.4 vs. 8.2 ± 0.3). There was no difference in terms of oocyte maturation, fertilization, and cleavage rates between the two groups. However, following embryo transfer, clinical pregnancy and implantation rates were significantly higher ($p < 0.05$) in the group from whom mature oocytes were retrieved (36.3% and 12.3%) than those of the group from whom immature oocytes only were collected (9.4% and 5.3%), although more embryos were transferred in the latter group (3.5 ± 1.6 versus 4.4

Table 27.1 Embryology and pregnancy outcome from natural cycle IVF combined with IVM treatment

Treatment cycles started (patients)	129 (129)
Treatment cycles completed (%)	123 (95.4)
No of mature oocytes retrieved (mean ± SD)	148 (1.2 ± 0.5)
No of immature oocytes retrieved (mean ± SD)	895 (6.9 ± 0.3)
No of oocytes fertilized (mean ± SD)	624 (4.9 ± 0.8)
No of oocytes cleaved (mean ± SD)	593 (4.6 ± 0.2)
No of embryos transferred (mean ± SD)	489 (4.0 ± 1.6)
No of clinical pregnancies (%)	36 (29.3)
No of embryos implanted (%)	51 (10.4)

Table 27.2 Embryology and pregnancy outcome from natural cycle IVF combined with IVM based on whether or not mature oocytes were retrieved from the leading follicles for women with regular menstrual cycles

	With mature oocytes retrieved from the leading follicles	Without mature oocytes retrieved from the leading follicles	Total
No of cycles completed (patients)	91 (91)	32 (32)	123 (123)
Age (mean ± SD)	35.5 ± 3.2	36.4 ± 2.1	36.9 ± 2.5
No of oocytes collected (mean ± SD)	773 (8.1 ± 0.4)	270 (8.2 ± 0.3)	1043 (8.1 ± 0.6)
No of oocytes matured in vivo (mean ± SD)	148 (1.6 ± 0.6)	0 (0.0 ± 0.0)	148 (1.2 ± 0.5)
No of in-vivo matured oocytes fertilized (%)	114 (77.0)	0 (0.0)	114 (77.0)
No of oocytes matured in vitro (%)	455 (72.8)	204 (75.6)	659 (73.6)
No of in-vitro matured oocytes fertilized (%)	346 (76.0)	164 (80.4)	510 (77.4)
No of embryos cleaved (%)	442 (96.1)	151 (92.1)	593 (95.1)
No of embryos transferred (mean ± SD)	358 (3.5 ± 1.6)	131 (4.4 ± 1.7)	489 (4.0 ± 1.6)
No of clinical pregnancies (%)	33 (36.3)[a]	3 (9.4)[b]	36 (29.3)
No of embryos implanted (%)	44 (12.3)[a]	7 (5.3)[b]	51 (10.4)

[a,b] At least $p < 0.05$ between columns

± 1.7). Importantly, it must be mentioned here again that 8 out of 32 patients in the group from which only immature oocytes were collected had already experienced premature ovulation at the time of egg collection.

When hCG was administered at the time of the leading follicles had reached <12 mm in diameter, 34.8% of patients (8/23), no mature oocytes were retrieved from the leading follicles (Table 27.3). Accordingly, failure rates for the mature oocytes retrieved were 25.6% (12/47), 18.2% (8/44), and 44.4% (4/9), respectively, when the size of the leading follicles reached 12–14 mm, 15–17 mm, and >17 mm in diameter, at the time of hCG injection. The pregnancy rate (20.0%) was significantly lower in the group from whom mature oocytes were retrieved where the size of the leading follicles had reached >17 mm in diameter at the time of hCG injection compared to others (33.3%, 40.0%, and 36.1%).

However, there is no significant difference in the pregnancy rates (12.5%, 8.3%, 12.5%, and 0.0%, respectively) among patients from whom only immature oocytes were retrieved when the size of leading follicles reached <12.0 mm, 12–14 mm, 15–17 mm, and >17 mm in diameter respectively, at the time of hCG injection. These are our preliminary data, and it is necessary to increase the number of patients in order to corroborate this finding.

POTENTIAL PROBLEMS DURING IVF/IVM TREATMENT

A number of problems arise in natural cycle IVF treatment alone, including an increased risk of empty retrieval during oocyte collection leading to cancellation of the treatment cycle. Although this problem does not occur in natural cycle IVF

Table 27.3 Analysis of mature and immature oocyte retrieval in terms of the size of leading follicles related to pregnancy outcome

Size of leading follicle (mm) at hCG injection	No of patients	No of patients (%)		No of patients (%)	
		Who had mature oocytes collected	Who become pregnant	Who had immature oocytes collected only	Who become pregnant
<12	23	15 (65.2)[a]	5 (33.3)[a]	8 (34.8)[a]	1 (12.5)[a]
12–14	47	35 (74.5)[b]	14 (40.0)[a]	12 (25.6)[b]	1 (8.3)[a]
15–17	44	36 (81.8)[b]	13 (36.1)[a]	8 (18.2)[b]	1 (12.5)[a]
>17	9	5 (55.6)[c]	1 (20.0)[b]	4 (44.4)[c]	0 (0.0)[a]
Total	123	91 (74.0)	33 (36.3)	32 (26.0)	3 (9.4)

[a,b,c] $p < 0.05$ in the same column

combined with IVM, there is the risk of premature ovulation, if we wait until the size of the follicles reaches more than 15 mm in diameter before administering an hCG injection; 15.1% (8/53) of patients had premature ovulation at the time of egg collection when the size of follicles had reached ≥15 mm in diameter (Table 27.3). However, the recovery rate of mature oocytes (81.8%) from the leading follicles was highest in the group where the size of the leading follicles reached 15–16 mm in diameter at the time of hCG injection. In addition, our experience indicates that although the quality of mature oocytes retrieved from the leading follicles was not different based on their morphology and fertilization rate as well as early embryonic development, the quality of immature oocytes was poor when the leading follicles reached >17 mm in diameter at the time of hCG injection. Furthermore, there was a higher risk of premature ovulation when the leading follicles reached >17 mm in diameter at the time of hCG administration. Therefore, the optimum size of follicles seems to be 12–16 mm in diameter when hCG is administered in order to maximize its efficiency of treatment, and at the same time to reduce the risk of premature ovulation from the leading follicles.

In addition, the recovery rate from the leading follicles at the time of egg collection is an important issue. Our recovery rate of mature oocytes from the leading follicles using a single-lumen aspiration needle (19G, Cook, Australia) was 74.0% (91/123). However, based on our experience, we recommend using a double-lumen needle first to aspirate the leading follicles, followed by flushing until the mature oocytes are removed from the leading follicles, and then changing to a single-lumen IVM aspiration needle to aspirate the small follicles. By following this procedure, the recovery rate of mature oocytes from the leading follicles will be significantly improved.

EMBRYO QUALITY FROM EGGS MATURED AT DIFFERENT TIMES

It has been demonstrated that the administration of hCG 36 h before harvesting immature oocytes improves the maturational and development competence of the oocytes, resulting in higher pregnancy rates[24,25]. This has been confirmed by several reports[22,26,27]. Interestingly, recent findings indicate that the time course and maturation rates are different when germinal vesicle (GV)-stage oocytes are divided into different groups based on the morphology of cumulus cells after hCG priming[28]. Cleavage and embryonic development rates are significantly different based on the maturation timing of oocytes in vitro, although there is no difference in the fertilization rate regardless of the maturation time of the oocytes (Table 27.2), suggesting that oocytes reaching metaphase II (MII) faster and have better embryonic developmental competence[29]. From the results of our study, it is hard to know which of the embryos implanted originated from in-vivo matured versus in-vitro matured oocytes. However, results from the present study clearly indicate that embryos produced from oocytes cultured 24 h for maturation are of better quality, as observed by morphology, and thus may have a higher implantation potential than those generated from the oocytes cultured 48 h for maturation. In addition, it is impossible to determine which of the embryos produced from in-vivo or in-vitro matured oocytes are implanted in natural cycle IVF combined with IVM. However, the results from natural cycle IVF combined with IVM treatment clearly indicate that there are embryos generated from implanted in-vitro matured oocytes.

CONCLUSIONS

The preliminary results from our study confirm that mature and immature oocyte retrieval followed by IVF and IVM is an efficient treatment for women with various causes of infertility. The results from this study also indicate that hCG should be given when the size of the leading follicles has reached 12–14 mm in diameter in order to maximize the mature oocyte recovery rate, which may relate directly to the pregnancy rate. In summary, the results from our study demonstrate that natural cycle IVF combined with IVM is an effective treatment in a selected group of women.

REFERENCES

1. Steptoe PC, Edwards RG. Birth after re-implantation of a human embryo. Lancet 1978; 312: 366.

2. Lopata A, Brown JB, Leeton JF et al. In vitro fertilization of preovulatory oocytes and embryo transfer in infertile patients treated with clomiphene and human chorionic gonadotropin. Fertil Steril 1978; 30: 27–35.

3. Johnston I, Lopata A, Speir A et al. In vitro fertilization: the challenge of the eighties. Fertil Steril 1981; 36: 699–706.

4. Jones HW Jr, Jones GS, Andrews MC et al. The program for in vitro fertilization at Norfolk. Fertil Steril 1982; 38: 14–21.

5. Beerendonk CCM, van Dop PA, Braat DDM et al. Ovarian hyperstimulation syndrome: facts and fallacies. Obstet Gynecol Surv 1998; 53: 439–49.

6. Tarlatzis BC, Grimbiziz G, Bontis J et al. Ovarian stimulation and ovarian tumours: a critical reappraisal. Hum Reprod Update 1995; 1: 284–301.

7. Duckitt K, Templeton AA. Cancer in women with infertility. Curr Opin Obstet Gynecol 1998; 10: 199–203.

8. Brinton LA, Moghissi KS, Scoccia B et al. Ovulation induction and cancer risk. Fertil Steril 2005; 83: 261–71.

9. MacDougall MJ, Tan SL et al. Comparison of natural with clomiphene citrate-stimulated cycles in *in vitro* fertilization: a prospective, randomized trial. Fertil Steril 1994; 61: 1052–7.

10. Thornton MH, Francis MM, Paulson RJ. Immature oocyte retrieval: lessons from unstimulated IVF cycles. Fertil Steril 1998; 70: 647–50.

11. Janssens RM, Lambalk CB, Vermeiden JP et al. In-vitro fertilization in a spontaneous cycle: easy, cheap and realistic. Hum Reprod 2000; 15: 314–18.

12. Nargund G, Watwestone J, Bland JM et al. Cumulative conception and live birth rates in natural (unstimulated) IVF cycles. Hum Reprod 2001; 16: 259–62.

13. Lukassen HGM, Kremer JA, Lindeman EJM et al. A pilot study of the efficiency of intracytoplasmic sperm injection in a natural cycle. Fertil Steril 2003; 79: 231–232.

14. Hiller SG. Current concepts of the role of FSH and LH in folliculogenesis. Hum Reprod 1994; 9: 188–91.

15. Baerwald AR, Adams GP, Pierson RA. A new model for ovarian follicular development during human menstrual cycle. Fertil Steril 2003; 80; 116–22.

16. Baerwald AR, Adams GP, Pierson RA. Charaterization of ovarian follicular wave dynamics in women. Biol Reprod 2003; 69: 1023–31.

17. Paulson RJ, Sauer MV, Francis MM et al. Factors affecting pregnancy success of human in-vitro fertilization in unstimulated cycles. Hum Reprod 1994; 9: 1571–5.

18. Chian RC, Buckett WM, Abdul Jalil AK et al. Natural-cycle in vitro fertilization combined with in vitro maturation of immature oocytes is a potential approach in infertility treatment. Fertil Steril 2004; 82: 1675–8.

19. Chian RC, Lim JH, Tan SL. State if the art in in-vitro oocyte maturation. Curr Opin Obstet Genecol 2004; 16: 211–19.

20. Franks S. Polycystic ovary syndrome: a changing perspective. Clin Endocrinol 1989; 31: 87–120.

21. Buckett WM, Bouzayen R, Watkin KL et al. Ovarian stromal echogenicity in women with normal and polycystic ovaries. Hum Reprod 1999; 14: 618–21.

22. Son WY, Yoon SH, Lee SW et al. Blastocyst development and pregnancies after in vitro fertilization of mature oocytes retrieved from unstimulated patients with PCOS after in vivo HCG priming. Hum Reprod 2002; 17: 134–6.

23. Yoon HG, Yoon SH, Son WY et al. Pregnancies resulting from in vitro matured oocytes collected from women with regular menstrual cycle. J Assist Reprod Genet 2001; 18: 249–53.

24. Chian RC, Gulekli B, Buckett WM et al. Priming with human chorionic gonadotropin before retrieval of immature oocytes in women with infertility due to the polycystic ovary syndrome. N Engl J Med 1999; 341: 1624–6.

25. Chian RC, Buckett WM, Tulandi T et al. Prospective randomized study of human cho-rionic gonadotrophin priming before immature oocyte retrieval from unstimulated women with polycystic ovarian syndrome. Hum Reprod 2000; 15: 165–70.

26. Nagle F, Sator MO, Juza J et al. Successful preg-nancy resulting from in-vitro matured oocytes retrieved at laparoscopic surgery in a patient with polycystic ovary syndrome. Hum Reprod 2002; 17: 134–6.

27. Lin YH, Hwang JL, Huang LW et al. Combination of FSH priming and hCG priming for in-vitro maturation of human oocytes. Hum Reprod 2003; 18: 1632–6.

28. Yang SH, Son WY, Yoon SH et al. Correlation between in vitro maturation and expression of LH receptor in cumulus cells of the oocytes col-lected from PCOS patients in HCG-primed IVM cycles. Hum Reprod 2005; 20: 2097–103.

29. Son WY, Lee SY, Lim JH. Fertilization, cleavage and blastocyst development accord-ing to the maturation timing of oocytes in in vitro maturation cycles. Hum Reprod 2005; 20: 3204–7.

CHAPTER 28

In-vitro maturation for fertility preservation

Hananel EG Holzer, Ri-Cheng Chian, William M Buckett, and
Seang Lin Tan

INTRODUCTION

Fertility preservation for females is a medical
issue of the utmost importance that has recently
gained attention by researchers, health-care
providers, and the public. Fertility preservation should be considered in cases of patients
with malignant diseases undergoing potentially
gonadotoxic treatments, patients with other
diseases undergoing similar treatments, such
as some cases of systemic lupus erythematosus
(SLE), and practically by all women at risk for
premature ovarian failure. Fertility preservation
may also be considered for women approaching
their fourth decade without a partner to start
a family but wishing to preserve their fertility
potential.

INDICATIONS FOR FERTILITY PRESERVATION

Patients undergoing potentially gonadotoxic treatments

In the modern era, cancer is considered as a
common lethal disease. It was estimated that in
2003, over 650 000 new cases of female cancer
were diagnosed in the USA. It is encouraging
that during the last three decades there has been
a tremendous improvement in the success rates
of cancer treatments and a continual rise in the
survival rates[1]. It is estimated that, in the foreseeable future, one in 250 people will be a cancer
survivor[2].

Unfortunately, the agents used for treatment
of many types of cancer, even though successful in up to 95% of patients, carry a considerable
risk for the future fertility potential. Patients (and
their families) are now seeking more than just
cure for their disease – they wish to have other
options to try to preserve their fertility potential
for a future normal healthy and fulfilling life.

The ovaries, containing a limited number
of germ cells, are prone to irreversible damage
as a result of chemotherapy[3]. The ovaries may
undergo follicular loss that may end up in a
complete absence of follicles and ovarian fibro-
sis, leading to premature ovarian failure, infertility, and a premature menopause[4,5]. The rates
of premature ovarian failure and infertility are
affected by many factors – particularly the age
of the woman at the time of treatment. Young
women and prepubescent girls are much more
likely to retain some degree of ovarian function
compared with women in their late 30s and 40s.
Other features which affect the rates of ovarian
failure are the type of disease, the duration of

treatment, and the combination of chemotherapeutic agents.

Some drugs present a higher risk for ovarian failure. Cyclophosphamide is the drug probably most associated with ovarian failure and subsequent infertility. Cyclophosphamide causes depletion of primordial follicles even at low doses, but the damage is dependent on both the dose and the cumulative dose given. Cyclophosphamide is used for treating both malignant diseases and non-malignant diseases such as SLE[5-8].

The patient's age correlates with the risk of premature ovarian failure. As age advances the ovarian primordial follicle pool declines and the woman has a shorter duration to ovarian failure after exposure to gonadotoxic drugs[9]. Even if the normal cycling pattern is resumed, patients who have been treated with gonadotoxic drugs are more prone to develop premature ovarian failure later in life[10-12].

Ionizing radiation also causes a reduction in the primordial follicle pool; oocytes are sensitive to radiation and show pyknosis, chromosome condensation, disruption of the nuclear envelope, and cytoplasmic vacuolization. These result in oocyte depletion and may cause ovarian failure and infertility[13,14]. The ovarian damage is dose related and the cut-off dose for ovarian damage depends on the age, extent, and type of radiotherapy. It was calculated that the threshold for destroying 50% of the oocytes is 200 cCy. Less than 150 cCy will have minimal or no deleterious effect in young women, whereas 250–500 cCy will cause infertility in about 60% of young women (aged 15–40 years) and in almost 100% of women over 40 years[13-15]. Oophorectomy (with or without uterine conservation) in women with borderline ovarian cancers will also lead to iatrogenic premature ovarian failure and infertility.

Patients with genetic abnormalities

Young patients with Turner's syndrome mosaics are destined to have premature ovarian failure and infertility. However, adolescent girls with Turner's syndrome mosaics may still have some follicles in their ovarian cortical tissue[16]. The follicles and/or oocytes retrieved may be preserved for future fertility. The issues of whether the oocytes retrieved from girls with Turner's syndrome have a normal chromosomal complement and of their fertility potential still need to be addressed.

The fragile-X premutation is also associated with premature ovarian failure[17], and female carriers should be advised of this risk and may consider fertility preservation. Obviously, any oocytes or embryos cryopreserved from these women would need to undergo some form of karyotypic evaluation (such as preimplantation genetic diagnosis or polar body testing) prior to embryo transfer.

Extending the fertile age span

In the last three decades, women have tended to delay childbirth and the mean age at first delivery continues to rise in most countries. However, advancing female age is associated with declining fertility, increased miscarriage rates, increased congenital and chromosomal abnormalities, and poorer obstetric and neonatal outcome[18]. These are due to decreasing numbers and quality of oocytes. Therefore, women in their thirties without a partner may consider fertility preservation. However, discussion of the psychologic and social issues arising from 'social' fertility preservation, although important, is well beyond the scope of this chapter.

OPTIONS FOR FERTILITY PRESERVATION

Various strategies for fertility preservation have recently been discussed in the medical literature and in the worldwide media. The strategies today could be regarded as either ovarian protection in vivo or extracorporal cryopreservation.

Nevertheless, most of these strategies should currently be regarded as still experimental.

Ovarian protection

Ovarian transposition

To avoid or to lower the radiation dose to the ovaries, the ovaries can be transposed out of the direct radiation field. Ovarian transposition should be considered prior to local radiotherapy in cancer patients younger than 40 years in whom gonadotoxic chemotherapy is not indicated. It necessitates a surgical procedure. Laparoscopic transposition is usually preferred[19].

GnRH analogs

Decreasing gonadal function by administering a GnRH analog during chemotherapy cycles may protect the ovaries against the sterilizing effects of chemotherapy; however, although animal studies and some human retrospective studies show some benefit, the mechanism of action is not clear[20]. Furthermore, the efficacy of GnRH analog in reducing ovarian damage is not yet clear.

Apoptosis

Apoptosis, the programmed cell death of the germ cells, may also have a role in chemo- and radiotherapy-induced cell depletion. Some experimental compounds may inhibit the chemotherapy- and radiotherapy-induced oocyte apoptosis. Unfortunately, treatments inhibiting apoptosis are still far away from clinical implementation[21,22].

Ovarian tissue cryopreservation

In cryopreservation of ovarian tissue, hundreds to thousands of immature oocytes may be preserved, and the primordial follicles seem much less susceptible to cryoinjury. However, at least two surgical procedures are needed: one for harvesting the ovarian tissue and at least a

second (or in some cases a second and a third) to transplant the cryopreserved ovarian tissue. Furthermore, in cases of transplantation to a heterotopic site (such as the forearm or the abdominal subcutaneous fat), an IVF procedure is needed as well. To date, less then a handful of pregnancies from transplanted ovarian tissue have been reported[23–25].

Although retransplantation of ovarian tissue carries the added benefit of re-instituting ovarian hormonal function as well as the possibility of future fertility, transplantation of the frozen–thawed ovarian cortex tissue strips back to the patient also carries the risk of re-seeding metastatic disease[26]. So far, ovarian graft life seems to be short lived, although the reasons for this are unclear. Possible causes for the poor ovarian function include cryoinjury, a depletion in the number of primordial follicles, and poor vascular perfusion of the transplanted graft.

As an alternative, the primordial follicles ideally could be cultured in vitro to mature oocytes. This would be a very attractive option as many hundreds of primordial follicles would be available, even from very small biopsy specimens. Unfortunately, however, in humans this technology still awaits further research and is far from clinical practice[27,28].

Embryo and oocyte cryopreservation after ovarian stimulation

Mature oocytes can be harvested from the ovaries after controlled ovarian hyperstimulation, allowing generation of embryos and their subsequent cryopreservation. This has the advantage that embryo cryopreservation and subsequent transfer is an established treatment for couples with infertility and is practised around the world.

However, there are two major drawbacks for the conventional IVF with ovarian stimulation and subsequent embryo cryopreservation. The first is the time interval needed for IVF; this ranges from 2 to 6 weeks, beginning at the patient's next menstrual period, which may sometimes be too long to wait prior to starting chemo- or radiotherapy due to the natural course of the malignant disease. The second is that ovarian stimulation is associated with relatively high estradiol levels that may not be safe in cases of estrogen-sensitive tumors such as breast cancer, or in women with a high likelihood of thromboembolism, as well as for other patients wishing to avoid ovarian stimulation.

To avoid the high estradiol levels associated with ovarian stimulation for cancer patients (particularly breast cancer), letrozole or tamoxifen plus low-dose FSH protocols have been used. These protocols are associated with lower peak estradiol levels, but do not totally avoid ovarian stimulation[29].

After collection of the mature oocytes, the oocytes can be fertilized using the partner's sperm. The resulting embryos will be frozen for future thaw and transfer. Transferring frozen-thawed embryos is an integral part of assisted reproductive technology (ART) programs. Survival rates per thawed embryos are 60–90% and the pregnancy rate per thaw is 20–25%[30,31]. When sperm is not available then oocyte cryopreservation may be considered; this will be discussed in the next section.

IN-VITRO MATURATION FOR FERTILITY PRESERVATION

Avoiding hormonal stimulation

Ovarian stimulation for collection of oocytes can be totally avoided by collecting immature oocytes. As discussed elsewhere in the book, in-vitro maturation (IVM) of oocytes collected via transvaginal ultrasound-guided aspiration has been performed since 1994; almost 1000 babies have been born and the clinical pregnancy rate is currently around 35% per cycle. Immature oocyte collection can be offered for cancer patients with no ovarian stimulation and thus with no concerns regarding aggravating hormone-sensitive

disease. The only hormonal treatment needed is a single injection of hCG 36 h prior to the collection to improve the IVM rate[32].

Timing of oocyte retrieval

For women undergoing immature oocyte retrieval for IVM, the collection can be performed during the follicular phase prior to ovulation for normal ovulating patients, and on almost any given day for PCOS patients. Thus, patients scheduled for therapy do not have to wait for the beginning of the next menstrual bleeding and then undergo ovarian stimulation. Patients with PCOS may have the collection at almost any given time 36 h after the hCG injection. Ovulating patients seen first during the follicular phase can have the collection soon after their initial visit. In the cases seen first during the luteal phase, due to lack of sufficient information on collections during the luteal phase, we tend to wait for the subsequent follicular phase. In the normal ovulating patient, a mature oocyte can be collected as well as immature oocytes; the presence of a dominant follicle does not hamper the maturation and developmental potential of the small antral follicles[33]. Therefore, collecting immature oocytes from unstimulated ovaries may save valuable time, time that may have critical importance for patients with malignant disease.

The short time needed may even enable more than one oocyte collection to be performed in the interval available before the gonadotoxic treatment is initiated. Typically this would be in women with breast cancer following surgery and prior to starting chemotherapy. The immature oocytes collected can be cryopreserved as immature germinal vesicle oocytes, or as in-vitro matured mature oocytes, or can be fertilized and cryopreserved as embryos.

Cryopreservation of immature oocytes

Immature oocytes as compared with mature oocytes have a smaller volume and no meiotic spindle, and the chromosomes are protected within a nuclear membrane. Therefore, it could be presumed that freezing of immature oocytes would yield better survival rates. Nevertheless, cryosurvival and subsequent maturation rates of immature oocytes have been disappointing so far. Pregnancies have been reported, but the overall experience is still poor[34–36].

Cryopreservation of mature oocytes

Conventional cryopreservation

Although the first live birth from a cryopreserved oocyte was reported almost 20 years ago[37], the overall results for mature oocyte cryopreservation have been discouraging. The oocytes are more vulnerable to the freezing process (slow freezing) than are embryos. Intracellular ice formation can cause membrane rupture, abnormal cortical granular reaction, zona hardening, and damage to the meiotic spindle and cytoskeleton. The meiotic spindle damage might result in chromosomal abnormalities. The reported survival rates for mature oocytes (collected from stimulated ovaries) are around 50%[38,39]. There are no data concerning rates of in-vitro matured oocytes surviving conventional oocyte cryopreservation (slow freezing).

Vitrification

Vitrification has been used successfully for the cryopreservation of human oocytes. Cryoprotectants in high concentration are used to induce a glass-like state; the cell is then rapidly frozen, avoiding the formation of intracellular ice. Live births after vitrification of oocytes have been reported, but there are still concerns about the effects of the high concentrations on the vulnerable oocytes[40,41].

Recently we have vitrified mature oocytes collected from stimulated ovaries in two studies. In the first study, 15 patients over-responding to ovarian stimulation underwent oocyte collection and oocyte vitrification, instead of cycle cancellation or converting to IVF. The oocytes were thawed and fertilized, and the subsequent embryos were transferred within the following few months. The oocyte survival, fertilization, and cleavage rates were 85.8%, 73.7%, and 82.5%, respectively. The clinical pregnancy and implantation rates were 46.7% and 22.4%, respectively. In the second study, 17 patients underwent ovarian stimulation for IVF. The collected oocytes were vitrified after collection. Within the following months the oocytes were thawed, fertilized, and transferred. The oocyte survival, fertilization, and cleavage rates were 89%, 72.5%, and 80.4%, respectively. The clinical pregnancy and implantation rates were 41.2% and 16.4%, respectively (McGill Reproductive Center, unpublished data). Thus oocyte vitrification seems to be a potentially promising technique with high oocyte survival rates. This technique should probably be implemented in fertility preservation programs for patients wishing to preserve their fertility and who do not have a partner.

Patients who cannot undergo ovarian stimulation or those who do not want to have ovarian stimulation have the option of immature oocyte collection from unstimulated ovaries. The immature oocytes will be matured in vitro and then vitrified for future use. However promising this option may be, the patients should be strongly advised of the experimental nature of this work.

Embryo cryopreservation after IVM

Patients who have a male partner and are wishing to preserve oocytes fertilized by their partner's sperm should undergo immature oocyte collection from unstimulated ovaries and then the oocytes would be fertilized utilizing ICSI. The resulting embryos would be vitrified or cryopreserved for a future transfer.

As noted above, embryo cryopreservation is an effective and reproducible treatment modality within conventional stimulated IVF. Similarly, many babies have been born following cryopreservation and subsequent thawing of embryos generated from IVM oocytes[42].

IVM FOR FERTILITY PRESERVATION – THE McGILL EXPERIENCE

We have recently reported the retrieval of immature oocytes from unstimulated ovaries of a cancer patient before gonadotoxic therapy for oocyte vitrification purposes. A 33-year-old stage II breast cancer patient was seen on day 10 of the menstrual cycle, hCG was given, and 19 immature oocytes collected on day 12. Six oocytes matured on day 13 and 11 more matured on day 14. Altogether, 17 mature oocytes were vitrified without any delay in chemotherapy[43].

Since that report, 32 patients with various malignant diseases have undergone 35 immature oocyte collections – 16 patients with breast cancer, 9 patients with Hodgkin's lymphoma, and 7 further patients with other malignancies (non-Hodgkin's lymphoma, anaplastic oligodendroglioma, Ewing's sarcoma, rhabdomyosarcoma, endometrial carcinoma, abdominal desmoid tumor, and desmoplastic ovarian tumor). The indications for immature oocyte collection without ovarian stimulation were at least one of the following:

(1) Hormone-sensitive disease

(2) Patient's request to avoid ovarian stimulation and

(3) Lack of sufficient time for an IVF cycle prior to starting chemo- or radiotherapy.

Of these patients 20 who underwent 23 oocyte collections without ovarian stimulation elected to have their oocytes cryopreserved, rather than generate embryos, because they did not have a partner. One patient had a partner but the couple chose not to use the husband's sperm for fertilization, and to cryopreserve oocytes. From these women, a total of 226 oocytes were collected; 18 were mature on the day of collection, 8 were at the metaphase I stage, and 200 were germinal vesicle oocytes. Of these oocytes, 143 were matured in vitro and a total of 160 mature oocytes were vitrified; the average maturation rate was 66.3% ± 30.5%.

The other 12 patients, with a partner, underwent 12 oocyte collections without ovarian stimulation. For these couples, a total of 97 oocytes were collected; 8 were mature on the day of collection and 89 were germinal vesicles (GV) oocytes. Sixty oocytes matured in vitro and the average maturation rate was 64.8% ± 27.8%. Following ICSI, 55 mature oocytes were fertilized, giving an average fertilization rate of 84.4% ± 15.9% and 53 resulting embryos were vitrified. To date, none of the cancer patients has returned for an embryo transfer.

CONCLUSIONS

Fertility preservation is of the utmost importance to patients undergoing gonadotoxic chemo- and/or radiotherapy, and also for patients facing the risk of premature ovarian failure as well as for others wishing to preserve their fertility potential.

The options vary between ovarian protection, ovarian tissue cryopreservation, and oocyte or embryo cryopreservation. Collection of immature oocytes from unstimulated ovaries followed by IVM of the oocytes does not carry the theoretic risk of re-instituting the metastatic malignant disease that transplanting ovarian tissue carries. Collection of immature oocytes from unstimulated ovaries followed by IVM of the oocytes can be performed for patients with a hormone-sensitive disease without risk of aggravating the disease. Collecting the immature oocytes does not require the same time needed for ovarian stimulation and the waiting time for the beginning of the next menstrual cycle. Thus precious time may be saved and therapy is not delayed.

Oocytes of patients without a partner should be vitrified after IVM and oocytes of patients with a partner should be fertilized after IVM and the resulting embryos then vitrified. However promising IVM of oocytes may seem, especially for patients for whom this may be the only safe procedure for preserving fertility, the patients and their families should be informed of the experimental nature of these treatments and of the lack of information concerning survival, fertilization, and pregnancy potential of oocytes frozen/vitrified after IVM.

REFERENCES

1. Jemal A, Murray T, Samuels A et al. Cancer statistics, 2003. Cancer J Clin 2003; 53: 5–26.

2. Bleyer WA. The impact of childhood cancer on the United States and the world. CA Cancer J Clin 1990; 40: 355–67.

3. Oktay K, Kan MT, Rosenwaks Z. Recent progress in oocyte and ovarian tissue cryopreservation and transplantation. Curr Opin Obstet Gynecol 2001; 13: 263–8.

4. Familiari G, Caggiati A, Nottola SA et al. Ultrastructure of human ovarian primodial follicles after combination chemotherapy for Hodgkin's disease. Hum Reprod 1993; 8: 2080–7.

5. Warne GL, Fairley KF, Hobbs JB et al. Cyclophosphamide induced ovarian failure. N Engl J Med 1973; 289: 1159–62.

6. Meirow D, Lewis H, Nugent D et al. Subclinical depletion of primordial follicular reserve in mice treated with cyclophosphamide: clinical importance and proposed accurate investigative tool. Hum Reprod 1999; 14: 1903–7.

7. Goldhirsh A, Gelber RD, Castiglione M. The magnitude of endocrine effects of adjuvant chemotherapy for premenopausal breast cancer patients. The International Breast Cancer Study Group. Ann Oncol 1990; 1: 183–8.

8. Koyama H, Wada T, Nishizawa Y et al. Cyclophosphamide-induced ovarian failure and its therapeutic significance in patients with breast cancer. Cancer 1977; 39: 1403–9.

9. Bines J, Oleske DM, Gobleigh MA. Ovarian function in premenopausal women treated with adjuvant chemotherapy for breast cancer. J Clin Oncol 1996; 14: 1718–29.

10. Byrne J, Fears TR, Gail MH et al. Early menopause in long-term survivors of cancer during adolescence. Am J Obstet Gynecol 1992; 166: 788–93.

11. Larsen EC, Muller J, Schmeigelow K et al. Reduced ovarian function in long term survivors of radiation and chemotherapy treated childhood cancer. J Clin Endocrinol Metab 2003; 88: 5307–14.

12. Huong DLT, Amoura Z, Duhaut P. Risk of ovarian failure and fertility after intravenous cyclophosphamide. A study in 84 patients. J Rheumatol 2002; 29: 2571–6.

13. Gosden RG, Wade JC, Fraser HM et al. Impact of congenital or experimental hypogonadotrophism on the radiation sensitivity of the mouse ovary. Hum Reprod 1997; 12; 2483–8.

14. Damewood MD, Grochow LB. Prospects for fertility after chemotherapy or radiation for neoplastic disease. Fertil Steril 1986; 45: 443–59.

15. Wallace WH, Thompson AB, Kelsey TW. The radiosensitivity of the human oocyte. Hum Reprod 2003; 18: 117–21.

16. Hreinsson JG, Otala M, Fridstrom M. Follicles are found in the ovaries of adolescent girls with Turner's syndrome. J Clin Endocrinol Metab 2002; 87(8): 3618–23.

17. Bretherick KL, Fluker MR, Robinson WP. FMR1 repeat sizes in the gray zone and high end of the normal range are associated with premature ovarian failure. Hum Genet 2005; 117(4): 376–82.

18. Heffner LJ. Advanced maternal age – how old is too old? N Engl J Med 2004; 351: 1927–9.

19. Tulandi T, Al-Sharani A. Laparoscopic fertility preservation. Obstet Gynecol Clin N Am 2004; 31: 611–18.

20. Blumenfeld Z, Eckmen A. Preservation of fertility and ovarian function and minimization of chemotherapy-induced gonadotoxicity in young women by GnRH-a. J Natl Cancer Inst Monogr 2005; (34): 40–3.

21. Tilly JL. Molecular and genetic basis of normal and toxicant induced apoptosis in female germ cells. Toxicol Lett 1998; 102: 497–501.

22. Morita Y, Perez GI, Paris F et al. Oocyte apoptosis is suppressed by disruption of acid sphingomyelinase gene or by sphingosine 1 phosphate therapy. Nat Med 2000; 6: 1109–14.

23. Oktay K, Buyuk F, Veeck L et al. Embryo development after heterotropic transplantation of cryopreserved ovarian tissue. Lancet 2004; 363: 837–40.

24. Donnez J, Dolmans MM, Demylle D et al. Livebirth after orthotopic tranplantation of cryopreserved ovarian tissue. Lancet 2004; 364: 1405–10.

25. Meirow D, Levron J, Eldar-Geva T et al. Pregnancy after transplantation of cryopreserved ovarian tissue in a patient with ovarian failure after chemotherapy. N Engl J Med 2005; 21: 353: 318–21.

26. Shaw JM, Bowles J, Koopman P et al. Fresh and cryopreserved ovarian tissue samples from donors with lymphoma transmit the cancer to graft recipients. Hum Reprod 1996; 11: 1668–73.

27. O'Brien MJ, Pendola JK, Eppig JJ. A revised protocol for in vitro development of mouse oocytes from primordial follicles dramatically improves their developmental competence. Biol Reprod 2003; 68: 1682–6.

28. Picton HM, Danfour MA, Harris SE et al. Growth and maturation of oocytes in vitro. Reprod Suppl 2003; 61: 445–62.

29. Oktay K, Buyuk E, Libertella N et al. Fertility preservation in breast cancer patients: a prospective controlled comparison of ovarian stimulation with tamoxifen and letrozole for embryo cryopreservation. J Clin Oncol 2005; 23: 4347–53.

30. Wang JX, Yapp YY, Mathews CD. Frozen-thawed embryo transfer: influence of clinical factors on implantation rate and risk of multiple conception. Hum Reprod 2001; 16: 2316–19.

31. Assisted Reproductive Technology in the United States: 2000 results generated from the American Society for Reproductive Medicine/Society for Assisted Reproductive Technology Registry. Fertil Steril 2004; 81: 1207–20.

32. Chian RC, Gulekli B, Buckett WM et al. Priming with human chorionic gonadotropin before retrieval of immature oocytes in women with infertility due to the polycystic ovary syndrome. N Engl J Med 1999; 341: 1624–6.

33. Chian RC, Buckett WM, Abdul Jalil C et al. Natural-cycle in vitro fertilization combined with in vitro maturation of immature oocytes is a potential approach in infertility treatment. Fertil Steril 2004; 82: 1675–8.

34. Toth TL, Lanzendorf SE, Sandow BA et al. Cryopreservation of human prophase I oocytes collected from unstimulated follicles. Fertil Steril 1994; 61: 1077–82.

35. Wu J, Zhang L, Wang X. In vitro maturation, fertilization and embryo development after ultrarapid freezing of immature human oocytes. Hum Reprod 2001; 121: 389–93.

36. Tucker MJ, Morton PC, Wright G et al. Clinical application of human egg cryopreservation. Hum Reprod 1998; 13: 3156–9.

37. Chen C. Pregnancy after human oocyte cryopreservation. Lancet 1986; 327: 884–6.

38. Fabbri R, Porcu E, Marsella T et al. Human oocyte cryopreservation: new prospectives regarding oocyte survival. Hum Reprod 2001; 16: 411–16.

39. Sonmezer M, Okatay K. Fertility preservation in female patients. Hum Reprod Update 2004; 10: 251–6.

40. Arav A, Yavin S, Zeron Y et al. New trends in gamete cryopreservation. Mol Cell Endocrinol 2002; 187: 77–81.

41. Yoon TK, Kim TJ, Park SE et al. Live births after vitrification of oocytes in a stimulated in vitro fertilization-embryo transfer program Fertil Steril 2003; 79: 1323–6.

42. Chian RC, Gulekli B, Buckett WM et al. Pregnancy and delivery after cryopreservation of zygotes produced by in vitro matured oocytes retrieved from a woman with polycystic ovarian syndrome. Hum Reprod 2001; 16: 1700–2.

43. Rao GD, Chian RC, Son W et al. Fertility preservation in patients undergoing cancer treatment. Lancet 2004; 363: 1829.

INDEX

Page numbers in *italics* indicate figures or tables.

T - #0056 - 111024 - C0 - 246/189/23 - PB - 9780367453244 - Gloss Lamination